Brain Injury Treatment
Theories and Practices

S0-BEG-461

Edited by
José León-Carrión, Klaus R. H. von Wild
and George A. Zitnay

Ψ Psychology Press
Taylor & Francis Group
HOVE AND NEW YORK

First published 2006 by Taylor & Francis

This edition published 2013 by Psychology Press
Psychology Press   Psychology Press
Taylor & Francis Group   Taylor & Francis Group
27 Church Road   711 Third Avenue
Hove   New York
East Sussex, BN3 2FA   NY 10017

Psychology Press is an imprint of the Taylor & Francis Group, an informa business

First issued in paperback 2013

Typeset in Times by RefineCatch Ltd, Bungay, Suffolk
Cover design by Jim Wilkie

British Library Cataloguing in Publication Data
A catalogue record for this book is available from the British Library

Library of Congress Cataloging in Publication Data
Brain injury treatment: theories and practices / edited by José León-
Carrión, Klaus R. H. von Wild, George A. Zitnay
    p. cm.
  Includes bibliographies references and index.
  ISBN 1-84169-572-6 (hbk)
    1. Brain damage—Patients—Rehabilitation.   I. León-Carrión,
José.   II. Wild, K. R. H. von (Klaus)   III. Zitnay, George A.
RC387.5.B745   2005
617.4′810443—dc22
                                         2004026204

ISBN 978-1-84169-572-3 hbk
ISBN 978-0-415-65370-1 pbk

Contents

11   Spasticity of cerebral origin   230

JOHN S. HONG AND CHRISTOPHER G. ZITNAY

12   Rehabilitation in water: A practical guide   250

GIANPIETRO SALVI, ANNAMARIA QUARENGHI, AND
PAOLA QUARENGHI

13   Neuropsychological assessment of persons with acquired brain injury   275

JOSÉ LEÓN-CARRIÓN, PAUL J. TAAFFE, AND JUAN MANUEL
BARROSO Y MARTÍN

From the series editor

Brain Injury Treatment: Theories and Practices is a truly international and interdisciplinary collaborative effort which brings together various approaches to rehabilitative intervention following CNS trauma. General care chapters range from pre-hospital patient management in the USA to organization of neurological intensive care units in Spain, to medical rehabilitation after intensive care in Italy, to issues unique to children and adolescents after brain injury. Unique treatment approaches such as electrical treatment of coma in Japan, the potential use of stem cells, the importance of including family members in treatment, rehabilitation in water, and the use of complementary medicine form the basis of chapters which offer varied and singular perspectives in dealing with patients. Finally, a number of chapters deal with issues of assessment in acquired brain injury, including estimates of response bias, consideration of affective factors, and methods and tools for establishing the validity of treatment outcome.

For the professional dealing with head injury, whether within a medical, psychological, or social context, this text provides an encyclopedic source of approaches, methods, and measures of effectiveness. One would be hard pressed to find a single reference which provides this range of viewpoints and similarly covers the international variety of approaches to rehabilitation after brain injury. The editors, Drs. León-Carrión, Zitnay, and von Wild, have faithfully presented the links between theory and methods of rehabilitation and it is expected that the reader will feel informed and delighted with the authors' presentations. We welcome this addition to our series and feel confident that health professionals and students will find it a valuable place in their library of references.

Linas A. Bieliauskas
Ann Arbor, March 2005

Contributors

Juan Manuel Barroso y Martín, Human Neuropsychology Laboratory, Department of Experimental Psychology, University of Seville, Spain.

E. O. Bixler, Professor, University Endowed Chair for Research, Department of Psychiatry, Pennsylvania State University, USA.

John Bruns, Jr, Clinical Assistant Professor, Department of Emergency Medicine, Mount Sinai School of Medicine, New York, USA.

Shane S. Bush, independent practice, Smithtown, NY, USA.

Elina Caminiti, Presidio Sanitario Austriliatrice, Acquired Brain Injury Rehabilitation Center, Torino, Italy.

Edwin Cooper, Visiting Associate Professor, Department of Neurosurgery, The University of Virginia Health System, and Associate Clinical, Professor, Department of Physical Medicine and Rehabilitation, The Brody School of Medicine, East Carolina University, USA.

María del Rosario Domínguez-Morales, Center for Brain Injury Rehabilitation (C.RE.CER.), Seville, Spain.

José María Domínguez-Roldán, Intensive Care Unit, Hospital Virgen del Rocio, Seville, Spain.

Erin Duncan, HealthSource NeuroRehabilitation, Warrenton, Virginia, USA.

Enrico Fiorio, Presidio Sanitario Ausiliatrice, Acquired Brain Injury Rehabilitation Center, Torino, Italy.

Claudio García-Alfaro, Hospital Virgen del Rocio, Seville, Spain.

John S. Hong, Research and Medical Director, John Jane Brain Injury Center, USA.

Andy Jagoda, Associate Professor, Department of Emergency Medicine, Mount Sinai School of Medicine, New York, USA.

Tetsuo Kanno, Professor and Chairman, Department of Neurosurgery, School of Medicine, Fujita Health University, Japan.

José León-Carrión, Professor, Center for Brain Injury Rehabilitation (C.RE.CER), and Human Neuropsychology Laboratory, Department of Experimental Psychology, University of Seville, Spain.

Andrea Maestri, Presidio Sanitario Ausiliatrice, Acquired Brain Injury Rehabilitation Center, Torino, Italy.

Michael F. Martelli, Director, Rehabilitation Neuropsychology, Concussion Care Center of Virginia Ltd., Tree of Life Llc. and Pinnacle Rehabilitation Inc.; Associate Clinical Professor, Virginia Commonwealth University and Medical College of Virginia, USA.

Tiziana Mezzanato, Presidio Sanitario Austriliatrice, Acquired Brain Injury Rehabilitation Center, Torino, Italy.

Eugene Mikhaelenov, NeuroBird, Seville, Spain/St. Petersburg, Russia.

M. A. Muñoz-Sanchez, Chief of the Emergency Department, Hospital Universitario de Traumatologica Virgin del Rocio, Sevilla, Spain.

Francisco Murillo-Cabezas, Head of Emergency and Critical Care Department, Hospital Universitario de Traumatología Virgin del Rocio, Sevilla, Spain.

Peter D. Patrick, School of Medicine, University of Virginia, USA.

Sean T. Patrick, NeuroPsych HealthCare, Charlottesville, Virginia, USA.

Claudio Perino, Presidio Sanitario Ausiliatrice, Acquired Brain Injury Rehabilitation Center, Torino, Italy.

Paolo Pietrapiana, Presidio Sanitario Ausiliatrice, Acquired Brain Injury Rehabilitation Center, Torino, Italy.

Treven C. Pickett, Ph.D., Defense and Veterans Brain Injury Center, Research Service, Richmond DVA Medical Center Department of PM & R, Virginia Commonwealth University – School of Medicine.

Annamaria Quarenghi, Psychiatrist, Centro di Riabilitazione Neuromotoria Clinica Quarenghi, San Pellegrino Terme (BG), Italy.

Paola Quarenghi, Physiotherapist, Centro di Riabilitazione Neuromotoria Clinica Quarenghi, San Pellegrino Terme (BG), Italy.

Roberto Rago, Presidio Sanitario Ausiliatrice, Acquired Brain Injury Rehabilitation Center, Torino, Italy.

Gianpietro Salvi, Neurologist, Centro di Riabilitazione Neuromotoria Clinica Quarenghi, San Pellegrino Terme (BG), Italy.

Paul J. Taaffe, Dominion Behavioral Healthcare, Richmond, Virginia, USA.

Dale F. Thomas, Research and Training Center, Stout Vocational Rehabilitation Institute, College of Human Development, University of Wisconsin, USA.

Antonio Vela-Bueno, Professor, Department of Psychiatry, Autonomous University, Madrid, Spain.

Davide Vernè, Presidio Sanitario Austriliatrice, Acquired Brain Injury Rehabilitation Center, Torino, Italy.

A. N. Vgontzas, Professor, Anthony Kales Endowed Chair in Sleep Disorders Medicine, Department of Psychiatry, Pennsylvania State University, College of Medicine, USA.

Walter Videtta, Hospital Prof. A Posadas, Buenos Aires, Argentina.

Olga Voronina, NeuroBird, Seville, Spain/St. Petersburg, Russia.

Klaus R. H. von Wild, Professor and Head Neurosurgical, Department for Neurosurgery and Early Neurotraumatological Rehabilitation, Clemens-hospital, Teaching Hospital, Westphalian Wilhelms University Munster, Germany.

Nathan D. Zasler, M.D., CEO and Medical Director, Concussion Care Centre of Virginia, Ltd., CEO and Medical Director, Tree of Life Services, Inc., Clinical Professor, VCU Department of Physical Medicine and Rehabilitation, Richmond, Virginia, Clinical Associate Professor, Department of Physical Medicine and Rehabilitation, University of Virginia, Charlottesville, Virginia, USA.

Christopher G. Zitnay, Medical Director, John Jane Brain Injury Center, USA.

George A. Zitnay, Professor, Virginia Neuro-Care, Inc., Virginia USA.

Tables and figures

Figures

Note

Any practice described in this book should be applied by the reader in accordance with the professional standard of care and unique circumstances of each patient. The authors, editor and publisher are not responsible for error or omissions or for consequences of the application of the book, and make no warranty, expressed or implied, on regards to the content of the book. Caution is especially urged when using drugs.

1 Prehospital management of traumatic brain injury

Andy Jagoda and John Bruns, Jr

Introduction

Traumatic brain injury (TBI) is a leading cause of death worldwide, particularly in those under the age of 40. Head injury and traumatic brain injury are two distinct entities that are often, but not necessarily, related. A *head injury* is best defined as an injury that is clinically evident upon physical examination and is recognized by the presence of ecchymoses, lacerations, deformities, or cerebral spinal rhinorrhea or otorrhea. *Traumatic brain injury* refers to an injury to the brain itself and can occur without external signs of trauma. Prehospital care providers must be prepared to diagnose not only head injuries but also TBI.

The incidence of TBI varies nationally and regionally. Regardless of the statistics reviewed, the true incidence most likely far exceeds the statistics reported in the literature. In the USA, approximately 1.6% of all emergency department (ED) visits are for a head injury. There are 444 new cases annually of TBI per 100,000,[1] with an estimated 98 per 100,000 hospitalization rate for TBI annually.[2] The incidence of head injury or TBI in individuals that do not seek medical care is not known, nor is the incidence of head injury assessed by prehospital care providers and not transported known. In a study from Colorado, the incidence of TBI was higher in rural than in urban populations and the mortality of rural patients was higher.[3] These findings are supported by similar results in an Australian study.[4] The mortality associated with TBI sustained in rural settings is partially due to delayed access to definitive care and emphasizes the critical role played by prehospital care providers in stabilizing these patients.

Prehospital providers are often the vital link between the injury and definitive care. They must make critical decisions regarding where, when, and how rapidly a patient is transported. They are additionally responsible for initiating interventions which can minimize mortality and morbidity.

As discussed in depth in other chapters in this book, when a head injury occurs there are primary injuries directly related to the trauma: skull fractures or blood vessel and parenchymal damage. Secondary injury refers to damage that results from neuronal death as a consequence of hypoxia, edema, and initiation of inflammatory cascades. Secondary injury greatly impacts outcome and can be minimized if proper resuscitative efforts are provided.[5]

Recognizing the important role prehospital providers play in the care of TBI patients, the US government provided a grant to the Brain Trauma Foundation to develop guidelines to assist prehospital care providers in assessing and managing the TBI patient. A task force of experts in the prehospital and in hospital trauma care was assembled in 1998 and the guidelines were published in 2000.[6] The task force systematically searched and pragmatically analyzed the scientific literature to develop evidence-based recommendations. The process clearly revealed a paucity of clinical research in prehospital care; therefore the document also presents areas in need of future research.

Prehospital systems

There is tremendous worldwide variability regarding access to, and the sophistication of, emergency medical service (EMS) systems. Prehospital providers range from physicians with critical care training to lay persons lacking any formal training. In the USA, there are approximately 600,000 prehospital providers. In general, they are paraprofessionals with varying degrees of training (Table 1.1). American EMS systems are state regulated

Table 1.1 General categories of prehospital care providers in the USA*

Category	Training and role
EMT-Ambulance (EMT-A)	Receive approximately 100 hours of first aid including certification in basic life support (BLS) and basic trauma life support (BTLS). In general, EMT-As are not able to start intravenous lines, initiate interventional procedures, or to give medications. The primary role of an EMT-A is to provide basic stabilization and transport
EMT-Intermediates (EMT-I) and EMT-Defibrillators (EMT-D)	EMT-As who have received an additional 20–50 hours of training, including training in the use of automatic defibrillators.
Paramedics (EMT-P)	Receive approximately 1000 hours of training in life support skills that are the equivalent of Advanced Cardiac Life Support (ACLS), Advanced Trauma Life Support (ATLS), Pediatric Advanced Life Support (PALS), and varying degrees of instruction on medical and surgical diseases. EMT-Ps are able to use manual defibrillators; intubate (in some systems using paralytic agents); establish intravenous access; use a limited number of intravenous and oral medications; and in some systems perform cricothyrodotomies and insert chest tubes.

* Due to the lack of national standards, there are many other classification systems in use, and the one presented here is a simplified model.

with guidance from the federal government.[7] There are three general categories of emergency medical technicians (EMTs). Some systems, however, especially those using aeromedical transport, utilize nurses who have completed additional course work in prehospital care designed by the Emergency Nurses Association. All EMTs must practice under the supervision of a physician medical director who is directly responsible for the quality of provided care. Prehospital care in some regions is dependent on volunteer services, while in other regions it is provided by paid civil servants. Non-municipal, private ambulance systems also exist.

A critical component in the training of all levels of US EMTs is working directly with nurses and physicians in the emergency department (ED). During this time the EMT learns the basic skills of physical diagnosis in a supervised setting and where EMT-Is and EMT-Ps learn to start intravenous lines and other procedures. The ED experience also provides the EMT with insight into the importance of their role in the emergency medical care team. All EMTs must participate in a set number of hours of continuing education each year and maintain up-to-date certifications.

In addition to communication and transportation resources, there are five key components to effective prehospital systems: (1) a standardized facilitated mechanism for public access, such as the 911 phone number in the USA or 118 in Italy; (2) trained dispatchers who receive call information and determine the type of response indicated; (3) trained responders who understand their emergency response system, including its limitations; (4) a physician medical director responsible for establishing policies and procedures that assist in decision making and resource utilization; (5) a quality assurance program that provides mechanisms for continuous assessment and implementation of necessary change.

A number of factors render the prehospital environment markedly different from that of the controlled intramural inhospital environment. Rescuer safely is paramount as a priority. Each patient encounter in the field begins with a scene assessment prior to approaching the patient, even if this delays the provision of life-saving interventions. The scene assessment also includes the mechanism of injury, the number and severity of patients involved, and the need for additional help. Exposure to toxic chemicals or fumes, fire, or the potential for violence, may impact patient access. Environmental factors may not only impact access, but often affect patient assessment. For example, hypothermia may affect pupillary reactivity and accuracy of pulse oximetry, bright ambient light may affect pupillary assessment, and ambulance movement can render assessments during transport difficult at best.

Other factors that impact the effectiveness of an EMS system include the political and geographical environment. In urban settings, hospital proximity often promotes short response times and a scoop and run policy. Urban EMS systems often have large call volumes, making accurate telephone triage critical, and congested streets and high-rise buildings may negate short distances and result in significantly delayed patient access and transport durations. The political climate in urban areas where a large number of hospitals compete for patients may also prevent the appropriate bypassing of one institution in favor of another, such as a trauma center. In rural communities where transport distances may be great, aeromedical utilization becomes important. If a trauma center is not proximate or if weather prohibits aeromedical transport, transport to the closest facility for initial stabilization is appropriate, with subsequent transfer based upon the patient's needs and stability.

Prehospital assessment of the TBI patient

Prehospital assessment of the TBI patient generally follows protocols well established by trauma courses such as the Basic Trauma Life Support Course and the Advanced Trauma Life Support Course.[8,9] Patient care at the scene begins with a primary survey which involves an evaluation of the airway, while maintaining cervical spine control. Breathing, the need for intubation or needle decompression of a pneumothorax and circulation, and fluid resuscitation are determined at this time (see management section below). A brief examination of the abdomen, pelvis, and extremities follows. A detailed head-to-toe evaluation is often best obtained during transport.

History

On the initial encounter, it is not possible to accurately determine the degree of brain injury that a head-injured patient has sustained (See Glasgow Coma Scale below). In patients who appear to have sustained a minor head injury, the only historical parameters proven to be useful in identifying patients with lesions requiring neurosurgical intervention are loss of consciousness (LOC) and amnesia.[10] The presence of either of these findings prompts the need for careful serial examinations and consideration for transport to a hospital with neurosurgical capabilities. Masters et al. retrospectively reviewed 22,035 head trauma cases and developed a risk categorization scheme.[11] The scheme was then prospectively validated in 7035 patients. The presence of LOC moved a patient from the low risk group to the moderate risk group with an associated increase in the incidence of clinically significant intracranial injury from 0% to 4%.

Although the mechanism of injury is interesting to obtain and may direct additional inquiries, there is no evidence that mechanism alone is predictive of an intracranial injury in blunt head trauma.[12,13,14] Patients with a history of a penetrating injury, or the potential for a penetrating injury such as a gunshot to the scalp, deserve special attention and should be transported directly to a trauma center even if the injury appears inconsequential.[15]

History of alcohol use, anti-coagulant therapy, hemophilia, or age over 60 years are additional historical findings that have been associated with an increased risk for an intracranial event. Although the literature provides only weak evidence, the elderly have higher rates of intracranial injuries,[16,17,18] and increased morbidity and mortality from TBI. In a prospective study, of the patients older than 60 with LOC or post-traumatic amnesia (PTA) and a GCS of 15 in the ED, 28% were found to have an intracranial lesion.[12] This was a significantly higher rate than for the younger cohorts in the same study. The increased incidence may be due in part to cerebral atrophy and stretching of bridging veins that tear, causing subdural hematomas. An extremely conservative approach is best when faced with an elder patient who has sustained head trauma. Prehospital care providers should take the aforementioned historical factors into consideration when determining the transport destination of potential TBI patients.

Physical

The extent of the physical examination performed on head-injured patients depends on the prehospital provider's level of training and expected transport times. Patient should be examined for signs of trauma including presence of open wounds, hemotympanum, and CSF rhinorrhea and otorrhea. All patients require a minimum assessment of: (1) blood pressure; (2) oxygenation; (3) pupils; (4) the Glasgow Coma Scale (GCS) score.

Blood pressure and oxygenation

Multiple studies demonstrate the association of hypoxemia and hypotension with poor outcomes in TBI patients.[5,19,20] Consequently, the cornerstone to providing prehospital care is to assess for these two factors and to initiate management as indicated. The Traumatic Data Coma Bank (TDCB) provides the best scientific evidence in which hypotension was defined as a single observation of < 90 mmHg SBP and hypoxemia defined as apnea, cyanosis, or a hemoglobin oxygen saturation < 90% in the field.[5] The TDCB found that hypotension and hypoxemia were predictors of a poor outcome independent of other major predictors, such as age, GCS score, intracranial diagnosis, and pupillary status. A single episode of hypotension was associated with a doubling of mortality and an increased morbidity when compared with a matched group of patients without hypotension. These findings have also been reported in the pediatric literature, although blood pressure must be adjusted for age.[20,21] Additionally, evidence supports the benefit of higher blood pressure in severe TBI patients being associated with improved outcomes.[22]

It is often difficult to independently assess hypotension and hypoxemia clinically, since decreased peripheral blood flow will result in decreased oxygen saturation when measured by pulse oximetry. However, in one field study documenting these assessment parameters, hypoxemia was found in 13 patients with no concomitant hypotension. Their outcomes were poor, supporting hypoxemia as an independent predictor of outcome. The precise definitions of hypotension and hypoxemia are unclear but their evidence indicates that both must be prevented or immediately corrected when present if TBI patient outcomes are to be maximized.

Pupils

Pupil size and reactivity may be affected by increased intracranial pressure. Therefore, the pupillary examination is a key component in prehospital assessment of the TBI patient. The examination consists of determining pupil size, symmetry, and reactivity to light. Intracranial hypertension resulting in uncal herniation may compress the third cranial nerve, reduce parasympathetic tone and result in a fixed, dilated pupil. Bilaterally dilated and fixed pupils are consistent with brain stem injury. However, hypoxemia, hypotension, and hypothermia are also associated with dilated pupil size and abnormal reactivity, making it necessary to resuscitate and stabilize the patient before accurate pupillary assessment can occur.[23]

The pupil examination is an important component of the prehospital evaluation of patients with head trauma. However, the ability of prehospital providers to perform accurate examinations and the diagnostic and management implications of their findings have never been systematically investigated. Regardless, serial evaluation of the pupils during transport remains a fundamental assessment parameter in that signs of intracranial hypertension may prompt critical temporizing interventions to lower intracranial pressure.

Glasgow Coma Scale (GCS)

The Glasgow Coma Scale (GCS) was created as a standardized clinical scale to facilitate the reliable interobserver neurologic assessments of head-injured patients in coma. The original studies utilizing the GCS score as a tool for assessing outcome required the presence of coma for at least six hours.[24,25,26] The scale was not designed to diagnose patients with mild (GCS 13–15) or moderate (GCS 9–12) TBI, nor was it intended to supplant a neurological examination. Instead, the GCS was originally developed as a simple assessment tool for serial TBI patient evaluations by relatively inexperienced care providers, and to standardize communication between inhospital care providers on rotating shifts. A single GCS score is of limited value, is insufficient to determine the degree of parenchymal injury after trauma and lacks prognostic value. However, serial GCS scores are a valuable clinical tool. A low GCS score that remains low, or a high GCS score that decreases, predicts poorer outcomes than high GCS scores that remain high, or a low GCS score that progressively improves.[13,14,26] To illustrate this, in their original paper Teasdale and Jennett present a patient who was admitted to the neurosurgical intensive care unit (NICU) with a GCS score of 14. The NICU chart reflected hourly scores of 14 for 3 hours, followed by a decline to 13 and then to 4, at which point the patient was taken to the operating room for craniotomy and subdural evacuation.[24]

From a prehospital perspective, the key to employing the GCS is in serial determinations. In one of the original multi-center studies validating the scale, approximately 13% of patients who ultimately were in coma had an initial GCS score of 15.[26] A single GCS determination is superfluous and cannot be used alone in either diagnosing or decision making in head injury.

Prehospital management of the TBI patient

The prehospital management of the TBI patient focuses on stabilizing and maintaining oxygenation and blood pressure. All head-injured patients have potential cervical injury and should be immobilized if there is cervical tenderness or pain, a neurologic deficit, altered mental status, or distracting injuries. A fundamental premise for emergency care is to anticipate and prepare for potential eventualities such as vomiting, seizures, and aberrations of blood pressure or oxygenation. Consequently, suction should be checked, emesis basins available, and consideration should be given for intravenous access, and to pulse oximetry, blood pressure, and cardiac monitoring. (See Figure 1.1.)

Airway

Ensuring a patent airway is the highest priority in all resuscitations. The airway must be secured and maintained throughout transport, and all airway maneuvers must be performed with consideration given to cervical spine stability. Indications for a field intubation include failure to protect the airway, failure to ventilate, and hypoxemia despite supplemental oxygen administration. It is reasonable to proactively secure the airway if it is anticipated that one of the above may occur during transport. This is particularly true in aeromedical transports. It has been reported that prehospital endotracheal intubation is associated with a decreased incidence of hypoxemia-related secondary brain insults.[20] In a retrospective case control study of 1092 patients with severe TBI, the outcome of patients endotracheally intubated in the field was compared to patients who were not intubated.[27] Paramedics were permitted to intubate only if patients were apneic, unconscious with ineffective ventilation, and had no gag reflex. Though the methodology was flawed, the study suggested that prehospital endotracheal intubation significantly improved survival.

The method of securing the TBI patient airway depends on the resources and skills of the EMS system. Emergency airway procedure options include oral endotracheal intubation, blind nasotracheal intubation, and induction/ neuromuscular blockade-assisted oral intubation. In a prospective randomized study of prehospital trauma patients with GCS scores less than 8, the nasotracheal intubation success rate was not shown to be significantly different than the success rate for neuromuscular blockade-assisted oral intubations using succinylcholine.[28] However, nasotracheal intubation may

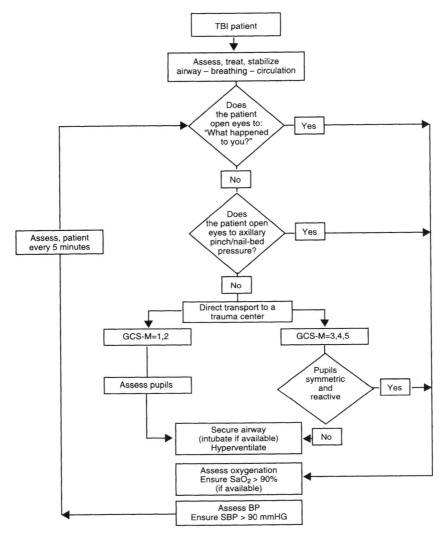

Figure 1.1 Algorithm for the prehospital management of traumatic brain injury.
Reproduced by permission of the Brain Trauma Foundation.

predispose patients to complications that may interfere with a successful
resuscitation such as epistaxis, intracranial intubation, and elevation of the
intracranial pressure. The emergency airway procedure of choice in the severe
head-injured patient must optimize intubation conditions, while minimizing
the adverse effects of intubation. Multiple studies have demonstrated the
safety of using short-acting neuromuscular blockade in the field to facilitate
intubation performed by prehospital care providers.[28,29,30,31,32,33] Many rapid-
sequence protocols recommend that lidocaine, 1.5 mg/kg, be given several

minutes before laryngoscopy. These protocols also recommend that other central nervous system protectants, such as fentanyl or thiopental, be given as part of the intubation protocol.[34,35] However, many of these agents decrease systemic blood pressure and subsequently cerebral perfusions, thus they must be employed judiciously.

Breathing/ventilation

Oxygen delivery must be maximized in the TBI patient in order to minimize secondary brain injury. Intubated patients should receive 100% oxygen, and non-intubated patients should receive supplemental oxygen via a non-rebreather mask at 12 to 15 liters per minute. In systems that carry pulse oximeters, the goal is to maintain the oxygen saturation at 100% throughout the prehospital course. Cerebral blood flow is low during the early post-injury hours and may be exacerbated by hyperventilation-induced vasoconstriction.[36] In a prospective, randomized clinical trial of severe head injury patients, it was demonstrated that early prophylactic hyperventilation to a $PaCO_2$ of 25 mmHg was associated with worse neurologic outcome at 3 and 6 months post-injury when compared to controls whose $PaCO_2$ was maintained at 35 mmHg.[37] Therefore, the goal of ventilation is to maintain adequate oxygenation without inducing hypocarbia, unless the patient exhibits clinical signs of intracranial hypertension. For EMS systems that do not carry pulse oximeters, it is recommended to ventilate adult severe TBI patients without evidence of herniation at a rate of 12 to 16 breaths per minute with a good chest rise with each ventilation.

Circulation

Similar to the detrimental effects of hypoxemia, hypotension is a critical factor associated with increased morbidity and mortality in head-injured patients. Blood pressure in the field should be monitored closely with the goals of avoiding hypotension (SBP < 90 mmHg in adults) and correcting it immediately. Generally, isotonic intravenous crystalloid administration has been the mainstay of prehospital treatment of hypotension. Of note, Vassar et al. reported that the prehospital administration of hypertonic (7.5%) saline to a subgroup of severe head-injured patients resulted in improved outcomes.[38] At the present time, the role of hypertonic saline is unclear and in need of additional study.

Herniation

The signs of cerebral herniation include a dilated, fixed pupil(s), extensor 4 posturing, or flaccid motor exam, and in severe TBI patients, a decrease in the GCS score of two or more points. Hyperventilation can decrease intracranial pressure by inducing vasoconstriction and is the recommended first line intervention for the field management of patients demonstrating signs of intracranial hypertension. Hyperventilation is continued if the signs of herniation resolve.

Mannitol does not have a defined role in the field management of patients with increased intracranial pressure. Its benefit in managing severe TBI is linked to its immediate plasma-expanding properties and to its delayed osmotic/diuretic action. Concern exists that these diuretic properties may cause hypovolemic hypotension. One pilot study has demonstrated that mannitol does not cause hypotension when given in the field.[39] However, no outcome data is available regarding mannitol use by prehospital providers. Consequently, its use is not recommended at this time.

Other prehospital treatment considerations

A potential pitfall in the management of the head-injury patient is to assume that trauma is entirely responsible for altered mental status. Consideration must be given to the reversible causes of altered mental status which include hypoglycemia, hypoxemia, hypotension, and drug toxicity. One case series demonstrated the potential mismanagement of trauma patients with unrecognized hypoglycemia and emphasizes the importance of a comprehensive approach to patient care.[40] Unfortunately, there is some evidence to suggest that hyperglycemia is associated with poor outcome in TBI patients.[41,42,43] Although cause and effect are not clear, the data questions the empiric use of dextrose in TBI patients with altered mental status. Ideally, EMS systems should utilize glucometers to assess the prehospital blood glucose concentration, and to avoid the unnecessary administration of dextrose in severe head-injured patients. In the absence of glucometers, empiric dextrose should be given if there is any question of the etiology of a patient's altered mental status.

Analgesia/sedation/neuromuscular blockade

Severe head-injured patients can experience episodes of agitation and combativeness, both of which tend to increase intracranial pressure. Therefore, as first line treatment for the prevention of increases in ICP, analgesics and sedatives should be utilized. These medications should have a short duration of action. Narcotic analgesics such as fentanyl, or a benzodiazepine such as midazolam, are typically employed. These agents help patients to tolerate diagnostic and therapeutic procedures without unacceptable agitation or intracranial hypertension. Use of these agents is relatively contraindicated in the hypovolemic, hypotensive patient. The GCS score should be determined before these agents are given. (See Table 1.2.)

Table 1.2 Clinical pearls in the prehospital management of head-injured patients

- Loss of consciousness and amnesia are the best historical predictors that a head-injured patient is sustaining a brain injury.
- Hypoxemia and hypotension are predictors of outcome in TBI patients and thus should be carefully monitored and treated appropriately.
- A single GCS score determination has no predictive value and thus the GCS must be repeated serially.
- Clinical signs of increased intracranial pressure include dilated fixed pupil(s) or extensor posturing and it is treated with hyperventilation.
- Patients with moderate or severe TBI should be transported to a hospital with neurosurgical monitoring capabilities.

Transport decisions

The overall goals of prehospital management of head-injured patients include rapid recognition and correction of life-threatening conditions, prevention of secondary brain insults, and transportation to the closest appropriate facility, which in the moderate or severe TBI patient must include 24-hour availability of neuro-imaging and neurosurgical capabilities, and intracranial pressure monitoring and treatment capabilities. Smith et al. demonstrated that patients initially treated in trauma centers had significantly less mortality than in non-trauma centers.[44] Another study compared the outcomes of injured patients before implementation of the American College of Surgeons Committee on Trauma guidelines for a level II trauma center with outcome after conversion to a level II trauma center.[45] For patients with closed head trauma, the survival was 15.4% before and 32% after meeting the criteria.

Severe TBI patients transported to trauma centers without prompt neuro-surgical care or intracranial pressure monitoring are at risk for a poor outcome. Acute subdural hematomas in severe TBI patients are associated with 90% mortality if evacuated more than four hours after injury, but only 30% mortality if evacuated earlier.[46] If subdural evacuation is initiated less than two hours post-injury, one study reported a 70% decrease in mortality.[47] To achieve this surgical window, 24-hour availability of CT scanning is mandatory. Intracranial pressure monitoring guides specific management to maintain cerebral perfusion and is recommended based on supporting scientific evidence in the *Guidelines for the Management of Severe Head Injury*.[48] Consequently, it is recommended that EMS systems operate under pre-established trauma transport protocols. Commonly accepted criteria for transport of head-injured patients to a trauma center include severity of injury, a respiratory rate < 10, systolic blood pressure < 90 mmHg, a GCS score < 12, and a penetrating mechanism of injury.

As previously discussed, it is often not possible for EMS personnel to accurately predict which head-injured patients have sustained a brain injury. Historical and physical information gathered at the scene may provide valuable information required to determine the appropriate transport destination of TBI patients. The hospital selected by the EMS provider can have a profound impact on outcome. An organized trauma system improves the outcome of patients with multi-system trauma. Therefore, all EMS systems should identify those institutions with the capabilities and resources to appropriately care for the injured.

Conclusion

In summary, the initial evaluation and treatment of the head-injured patient entail a careful primary and secondary trauma survey focusing on oxygenation, blood pressure, pupils, and the Glasgow Coma Scale score. Strict attention to the cervical spine and rapid sequence endotracheal intubation are recommended when airway control is required. Sedation, with or without a short-acting pharmacologic paralytic agent, may be needed in the agitated, combative head-injured patient once reversible causes of agitation, such as hypoglycemia, hypotension or hypoxemia, have been addressed. The field management of intracranial hypertension is through hyperventilation which is continued only as long as clinical signs are present. Hypotension is managed with isotonic fluid bolus infusions. Patients with severe TBI should be transported to a trauma center with dedicated neurosurgical capabilities. Patients with a moderate TBI should be transported to a trauma center with access to neurosurgical services. Transport decisions can be difficult in those patients with a head injury of undetermined severity; i.e. those patients with a GCS above 12, since the clinical course is unpredictable. It is best to transport these patients to centers with higher instead of lower levels of trauma care.

References

1. Jager, T., Weiss, H., Coben, J., & Pepe, P. (2000). Traumatic brain injuries evaluated in U.S. emergency departments, 1992–1994. *Acad. Emerg. Med., 7*, 134–140.
2. Thurman, D., & Guerrero, J. (1999). Trends in hospitalization associated with traumatic brain injury. *J. Am. Med. Assoc., 282*, 954–957.
3. Gabella, B., Hoffman, R., Marine, W., & Stallones, L. (1997). Urban and rural traumatic brain injuries in Colorado. *Ann. Epidemiol., 7*, 207–212.
4. Woodward, A., Dorsch, M., & Simpson, D. (1984). Head injuries in country and city: a study of hospital separations in South Australia. *Med. J. Austral., 141*, 13–17.
5. Chestnut, R. M., Marshall, L. F., Klauber, M. R., et al. (1993). The role of secondary brain injury in determining outcome from severe head injury. *J. Trauma, 34*, 216–222.
6. Brain Trauma Foundation (2000). *Guidelines for prehospital management of traumatic brain injury*. New York: Brain Trauma Foundation Press.
7. Snyder, J., Baren, J., Ryan, S., et al. (1995). Emergency medical service system development: results of the statewide emergency medical service technical assessment program. *Ann. Emerg. Med., 25*, 768–775.

8. Campbell, J. (1995). *Basic trauma life support* (3rd ed., pp. 23–46). Englewood Cliffs, NJ: Brady/Prentice Hall.
9. American College of Surgeons (1993). *Advanced trauma life support* (3rd ed.). Chicago, IL: First Impression.
10. Gottesfeld, S., & Jagoda, A. (2000). Mild head trauma: appropriate diagnosis and management. *Emerg. Med. Pract., 2*, 1–24.
11. Masters, S. J., McClean, P. M., Arcarese, J. S., et al. (1987). Skull X-ray examination after head trauma. *N. Engl. J. Med., 316*, 84–90.
12. Jeret, J. S., Mandell, M., Anziska, B., et al. (1993). Clinical predictors of abnormality disclosed by computed tomography after mild head trauma. *Neurosurgery, 32*, 9–15.
13. Shackford, S. R., Wald, S. L., Ross, S. E., et al. (1992). The clinical utility of computerized tomographic scanning and neurologic examination in the management of patients with minor head injuries. *J. Trauma., 33*, 385–389.
14. Stein, S. C., O'Malley, K. F., & Ross, S. E. (1991). Is routine computerized tomography scanning too expensive for mild head injury? *Ann. Emerg. Med., 20*, 1286–1292.
15. Anglin, D., Hutson, H., Luftman, J., et al. (1998). Intracranial hemorrhage associated with tangential gunshot wounds to the head. *Acad. Emerg. Med., 5*, 672–678.
16. Borczuk, P. (1995). Predictors of intracranial injury in patients with mild head trauma. *Ann. Emerg. Med., 25*, 731–736.
17. Schynoll, W., Overton, D., Krome, R., et al. (1993). A prospective study to identify high-yield criteria associated with acute intracranial computed tomography findings in head injured patients. *Am. J. Emerg. Med., 11*, 321–326.
18. Nagurney, J., Borczuk, P., & Thomas, S. (1998). Elder patients with closed head trauma: a comparison with non-elder patients. *Acad. Emerg. Med., 5*, 678–684.
19. Fearnside, M. R., Cook, R. J., McDougall, P., et al. (1993). The Westmead Head Injury Project outcome in severe head injury. A comparative analysis of prehospital, clinical and CT variables. *Br. J. Neurosurg., 7*, 267–279.
20. Kokska, E. R., Smith, G. S., Pittman, T., & Weber, T. R. (1998). Early hypotension worsens neurological outcome in pediatric patients with moderately severe head trauma. *J. Pediatr. Surg., 33*, 333–338.
21. Pigula, F. A., Wald, S. L., Shackford, S. R., et al. (1993). The effect of hypotension and hypoxemia on children with severe head injuries. *J. Pediatr. Surg., 28*, 310–314.
22. Silverston, P. (1989). Pulse oximetry at the roadside: a study of pulse oximetry in immediate case. *Br. Med. J., 298*, 711–713.
23. Meyer, S., Gibb, T., & Jurkovich, G. (1993). Evaluation and significance of the pupillary light reflex in trauma patients. *Ann. Emerg. Med., 22*, 1052–1057.
24. Teasdale, G., & Jennett, B. (1974). Assessment of coma and impaired consciousness: a practical scale. *Lancet, 4*, 81–83.
25. Teasdale, G., & Jennett, B. (1976). Assessment and prognosis of coma after head injury. *Acta Neurochir., 34*, 45–55.
26. Jennett, B., Teasdale, G., Galbraith, S., et al. (1977). Severe head injuries in three countries. *J. Neurol. Neurosurg. Psych., 40*, 291–298.
27. Winchell, R. J., & Hoyt, D. B. (1997). Endotracheal intubation in the field improves survival in patients with severe head injury. *Arch. Surg., 132*, 592–597.
28. Rhee, K. J., & O'Malley, R. J. (1994). Neuromuscular blockade-assisted oral

intubation versus naso-tracheal intubation in the prehospital care of injured patients. *Ann. Emerg. Med., 23*, 37–42.

29. Syverud, S. A., Borron, S. W., Storer, D. L., et al. (1998). Prehospital use of neuromuscular agents in a helicopter ambulance program. *Ann. Emerg. Med., 17*, 236–242.

30. Sing, R., Reilly, P., Rotondo, M., et al. (1996). Out-of-hospital rapid-sequence induction for intubation of the pediatric patient. *Acad. Emerg. Med., 3*, 41–45.

31. Ma, O. J., Atchley, R., Hatley, T., et al. (1998). Intubation success rates improve for an air medical program after implementing the use of neuromuscular blocking agents. *Am. J. Emerg. Med., 31*, 228–233.

32. Hedges, J., Dronen, S., Feero, S., et al. (1988). Succinylcholine-assisted intubations in prehospital care. *Ann. Emerg. Med., 17*, 469–472.

33. Brownstein, D., Shugerman, R., Cummings, P., et al. (1996). Prehospital endotracheal intubation of children by paramedics. *Ann. Emerg. Med., 21*, 664–668.

34. Walls, R. (1993). Rapid-sequence intubation in head trauma. *Ann. Emerg. Med., 22*, 1008–1013.

35. Walls, R., & Murphy, M. (2000). Increased intracranial pressure. In R. Walls (Ed.), *Emergency airway management* (pp. 159–163). Philadelphia, PA: Lippincott, Williams & Wilkins.

36. Marion, D., Darby, J., & Yonas, H. (1991). Acute regional cerebral blood flow changes caused by severe head injuries. *J. Neurosurg., 74*, 407–414.

37. Muizelaar, J., Marmarou, A., Ward, J., et al. (1991). Adverse effects of prolonged hyperventilation in patients with severe head injury: a randomized clinical trial. *J. Neurosurg., 75*, 731–739.

38. Vassar, M. J., Perry, C. A., & Holcroft, J. W. (1993). Prehospital resuscitation of hypotensive trauma patients with 7.5% NaCl versus 7.5% NaCl with added dextran: a controlled trial. *J. Trauma., 34*, 622–632.

39. Sayre, M., Daily, S., Stern, S., et al. (1996). Out-of-hospital administration of mannitol to head-injured patients does not change systolic blood pressure. *Acad. Emerg. Med., 3*, 840–848.

40. Luber, S., Brady, W., Brand, A., et al. (1996). Acute hypoglycemia masquerading as head trauma: a report of four cases. *Am. J. Emerg. Med., 14*, 543–547.

41. Robertson, C., Goodman, J., Narayan, R., et al. (1991). The effect of glucose administration on carbohydrate metabolism after head injury. *J. Neurosurg., 74*, 43–50.

42. Lam, A., Winn, H., Cullen, B., & Sundling, N. (1991). Hyperglycemia and neurological outcome in patients with head injury. *J. Neurosurg., 75*, 545–551.

43. Young, B., Oh, L., Dempsey, R., et al. (1989). Relationship between admission hyperglycemia and neurologic outcome of severely brain injured patients. *Ann. Surg., 210*, 466–472.

44. Smith, J., Martin, L., Young, W., et al. (1990). Do trauma centers improve outcome over non-trauma centers? The evaluation of regional trauma care using discharge abstract data and patient management categories. *J. Trauma., 30*, 1533–1538.

45. Norwood, S., Fernandez, L., & England, J. (1995). The early effects of implementing American College of Surgeons Level II criteria on transfer and survival rates at a rurally based community hospital. *J. Trauma., 39*, 240–245.

46. Seeling, J. M., Becker, D. P., Miller, J. D., et al. (1981). Traumatic acute subdural hematoma. Major mortality reduction in comatose patients treated within four hours. *N. Engl. J. Med., 304*, 1511–1518.

47. Haselberger, K., Pucher, R., & Auer, L. M. (1988). Prognosis after acute subdural or epidural hemorrhage. *Acta Neurochir., 90*, 111–116.
48. Brain Trauma Foundation (1995). *Guidelines for the management of severe head injury*. New York: Brain Trauma Foundation.

Appendix: Explanation of the algorithm for prehospital assessment and treatment of traumatic brain injury

The Emergency Medical Services (EMS) task force used a consensus method to develop an algorithm based on the scientific evidence contained in *Guidelines for Prehospital Management of Traumatic Brain Injury*. The algorithm can be used as a framework to assess, treat and transport the patient with traumatic brain injury (TBI). Individual and regional circumstances may require prehospital healthcare providers to modify the algorithm, because it may not be appropriate for all patients and locations. The following points provide more detail for summaries of the steps in the graphic algorithm:

1   The healthcare provider's first priority in assessing, stabilizing, and treating a TBI patient is to follow basic resuscitation protocols that prioritize airway, breathing, and circulation assessment and treatment.

   Following stabilization of airway, breathing and circulation, the healthcare provider assesses the patient by first asking him or her, "What happened to you?"

   If the patient opens his or her eyes, the provider then asks the questions in the verbal and motor sections of the Glasgow Coma Scale (GCS) to determine the total score. Patients with a GCS score of 9 to 13 (moderate TBI) and patients with a GCS score of 3 to 8 (severe TBI) should be transported to a trauma center.

2   If the patient does not open his or her eyes, the healthcare provider applies blunt pressure to the nail bed or pinches the anterior axillary skin to elicit eye opening.

3   If the patient opens his or her eyes with nail-bed pressure or axillary pinch, the healthcare provider assesses the verbal and motor sections of the GCS to determine the total score.

4   Patients who are unresponsive with a GCS score of 3 to 8 should be transported to a trauma center with the following TBI capabilities:

   • 24-hour CT scanning capability
   • 24-hour available operating room and prompt neurosurgical care
   • The ability to monitor intracranial pressure and treat intracranial hypertension as delineated in the *Guidelines for the Management of Severe Head Injury*.

5   Patients with a GCS score of 14–15 can be transported to a nontrauma center hospital, which has the basic emergency department capabilities for immediate resuscitation of the critically injured.

6 If the patient does not open his or her eyes with nail-bed pressure or axillary pinch, he or she should be transported directly to a trauma center described above.

7 For unresponsive patients who respond to nail-bed pressure with extensor posturing or who are flaccid, the healthcare provider should secure the airway (intubate, if available) and hyperventilate (20 bpm in an adult, 30 bpm in a child, and 35 bpm in an infant).

8 For unresponsive patients who respond to nail-bed pressure or axillary pinch with abnormal flexion or a higher GCS motor response, but have asymmetric and/or dilated and fixed pupil(s), the prehospital healthcare provider should hyperventilate at the rates described above.

9 All TBI patients should have their oxygenation assessed at least every 5 minutes and their O_2 saturation maintained at > 90%. Systolic blood pressure should also be measured, and maintained greater than 90 mmHg in adults and for ages 12–16; 80 mmHg for ages 5–12; 75 mmHg for ages 1–5; and 65 mmHg for infants less than 1 year of age.

10 Because the patient's neurological status may change, the healthcare provider should fully assess the patient every 5 minutes and treat or modify treatment as appropriate.

2 Mild brain injury

Detecting high-risk patients

M. A. Muñoz-Sanchez, F. Murillo-Cabezas, and J. Léon-Carrión

Introduction

Given that the goal of medical attention for patients with mild head injury (MHI) is the same as that for patients with severe head injuries, that is, to achieve optimum results avoiding secondary brain damage, strategies that will facilitate the early detection of patients with asymptomatic or scarcely symptomatic intracranial damage must be developed.

There is no doubt that the safest and earliest way to detect potentially severe head injuries is verifying, by computerized tomography (CT), the existence of clinically silent intracranial lesions (IL). However, because of the large number of patients, we need an optimized strategy for patients' assistance that will deal with the risk of neurological complications in a small number of patients and the high cost of neuroimaging studies in all patients with an MHI.

The indiscriminate use of CT scans for the study of any cranial blow is not the most efficient attitude, nor the most effective measure. As demonstrated in a study by Stiell et al.[1] carried out in seven Canadian hospitals, the greatest number of diagnostic omissions of intracranial lesions among mild brain injuries was found in the hospitals in which a greater number of CT scans were solicited for these patients. Despite this, we must consider not only the cost of these examinations, but also the cost derived from their lack of use. On the other hand, the diagnostic tools available are determinant in the choice of the most adequate algorithm of medical care.

The first obstacle that we find is a conceptual one. The definition of head injury as "a physical damage to, or a functional impairment of, the cranial contents from an acute mechanical energy exchange, excluding birth trauma" seems to be too strict since it would only include patients with a loss of consciousness, expressing global and transitory cerebral dysfunction, with post-traumatic amnesia or neurological disorders. However, a large group of patients with only an intense holocranial headache or repeated vomiting would be excluded, according to this definition. For that reason, certain authors, such as Jennet[2] include these two symptoms in the concept of head injury. These conceptual differences, among other reasons, explain the variable incidence of MHI that ranges from 123–377/100,000 inhabitants/ year.

On the other hand, there exist important differences in the management of these patients, even in the same country or territory. These differences are sometimes based on the availability of diagnostic resources (X-ray, CT scan, etc.) or on the financing system of the public or private healthcare systems, but the true reasons for these differences do not always justify the differences. However, the necessity of clear criteria for medical care to these patients, especially for detection in patients that seem to have only a mild injury, is of unanimous interest.

The deterioration of brain injuries initially classified as mild is of quantitative and qualitative importance. These injuries form approximately 10% of the total amount of brain injuries finally classified as severe. In regard to the impact on mortality, we must remember that authors such as Klauber et al.[3] have established that the interhospital differences documented for the lethalness of severe brain injury have a statistically significant correlation with greater mortality among the initially mild brain injuries, and not with worse outcome for the initially severe brain injuries.

Many studies in the literature[4–24] have analyzed the factors that could be considered risk markers in an MHI, that is, the signs and symptoms of an apparently mild head injury associated with the presence or development of traumatic intracranial damage that initially have a null or scant clinical expression. However, predicting that patients will present acute intracranial traumatic lesions is not easy since there is no group of clinically proven markers that can identify all the patients that have asymptomatic or scarcely expressive brain lesions.

Risk factors

Past medical history

The use of anticoagulant drugs and alcohol abuse are considered risk factors to the extent that certain special guidelines are advised, like those of the Italian Neurological Society,[4] for urgent CT and hospitalization for patients with a head injury, a Glasgow Coma Scale (GCS) score of 15 and the previously mentioned past case history. The results of our studies agree with the data concerning the use of anticoagulant medication.[5] In regard to alcohol abuse, we have not encountered a greater incidence of intracranial lesions among alcoholic patients, but a greater risk for trauma and more difficulties in the initial clinical evaluation.

Level of consciousness

This is the most relevant clinical sign and the basis for the classification of head injury (HI) severity. The classification of the severity of head injury is controversial. While all HI with a score on the Glasgow Coma Scale of less than 9 points are considered severe, the score that defines the limit between mild and moderate is changing, because of recent reports during the 1990s. In 1989, the Committee on Trauma of the American College of Surgeons[6] classified as mild those head injuries with scores between 13 and 15 on the GCS. Later reports, such as those of Stein and Ross[7] in 1990, Borczuk[8] in 1995, and, more recently, Culota et al.[9] in 1996, reveal with computerized tomography that the MHI with a score of 13 on the GCS present a rate of intracranial abnormalities ranging between 28% and 32%. Considering that 8% to 13% of patients required neurosurgical treatment, the authors advise that a 13-point score be considered a moderate head injury. Classification of the severity of the head injury would be as expressed in Table 2.1. At present,

Table 2.1 Head injury classification

	Degree 0	Degree 1	Degree 2	Degree 3
Glasgow scale	15	14–15	9–13	< 9
Loss of consciousness	No	Transitory	–	–
Superior functions	Normal	Altered	–	–
Amnesia	No	Yes	–	–
Headaches	No	Yes	–	–
Vomiting	No	Yes	–	–
Agitation	No	Yes	–	–
Cranial fracture	No	Yes	–	–
Convulsion	No	No	Yes	–
Focal signs	No	No	Yes	–
Complementary studies				
AP, L X-ray	Yes*	Yes	–	–
Cervical L X-ray	a, b, c	a, b, c	Yes	–
CT scan	No	d		
Neurosurgery consulting	No	If deterioration	Yes	Yes
ICP monitoring	No	No	Some	Yes
Destination				
Discharge to home	Yes	–	–	–
Admission to observation	No	Yes, 24 h	Yes, 24–48 h	–
Admission to ward	–	CT lesion	After observation	–
Admission to ICU	–	–	Yes, IL	Yes

a, spontaneous pain or with palpation; b, fall or dive; c, overturning or fall of a vehicle; d, deterioration, cranial fracture, GCS of 14, anticoagulant drug; IL, intracranial lesion. * See text.

however, this classification seems too extensive and certain authors suggest a separation of the brain injuries with a score of 14 from the group of mild brain injuries.[9]

Table 2.1 shows a fourth group of head injuries classified as banal head injury. The Glasgow Coma Scale is not useful in differentiating between banal and mild head injuries, since a score of 15 may apply to either group. The answer to this question is not a trivial or semantic matter. It will have extremely important and direct consequences on our medical decisions concerning the patient. Remember that a patient suffering a banal blow can and should be sent home.

A banal blow to the skull would be that in which the patient has no symptoms at the moment of the accident nor when seen at the hospital. Some authors, however, include patients with unspecific symptoms, such as non-holocranial and non-progressive headaches or dizziness. Other authors more cautiously demand that no bone damage exists.[10]

Age

In relation to age, most of the authors agree. The possibility of an intracranial hematoma in an MHI is two to three times greater in an adult than in a child. If the patient is over 60, the relative risk of neurologic deterioration is much higher, according to Borczuk,[8] and French and Dublin,[11] and even ten times greater according to Jones and Jeffreys.[12] From our experience, in a series of 5098 head injuries with a GCS of 14–15, the probability for the development of a brain lesion in a child (< 14 years) is three times lower (see Table 2.2) than that of an adult (> 14 years). The odds ratio for an adult over 54 years of age resulted in 2.22 (see Table 2.3), reaching levels even six times greater after excluding fractures as confounding variables (see Table 2.4).

Loss of consciousness/amnesia

The transitory loss of consciousness (LOC) and post-traumatic amnesia (PTA) are considered high risk variables. The transitory loss of consciousness is, according to Moran et al.[13] a clinically independent predictor of anomalies

Table 2.2 Age–severity

| Age (years) | Intracranial lesion | | |
	Yes	No	Total
< 14	16	1880	1896
> 14	87	3114	3201
Total	103	4994	5097

$p < 0.001$; odds ratio, 3.22 (1.9–5.47).

Table 2.3 Age–severity

Age (years)	Intracranial lesion		
	Yes	No	Total
< 54	74	4259	4333
> 54	29	735	764
Total	103	4994	5097

$p < 0.001$; odds ratio, 2.22 (1.46–3.39).

Table 2.4 MHI without cranial fracture: age–severity

Age (years)	Intracranial lesion		
	Yes	No	Total
< 54	17	4183	4200
> 54	18	723	741
Total	35	4906	4941

$p < 0.001$; odds ratio, 6.13 (3.11–11.59).

in the CT scan. Amnesia lasting more than 5 minutes is also associated with greater risk, increasing the positive predictive value to 60% when agitation co-exists, according to Duus et al.[14]

Cephalagia (headache)/vomiting/agitation

If we only include the loss of consciousness as an expression of global brain dysfunction, and amnesia as a clinical correlate of the loss of consciousness recovered, an important group of patients that have only symptoms of intense, persistent headache and/or repetitive vomiting and or/agitation would be excluded from the definition of brain injury.

Many authors, including our study group, consider that the presence of at least one of the referred symptoms is sufficient to differentiate a banal blow from a head injury (please refer to Table 2.1), since its presence seems to be associated with the increase in the risk of neurological deterioration. The relative risk of neurologic deterioration for headaches and vomiting, published by Lee et al. in 1996,[15] is of 7% and 15% respectively. The absolute risk for the development of intracranial complications related to agitation, according to Duus et al. in 1993,[14] is of 16.7%.

Focal neurological signs

These are classified as high risk clinical variables, especially if associated with cranial fracture and an age > 60 years, according to the studies by Borczuk,[8] or with the co-existence of agitation, according to Duus et al.[14] Thus, the presence of focal signs classifies the patients directly as having a moderate brain injury, as can be seen in Table 2.1.

Skull fracture

The risk related to a skull fracture is controversial. For certain authors, such as Jennett,[10] Jones and Jeffreys,[12] Moran et al.,[13] or Mendelow et al.,[16] the detection of this lesion in an MHI is even more relevant than the loss of consciousness or transitory amnesia. Moran et al.[13] consider it an important predictor of positive cerebral CT scan in their publication in 1994. Other authors, such as Feuerman, Cooper, Murshid, or Duus,[17-20] do not consider fractures as variables of risk. It should be pointed out, however, that Murshid's series with 566 cases and 22% of CT scans done, as well as Feuerman's series with 373 cases of MHI and 34% scanned, and Cooper's series on 207 patients with intracranial hemorrhagic lesions and head injury of varying severity, are all retrospective studies. The total amount is no more than 1442 patients with mild head injury alone, including Mendelow et al.'s retrospective study,[21] and much less than the 36,637 MHI admitted to the primary surgical ward, documented by Mendelow in his publication of 1983.[16]

Duus et al.'s retrospective study of 1876 cases[14] cannot be comparatively evaluated since skull X-rays were not carried out and the study excludes patients with clinical evidence of basilar or depressed fractures.

In our prospective study on 1293 cases of MHI attended in the first semester of 1995 in our Emergency Department,[22] the presence of skull fracture was associated with an intracranial lesion in 32 cases (45% of the patients). Due to this, we consider it a factor of primordial relevance. If we distribute the sample into different age groups, the majority of the tomographic abnormalities appear in adults, with a statistically significant difference ($p < 0.001$) in comparison to children.[23] We agree with those authors that consider a fracture in a child with MHI of less clinical importance than in adults, except for depressed fractures that imply surgical treatment.

On the contrary, a fracture in an adult involves a considerably greater risk for the development of intracranial lesions. Summarizing, notwithstanding the existing controversy, there are an increasing number of studies that document a statistically significant association between cranial fracture in mild brain injury and brain lesion.

Biochemical markers

Two substances have been studied as possible markers of brain lesion in mild brain injury: the Beta-endorphins and protein S100. Pasaoglu et al.,[24] after determining Beta-endorphin levels in the CSF of a group of patients with brain injury of varying severity, conclude that, although high, the levels are not useful for establishing outcome given that the authors' values do not correlate with the Glasgow Coma Scale. According to Ingebrigtsen and Romner,[25] the study of protein S100 seems to be more promising given that, during the immediate post-traumatic phase of patients with GCS scores of 14–15 and normal CT scans, an increase of this protein in those patients with cerebral lesions found in magnetic resonance imaging (MRI) was observed.

Guidelines for the management of mild head injury

Triage

The management of an MHI starts in the emergency room with a history and physical examination. This permits an initial triage in which HI are classified as banal in asymptomatic patients with a GCS score of 15 and no loss of consciousness or amnesia. If the patient presents a transitory loss of consciousness, post-traumatic amnesia, a strong holocranial headache, repeated vomiting, cranial fracture, agitation, or 14 points on the GCS, he or she will be included in the category of MHI. The head injury will be considered moderate in the case of post-traumatic seizure, any focal neurological sign or a GCS score between 13 and 9.

Complementary studies

Assuming that the presence of a cranial fracture is an independent predictor of pathological findings in the CT scan of mild brain injury, is it reasonable to have an X-ray done for all cranial blows? In general, we consider this study necessary for asymptomatic cranial blows alone (head injury 0 from Table 2.1) if the patient presents: alcohol or drug abuse, the suspicion of a skull fracture (depression, and so forth) or a lesion of the cranial base (loss of SCF through the nose or ear, hemotympanus, Battel's sign, periorbital hematoma), an extensive or open scalp injury, facial trauma, age < 2 years or the suspicion of child abuse.[26]

This attitude is motivated by the number of fractures documented among banal blows that occur independently of the situations or characteristics mentioned. On the other hand, due to the low cost of the examination, the higher rate of fractures (between 6% and 10%) and mainly to its value as a marker of severity, simple X-rays are taken for all mild head injuries (head injury 1 of Table 2.1), that is, symptomatic blows. In conclusion, the indications for cranial roentgenograms increase, including Masters et al.'s moderate risk[27] plus a criterion from Jennett: scalp injury.

CT scan

In regard to CT scan indications, all moderate and severe head injuries should have an urgent CT done. This does not apply to MHI. While certain authors, such as Stein and Ross,[7] consider an urgent CT scan to be imperative in any case with MHI loss of consciousness or amnesia, others, such as Duus et al.[20] believe that no neuroimaging studies are necessary. Others, such as Feuerman et al.[17] are less radical and advise a tomography in MHI with 14 points, and with 15 points only in the presence of a mental disorder or neurologic deficit. The strategy that facilitates the most efficient identification of all the tomographic anomalies should undoubtedly be decided upon by each hospital, since the number of diagnostic tools and the number of beds for hospitalization will be of determinant value for the optimal algorithm of medical care.

In our department, where we receive 215 MHI/month, having two scanners and a small number of hospital beds, we have chosen to limit the urgent CT scans in MHI to patients that present a skull fracture, neurologic deterioration, 14 points on the GCS or the ingestion of anticoagulant drugs. This strategy has enabled the early identification of a group of mild brain injuries, potentially severe, without overwhelming the neuroradiology section, and avoids unnecessary hospitalizations.

Destination

After the patient's case history is noted down and physical and radiological examinations given, we make a crucial decision: either to discharge the patient from the hospital or to admit her or him. Although there is no general consensus among the authors, neither are there any important disagreements among the different criteria for admission. There do exist certain aspects to be clarified. If there is no associated extracranial lesion justifying admission to the hospital, no alcohol or drug abuse interfering with the neurological examination, and a responsible adult is available to observe the patient at home, we may then safely discharge all patients that were asymptomatic at the moment of the blow and when seen at the hospital, with 15 points on the GCS and a normal neurologic examination.

Certain authors,[2] ourselves included,[26] demand radiologic evidence of a lack of fracture. Others,[7] after carrying out a CT scan, limit the discharges from the hospital to those under 60 years of age and with a normal CT scan, but then discharge symptomatic MHI with amnesia or loss of consciousness.

If the circumstances first established are present, then we discharge all asymptomatic patients with a score of 15 points and no skull fracture. Following these guidelines – discharging all banal HI and keeping under hospital observation the MHI – of the 5098 patients assisted in one year in our emergency department (ED), 54% were discharged directly from the ED after being classified as banal blows, that is, asymptomatic and without fractures. The remaining 46% were considered MHI, based on the presence of symptoms (loss of consciousness, amnesia, and so forth), clinical signs (confusion, agitation, 14 points on the GCS) or skull damage, and left under observation in the ED for a 24-hour period.

Only 1.8% of the patients with cranial blows were hospitalized in hospital wards due to the brain injury. Eleven patients required surgery for intra-cranial hematomas; ten belonged to the group with cranial fractures. Only four patients died: three of extracranial causes (two due to severe extracranial lesions, hepatic rupture and tetraplegia after a fracture of C4, associated with mild brain injury; one due to sepsis) and one death after a post-operative relapse of an intracranial lesion, a subdural hematoma, in a patient undergoing anticoagulant therapy.

An aspect that is poorly emphasized in the clinical practice guidelines is "safety": that is, the number of undetected intracranial lesions. In our hos-pital, all patients receiving assistance in the emergency department were followed up after discharge from this area. We observed that 17 of the 1011 patients initially sent home during the first four months of 1995 came back to the ED, some because symptoms had appeared and others because mild symptoms had increased. Of these patients, 3 were discharged to their homes and 14 were admitted for a 24-hour period of observation, but all were sub-sequently discharged. Only one patient presented an intracranial lesion, a subdural hematoma not initially detected but, because of its small volume and the lack of clinical expression, hospital admission was not necessary. Of the 853 MHI observed for a 24-hour period, 5 came back because symptoms persisted. After another 24-hour period of observation, they were all dis-charged with no changes in the diagnosis or treatment.

Concluding remarks

The use of algorithms which can adequately assess risk factors in mild head injuries constitutes a reasonable strategy for discriminating among apparently mild cranial blows in those who have a probability of suffering neurological deterioration during the first 48 hours post-injury.

Based on our results and, although an optimal and universally accepted strategy to assist MHI does not exist, we consider our guidelines to be safe and adequate. In any case, a substantial reduction in mortality and morbidity could be achieved by paying more attention to injuries that are initially of mild severity.

References

1. Stiell, I. G., Wells, G. A., Vandemheen, K., et al. (1997). Variation in ED use of computed tomography for patients with minor head injury. *Ann. Emerg. Med., 30,* 14–22.
2. Jennet, B. (1989). Some international comparisons. In H. S. Levin, H. M. Eisenberg, and A. L. Bendon (Eds.). *Mild head injury* (p. 23). New York: Oxford University Press.
3. Klauber, M. R., Marshall, L. F., Luerssen, T. G., Frankowski, R., Tabaddor, K., & Eisenberg, H. M. (1989). Determinants of head injury mortality: importance of the low risk patients. *Neurosurgery, 24,* 31–36.

4. The Study Group on Head Injury of the Italian Society for Neurosurgery (1996). Guidelines for minor head injured patient management in adult age. *J. Neurosurg. Sci., 40*, 11–15.

5. Saab, M., Gray, A., Hodgkinson, D., & Irfan, M. (1996). Warfarin and apparent minor head injury. *J. Accid. Emerg. Med., 13*, 208–209.

6. Committee on Trauma, American College of Surgeons (1989). Head trauma in advanced trauma life support program. *Am. Coll. Surgeons, 133*.

7. Stein, S. L., & Ross, S. E. (1990). The value of computed tomographic scans in patients with low risk head injuries. *Neurosurgery, 26*, 638–640.

8. Borczuk, P. (1995). Predictors of intracranial injury in patients with mild head trauma. *Ann. Emerg. Med., 25*, 731.

9. Culotta, V. P., Sementilli, M. E., Gerold, K., & Watts, C. C. (1996). Clinical heterogeneity in the classification of mild head injury. *Neurosurgery, 38*, 245–250.

10. Jennett, B. (1980). Skull X-ray after recent head injury. *Clin. Radiol. 31*, 463.

11. French, B. N., & Dublin, A. B. (1977). The value of computerized tomography in the management of 1000 consecutive head injuries. *Surg. Neurol. 7*, 171.

12. Jones, J. J., & Jeffreys, R. V. (1981). Relative risk of alternative admission policies for patients with head injuries. *Lancet, 2*, 850–853.

13. Moran, S. G., McCarthy, M. C., Uddin, D. E., & Poelstra, R. J. (1994). Predictors of positive CT scans in trauma patients with minor head injury. *Am. Surg., 60*, 533–535.

14. Duus, B., Boesen, T., Kruse, K. V., & Nielsen, K. B. (1993). Prognostic signs in the evaluation of patients with minor head injury. *Br. J. Surg., 80*, 988–991.

15. Lee, S. T., Liu, T. N., Wong, C. S., Yeh, Y. S., & Tzaan, W. C. (1995). Relative deterioration after mild head injury. *Acta Neurochir. (Wien), 135*, 136–140.

16. Mendelow, A. D., Teasdale, G., Jennett, B., Bryden, J., & Hessett, C. (1983). Risk of intracranial hematoma in head injured adults. *Br. Med. J., 287*, 1173–1176.

17. Feuerman, T., Wackym, P. A., Gade, G. F., & Becker, D. P. (1988). Value of skull radiography, head computed tomographic scanning and admission OFR observation in case of minor head injury. *Neurosurgery, 22*, 449–453.

18. Cooper D. R., & Ho, V. (1983). Role of emergency skull X-ray films in the evaluation of head injured patients: a retrospective study. *Neurosurgery, 130*, 136.

19. Murshid, W. R. (1994). Role of skull radiography in the initial evaluation of minor head injury: a retrospective study. *Acta Neurochir. (Wien), 129*, 11.

20. Duus, B. R., Lind, B., Christensen, H., & Nielsen, O. A. (1994). The role of neuroimaging in the initial management of patients with minor head injury. *Ann. Emerg. Med., 23*, 1279–1283.

21. Mendelow, A. D., Campbell, D. A., Jeffrey, R. R., et al. (1982). Admission after mild head injury: benefits and costs. *Br. Med. J., 285*, 1530–1532.

22. Muñoz-Sanchez, M. A., et al. (1997). High risk cranioencephalic trauma: assistance recommendations. *Med. Intensiva, 21*, 378.

23. Muñoz-Sanchez, M. A., Murillo-Cabezas, F., & Cayuela-Domínguez, A., et al. (2005). The significance of skull fracture in mild head trauma differs between child and adults *Child Nerv Syst, 21* (2): 128–32.

24. Pasaoglu, H., Inci Karakucuk, E., Kurtsoy, A., & Pasaoglu, A. (1996). Endogenous neuropeptides in patients with acute traumatic head injury, I: Cerebrospinal fluid beta-endorphin levels are increased within 24 hours following the trauma. *Neuropeptides, 30*, 47–51.

25. Ingebrigtsen, T., & Romner, B. (1996). Serial S-100 protein serum measurements related to early magnetic resonance imaging after minor head injury. Case report. *J. Neurosurg., 85*, 945.
26. Muñoz-Sanchez, M. A., & Murillo-Cabezas, F. (1996). Potentially severe craneoencephalic trauma. In A. Net and L. Marruecos-Sant (Eds.), *Traumatismos craneoencefálicos graves* (p. 60). Barcelona: Springer-Verlag.
27. Masters, S. J., McClean, P. M., Arcarese, J. S., et al. (1987). Skull X-ray examinations after head trauma. Recommendations by a multidisciplinary panel and validation study. *N. Engl. J. Med., 316*, 84–91.

3 Organization of neurological intensive care units

José María Domínguez-Roldán,
Claudio García-Alfaro, and
Walter Videtta

History of the development of intensive care units

The grouping of critically ill patients with poor prognosis was one of the care strategies that developed at the time of great military conflicts. Centralizing high-risk patients with qualified caregivers and with the technological resources directed towards the treatment of these patients began to be an essential part of the organization of daily hospital medical care. As a result of this the first organized areas of intensive treatment for critical patients appeared in the 1960s.

It was during the great polio epidemics of the 1950s and 1960s that the need to centralize patients developing respiratory complications became urgent. Even in these early stages of intensive care unit (ICU) development, assisted ventilation stood out as one of their most relevant features.

There were various factors underlying the emergence of the first intensive care units: the most important being the need to centralize patients requiring highly complex care together with the specific technological resources used in their treatment. To this was added the need to group together nursing and medical personnel with specialized training and knowledge in the care of critical patients.

The first intensive care units were concentrated in a fairly reduced number of countries and institutions. Initially their focus was on the care of a small percentage of patients often so critically ill that survival was considered a huge success.[1] Today, intensive care units are considered a basic necessity in any hospital offering medium to highly complex care.[2] In some countries they have been in place for 30 years.[3,4]

Both the experience obtained during World War II together with specific studies demonstrated that the organized concentration of patients with the right equipment and human resources significantly reduced intrahospital complications and mortality.[5] Civil disasters, such as the 1942 fire in Coconut Grove and Boston in 1942, were similar experiences corroborating the war-time findings. The appearance of polio in Denmark and New England during the late 1940s and early 1950s triggered the use of artificial respirators in intensive care settings. This was an historic milestone in the development of intensive care units. Later on, during the 1960s, coronary units in Toronto, Kansas, and Philadelphia demonstrated their efficiency by reducing morbidity and mortality related to acute myocardial infarction.[6] This gave a new momentum to the implementation of treatment units for the critically ill. As an outcome of this, differentiated types of critical patients were then grouped together, such as groups of coronary patients, or those needing critical postoperative care or mechanical ventilation.

The need to group critically ill patients together was not, however, the only underlying factor in the emergence of intensive care units. Many ICUs branched off from the various activities that were part of postsurgical reanimation units, which managed the care of patients following highly complex surgery. From 1863, when the first postsurgical reanimation units appeared in the UK, until our time, the development of intensive care units linked to postoperative care has grown in exponential terms.[7] At the same time, the success that postoperative ICUs have generated in the survival rate of severe trauma surgical patients has greatly benefited the evolution of high complexity surgery.

As a result of the different experience obtained from wartime and civil events, the hospital rooms dedicated to assisting patients in critical condition began to evolve towards today's intensive care units, owing more to necessity than to pre-planned efforts.

Although the number of intensive care units grew very slowly during the 1950s and 1960s, it was during these decades when critical patient care, as a result of societal demands, began to become a generalized practice. At the same time, the benefits of the ICU, mainly focused on postoperative care, became extensive to patients with severe trauma, patients with acute respiratory insufficiency, patients with neurological processes, and those with coronary pathologies. In this context, and during the past 15 to 20 years, with the increase of life expectancy and a relative lesser effect from epidemics, emerging pathologies such as traumatic brain injury and cerebrovascular pathology have become more and more important and have led towards new developments.

Another factor underlying the implementation of intensive care units is the diverse origin and later organization of the medical professionals who were involved in the process. Thus, critical care medicine can be affiliated with different areas (medical or surgical), and in some countries critical care medicine has become an independent medical discipline. In Scandinavian countries and the UK for example, intensive care units developed within specialized anesthesiology. In Germany, anesthesiologists are commonly in charge of surgical intensive care units while physicians specializing in internal medicine are in charge of medical intensive care units. In Italy, intensive care units have developed within the fields of anesthesiology and reanimation. In Spain, Portugal, Belgium, New Zealand, Australia and Latin American countries, critical care medicine has become a primary and independent specialty. All of these countries require that physicians receive significant training in anesthesiology and internal medicine as well as acquiring considerable experience in different types of intensive care units. In the USA, critical care medicine is implemented by specific specialists. There are surgeons in charge of surgical intensive care units,[8] pneumologists are in charge of intensive care units assisting patients with respiratory pathologies,[9] neurosurgeons are in charge of patients with traumatic brain injury, neurologists for stroke patients and plastic surgeons for patients with severe burns.[10–11] In general, pediatricians with intensive care unit training manage critical pediatric patients in the ICU.[12]

After several years working on the matter, the American Board of Medical Specialties (ABMS) identified critical care medicine as an independent medical discipline. During September 1980, all members of the ABMS to which all primary and associated councils belong, unanimously approved critical care medicine as a specific area of medical practice, affording this discipline a unique status in the USA as a multidisciplinary subspecialty. It was formally defined as follows:

> Critical Care Medicine is a multidisciplinary effort that crosses traditional department and specialty borders in the same way that the problems found in critical patients require diverse aspects of many different specialties. The critical care physician is a specialist with a necessarily wide spectrum of knowledge, spanning all aspects of management of a critical patient and whose base of operation is the intensive care unit. A physician specializing in intensive care must have completed training in a primary specialty, and in addition, is trained and involved in all aspects of management of the critically ill patient, and works in concert with the various specialties on the patient care team in the ICU to utilize recognized techniques for vital life support, to teach other physicians, nurses, and health professionals the practice of intensive care and to foster research. Thereby, critical care medicine is a multidisciplinary specialty, based in intensive care units, and having as its core objective the care of critically ill patients.

At major medical centers, critical care specialists are usually a part of larger departments and interact with emergency specialists. Emergency departments are thus configured, focusing efforts on reanimation and the initial treatment of potentially life-threatening acute pathologies before patients are taken to the operating room, intensive care unit or other treatment facilities. We can see how emergency and critical care medicine (both relatively new specialties) are therefore superposed, one upon the other, working in close cooperation on a daily work basis as well as in the ongoing training of the specialists in the two disciplines. This constitutes another aspect in the activities of physicians in intensive care units, as their efforts become interdisciplinary.

Intensive care units can be classified at different levels according to their capacity to monitor, diagnose, and treat the patient. This is conditioned both by the population it will be serving and by the type of pathology it is dedicated to. Nonetheless, there is a generally accepted classification of intensive care units based on the technological and human resources assigned to the unit. There are three levels:

- *Level 1*: there is a medical director of the ICU, although not exclusively dedicated to the unit. Immediate care is usually provided by other physicians who are commonly on call. Also the proportion of nurses per patient is low.
- *Level 2*: the ICU medical director dedicates his or her time fully or partially to the unit. The nurse/patient ratio is 1:3 to 1:2.
- Level 3: The medical director of the intensive care unit is dedicated full time to the unit. All continuous medical care is provided by specialists in critical care medicine. The nurse/patient ratio is high, usually 1:1. These intensive care units are usually located in academic institutions and are dedicated to education and research.

The trend in recent years is for hospitals with Level 3 intensive care units also to have other units with less intense levels of observation, equivalent to Levels 1 and 2. The stratification of the different levels of observation and treatment generally varies depending on the different types of pathologies being treated as well as on the evolution of the individual patient. Intermediary care units (Levels 1 and 2), also known as "step-down" units, provide treatment for patients that do not require highly complex monitoring and/or treatment, but do need more care and observation than can be provided in a general ward.

Neurological intensive care

Intensive care for patients with neurological illnesses started to develop together with intensive therapy when it became necessary to provide respiratory care for polio patients.[4] Later on, neurological pathologies treated in intensive care units were not limited to acute neuromuscular weakness such as Guillain-Barré syndrome or myasthenia gravis which required respiratory support. ICU treatment became extensive to patients with central nervous system dysfunction who, due to the severity of their condition or the need for medical or surgical therapy in order to improve prognosis, could directly benefit from care in an intensive care unit.

Today there is a wide range of services offered by intensive care units to patients suffering a severe neurological condition as can be seen in Table 3.1.

The demand for the implementation of neurological intensive care units has been characterized by several factors that are presented in Table 3.2. Social demand has been the main determining factor in the development of neurological intensive care units. The number of neurological patients that

Table 3.1 Neurological pathologies more frequently admitted in ICU

1. Traumatic brain injury
2. Intracerebral hemorrhage
3. Subarachnoid hemorrhage
4. Encephalitis
5. Central nervous system vasculitis
6. Myasthenia gravis
7. Guillain-Barré syndrome
8. Cervical or thoracic level acute spinal cord injury
9. Meningitis and meningeal-ventriculitis
10. Status epilepticus
11. Ischemic stroke
11. Other

Table 3.2 Factors underlying the creation of neurological intensive care units

1. A growing demand for ICU treatment of neurological patients
2. Increasing therapeutical possibilities of improving prognosis of neurological illnesses
3. Development of specific techniques for monitoring phenomena related to severe neuropathology
4. Progressive development of a specific scientific discipline encompassing severe neuropathology

needed the specialized care which the ICU provides increased significantly. In the early 1970s, the monitoring and diagnostic techniques needed in critical care could be superposed, in most cases, on those used with non-neurological critical patients. Subsequent technological advancements brought the development of specific neuromonitoring and neurodiagnostic techniques for this subgroup of patients. The progressive implementation of computerized axial tomography (CT scan) is a good example of this. The progressive refining of CT scan image definition allows for ever more precise and reliable diagnoses of structural lesions. The monitoring of intracranial pressure has become the most widely used technique when dealing with patients suffering severe head injury.

A neurointensivist is a critical care physician with the combined knowledge of medical care of neurological diseases and critical care techniques. Both critical care of neurological and neurosurgical patients and critical care medicine were born from practical necessity. Their origin can be traced back to the birth of intensive care units themselves given that it was a neurological illness which gave rise to ICUs. Neurological and neurosurgical critical care gradually developed as a subspecialty directed towards clinical and physiopathological nervous system specialists.

Neurocritical care requires a convergence of knowledge from various medical disciplines: internal medicine, neurology, anesthesiology, neurosurgery and critical care medicine. However, the area of expertise must extend to neuroanatomy and neurophysiology, and focus on the knowledge of brain physiopathology and associated techniques in monitoring intracranial pressure, cerebral perfusion pressure, cerebral blood flow and cerebral metabolism. In the late 1960s, there was an increase in the number of aggressive surgical operations. At the same time innovative recording and monitoring techniques began to be used in recovery rooms and large intensive care units. As the number of surgical patients needing intensive care increased, accommodating patients with acute illnesses, such as brain and spinal cord trauma, neuromuscular illness, stroke, and so forth, began to be a problem. As a result, intensive care areas were organized within neurological and neurosurgical wards.

The first modern neurointensivist programs were developed in the mid-1970s and have widely spread over the past ten years. According to Ropper, in 1992[13] there were 25 neurological intensive care units with 6 beds each, with full-time medical directors in academic institutions in the USA, and twice the space of special areas in intensive care units in academic hospitals. At the same time in Europe there were 50 neurological intensive care units, either in place or in progress. Intermediary intensive care units and stroke units appeared later, probably branching off from neurological intensive care units with some differences as to the level of complexity but with the same goal of providing acute care. These units are a response to the special needs of these patients, more than can be provided in recovery rooms or general wards. Pathologies requiring a patient's admission to a neurological intensive care unit are varied, ranging from those that require minimal monitoring to more severe pathologies, such as brain trauma, which require more specific monitoring (Table 3.1).

Care management of patients with traumatic brain injury

The study of the methodology of care for patients with severe trauma led to research which could demonstrate how these patients would benefit from care management (patients with severe trauma in general and patients with brain trauma in particular). At the end of the 1970s, several researchers strove to demonstrate the efficiency of trauma systems. Early studies showed that those areas lacking an organized system of trauma care had an excessive number of deaths or a high number of potentially preventable deaths.[14–17]

The methodology used in these studies was initially criticized by some authors.[18] Nonetheless, later studies proved time and again the beneficial results of managed care with regard to higher survival rates and lower morbidity. These later studies compared the prognosis of accident patients in areas in which an organized trauma care system had been implemented with patients' prognosis in areas in which there was not.[19–21] In addition, according to the Brain Trauma Foundation, in the chapter on "Trauma Systems and the Neurosurgeon" of the *Guidelines for the Management of Severe Head*

Injury, there are no published data suggesting better outcomes in areas or regions lacking an organized care system than in those areas which do provide organized care management.

Achieving better outcomes in the care of patients with traumatic brain injury depends on a great number of variables. We would highlight the following: the existence of an integrated system of trauma patient care; the presence of neurosurgeons specialized in assisting patients with traumatic brain injury; the availability of a trauma surgeon; and the availability of physicians trained in emergency and critical care medicine with a special focus on this type of pathology. In cases where the patient suffers multiple injuries, the trauma surgeon, the neurosurgeon, and the intensivist should decide which injuries would be necessary to treat first. Obviously, in cases where the patient suffers an isolated brain or spinal cord trauma, the neurosurgeon and the intensivist have complete responsibility.

The neurosurgeon[22] as well as the intensivist, the emergency physician, and the trauma surgeon should participate in the design of prehospital care as well as in the training of the staff providing prehospital care and those assisting patients in the emergency room. They should also ensure that the appropriate diagnostic systems (e.g., CT scan), an operating room with trained professionals, as well as beds in the ICU are available 24 hours a day, year round. The neurosurgeon, the intensivist, and all members of the critical care team should participate in the revision of the system and on all proposed changes.

All care provided to the patient with traumatic brain injury during the prehospital stage and in the emergency room has great impact on the patient's future morbidity and mortality. Many different specialists (i.e., emergency physicians, general surgeons, neurosurgeons, trauma surgeons, anesthesiologists, and intensivists) intervene during the first hours of neurotrauma care. Given that treatment of central nervous system injury must be correctly performed and that this involves many different specialists, it is important that step-by-step procedures and guides be used.[23]

The organization of a neurocritical care unit is based on structural and organizational aspects whose final result is an increase in the survival rate of brain trauma patients and improved functional abilities of survivors. To accomplish these results, the organizational structure of a Level 3 intensive care unit should be followed. This requires a full-time medical director and continuous and permanent patient care provided by highly qualified neurointensivists. During the acute phase, the nurse/patient ratio should be 1:1. The recommended techniques for caring for these patients should be available 24 hours a day and are presented in Table 3.3. Obviously, not all neurointensive care units are currently so equipped, and those that are do not apply these techniques to all patients. Nor are all monitoring and diagnostic techniques equally advantageous in the care of brain trauma patients during the acute phase. Although it is difficult to define which minimum requirements would be necessary to certify an intensive care unit as a reference for the treatment

Table 3.3 Neuromonitoring and neurodiagnostic techniques for patients with severe brain trauma

1. Computerized axial tomography
2. Continuous monitoring and recording of intracranial pressure
3. Continuous monitoring of cerebral perfusion pressure
4. Monitoring of jugular oxygen saturation
5. Transcranial Doppler sonography
6. Regional cerebral oxygen saturation (near-infrared spectroscopy)
7. Partial tissular pressure of cerebral oxygen
8. Cerebral microdialysis

of trauma patients, there seems to be a general consensus that at least the three first techniques shown in Table 3.3 should be used and available 24 hours a day for neurotrauma patients. This claim is supported by the success of two major breakthroughs over the last decades not previously discussed here. One is the surgical evacuation of postraumatic intracranial hematomas and the other being the specific treatment of intracranial hypertension (so frequent in patients with severe brain injury), resulting in lower mortality.

The negative effect of the development of a sudden increase in intracranial mass (as in the case of post-traumatic intracranial hematoma) on the prospects of survival and recovery of patients is not questioned. On one hand, the hematoma can cause intracranial pressure to increase to such a degree as to compromise cerebral perfusion pressure and cerebral blood flow, both global and regional. On the other hand, because of the compartmentalization of intracranial structures (delimited by borders such as the falx cerebri or the tentorium cerebelli), the uncontrolled and acute increase of intracranial mass generates wedges of pressure with serious life-threatening effects, mainly represented by herniation of the brain (uncal or subfacial).

Most deaths of intracranial origin in brain injury patients are owing to uncontrollable intracranial hypertension causing cerebral circulatory arrest. It is therefore apparent that any measure designed to identify and treat intracranial hypertension is beneficial to the evolution of patients suffering this type of injury.

It is important to note the importance of objectivity and low interobserver variability when registering the severity of brain injury. In order to accomplish this, scales for evaluating the different levels of neurological damage should be used, as well as accepted clinical evaluation strategies for this type of patient. For the patient with brain trauma, the most widely accepted scale is the Glasgow Coma Scale presented in Table 3.4. Aside from this, the evaluation protocols of instrumental tests, such as the CT scan (see Tables 3.5, 3.6, 3.7) are strategies that optimize trauma patient care.[24,25]

Although a neurological injury is the basis for admitting patients into a neurotrauma intensive care unit, in most cases patients also present traumatic lesions in other parts of their bodies. Data from the neurotrauma ICU of the

Table 3.4 Glasgow Coma Scale

Eyes open	
Spontaneously	4
To verbal commands	3
To noxious stimuli	2
No eye opening	1
Verbal response	
Fully oriented and converses	5
Disoriented and converses	4
Voices inappropriate words	3
Makes incomprehensible sounds	2
No verbal response	1
Motor response	
Obeys verbal commands	6
Localizes to noxious stimuli	5
Normal flexion to noxious stimuli	4
Abnormal flexion to noxious stimuli	3
Extension to noxious stimuli	2
No response to noxious stimuli	1

Table 3.5 Indicators for cranial CT scan in the acute phase of head trauma

1. Consciousness level below 14 points on the Glasgow Coma Scale
2. Ear discharge of blood and/or cerebrospinal fluid
3. Open skull fracture
4. Motor asymmetry in clinical exploration
5. When, due to other lesions, sedation or muscular relaxants are administered to the patient

Maryland Institute of Emergency Medical Services Systems (MIEMSS) of the University of Maryland showed that a large proportion of patients admitted over a period of 5 months presented systemic injuries, and that other critical patients presented a wide variety of potential and acute complications.[25] In fact, the team in Maryland found the correlation of the level of life support with the frequency with which non-neurological complications were encountered to be very similar to the general population of trauma patients.

Due to this, the management of severe head trauma patients presenting other lesions as well demands not only neurological treatment knowledge, but that of several other areas of modern medicine. During the last few decades, critical care medicine has developed multiple forms of monitoring and a new way of understanding the physiopathology of each patient. As critical care medicine has advanced, and the complexity of severe trauma patients has increased, it has become more and more difficult to apply traditional concepts in deciding who is in charge of the patient and what role to assign to the different specialties in the treatment of critical patients. Recognizing trauma

Table 3.6 Protocol for reading and interpretation of CT scan in the acute phase of head trauma

Computerized axial tomography reading
1. Potentially evacuable space-occupying lesions
       Subdural hematoma
       Extradural hematoma
       Hemorrhagic contusion/intraparenchymatous hematoma
       *Analyze: volume, location
2. Hypodense space-occupying lesions
       Simple contusion
       Hemispheric swelling
       Vascular distribution hypodensities
3. Signs of diffuse axonal lesion
       Corpus callosum lesion
       Mesencephalic/brainstem lesion
       Basal ganglia lesion
       Intraventricular hemorrhage
       Subarachnoid hemorrhage
4. Signs of increased cerebral volume
       Compression/absence basal cisterns
       Compression/absence fourth ventricle
       Compression/absence third ventricle
       Diminished size lateral ventricles
       Disminished perihemispheric cerebrospinal fluid

Interpretation of computerized axial tomography
1. Endocranial hypertension
       Large volume space-occupying lesions (> 25 ml)
       Signs of increased cerebral volume
2. Clinically significant compromise of structures
       Signs of uncal herniation
       Significant midline displacement
       Signs of subfacial herniation
       Midline shift
       Bihemispheric lesions
       Mid-brain lesions
       Signs of diffuse axonal lesion
3. Risk of compression of vascular structures
       Signs of subfacial herniation
       Signs of uncal herniation

as a nosologic entity and applying a systematic approach has contributed to decreased mortality and morbidity from a multidisciplinary point of view; the same generally occurs with all critical patients. Critical patients present a wide variety of needs requiring specific training in understanding each problem, in applying technology, and in performing specific treatment procedures.

Intensive care is a term that in an operative way signifies close observation of the patient, multiple monitoring and the possibility of continuously applying different techniques. The type of critical problems that a specific

Table 3.7 Classification of computerized axial tomography findings according to recordings of the traumatic coma data bank

---

Type I diffuse injury
   No observed intracranial pathology in the CT

Type II diffuse injury
   Cisterns present with shift of midline 0–5 mm. Absence of hyperdense or mixed lesions > 25 ml. Possible presence of bone fragments or foreign objects. Subarachnoid hemorrhage is also possible

Type III diffuse injury
   Cisterns compressed or absent; shift of midline 0–5 mm. Absence of hyperdense or mixed lesions > 25 ml

Type IV diffuse injury
   Shift of midline 0–5 mm. Absence of hyperdense or mixed lesions > 25 ml

Non-evacuated space-occupying lesion
   Any evacuated or considered evacuable lesion

Evacuated space-occupying lesion
   Any non-evacuated hyperdense or mixed lesion > 25 ml

---

population presents, the different types of monitoring and the different therapeutical interventions required, define the professional profile of the intensive care unit staff. They will also directly affect the type of equipment that each specific unit needs. Today and in the past, a different array of economic and financial elements, as well as the legal environment, greatly influence the training of professionals, and the equipment they use. These elements should be taken into account when deciding what type of intensive care unit is to be installed, and which monitoring techniques, technology, and personnel will be available when designing a unit.

Defining the role of the neurosurgeon, the anesthesiologist, and the intensivist in an intensive care unit has always been controversial. In 1989, Pitts[26] stated that the role of the neurosurgeon in the ICU was yet to be defined. Today the role of the neurosurgeon varies depending on the particular region or hospital. Opinions vary among neurosurgeons and other specialists concerning the status of a neurosurgeon in critical care. This subject even became a hot topic with political connotations in the world of medicine.

As in other areas of medicine undergoing continual change, neurosurgeons should form their own opinion and take a position as to what they believe their role in the ICU.[26]

Care management of patients with cerebrovascular pathology

Patients with acute cerebrovascular pathologies, including subarachnoid hemorrhage, intracerebral hematomas, and ischemic stroke are seen with increasing frequency in the ICU. There are two main reasons for this: the first is the change developed countries are undergoing in their population pyramids, with a progressive increase in the elderly population, a segment where cerebrovascular pathology is common; the second is the fact that in recent years significant advances have been wrought in the management and use of diagnostics and therapy for this type of disease.

Recent studies have shown that some countries present a larger number of patients going into intensive care units with cerebrovascular pathologies than with neurotrauma pathologies.

The diagnosis and treatment approach of spontaneous subarachnoid hemorrhage and its most frequent cause, Willis circle aneurysm, has experienced significant growth and momentum in recent years. Currently, the diagnosis of a cerebral circulatory aneurysm can be accomplished using not only techniques like conventional arteriograms, but also with more precise techniques with lower morbidity such as digital substraction angiography, the helicoidal CT scan, or nuclear magnetic resonance, which obtain significant diagnostic results. Along the same line, the development of new techniques, such as excluding the aneurysm from circulation by techniques different from those used in classic surgery, has proved to be a significant advance in favor of these patients. Excluding the aneurysm from circulation by placing intra-neurysmatic coils, or "balloons", favors early intervention in this type of pathology, thereby decreasing morbidity and mortality secondary to one of the most frequent complications in these patients: the rebleeding of the aneurysm.

Another complication determining prognosis of patients with spontaneous subarachnoid hemorrhage is vasospasm, causing severe areas of cerebral ischemia which can lead to the patient's death, or in some instances to the development of severe neurological deficits following recovery from an acute phase. In recent years, the treatment and prophylaxis of cerebral vasospasm have improved owing to the development of certain drugs, such as nimo-dipine, which limit the extent of brain damage in these patients. Improvement has also been achieved through direct action (after catheterism) on the spastic vascular area with either mechanical angioplasty or chemical angioplasty or a combination of both techniques on the same patient.

Researcher and clinical interest concerning patients presenting intracerebral hemorrhagic pathology has also significantly increased. Studies have been carried out in recent years with the goal of establishing the best surgical strategy for the evacuation of hematomas, or of discovering if the effects of fibrinolitic substances on hematomas can help to improve classic surgical evacuation. This is also true with regard to the treatment approach of arterial hypertension, often present in patients with cerebral hemorrage. As with brain trauma patients, scales for the clinical evaluation of the severity of neurological damage in patients with stroke, and assessment scales for diagnostic images (Tables 3.8–3.11), will be able to improve the evaluation of brain damage in stroke patients.[27,28]

Table 3.8 CT reading of ischemic stroke in late phase

Focal hypodensity
• Middle cerebral artery: subcortical, cortical cort/subcortical
• No middle cerebral artery
• Watershed infarct

Size of cerebral infarct
• Small/medium/large

Hemorrhagic transformation
• None
• 1. Petechial (types I and II)
• 2. Parenchymatous (types I and II)

Mass effect
• None/slight/moderate/severe

Table 3.9 CT reading of ischemic cerebrovascular arrest – early phase early hypodensity

• Lack of definition of insular lobe margins
• Hypodensity of lentiform nucleus, others
• Early mass effect: none/slight/moderate/severe
• Effacement of cortical sulci, or of the lateral ventricular body, compression of fourth ventricle
• Hyperdensity mid-cerebral artery: none/proximal/lateral/complete

Table 3.10 Fisher CT grading scale of subarachnoid hemorrhage

Grade	Findings
I	No SAH detected
II	Layer < 1 mm in basal cisterns
III	Layer > 1 mm in basal cisterns
IV	Intraventricular or intracerebral clot

Table 3.11 Hunt–Hess clinical classification of subarachnoid hemorrhage (SAH)

Grade 0	Unruptured aneurysm, asymptomatic
Grade 1	Asymptomatic aneurysm or mild cephalea or slight nuchal rigidity
Grade 2	Moderate to severe cephalea, nuchal rigidity; or CN palsy
Grade 3	Lethargy or confusion; mild focal deficit
Grade 4	Stupor, moderate to severe hemiparesis
Grade 5	Deep coma, decerebrate rigidity, moribund appearance

The development of stroke units

In the 1960s, at the same time that coronary units were being successfully implemented and proving to be useful, the first intensive care stroke units appeared in the USA. Some stroke units were designed and implemented using coronary units as a model, and patients were admitted during the acute phases of stroke. The monitoring of patients during the pioneering stages of stroke units included monitoring of vital signs, arterial pressure measurement, ECG, laboratory analysis, radiology, and, in some cases, EEG. These stroke units probably contributed to reducing the number of complications[29] and to improving diagnostic precision.[30,31] It is also probable that stroke units, as in the case of coronary units, aided in the development of acute phase stroke research and education.[32]

As more and more patients treated in stroke units survived, there was a logical increase in the number of patients with physical and neuro-psychological disabilities. This meant that along with the development of stroke units it became necessary to develop specific rehabilitation units for this type of patient. Stroke units specializing in rehabilitation appeared during the 1970s. Patients would be cared for in rehabilitation units after overcoming the acute stage of stroke and emphasis was placed on mobility and rehabilitation in the early stages. Isaacs[33] evaluated five years of stroke unit implementation within a geriatric department and concluded that the unit proved its worth. He found this to be especially true in relation to the unit's focus on an interdisciplinary approach and in facilitating education. In a different non-randomized study, Feigenson et al.[34] found beneficial results on the functional prognosis of patients.

From the combination of features of both types of units, the concept of stroke units emerged in areas other than intensive care units, such as in diagnosis, prevention of complications, research, and training of personnel dedicated to the care of patients with cerebrovascular pathology. Mobility and early rehabilitation were added later, as well as the creation of multidisciplinary teams and the involvement of patients' families.[35]

With the advent of new treatment modalities directed towards the treatment of ischemic stroke, especially with regard to aspects related to the reopening of acutely clogged arteries, the usefulness of stroke units was again made clear.[36]

Stroke is an emergency which can occur at any time, 24 hours a day. Emergency areas and intensive care units are hospital services available 24 hours a day, 365 days a year. It is only logical that stroke units should therefore be designed within already existing structures and organizational systems, such as those found in neurocritical care units.

Although there are still pending issues and some argument in relation to stroke units, there is an abundance of information regarding ischemic stroke patients treated in stroke units which shows they generally have a better prognosis than those treated in a conventional way or in other areas.[37]

The meta-analysis of randomized trials also showed that stroke unit treatment reduced hospitalization time, the degree of dependence, and mortality.[38] These studies reveal better prognosis at 6 and 12 months as well as at 5 years.[39] The improved functional outcome achieved during the first weeks continues to show 5 years later. A recent study on a small sample using the Barthel Index score showed this same tendency 10 years post-treatment. It therefore seems that standardized treatment and a rehabilitation program during the acute phase of stroke are the principal contributing factors for improved prognosis. The differences between the treatment and rehabilitation programs implemented in these stroke units need to be elucidated, and a comparison of different stroke unit models must be done, in order to determine which are more effective.

Emergency medical services channeled towards a system that can respond to the necessities of people suffering cerebrovascular pathology in its acute and hyperacute phases, requires ample vision, and must focus beyond emergency service. Implementation of such a system must focus on integrating the different services involved in the initial care of these patients. The cooperation and coordination of different services and departments within a hospital become paramount. In these efforts, a leader, knowledgeable in the pathology and with the authority to coordinate resources and give orders, must be designated. The system that a given hospital adopts would depend on its own institutional characteristics and on the peculiarities of the local or regional communities it serves. The National Institute for Neurological Disorders and stroke (NINDS) study, for example, was carried out through the coordinated efforts of emergency medical services and community hospitals.

Raising the level of public awareness and the ability of the general population to recognize the symptoms related to stroke as an emergency, and therefore to immediately notify emergency services, is crucial. Immediate care in stroke is of vital importance. The task of educating the public can be carried out through different institutions and agencies within each country, with scientific associations playing an important part. Through all possible means, scientific associations should spread the knowledge of what stroke is, how to recognize the symptoms, and what steps must be taken when it occurs. A national emergency telephone number should be provided to facilitate a stroke patient's immediate admission into treatment services. This number should be easy to remember and toll free. Countries such as the USA and Spain have implemented this system with positive results.

The prehospital stage of the initial treatment of stroke is made up of the following basic features or components. The operator receiving the emergency call should be able to recognize stroke symptoms and give these calls priority. The treatment team should establish the time of onset, communicate with the hospital that will receive the patient, initiate treatment, and safely transport the patient to the hospital. Efforts should be coordinated in such a way as to establish continuity in the care of the patient through the different stages of the medical care system.

The initial treatment of stroke shares some points in common with any other emergency. One of these is the "ABCs" of reanimation of critical patients. First, clear air passages and ensure ventilatory function. This would be followed by maintaining adequate cerebral perfusion and the normalization of blood flow. Following this, neurological evaluation should take place (point D or disabilities). Medical strategies to be followed after an initial evaluation are well defined in protocols and recommendations from several organizations. These highlight not only the therapeutic objectives for each phase of the disease, but also recommendations for treatment of the different periods.

Some of these tasks are repeated in the emergency room, during imaging and upon admittance to the ICU or operating room. The tasks of each link in the chain of initial care should be carried out in concordance with pre-established protocols in such a way as to facilitate the work to be performed by the team acting in the subsequent stage.

The idea of opening an occluded cerebral artery prompted the use of fibrinolitic drugs to assist in the effort of restoring cerebral blood flow to a threatened area. There were several drugs used: intravenous administration of streptokinase, urokinase, and rt-PA.[40-45]

The NINDS carried out a trial on rt-PA versus placebo administered during the first 3 hours following onset of neurological symptoms and concluded that 30% more of the patients benefited from this fibrinolitic drug, with no or minimal sequelae, allowing them to live independently. Based on the results of these findings, the Food and Drug Administration (FDA) approved its use in the USA and in September 1996 the *Thrombolitic Therapy Guidelines for Acute Stroke* (a supplement to the *Guidelines for Care Management of Patients with Acute Ischemic Stroke*) were published.

In order to implement fibrinolitic protocols in an institution, a stroke team must be organized. Algorithms and flow charts should be created in order to anticipate all possible situations and leave no alternatives to chance. All personnel involved in the admission, classification, and treatment of these patients should be properly trained (including telephone operators, receptionists, nursing personnel, paramedics, laboratory technicians and hemotherapy personnel, CT scan technicians, radiologists, neurologists, intensive therapists, emergency physicians, neurosurgeons, pharmacists, and so forth).

For best results, it is recommended that teams perform within specific time periods, set forth by the National Institute of Health (NIH) in the USA, as follows. From the medical center door to:

1   Patient evaluation by a physician, 10 minutes.
2   Notification of the stroke team, 15 minutes.
3   CT scan, 25 minutes.
4   Interpretation of CT scan, 45 minutes.
5   Initiation of fibrinolitic drug administration, 60 minutes.
6   Bed and monitored, 3 hours.

The NIH Stroke Scale (NIHSS) should be part of the examination of a stroke patient. It has been noted that patients with a low score on the NIHSS, probably equal to or less than 4 (all researchers do not agree on this), do not benefit from the use of rt-PA, given that their natural evolution is favorable. Nor is rt-PA administration beneficial to patients with a high NIHSS score, given that these patients may present a higher incidence of symptomatic intracerebral hemorrhage as a complication from the use of rt-PA.

The training of physicians responsible for including patients in these protocols, as well as those responsible for the reading of CT scans is crucial. This is especially true since early damage compatible with ischemia compromising over one-third of the middle cerebral artery is highly predictive of complications such as symptomatic cerebral hemorrhage or the development of severe cerebral edema.

The moment of onset of neurological symptoms should be precisely determined. In any patient awakening with neurological symptoms, the moment of onset should be considered the last moment the patient was seen neurologically intact. The criteria for meeting inclusion in or exclusion from fibrinolitic treatment must be strictly followed.

Other pathologies in neurological intensive care

Another common cause for admittance to the ICU is status epilepticus, owing to several reasons. Aside from requiring mechanical ventilation, status epilepticus is per se, a deleterious situation for the brain itself, which can be associated with a focal neurological deficit, intellectual deterioration, chronic epilepsy, and high mortality.

The first line of treatment of status epilepticus is effective in 70% to 80% of cases. However, in cases where this is not effective, the patient should be transferred to an intensive care unit, where different monitoring techniques can be implemented and more aggressive treatment, such as any necessary use of anesthetics, can be provided.[46] An article by Walker et al.,[47] reports how the evolution of patients diagnosed with status epilepticus and treated in a neurological intensive care unit was monitored during several months. The goal of this study was to identify: (1) deficiencies in the diagnosis of status epilepticus; (2) why the first line of treatment failed; (3) the effectiveness of implemented therapies. It was found that only 54% of patients presented status epilepticus, and that the dosage of diphenylhydantoin was inadequate in 44% of patients with regard to the dosage recommended in other studies.[48, 49] It was also found that only 50% of patients were intubed before being transferred.

The high incidence of pseudostatus epilepticus diagnosed as refractory status epilepticus reported in literature,[50] was also found in this study. This is in part due to the fact that many patients presenting pseudostatus have been previously diagnosed with epilepsy and in part due to failure to do the necessary encephalograms. In this study, as in others,[51,52] the most frequent etiology of status epilepticus was the abandonment or interruption of antiepileptic drugs (21% of cases).

Should the first line of treatment fail, the patient's transfer to an intensive care unit is mandatory given the advanced state of status epilepticus: rabdomiolysis, renal dysfunction, hyperthermia, cardiological arrhythmia, arterial hypertension, acute pulmonary edema, hepatic dysfunction, and disseminated intravascular coagulation.[53, 54]

Orotracheal intubation and mechanical respiratory care are frequently necessary when treating status epilepticus as this permits the use of second- and third-line medication in a safer way. Several studies reveal the deficiencies in the diagnosis and first initial treatment of status epilepticus patients, as well as the importance of early derivation and the role of the neurointensivist. Refractory status epilepticus treated in a neurological intensive care unit generally has a good prognosis and fewer complications.

There are other neurological diseases that, although they do not affect the central nervous system, may require treatment in a neurological intensive care unit. This is especially true in the case of neurological illness of a neuromuscular nature which frequently require intensive care owing to the respiratory insufficiency they provoke. Myasthenia gravis, Guillain-Barré syndrome, and spinal trauma are examples of these diseases.

It is important to mention that the intensive care unit can in turn be a generating mechanism of neuromuscular disease. During the course of the last two decades a significant percentage of patients with no previous history of neuromuscular disease was found to develop neuropathies or myopathies during their stay in intensive care units. These were associated with mechanical ventilation, sepsis, multisystemic failure, and the administration of different drugs. These clinical patterns, which as a group are known as neuropathies and myopathies of the critically ill patient, prolong the patient's stay in therapy, impede weaning from the respirator, and increase morbimortality.

Neuropathy of the critical patient occurs in 70% of patients who suffer sepsis and multisystemic failure during mechanical ventilation. When the primary cause of admission to the intensive care unit is overcome, followed by the aggregate complications, extubation cannot be carried out due to muscular weakness. Patients generally require increased duration on mechanical ventilation and intensive care unit stay. The mortality rate of the group developing neuropathy is near 50%, while those that survive frequently recover very slowly and suffer motor sequelae.

General management of neurological intensive care units

The answer to the question of who should be in charge of managing neurological intensive care units or who should be in charge of neurosurgical patients in the ICU is still controversial. Neurosurgeons themselves and other specialists agree that the neurosurgeon is the best prepared in the different aspects concerning knowledge of critical care. Neurosurgeons invest a great amount of time during their residency and in their medical practice with critical patients and customarily manage constantly changing patients. Neurosurgeons can direct or be essential members of the ICU team. On the other hand, the neurosurgeon is well aware of what took place during surgery (retraction, resection, vascular manipulation) and, therefore, the postoperatory problems that may present.

Some neurosurgeons have expressed the feeling that they are merely "technical operatives",[55] although the truth is that perhaps such an extreme point of view is not really representative of most. The patient will benefit more from specialists working together as a team. This concept is true both in surgery and in other areas, but is particularly so in the ICU. Patients should be managed by a group of specialists, and each member of the team should offer the best of himself or herself in order to achieve excellence in critical care. The practice of critical care medicine should take maximum advantage of the best that each specialist can provide in patient care, in training residents, and in research in order to better understand the physiopathology of the illness and its treatment.[56]

Specialists in many different fields can be in charge of managing intensive care units. In a survey on traumatic brain injury in 35 intensive care units in the UK and Ireland,[57] 23 (66%) were directed by anesthesiologists, 8 (23%) by neurosurgeons, and 4 (11%) by other medical specialists. On the other hand, in a survey on acute traumatic brain injury in 261 acute care centers in the USA,[58] most (27%) were directed by an intensivist, 24% by a neurosurgeon or neurologist and 21% by a general surgeon. In Argentina most intensive care units are managed by intensivists.

The head of the ICU should be a competent physician, an able administrator, an inquisitive researcher, and should be available at all times. In the case of a neurosurgeon or an anesthesiologist, these activities should be not be superimposed on the obligations of the operating room. In addition, in order to manage an ICU with a high level of efficiency and sophistication, the ICU equipment must be well oiled, taking into account a novel economic, financial, and legal framework.

In deciding who is to be in charge of the ICU, all of the preceding factors must be taken into account. The neurosurgeon should be a member of the team, although whether or not he or she will be in charge of the unit will vary widely depending on the different intensive care units, hospitals and regions, even within the same country. Perhaps the matter does not depend so much on which specialist should be in charge, but rather on taking into account: (1) the fundamental needs of the patient; (2) the tasks that the patient's care requires; (3) the time these tasks require; and then decide who is in the best position to carry them out. In the case of intensivists, in most countries they come from many different medical specialties, and they must acquire training in specific problems, although undoubtedly, always primarily within the ICU and at the patient's bedside.

Monitoring and observation are fundamental elements in the management and prognosis of the critically ill patient in general, and particularly true in the case of trauma patients. Although constant technological developments allow for better and more sophisticated equipment for observing the patients and the multiple physiological variables, the critical nursing care received in the intensive care unit can be considered the key element in monitoring the trauma patient. Neurological intensive care unit teams must always include nursing personnel specially trained in the care of critically ill patients, with particular emphasis on neurocritical patients. This group of health professionals is the main pillar and backbone of the neurological ICU.

Although it is difficult to define a generalized appropriate study plan, it is necessary to outline a basic profile for critical care nurses. This nonetheless runs the risk of being restrictive and should be adapted to the size of the ICU and to the type of prevailing pathologies and operations carried out in each specific ICU.[59]

Two years of professional experience in general nursing practice, and practice and rotation in a general ICU, could constitute the prerequisites towards specific training in critical care medicine. A continuous training program could be implemented simultaneously with routine nursing tasks (in-service education). Education and training should be guided by an official curriculum with a detailed catalogue of the theoretical and practical objectives to be achieved. This curriculum would vary from country to country, with general similarities and particular differences. The prerequisite professional experience in Germany for example, requires at least 240 hours of theoretical study, 480 hours of practice, 2 years experience in general nursing and 6 months prior experience in the ICU.

In small hospitals or in multipurpose intensive care units, critical care nurses would need professional experience vouching for a multidisciplinary education. In large hospitals and in those which include specialized intensive care units, it is advisable that critical care nurses rotate between the different ICUs.

Control of the quality of education can be assured by means of exams. In addition, it is important that the quality of education be controlled in the institutions offering training in this field. Practical examinations should also be carried out during the educational process.

Given that critical care medicine is constantly evolving, specialized ongoing education and training should continue even once initial training has been completed. This can be achieved through different means: (1) attending congresses, seminars, and regional and interregional work groups; (2) national and international nursing exchange programs; (3) the creation of special research groups, which would motivate and promote knowledge. Educational institutions must be accredited. The Canadian Association of Nursing and Neurosciences offers a Certification Programme. The Canadian Nursing Association has designated neuroscience nursing as a specialized nursing field. There are educational programs which teach the theoretical and practical knowledge of the general medical, neurological, and psychological aspects of patient care.

Nurses were initially in charge of intermittent clinical monitoring of patients. There should be an adequate nurse/bed ratio and nurses should be trained in the use of the different monitoring systems. The monitoring equipment and computers are of immense value to nurses and greatly facilitate their tasks,[60] allowing more time for the specific care of the patient.

Implementing the concept of teamwork is of the utmost importance. Orders given to the nursing team should be clear and should not reveal any conflict that may exist at times among the different physicians treating the same patient. Frequently, measures are suggested or orders given that are different from those given by the ICU professional. These differences should be resolved before the nursing team carries out orders. The head of the ICU must coordinate all efforts and maintain fluid communication lines between all parts involved in order to avoid any confusion.

Cerebral monitoring techniques in the critical patient

The term "monitor" comes from the Latin *moneare*, meaning "one that warns". The principal reason for the existence of neurological intensive care units is monitoring. By allowing the early detection of, at times deadly, intracranial and systemic phenomena, a rapid diagnosis may be found while these are still in a reversible stage.[61-63]

Intensive care units provide a continuum to the care and treatment of the patient. The permanent nature of intensive care ties the activities of intensive care units to one of the most beneficial activities in the management of the critical patient, continuous and permanent monitoring. On the other hand, the ongoing development of neurointensive medicine has been possible in large part owing to the parallel development of diverse neurofunction monitoring techniques. In order to detect potential dangers, the person in charge of monitoring in the intensive care unit should maintain an attitude of constant scrutiny and observation. This person should know when any changes should be communicated to those who must make decisions, who will react quickly and propose a course of action. When referring to monitoring techniques in the ICU, there is always an implied reference to a monitoring system. The system must act as a servomechanism that feeds the information received back into the same system.

Monitoring in the early stages of neurological intensive care units was carried out as intermittent observations, or "neurochecks", and not considered a continuous activity. On the other hand, in the early years, monitoring was basically clinical and not instrumental and was generally relegated to nurses. Even under the best circumstances, observations were intermittent and highly subjective. Often, deterioration in the patient's state cannot be anticipated with this type of monitoring. Contrary to the objectives of monitoring systems, observation can only give us warning when clinical deterioration has already begun and when physiological changes are no longer reversible. The limitations of this type of monitoring system increase when patients receive opioid analgesics, sedation and/or muscular relaxants, or barbituric coma.[64]

A variety of important bedside neurophysiological monitoring methods has been introduced in the last years. These methods, studied in clinical research and published in research papers and publications, are shown in Table 3.3. Continuous electroencephalogram monitoring was added to the monitoring of intracranial pressure, cerebral oxygen consumption, multimodal evoked potentials, and transcranial Doppler sonography. Given that each of these techniques evaluates different intracranial phenomena, the information they provide is complementary each to the other. The use of real time monitoring systems is part of the normal management of patients in neurological intensive care units. Neurointensivists and other members of the ICU team must be familiar with the different monitoring techniques and equipment.

It is difficult to establish the definitive role of each of these techniques in managing the neurocritical patient.[65–67]

Many monitoring techniques are still being studied in order to definitely establish their validity. Even so, the different monitors are still used and being improved with time and experience.

Monitoring of intracranial pressure

Increased intracranial pressure is very frequent in patients suffering acute traumatic brain injury, with an incidence of 30–70% of patients. The importance of increased intracranial pressure is mainly due to two factors: to the displacement of encephalic mass within the intracranial compartments, and to the negative effects of the increase of intracranial pressure on cerebral perfusion. There are three mechanisms frequently implicated in the increase of intracranial pressure following brain trauma: the appearance of hemorrhagic intracranial lesions, with space-occupying lesions; the increase of water content in the brain tissue (edema or brain swelling), and the increase of cerebral intravascular blood volume. These three mechanisms can present individually or in combination. The final consequence is the increase of the normal intracranial volume contained within a rigid enclosure, the skull. As a consequence of this, the intracranial pressure is raised.

Direct measurement of intracranial pressure is the best way to evaluate any changes in it. Different technical devices such as hydrostatic, pneumatic, and fiber optic systems have been developed in recent years to measure intracranial pressure. There has been some dispute concerning which is the most appropriate intracranial compartment for measuring intracranial pressure. Intraventricular, intraparenchymatous, subarachnoid, subdural and epidural locations have all been used. Not only has the optimum locus for the sensor been debated, but the required exactness of the measurement, the stability of the system and the complications generated by each measuring system as well. Traditionally, the intraventricular locus has been the most commonly used as a reference for assessing the precision of measurement of intracranial pressure in comparison with other compartments. The greatest equivalence with intraventricular pressure has been found with intraparenchymatous and subdural pressure transducers. The main complications from stemming from the use of intracranial pressure devices are: infection, hemorrhage, and obstruction. Intraventricular systems are those most commonly accompanied by infection. Nonetheless, a clear line must as yet be drawn between system contamination and real infection. The choice of the most appropriate device for the monitoring of intracranial pressure will depend on four variables: precision of measurement, medical experience in interpreting the measured values, cost and morbidity.

From the physiopathological point of view, the direct influence of the intracranial pressure wedges, together with the progressive decrease in cerebral perfusion pressure are the two most relevant mechanisms of the increase of intracranial pressure. The first is the pressure gradient generated from the encephalic areas with greatest hypertension, with the resulting displacement of cerebral structures within the skull (herniation, displacement of mid-cerebral structures or compression of vascular structures). The second is the negative influence on the cerebral perfusion pressure of the increase in intracranial pressure. Cerebral perfusion pressure is the difference between the mean arterial pressure and the intracranial pressure and is directly related to cerebral blood flow. Decreases in cerebral perfusion pressure bring about cerebral ischemia, with serious clinical consequences. It has been widely shown that the probability of a favorable clinical evolution is inversely proportionate to the time that the intracranial pressure remains above 20 mmHg (considered a pathological value).[68–73]

A study by Saul and Ducker in 1982[74] demonstrated that endocranial hypertension treatment lowers mortality. This study showed that in a group of patients in which endocranial hypertension treatment was begun at an intracranial pressure near 15 mmHg, mortality was lower than in a group in which treatment was begun when the intracranial pressure level was greater than 20 mmHg. Eisenberg et al. in a 1988 study,[75] found the same beneficial effects from the control of intracranial pressure.

Electroencephalography (EEG) and multimodal evoked potentials

Both EEG and multimodal evoked potentials are extraordinarily useful neurocritical patient monitoring methods, especially when the patient is under the effects of neurodepressant drugs.

Electroencephalography has been extensively used in the follow-up of patients with head injury and has proven to be very advantageous in predicting a poor evolution. The prognosis of patients with low amplitude EEG recordings and slow rhythms is significantly worse than patients showing a predominant alpha rhythm. Predicting a favorable evolution of a patient is less precise than predicting a poor evolution. Among other reasons, this is due to the fact that the EEG does not present specific patterns for severe cerebral compromise. There are no EEG measurements characteristic of a fall in cerebral perfusion pressure. The ability of the EEG to detect changes in cerebral perfusion is rather belated when compared to other neuromonitoring methods. Nonetheless, there are certain types of EEG recordings that can facilitate predicting a good prognosis. The reactivity of EEG recordings to stimuli, such as auditory stimuli, has been identified as a factor indicative of good prognosis in patients with head injury and other kinds of acute pathology such as ischemic-anoxia encephalopathy. Computer analysis of condensed EEG recordings, known as "compressed spectral array", converts the information received from a classic EEG into a recording of dominant frequencies in time.

Somesthetic (electrical stimuli applied to the nerves of extremities), auditory and visual stimuli are the three most commonly used stimuli for evoked potential recordings. Somesthetic stimuli explore the different pathways through which an electrical stimulus is transmitted. An initial wave, generated by the brachial plexus (if the stimulus was made on the upper extremity) is followed by those generated in the superior cervical column, dorsal nuclei and primary parietal sensory cortex. In the case of auditory potentials, the stimulus is an auditory "click" stimulating the eighth cranial nerve, the evoked potential then travels through the cochlear nucleus, superior olive complex, the lateral lemniscus and the inferior colliculus. The presence of an I wave assures the integrity of the peripheral auditory structures. Visual evoked potentials explore the integrity of the retina, optic nerve, chiasma, and occipital cortex. Visual evoked potentials are usually applied together with auditory and somatosensorial evoked potentials, but are generally less useful. The greatest advantage of monitoring evoked potentials is that they are resistant to the influence of pharmacological agents such as barbiturates.

The predictive value of somatosensorial potentials in patients with head trauma can be superior to that of an EEG. This is due to the fact that many extraneurological factors have less of an influence on evoked potentials than they do on an EEG. Many studies have found that significantly pathological somesthetic potentials correlate with a poor clinical evolution. Conflicting results have been found regarding the predictive value of auditory evoked potentials. Whereas some studies find a good correlation between auditory evoked potentials and the prognosis of a patient with brain trauma, other studies do not.[76–79]

Comparative studies between somesthetic and auditory potentials have shown the somesthetic potentials to be superior. This is most probably owing to the fact that somesthetic potentials present several components which include the peripheral nerve all the way to the cerebral cortex, whereas the upper level of auditory signal processing is the brain stem.

Monitoring for cerebral blood flow (CBF) estimation and cerebral metabolic activity

In most cases of acute brain injury, modifications in cerebral blood flow are produced. Monitoring of these changes can at times be highly important in establishing the physiopathology of the brain lesion. At other times, modifying CBF becomes a therapeutic objective. Changes in CBF occurring during the acute phase of traumatic brain injury (TBI) cause relevant alterations in the delivery of oxygen to the brain. Due to this, the quantification of CBF is an important contribution to the management of patients with severe traumatic head injury. However, owing to the technological requirements necessary for the direct measurement of CBF (the nitrous oxide method; Xenon 133), continuous bedside monitoring of CBF is not currently possible. Instead, most neurological intensive care units make indirect estimations of CBF using such techniques as transcranial Doppler sonography or monitoring of the oxygen saturation in the bulb of the internal jugular vein.

Transcranial Doppler sonography, developed by Aaslid and based on the Doppler effect, allows us to measure the blood flow velocity at the base of the skull. In addition, using transcranial Doppler sonography we can record the blood flow velocity over time on a graphic scale called a sonogram. A bidirectional flowmeter of 2 MHz which emits pulsed sound through a piezo-electric crystal is used in these studies. To gain sonographic access to Willis's polygon, so called "sonic windows" are used. These are cranial regions whose structural characteristics present greater transparency for ultrasounds. The most widely used are the temporal, ophthalmic, and foramen magnum windows. Identification of the explored arteries is done through three factors: depth of the artery, presence of anterograde flow (arterial flow towards the probe) or retrograde flow (arterial flow away from the probe), and by the response of arterial flow after compression of the two carotids.

Three fundamental facts are obtained from the sonographic signal. These are:

1   Morphology of the sonogram.
2   Values (in centimeters performance second) of the systolic, diastolic and mean velocities.
3   Estimation of cerebrovascular resistance through Gosling's pulsatility index or Pourcelot's resistance index.

The high incidence of changes in intracranial pressure, and the consequential changes in CBF, following spontaneous cerebral hemorrhage and trauma is a well-known fact. Change in CBF is conditioned by changes in the intracranial pressure. This is owing to the fact that alterations in intracranial pressure determine changes in cerebrovascular resistance, which then modify CBF. This in turn determines changes in blood flow velocity in the arteries at the base of the skull. Aside from intracranial pressure there are other factors, such as changes in cerebral oxygen consumption, changes in vascular response to carbonic anhydride, vasospasm due to subarachnoid hemorrhage, and so forth, which determine changes in blood flow velocity. During the first 24 hours post-trauma, patients with severe traumatic head injury often have low-speed sonographic recordings. This can be due to various factors including hypovolemia secondary to the trauma, a decrease in cerebral oxygen consumption, and endocranial hypertension. Such a sonographic pattern, especially when it is due to endocranial hypertension evolving with an increase in the pulsatility index beyond the normal limits, tends to correspond with a clinical pattern of cerebral hypoperfusion. An increase in the mean velocity, and a decrease in the pulsatility index during the days following the trauma, are indicative of a good prognosis.

A decrease in the intracranial arterial blood flow velocity following head injury can be owing either to a decrease in CBF secondary to a decrease in cerebral metabolism, or to an increase in intracranial pressure. An inverse correlation between the severity of injury and the mean velocity of the midcerebral artery has been shown.[80] Nonetheless, the mean blood flow velocity does not generally show a significant decrease until the cerebral perfusion pressure begins to fall below normal limits. There is, however, a close correlation between the pulsatility index and intracranial pressure. An increase in intracranial pressure determines a parallel increase in the pulsatility index due to a reduction in diastolic velocity. When intracranial pressure begins to rise uncontrollably, a systolisized sonographic pattern is recorded. This pattern shows a decrease in the mean velocity and an increase in the pulsatility index. When the value of the cerebral perfusion pressure nears the value of the mean arterial pressure, the anterograde flow of the diastolic phase ceases and retrograde flow is observed. This sonographic pattern is known as reverberant flow and is indicative of cessation of cerebral blood flow. In more advanced stages of cerebral circulatory arrest, the diastolic wave disappears, with only the systolic component remaining. The final process of cerebral circulatory arrest is accompanied by the impossibility to record any signal at all from the arteries of the base of the skull.[81-84]

In the case of pathological cerebrovascular hemorrhage, the changes observable through transcranial Doppler sonography can be superposed on those which are found in patients with acute endocranial hypertension from other causes, such as head trauma. In the acute phase of spontaneous subarachnoid haemorrhage as well as in cases of large intracerebral hematomas, a hemodynamic pattern of reduced CBF is detected through transcranial Doppler sonography.

Vasospasm, so frequently found in the weeks following the appearance of subarachnoid haemorrhage, can be inferred through the use of a sonograph. A significant increase in the mean velocity at the level of the artery where the vasospasm develops, accompanied by a decrease in the pulsatility index, translates into the existence of a narrowing at the level of the arteries at the base of the skull and of a vasodilatation of microcirculation compensating for the potential decrease of blood flow caused by the vasospasm.

Measurement, whether continuous or discontinuous, of oxygen saturation at the level of the bulb of the internal jugular vein is a frequently used technique in monitoring neurocritical patients. If it is assumed that the arterial oxygen content, the concentration of hemoglobin and the position of the dissociation curve of the hemoglobin are constant, then the relation between cerebral oxygen requirements and CBF will vary proportionately with the venous oxygen content, and therefore with the oxygen saturation of jugular venous hemoglobin (SjO2). Thus, monitoring of SjO2 becomes a useful element in estimating the balance between cerebral oxygen requirements and cerebral blood flow.

The end of the catheter should be situated below the bulb of the internal jugular vein in order to minimize extracranial contamination from the pterygoid and facial veins. The position of the catheter should be checked with a lateral X-ray, to verify that the end of the catheter is above the lower edge of the first cervical vertebra. There are several ways that the data received following the positioning of the catheter in the internal jugular vein can be used. One of these is the direct measurement of venous oxygen saturation. Normal parameters are between 50 to 55% at the lower limit and 75% at the upper limit (65% as the average value). When saturation exceeds 75%, the patient is considered to present relative hyperemia (high CBF in relation to oxygen extraction, which in turn can be normal or low). In patients in which high extraction indicates low jugular extraction, it is considered that there is a low CBF in relation to oxygen consumption.

Some authors prefer the arteriojugular differences in oxygen content to calculate the amount of oxygen extracted from cerebral circulation. Another way to express cerebral oxygen extraction when using data obtained from jugular oxygen saturation is the Oxygen Extraction Rate formula. Other parameters have also been employed, such as the Oxygen/Lactate Index, cerebral glucose consumption, and so forth. However, SjO2 continues to be the most currently used parameter in management of patients with traumatic head injury. Due to its continuous monitoring and direct reading capabilities, it can be used as an efficient method for the detection of jugular desaturation episodes (compatible with cerebral hypoperfusion episodes), or of saturation above normal parameters (compatible with low perfusion or hyperemia).

Persistent neurological dysfunction is the main cause of morbimortality in intensive care units and has serious long-term effects on quality of life and in care costs. The improvement in the monitoring and assessment of central nervous system injury is a vital part of the effort to improve the outcome of patients in the intensive care unit.

No one piece of equipment, no matter how sophisticated, constitutes of itself a monitoring system. There have been remarkable advances in signal detection and the way these signals can be viewed. This fact has greatly improved the capacity to observe and recognize diverse physiopathological events. These steps and those that follow will ultimately depend on the training, abilities, and dedication of neurological intensive care unit teams. These professionals must be highly competent in the use of the equipment, clearly communicate observations, implement appropriate action, and subsequently observe the response to the measures taken. In the last analysis, it is this human component which ultimately determines the success of a monitoring system. This team of human "equipment" must be as carefully maintained as the most sophisticated equipment found in the intensive care unit.

Evaluating the efficiency of neurological intensive care units

It is a well-known fact that mortality and morbidity in intensive care units, and in particular in neurointensive care units, are higher than in general hospital wards. Given this high mortality, it is both appropriate and sensible to measure outcomes.[85] However, mortality can be the expression of many other factors other than inefficient or ineffective care in the ICU.

It is difficult to establish standards for analyzing outcome in intensive care units. This not only depends on equipment, unit staff, and the care process (type, capacity, and amount of time of care), but also on populational characteristics. The population of patients in a major medical center is quite different from that of a local or regional hospital. Admission criteria to the ICU can be very diverse, although pre-existing illnesses and the current illness must also be considered. Intensive care units with a high admission rate of elderly patients have a high proportion of high-risk patients. In such cases a higher mortality rate is therefore to be expected.

There are various issues concerning the level and quality of care that patients with neurological and acute neurosurgical illnesses receive, both within and outside of non-specialized intensive care units. The general ICU treats a great variety of cases and rarely boasts of medical or (even less frequently) nursing staff specially trained in the care of neurocritical patients. In neurological and neurosurgical wards, the nurse/bed ratio is usually inadequate to the needs of patients with acute illness who do not meet criteria for admission to the ICU. The necessary equipment for monitoring the different physiological variables is not available, either in the necessary amount or quality, and nurses are generally not trained in their use.

There is growing evidence that the process in which care is offered to patients is more important than the actual physical area of the unit where care takes place. This is applicable to multipurpose ICUs and in many aspects to neurological intensive care units as well.[86] In a prospective study by Knaus et al.[87] which included 5030 patients in general intensive care units of major medical centers in the USA, a significant variation was found in the mortality rate. The differences in the mortality rate were related more to the coordinated efforts and interaction of ICU staff than to the administrative structure, specialized treatment or the level of training. Indredavik et al.[88] carried out a study focused on stroke units, in which they compared stroke patients hospitalized in stroke units to stroke patients hospitalized in general wards. The findings in this study revealed significant differences in: lower early mortality, a lower percentage of chronically hospitalized patients, and a higher percentage of patients discharged from hospital and returning to their homes. Other randomized studies[89,90] revealed that patients admitted to stroke units presented a lower mortality at 17 weeks and after the first year than stroke patients not treated in stroke units. A recent meta-analysis[91] analyzing ten studies that included patients treated in stroke units and by mobile stroke teams, showed 28% lower early mortality and 21% lower late mortality in comparison with patients who were not managed in this way. In contrast to this, an earlier study in Canada[92] found no greater benefit for patients in stroke units. In these hospitals, however, all of the patients with this pathology were treated by stroke teams in different places of hospital confinement. This supports the hypothesis that outcome depends more on the nature of care than on the particular physical structure in which care takes place.

In a retrospective study by Wärme et al.,[93] findings showed that the introduction of a neurosurgical intensive care unit was associated with an increase in good outcome, by 15–52%. This improvement was even more marked for patients with a motor response score greater than or equal to 4 on the Glasgow Coma Scale. A characteristic of these intensive care units was that well-trained personnel provided organized and continuous care. Quality care is possible if comprehensive management of diverse illnesses and acute situations is planned, as well as by implementing planning maps or critical care pathways. These would be co-coordinated by the different medical and non-medical professionals involved in the patients' care.[94, 95] A work methodology emphasizing communication and coordination between physicians and nursing staff should be implemented.[96]

In the decision-making process, an multidisciplinary approach to the problem must be made.[97] During the acute phase of the illness, a daily plan with expected results should be drawn up. Care maps describe planned interventions and actions through the course of time.[98] In addition, maps describe the indicators for measuring quality and good outcome, which in turn make it possible to continue with new initiatives to improve on what has already been achieved.[99]

Score systems are used with the aim of quantifying cases and use the scores to estimate outcome. Score systems are generally used to measure mortality after stay in the ICU and before discharge from the hospital. In the 1970s Knaus developed APACHE (acute physiology and chronic health evaluation), a score system which scores the severity of an acute illness by the measure of the alteration of the affected physiological variables. Score systems fulfill various functions:

1   *Comparative audit*: the comparison between actual and expected outcome for a given group of patients can be used to compare between different intensive care units and health providers. The differences in mortality rates indicate a need to investigate local problems or characteristics.

2   *Evaluation of research*: given the heterogeneity of populations in intensive care units, scores allow us to obtain a more homogeneous subgroup of patients and thereby better to isolate and discern the influence of a given intervention in a study.

3   *Individualized clinical management of patients*: although first generation scores were conceived to measure outcome, obtaining second and third generation scores is encouraged in order to guide clinical care and treatment. Currently available scores allow us to determine general probabilities, although not for any given individual.

Score systems can be generic or specific. Specific score systems can be used for certain patient types, whereas generic score systems can be used for virtually all types of patients. Score systems should be either anatomical or physiological. Anatomical systems evaluate the extent of injury whereas physiological systems evaluate the impact of injury. Anatomical score systems are fixed, while physiological systems are variable and can change according to the physiological response to injury during treatment. Score systems were first developed for trauma patients. The AIS (1969), Burns Score (1971), and ISS (1974) are all anatomical score systems. The physiological score systems are: Trauma Index (1971), GCS (1974), Trauma Score (1981), and Sepsis Score (1983). The latest score systems developed in intensive care units are of the generic type. Two approaches were used in their development: one to measure the severity of the illness by the intensity of treatment; the other to measure severity through the physiological characteristics and measurements of the patient. These systems are the Therapeutic Intervention Scoring System (TISS), and the APACHE II and Simplified Acute Physiology Score (SAPS) respectively.

The selection of a particular score system depends on the proposed use. The main criteria for selection should be the precision of the score and the calibrations and discriminating power of the mathematical equation used to estimate the result. In several countries, APACHE II has been the most widely used and proven score.

The Glasgow Coma Scale (GCS) is commonly used in intensive care units. It helps to avoid describing the patient's neurological level in words as it is assumed that colleagues understand its meaning. The GCS evaluates the best motor, verbal, and ocular response, going from 3 to 15 points, and is the most widely used scale for acute neurological dysfunctions.[100] The main benefits of the GCS are its simplicity, replicability, and reliability. The main utility of the Glasgow Coma Scale is its use with traumatic brain injury patients as it permits a clinical classification according to slight, moderate, and severe injury. The usefulness of the GCS is clearly limited, however, in intubated patients and in those with ocular and facial trauma.

References

1. Eidelman, B. H., Obrist, W. D., Wagner, W. R., Kormos, R., & Griffith, B. (1993). Cerebrovascular complications associated with the use of artificial circulatory support services. *Neurol. Clin., 11*, 463–474.
2. Safar, P., & Grenvick, A. (1977). Organization and physician education in critical care medicine. *Anesthesiology, 47*, 82.
3. Ibsen, B. (1954). The anesthetist's viewpoint on treatment of respiratory complications in poliomyelitis during the epidemic in Copenhagen. *Proc. R. Soc. Med., 47*, 72.
4. Sadove, M. S., et al. (1951). An ideal recovery room. *Mod. Hosp., 76*, 88.
5. Dunn, F. E., & Shupp, M. G. (1943). The recovery room: a wartime economy. *Ann. J. Nurs., 43*, 279.
6. Hilberman, M. (1975). The evolution of intensive care units. *Crit. Care. Med., 3*, 159.
7. Fein, A., & Spanier, A. H. (1991). Organization and management of critical care units. In J. M. Rippe et al. (Eds.), *Intensive care medicine*. (2nd ed.). New York: Little, Brown.
8. Kinney, J. M. (1966). The intensive care unit. *Bull. Am. Coll. Surg., 51*, 201.
9. Rogers, R. M., Weiler, C., & Rupponthal, B. (1972). Impact of the respiratory intensive care unit on survival of patients with acute respiratory failure. *Chest, 62*, 94.
10. Artz, C. P., Mancrief, J. A., & Pruitt, B. A. (Eds.) (1997). *A team approach*. Philadelphia, PA: W. B. Saunders.
11. Boswick, J. A. (1978). Symposium on burns. *Surg. Clin. N. Am., 58*, 1105.
12. Bachman, L., et al. (1967). Organization and function of an intensive care unit at a children's hospital. *Anesth. Analg., 46*, 570.
13. Ropper, A. H. (1992). Neurological intensive care. *Ann. Neurol., 4*, 564.
14. Ropper, A. H. (1993). Introduction to critical care in neurology and neurosurgery. In A. H. Ropper (Ed.), *Neurological and neurosurgical intensive care* (3rd ed.). New York: Raven.
15. West, J., Trunkey, D., & Lim, R. (1979). System of trauma care. A study of two countries. *Arch. Surg., 114*, 455.
16. Kreis, D., et al. (1986). Preventable trauma deaths: Daude County, Florida. *J. Trauma, 26*, 649.
17. Campbell, S., Walkins, G., & Kreis, D. (1989). Preventable deaths in a self-designated trauma system. *Ann. Surg., 55*, 478.
18. Wilson, D., McElligott, J., & Fielding, L. (1992). Identification of preventable trauma deaths: confounded inquiries? *J. Trauma, 32*, 45.
19. Roy, P. (1987). The value of trauma centers: a methodologic review. *Can. J. Surg., 30*, 7.
20. Mendeloff, J., & Cayten C. (1991). Trauma system and public policy. *Ann. Rev. Pub. Health, 12*, 401.
21. Bullock, R., et al. (1995). Trauma system and the neurosurgeon. In: Brain Trauma Foundation, (Eds.), *Guidelines for the management of severe head injury*. New York: Brain Trauma Foundation.
22. American College of Surgeons Committee on Trauma (Eds.) (1993). *Resources for optimal care of injured patients*. Chicago, IL: American College of Surgeons.

23. Winston, S. R. (1996). Neurosurgical intensive care for severe head injuries. *Iowa Med., 83*, 17.
24. Marshall, L. F., et al. (1991). A new classification of head injury based on computerized tomography. *J. Neurosurg., 75*(suppl), S14.
25. Teasdale, G., & Jennet, B. (1974). Assessment of coma and impaired consciousness: a practical scale. *Lancet, 2*, 81.
26. Pitts, L. H. (1989). Neurosurgical critical care: who's in charge? *Clin. Neurosurg., 35*, 55.
27. Fisher, C. M., Kristler, J. P., & Davis, J. M. (1980). Relation of cerebral vasospasm to subarachnoid hemorrhage visualized by computerized tomographic scanning. *Neurosurgery, 6*, 1.
28. Hunt, R. E., & Hess, R. M. (1968). Surgical risk as related to time of intervention in the repair of intracranial aneurysms. *J. Neurosurg., 28*, 14.
29. Drake, W. E., et al. (1973). Acute stroke management and patient outcome: the value of neurovascular care units. *Stroke, 4*, 933.
30. Kennedy, F. B., Pozen, T. J., & Gabelman, E. H. (1970). Stroke intensive care – an appraisal. *Am. Heart. J., 80*, 188.
31. Norris, J. W., & Hachinski, V. C. (1986). Stroke units or stroke centres. *Stroke, 49*, 360.
32. Haerer, A. F., Smith, R. R., & Currier, R. D. (1969). Stroke unit: review of the first 100 cases. *J. Miss. State Med. J., 10*, 237.
33. Isaacs, B. (1977). Five years experience of a stroke unit. *Health Bull., 35*, 98.
34. Feigenson, J. S., Gitlow, H. S., & Greenberg, S. D. (1979). The disabilited oriented rehabilitation unit – a major factor influencing stroke outcome. *Stroke, 10*, 5.
35. Von Arbin, M., et al. (1980). A study of stroke patients treated in a non-intensive stroke unit or in general medical wards. *Acta Med. Scand., 208*, 81.
36. Hacke, W., Schwab, S., & de Georgia, M. (1994). Intensive care of acute ischemic stroke. *Cerebrovasc. Dis., 4*, 385.
37. Indredavik, B., et al. (1999). Stroke unit treatment 10-year follow-up. *Stroke, 30*, 1524.
38. The Stroke Triallist Collaboration (1997). Collaborative systemic review of the randomized trials of organised inpatient (stroke unit) care after stroke. *Br. Med. J., 314*, 1151.
39. Indredavik, B., et al. (1997). Stroke unit treatment: long-term effects. *Stroke, 28*, 1861.
40. Donnan, G. A., et al. (1995). Trials of streptokinase in severe acute ischaemic stroke. *Lancet, 345*, 578.
41. Hommel, M., et al. for the MAST Study Group (1994). Termination of trial of streptokinase in severe acute ischaemic stroke. *Lancet, 345*, 56.
42. Fletcher, A. P., et al. (1976). A pilot study of urokinase therapy in cerebral infarction. *Stroke, 7*, 135.
43. Adams, H. P., et al. (1996). Guidelines for thrombolytic therapy for acute stroke: a supplement to the guidelines for the management of patients with acute ischemic stroke. *Circulation, 94*, 1167.
44. The National Institute of Neurological Disorders and Stroke rt-PA Stroke Study Group (1995). Tissue plasminogen activator for acute ischemic stroke. *N. Engl. J. Med., 333*, 1581.
45. Fustinoni, O., & Goldemberg, F. (In press). Ischemic stroke: general treatment.

In Sociedad Argentina de Terapia Intensiva (Eds.), *Manual of intensive therapy*. Buenos Aires: Editorial Médica Panamericana.

46. Walker, M. C., et al. (1996). Diagnosis and treatment of status epilepticus on a neurological intensive care unit. *Q. J. Med., 89*, 913.
47. Walker, M. C., Smith, J. M., & Shorvon, S. D. (1995). The intensive care treatment of convulsive status epilepticus in the UK. *Anaesthesia, 50*, 130.
48. Delgado-Escueta, A. V., & Enrile-Bacsalm, F. (1983). Combination therapy for status epilepticus: intravenous diazepam and phenytoin. *Adv. Neurol., 34*, 477.
49. Wilder, B. J. (1983). Efficacy of phenytoin in treatment of status epilepticus. *Adv. Neurol., 34*, 441.
50. Howell, S. J., Owen, L., & Chadwick, D. W. (1989). Pseudostatus epilepticus. *Q. J. Med., 71*, 507.
51. Lowenstein, D. H., & Alldredge, B. K. (1993). Status epilepticus at an urban public hospital in the 1980s. *Neurology, 34*, 483.
52. Barry, E., & Hauser, W. A. (1994). Status epilepticus and antiepileptic medication levels. *Neurology, 44*, 47.
53. Aminoff, M. J., & Simon, R. P. (1980). Status epilepticus: causes, clinical features and consequences in 98 patients. *Am. J. Med., 69*, 657.
54. Fisher, S., Zatucchi, J., & Greenberg, J. (1977). Disseminated intravascular coagulation in status epilepticus. *Thromb. Haemost., 38*, 909.
55. Sugerman, P. (1982). Surgeons and the surgical intensive care unit. *Arch. Surg., 117*, 391.
56. Modell, J. H. (1982). Critical care medicine and the surgical intensive care unit. A balanced view. *Arch. Surg., 117*, 265.
57. Matta, B., & Menon, D. (1996). Severe head injury in the United Kingdom and Ireland: a survey of practice and implications for management. *Crit. Care Med., 24*, 1744.
58. Ghajar, J., et al. (1995). A survey of critical care management of comatose, head injured patients in the United States. *Crit. Care Med., 23*, 560.
59. Burchardi, H., & Atkinson, B. L. (1990). Education and training. In R. D. Miranda and A. W. Loirat (Eds.) *Management of intensive care: Guidelines for better use of resources*. Dordrecht: Kluwer Academic.
60. Welleck, C. (1975). The neurosurgical nurse and computer work together. *J. Neurosurg. Nursing, 7*, 102.
61. Domínguez-Roldán, J. M., Murillo, F., & Muñoz, A. (1997). Interventions in the acute phase of severe brain-injured patients. In *Neuropsychological rehabilitation* (p. 127). Delray Beach, FL: St. Lucy Press.
62. Jordan, K. G. (1995). Neurophysiologic monitoring in the neuroscience intensive care unit. *Neurol. Clin., 13*, 579.
63. Domínguez-Roldán, J. M., Madrazo, J., & Lagos, R. (1999). Techniques in the neurodiagnosis of patients in ICU. In F. Barranco, et al. (Eds.), *Principles of urgency, emergency and intensive care units* (p. 605). Granada: Alhulia.
64. Jordan, K. G. (1993). Continuous EEG and evoked potential monitoring in the neuroscience intensive care unit. *J. Clin. Neurophysiol., 10*, 445.
65. Domínguez-Roldán, J. M., & Gracia, R. M. (2000). Neuromonitoring. In J. Pacin et al. (Eds.), *Terapia intensiva*. Buenos Aires: Panamericana.
66. Cruz, J. (1993). Combined continuous monitoring of systemic and cerebral oxigenation in acute brain injury. Preliminary observations. *Crit. Care Med., 21*, 1225.

67. Martin, N. A., et al. (1992). Posttraumatic cerebral arterial spasm: transcranial Doppler ultrasound, cerebral blood flow and angiographic findings. *J. Neurosurg., 77*, 575.
68. Narayan, R. K., et al. (1982). Intracranial pressure: to monitor or not to monitor? A review of our experience with head injury. *J. Neurosurg., 56*, 650.
69. Jordan, K. G. (1990). Continuous EEG monitoring in the neurological intensive care unit. *Neurology, 40*(suppl. 1), 180.
70. Domínguez-Roldán, J. M., et al. (1999). Changes in the intracranial pulse pressure waveform associated with brain death. *Transplant Proc., 31*, 2597.
71. Johnston, I. H., Johnston, J. A., & Jennet, B. (1970). Intracranial pressure changes following head injury. *Lancet, 2*, 433.
72. Marshall, L. F., Smith, R. W., & Shapiro, R. (1979). The outcome with aggressive treatment in severe head injuries. Part II: acute and chronic barbiturate administration in the management of severe head injury. *J. Neurosurg., 50*, 26.
73. Miller, J. D., et al. (1981). Further experience in the management of severe head injury. *J. Neurosurg., 54*, 289.
74. Saul, T. G., & Ducker, T. B. (1982). Effect of intracranial pressure monitoring and aggressive treatment on mortality in severe head injury. *J. Neurosurg., 56*, 498.
75. Eisenberg, H. M., et al. (1988). High-dose barbiturate control of elevated intracranial pressure in patients with severe head injury. *J. Neurosurg., 6915*.
76. Karnaze, D. S., Weiner, J., & Marshall, L. (1985). Auditory evoked potentials in coma after close head injury: a clinical–neurophysiologic coma scale for predicting outcome. *Neurology, 35*, 1122.
77. Becker, D. P., Gade, G. F., & Miller, J. D. (1990). Prognosis after head injury. In J. R. Youmans, (Ed.), *Neurological surgery* (3rd ed., p. 2194). Philadelphia, PA: W. B. Saunders.
78. Dauch, W. A. (1991). Prediction of secondary deterioration in comatose neurolsurgical patients by serial recording of multimodality evoked potentials. *Acta Neurochir. (Wien), 111*, 84.
79. Alster, J., Pratt, H., & Feinsod, M. (1993). Density spectral array, evoked potentials, and temperature rhythms in the evaluation and prognosis of the comatose patient. *Brain Inj., 7*, 191.
80. Chan, K. H., Miller, J. D., & Dearden, N. M. (1992). Intracranial blood flow velocity after head injury: relationship to severity of injury, time, neurological status and outcome. *J. Neurol. Neurosurg. Psychiat., 55*, 787.
81. Domínguez-Roldán, J. M., et al. (1995). Changes in the Doppler waveform of intracranial arteries in patients in brain death status. *Transpl. Proc., 27*, 2391.
82. Domínguez-Roldán, J. M., et al. (2000). Transcranial Doppler sonography: its usefulness in the diagnosis of cerebral circulatory rest accompanying brain death. *Med. Intens., 24*, 151.
83. Domínguez-Roldán, J. M., & Barrera-Chacon, J. M. (1999). Diagnosis of whole brain death. *Organs Tissues, 2*, 103.
84. Domínguez-Roldán, J. M., et al. (1995). Study of blood flow velocities in the middle cerebral artery using transcranial Doppler sonography in brain-dead patients. *Transpl. Proc., 27*, 2395.
85. Gunning, K., & Rowan, K. (1999). Outcome data and scoring systems. *Br. Med. J., 319*, 241.
86. Miranda, R. D., & Langrehr, D. (1990). National and regional organisation. In

R. D. Miranda, & A. W. Loirat (Eds.), *Management of intensive care: Guidelines for better use of resources.* Dordrecht: Kluwer Academic.

87. Knaus, W. A., et al. (1986). An evaluation of outcome from intensive care in major medical centers. *Ann. Intern. Med., 10,* 410.

88. Indredavik, B., et al. (1991). Benefit of a stroke unit: a randomized controlled trial. *Stroke, 22,* 1026.

89. Strand, T., et al. (1985). A non-intensive stroke unit reduces functional disability and the need for long-term hospitalization. *Stroke, 16,* 29.

90. Garraway, W. M., Akthar, A. J., & Presscott, R. J. (1980). Management of acute stroke in the elderly: follow-up of a controlled trial. *Br. Med. J., 281,* 827.

91. Langhorne, P., et al. (1993). Do stroke units save lives? *Lancet, 342,* 395.

92. Wood-Dauphinee, S., et al. (1984). A randomized trial of team care following stroke. *Stroke, 15,* 864.

93. Wärme, P. E., Bergström, R., & Persson, L. (1991). Neurosurgical intensive care improves outcome after severe head injury. *Acta Neurochir., 110,* 57.

94. Health Services Research Group (1992). Quality of care: 2. Quality of care studies and their consequences. *Can. Med. Assoc. J., 147,* 163.

95. Health Services Research Group (1992). Quality of care: 1. What is quality and how can it be measured? *Can. Med. Assoc. J., 146,* 2153.

96. Mosher, C., et al. (1992). Upgrading practice with critical pathways. *Am. J. Nurs., 92,* 41.

97. Young, G. B. (1994). Planning care for neurology and neurosurgery patients with critical illnesses. *Can. J. Neurol. Sci., 21,* 295.

98. Zander, K. (1991). Care maps: the core of cost/quality care. *New Definition, 6,* 1.

99. Zander, K. (1992). Qualifying, managing and improving quality: how care maps link CQI to the patient. *New Definition, 7,* 1.

100. Jennett, B., & Teasdale, G. (1977). Aspects of coma after severe head injury. *Lancet, 878,* 81.

4   Current concepts and strategies on early neurorehabilitation for patients with traumatic brain injury (TBI)

A model project according to the guidelines of the German Task Force on Early Neurological–Neurosurgical Rehabilitation

Klaus R. H. von Wild

Introduction

The last 25 years have seen dramatic changes in the care and treatment of patients with traumatic brain injury (TBI). These changes have impacted on both the acute care as well as the post-acute rehabilitation by lowering the mortality rate and increasing the number of persons that require longer term neurorehabilitation. The treatment of head-injured patients has increasingly occupied the neurosurgery area.[1-4] While earlier the focus was on the purely clinical aspects, for example, concerning suitable therapy concepts for acute care and intensive medical treatment, the interest is now concentrated on outcomes and therapeutic approaches in the clinical research of pathophysiological and post-traumatic changes. How can imminent secondary and tertiary damage be avoided or recognized early on and subsequently minimized? This is the starting point for rehabilitation research in the neurotraumatology field.[4-8] However, in respect to the so-called "evidence-based" concepts for post-traumatic rehabilitation, prospective controlled clinical trials are still lacking in neurorehabilitation.[1] This is why there are so few standards for management in post-traumatic rehabilitation although there is a lot of experience and expert opinion documented in the literature over the last 100 years – along with expert opinions in this field which provide for some algorithms and options.[1,9-12] Cognitive impairment and neuropsychological disabilities determine the final performance capacity and the degree of the handicap of the patients with TBI. In contrast to the TBI patient, sensory-motor disabilities are the major handicap in persons with spinal cord injury (SCI), which differs according to the stages of the transsection syndrome, many of these patients can look after themselves because of the intact cognitive and neurobehavioral functions.[13,14]

Neurorehabilitation is primarily based on the prevention, diagnosing and treating post-traumatic complications and defining specific strategies in respect to the various impairments that decrease functional ability. The ultimate goal is the achievement of the patients' functioning in society.

Neurorehabilitation was introduced into the acute treatment of TBI as a highly specialized multidisciplinary therapeutic concept.[9–11] Its target is to minimize secondary brain damage and, at the same time, to restore and improve impaired brain functions in respect to sensory motor, mental and cognitive capacity.

However, the economic and cultural aspects must also be considered in the planning stage, at least in regard to public healthcare and, even more importantly, in respect to the family's needs and wishes.

Historical remarks

The obligation of a state to reintegrate the sick and injured into social and vocational life and the commitment to give these people support was first defined in the French constitution in the wake of the enlightenment of the French Revolution and the accompanying upheavals of social conditions, resulting in the emergence of early models of social medicine in the modern-day sense of the term. The desire and requirement for rehabilitation (Latin: *habilis* and *habilitare*) in the context of "apt" and "appropriate" is, in terms of the person with disability, defined by the ICIDH-2 of the World Health Organization (WHO).[15]

History teaches us that progress and renewal always emerge in a society only as a response: in other words, as a direct reaction to specific demands of a certain limited time span, depending on regional, continental, and now – in these days of globalization – worldwide requirements and challenges. An exemplary case in this regard is the history of modern neurological rehabilitation in connection with neurotraumatology over the past 100 years. First, it was an immediate reaction to the events of World Wars I and II for the acute care and rehabilitation of both military and civilian victims,[16,17] while today it is for the victims of road traffic crashes, personal violence and child abuse, sports-related accidents, or in accidents occurring at work or in the household. Technological advances in the areas of implantable microelectronics, computer technology and telecommunications, and also the availability of novel, constantly improved materials have revolutionized the diagnosis and therapy in neurotrauma over the past three decades.[18] These changes have improved the entire spectrum of traumatic, central and peripheral nervous system injury care from acute medical-surgical management to the development of novel post-acute rehabilitation programs in the community.

Our ideas and concepts of post-traumatic rehabilitation of sensory-motor disorders today are essentially based on the fundamental rules formulated by

Ottfrid Foerster (1873–1941) regarding exercise therapy for peripheral pareses and for central motor disorders, differentiating between the spastic and the paretic component.[19,20] Today we know that motor skills can be improved only by specifically targeted exercises. By the close of the "Decade of the Brain" in the 1990s, the use of state-of-the-art neuroimaging procedures was evidence of the importance of the sensory-motor network in the reorganizational ability of the brain. This was already sketched out as a model by Foerster in 1916, in the form of a *central network of sensitive and motor cerebral fields* with diffusely distributed cortical systems of the formulation of the will and a spatial presentation on the environment.

In much the same sense, the great neuropsychologist Alexander R. Luria (1902–1977) saw the activity of the *nervous system as a social organ* with coordinated and adaptable cooperation between various segments of the nervous system and, consequently, constant results are always yielded under varying historical, cultural and social conditions.[21,22] It is essentially the cognitive impairment and neuropsychological disability that ultimately determine the final degree of the handicap and the performance capacity in TBI.[23–26]

At the beginning of this century, Kurt Goldstein (1878–1965), who worked in Frankfurt am Main, had already defined patients' enormous emotional crises after severe TBI as catastrophic reactions. He introduced neuropsychological therapeutic concepts into rehabilitation to create an individual replacement strategy for the person with TBI according to their impairments.[27,28] Today our concepts of post-traumatic neuropsychological rehabilitation are mainly based upon the realization of his principles as formulated by Christensen and Caetano (1996):

• respect for the uniqueness and variability of functional systems
• support and enhancement of functional reorganization
• creation of new and purposeful tasks and assignments
• feedback of strengths and weaknesses to the patients provided in a supportive and educational milieu by trained therapists.[25]

Spectrum of neurorehabilitation

In 1993, as a measure to underscore the spectrum of services provided in neurorehabilitation, the special conditions, complexity and temporal dynamics of neurorehabilitation measures, the phrase "spectrum of neurological-neurotraumatological rehabilitation" was coined[29] similar to the characteristics of Frauenhofer (Figure 4.1).

The spectrum of neurorehabilitation starts at the site of the accident. The special circumstances of the accident, the primary and secondary injuries that may have already occurred, the type and extent of the combined injuries, the time interval, and also the type and extent of the emergency and resuscitation measures provided at the site determine outcome. A major aspect of

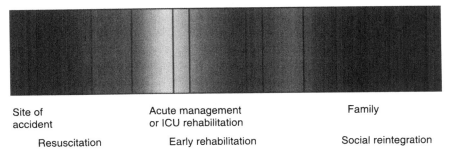

| Site of accident | Acute management or ICU rehabilitation | Family |

| Resuscitation | Early rehabilitation | Social reintegration |

Figure 4.1 Spectrum of neurological–neurosurgical rehabilitation.

the spectrum is emergency admittance to a trauma hospital; the diagnosis, the operating theatre and/or intensive care therapy, where early rehabilitation begins the final reintegration of the patient into society. At the end of that process the reintegration of the person with TBI back into their family, society, and professional life constitutes the ultimate aim of our holistic rehabilitation concept. Targets of neurological–neurosurgical early rehabilitation are defined as follows:

- Verification of rehabilitation potential
- Preservation of the plasticity of the brain
- Support of spontaneous remission
- Avoidance of continuing damage to the brain
- Diagnosis and treatment of secondary complications (e.g. hydrocephalus) and tertiary complications (e.g. contractures).

Epidemiology

When planning services for persons with TBI or SCI, the incidence level should be considered as well as post-traumatic rehabilitation – the data regarding the severity of the primary brain damage and the acute medical management provided to the patient. However, the variety in the collected data and the problems concerning initial assessment and definition of trauma severity is well known and was recently underlined in the report by Murray from the EBIC Survey in Head Injury.[4] The GCS has been accepted throughout the world for classification of TBI as well as the GOS in respect to the final outcome,[1,2] whereas for multi-organ lesions concomitant with TBI, the AIS and ISS have been accepted for scoring.[30–35]

The incidence of TBI in Europe and USA, as in other developed countries, is reported to be about 300/100,000 population/year, which has been confirmed in our previous studies in respect to ICU treatment.[36–39] The incidence of TBI with concomitant organ lesion (polytrauma)[24,38,40] is 70%, which is important in respect to both the functional impairments and secondary, tertiary complications during the phase of early and late rehabilitation.[36] In our survey, TBI mortality in hospitals was 19.2% within the first 10 days and 25.3% within the first month. Bouillon and co-workers reported an overall mortality of 93% in severe isolated TBI with concomitant lesions for polytrauma cases within the first week.[39]

From these figures and our own studies[35] we may calculate the necessity for neurorehabilitation in a total of 55% of all TBI patients admitted to the ICU at an average age of 43 years. The proportion of children up to 10 years of age as well as that of youths up to 18 years of age, was in both cases of our own series only 6.6%. The proportion of patients over 60 years of age was 25% of all cases. In contrast to the figures that have been published some years ago, we did not observe an essentially poorer outcome in polytraumatized patients in respect to the GOS and the FIM [3,41]), as was clearly demonstrated by Erika Ortega Suhrkamp for isolated TBI and HI with concomitant organ lesions after early rehabilitation as reported during the WFNS Conference on neurosurgical rehabilitation in Münster, August 2000.

According to B. Jennett (VS conference, London, 1995), only about 50% of patients vegetative at one month are still vegetative at three months, and a third at six months.

Coma Remission Scale

Early rehabilitation starts when the patient with head injury has been stabilized, is seen to be breathing spontaneously, with an ICP within the normal range, and when the threatening local and/or systemic infections are not complicating the clinical course. In connection with the early rehabilitation phase, the course of rehabilitation can only be adequately recorded with the aid of scales and scores, in which the day's best performance should be defined by the team and assessed.[11,41,42] The Coma Remission Scale (CRS) (see Tables 4.1 and 4.2) which was published in 1993[10] is based on the GCS, and therefore comparable to initial scores. However, two items were added to describe cognitive and neurobehavioral functions and recovery in the early stage when FIM, Barthel and DRS are not applicable.[43]

Patients who have recovered from coma and vegetative status or from the minimal responsive state within an average period of three months can now participate in a regular program of therapy with a discernible learning effect. After the patients have regained a certain degree of independence in their everyday skills enabling them to take care of their personal hygiene and eat and drink without assistance, they may be transferred to special facilities for post-acute or long-term rehabilitation.[44]

In post-acute rehabilitation the patients learn to become more independent, to accommodate functional limitations posed by their impairments by using new strategies (e.g., in TBI compensation of impaired memory, keeping a memory notebook, using preserved reading and writing skills and computerized technology). However, these rehabilitation programs[10,14,23,24] may not be trauma specific compared to the early rehabilitation programs, which

Table 4.1 Coma Remission Scale (CRS) (Voss, von Wild, & Ortega-Suhrkamp, 1993, pp. 112–120)

	Patient name:	
	Date:	
	Investigator (initials):	

1. Arousability/attention (to any stimulus)

Attention span for 1 minute or longer	5	
Attention remains on stimulus (longer than 5 sec)	4	
Turning towards a stimulus	3	
Spontaneous eye opening	2	
Eye opening in response to pain	1	
None	0	

2. Motoric response (minus 6 points from max. attainable sum if tetraplegic)

Spontaneous grasping (also from prone position)	6	
Localized movement in response to pain	5	
Body posture recognizable	4	
Unspecific movement in response to pain (vegetative or spastic pattern)	3	
Flexion in response to pain	2	
Extension in response to pain	1	
None	0	

3. Response to acoustic stimuli (e.g. clicker) (minus 3 points from max. attainable sum if deaf)

Recognizes a well-known voice, music, etc.	3	
Eye opening, turning of head, perhaps smiling	2	
Vegetative reaction (startle)	1	
None	0	

4. Response to visual stimuli (minus 4 points from max. attainable sum if blind)

Recognizes pictures, persons, objects	4	
Follows pictures, persons, objects	3	
Fixates on pictures, persons, objects	2	
Occasional, random eye movements	1	
None	0	

5. Response to tactile stimuli

Recognizes by touching/feeling	3	
Spontaneous, targeted grasping (if blind), albeit without comprehension of sense	2	
Only vegetative response to passive touching	1	
None	0	

6. Auditory response (tracheostoma = 3 if lips can be heard to utter guttural sounds/seen to mime "letters")

At least one understandably articulated word	3	
Unintelligible (unarticulated) sounds	2	
Groaning, screaming, coughing (emotional, vegetatively tinged)	1	
No phonetics/articulation audible/recognizable	0	
Sum score:		
Max. attainable score (of 24) for this patient		

Table 4.2 Coma Remission Scale (CRS) guidance

1. Arousability/attention

5 pts: Patient can direct his/her attention towards an interesting stimulus for at least 1 minute (perceivable by vision, hearing, or touching; stimulus: persons, objects, noises, music, voices, etc.) without being diverted by secondary stimuli.

4 pts: Attention fixed to a stimulus for a discernible moment (fixation with the eyes, grasping, and feeling or "pricking up of ears"); patient is, however, easily diverted or "switches off".

3 pts: Patient turns to source of stimulus by moving eyes, head, or body; patient follows moving objects. Vegetative reactions should also be observed (patient capable only of vegetative reaction).

2 pts: Spontaneous opening of eyes without any external stimulus, e.g. in connection with a sleep–waking state rhythm.

2. Motoric response

6 pts: Patient spontaneously grasps hold of held out everyday objects (only if patient's vision function is intact, otherwise lay object on back of patient's hand) OR patient able to respond to such gestures with an invitational character only with a delay or inconsistently, yet adequately, due to paralysis or contraction.

Note regarding the following items (use of pain stimuli):

The pain stimuli must be applied to the various limbs and to the body trunk, since there may be regional stimulus-perception impairments; pain stimuli can take the form, e.g., of a gentle twisting pinch of a fold of skin, pressure applied to a fingernail fold, tickling of the nose.

5 pts: Patient responds to pain stimuli defensively after localization, by a targeted and adequate measure, e.g., pushing away, sweeping motions of the hand, etc.

4 pts: The patient should be seated upright: tests for the sense of balance and/ or posture by slight pushes applied to the body (corrective movements of trunk or extremities).

3 pts: Untargeted withdrawal from pain stimulus or merely vegetative reactions (tachycardia, tachypnea, agitation) or increase of spastic pattern.

2 pts: Strong, hardly resolvable flexion, especially in the arms/elbows. Legs may stretch out.

1 pt: Typical "decerebrate rigidity" with spastic extension of all extremities, in many cases opisthotonus (dorsal overextension/hyperlordosis).

3. Response to acoustic stimuli (tests as a rule to be carried out beyond patient's field of vision!)

3 pts: Patient can recognize voices or music, i.e., he or she is able either to name the stimulus or to react in a differentiated manner (e.g., to certain pieces of music or persons with pleasure or defensively).

2 pts: Patient only opens eyes, fixates or turns to source of stimulus with his/ her head, in some cases accompanied by emotional expressions such as smiling, crying.

1 pt: Rise in pulse and/or blood pressure, perspiration or agitation, excessive twitching of the body, slight triggering of eye blinking.

Note: Similar to the procedures applied when testing the motor responsiveness by the application of pain stimuli, the use of a clicker held directly next to each of the patient's ears (bilateral testing) suggests itself as the relatively strongest non-pain-involving stimulus for items 1 and 2. If the response is positive, the patient can be assumed to still be in possession of his/her hearing and the stimuli can be made more manifold.

4. Response to visual stimuli (must be presented without speaking or any other form of comment)

4 pts: Patient recognizes pictures, objects, portraits of familiar persons.

3 pts: Follows pictures, etc. with the eyes without any sign of recognition or questioning, inconsistent recognition.

2 pts: Fixates moving pictures or objects without being able to follow them properly, or when picture/object moves outside patient's field of vision patient makes no attempt to keep track.

5. Response to tactile stimuli

3 pts: Patient capable of feeling and recognizing objects, hands of other persons, etc. even if his/her sense of vision is absent and the objects must be placed on the skin/in the hands; adequate response to stimuli in the area of the mouth/face (edible/inedible, e.g. response to a kiss).

2 pts: Touches, feels, and grasps targetedly, but without an adequate reaction.

1 pt: Unspecific response to stroking and touch (vegetative signs such as agitation, raised pulse).

---

6. Auditory response

3 pts: Patient is capable of expressing an intelligible word, even if this is not related to the context or situation. Names also count as words here.

2 pts: Patient utters unintelligible sounds, e.g. slurred, also repetition of syllables or similar ("ma-ma", "au").

Total score: In the event that certain channels of sense or motor systems are completely absent ("blind", "deaf", "plegic"), the point scores of the respective category must be subtracted from the maximum attainable score, e.g. 12/21 points instead of 12/24 points.

---

have to take into account all the early, secondary and tertiary trauma-related complications.

Standards

Some years ago a transdisciplinary neurological–neurosurgical working group was started on early rehabilitation affiliated with the German Ministry of Labour and Social Affairs (Phase II). The task force consists of physicians active in the neurorehabilitation area. We have elaborated certain indicative values and guidelines for the therapeutic area of early rehabilitation and published a quality management paper regarding the structures and process, and the quality of the results that may be anticipated.[11]

Our own post-traumatic early rehabilitation measures at Clemenshospital in connection with our neurosurgical acute care clinic are based on these guidelines, which we first published in 1993.[10] Virtually all new facilities and treatments in Germany are developed on the basis of these guidelines. Critical analysis over the years has shown them to be reliable. Per-patient costs are calculated at €500/patient/day, which corresponds mainly to the number and qualifications of the transdisciplinary personnel (Table 4.3, Figure 4.2) and the diagnostic and therapeutic equipment calculated for a minimum of 20 patients as follows per patient: These disciplines include rehabilitation nursing 1:0.4, physiotherapy and occupational therapy 1:3 each, physical therapy 1:10, speech-language therapy 1:6, cognitive rehabilitation 1:6, music therapy 1:12, electroneurophysiology 1:12, social work 1:12; diet, pharmacy, and religious counselling.

The unit is calculated with a special design (see Table 4.4 and Figures 4.3 and 4.4).

Multidisciplinary team

The objective of early rehabilitation departments is to provide comprehensive rehabilitation treatment to patients (Figure 4.4) on the basis of residual plasticity and regeneration capacities, to preserve and enhance the remaining brain functions or else to elaborate substitute strategies; to recognize and pre-

Table 4.3 The multidisciplinary neurorehabilitation team (20 beds)

- 1 medical director (neurosurgeon/neurologist)
- 2 consultants (neurosurgeon/ neurologist)
- 4 interns
- 2 neuropsychologists
- 1 speech therapist
- 1 music therapist
- 1 social worker
- 1 technical assistant
- 6 physiotherapists
- 6 occupational therapists
- 1 masseuse, 1 masseur
- 1 secretary

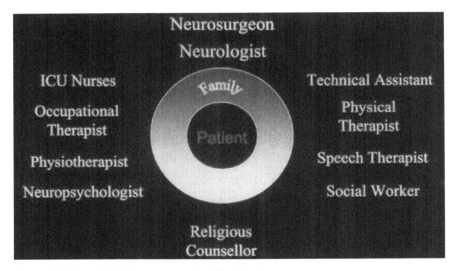

Figure 4.2 Interdisciplinary neurorehabilitation team.

Table 4.4 Design of an early neurorehabilitation unit

- 20 beds (1 and 2 bedrooms), neurosurgical and intensive care monitoring
- 1300–1500 m^2 area
- All patient rooms, medical care, nursing staff, diagnostic and therapeutic facilities on the same floor (see Figures 4.3, 4.4)
- Medical consultant service available within 30 min, 24 h/day
- Permanent X-ray and laboratory service nearby

vent secondary and tertiary damage, i.e., treat such damage in a transdisciplinary, multidisciplinary manner (hydrocephalus, subdural effusions, cerebral abscess, CSF fistulae, sinus-cavernous fistulae, plastic skull reconstruction as well as heterotopic ossifications, decubitis ulcers, and venous thromboses);

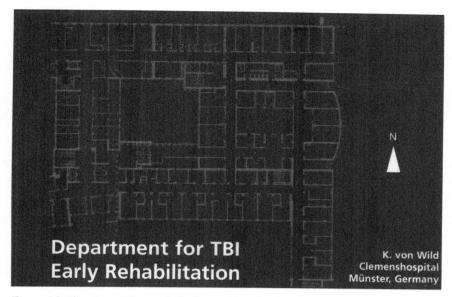

Figure 4.3 Site plan of the newly built special unit related to the central staircase and elevators (left) and X-ray department (top). The ward is connected to the central therapeutic area by two short accesses.

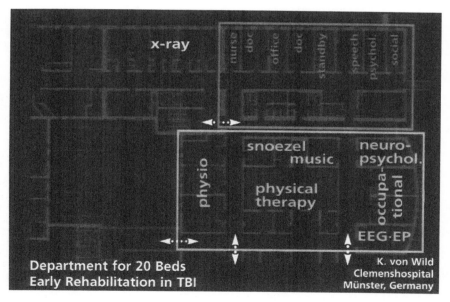

Figure 4.4 Design of the unit for early neurorehabilitation for the TBI neurosurgical department, Clemenshospital.

and also to intervene in the event of contractures, e.g., with botulinum toxin Type A (Botox®, Merz und Co. Frankfurt, Dyport®, Ipsen-Pharma, Ettlingen). Appropriate treatment and therapy should commence as early as possible depending upon the condition and needs of the individual patient. Central respiratory and swallowing disorders are typical in the comatose, severely cognitively handicapped patients and in patients in the vegetative state; aspects that demand special diagnostic and therapeutic techniques and procedures. These complications require a multidisciplinary team.

Admission to our early rehabilitation unit was possible in 27% of patients within 10 days and three-quarters within 20 days respectively after the traumatic impact. The initial GCS of these patients admitted for the last 5 years is listed in Table 4.5.

The early outcome of our 327 patients at time of referral for further treatment is listed in Figure 4.5.

The GOS of our patients changed during the follow-up period of more than 6 months (mean 30 months) in all groups with late improvement over time, independent of the age of the patients (Figure 4.6).

Table 4.5 Initial GCS of 327 patients after TBI, admitted to the early rehabilitation unit

GCS	3–8	$n = 205$ (63%)
GCS	9–12	$n = 78$ (24%)
GCS	13–15	$n = 44$ (13%)

All patients were treated according to the standardized protocol.

One-quarter of patients were < 30 and one-third were > 60 years

GCS	N	GOS 1	GOS 2	GOS 3	GOS 4	GOS 5
3	57	6	19	30	0	2
4	10	0	0	8	1	1
5	53	2	0	34	14	3
6	21	1	0	12	5	3
7	31	0	0	12	12	7
8	33	1	0	17	10	5
9	22	0	0	10	8	4
10	16	0	1	5	7	3
11	12	1	0	3	4	4
12	28	0	0	9	7	12
13	22	1	0	3	8	10
14	1	0	0	0	0	1
15	21	0	0	4	6	11
Gesamt	327	12	20	147	82	66

Figure 4.5 Early outcome on 327 patients with TBI. Comparison of initial DGC and GOS at the end of early rehabilitation (mean stay, 46 days).

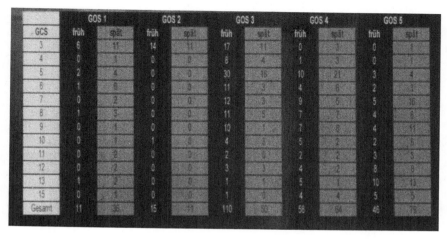

Figure 4.6 Comparison of the early and late outcome after early rehabilitation (GOS) with the initial GCS at the time after the impact.

Technology and quality of life

The technological advances in neurosurgery and neurointensive care along with advances that have been made in the areas of microelectronic, computer technology and telecommunication, plus the availability of neuromodulation and implants, have no less than revolutionized neurotraumatological diagnosis and therapy throughout the second half of this century. Neurosurgeons and neurologists have reacted accordingly by founding special task forces – like the novel rehabilitation committee of the World Federation of Neurological Surgeons. Therefore, we are focussing our interest on epidemiological data, education and training on the one hand, and on quality management procedures with randomized controlled studies and analyses of daily practice on the other.

However, the term *quality of life* in respect to final outcome after rehabilitation for persons with TBI is just being defined, with working groups from the Euroacademia Multidisciplinaria Neurotraumatologica (EMN), with support from the National Brain Injury Research, Treatment and Training Foundation (NBIRTT) in the USA. Under the chairmanship of Edmund Neugebauer from Cologne (International Task Force on QoL 1999)[45] and Professor Jean-Luc Truelle from France, a new Quality of Life Tool in TBI is being developed. When looked at from this new point of view, it seems logical – indeed even imperative – for neurosurgeons to intensely devote our attention to aspects of post-traumatic neurorehabilitation now that patients survive their brain damage and spinal cord lesions, due to the increasing progress that has been attained.

Today there are a number of possibilities for surgical treatment that complement neurorehabilitation concepts and these shed light on new paths in functional rehabilitation: for example, non-destructive interventions and neuromodulation to arouse patients in persistent coma or, respectively, stimulating patients with vegetative syndrome (VS) to voluntary attention and, in the case of central motor disorders, facilitating self-supplied impulses by implanting indwelling electrodes. Also, concepts for stimulation by neuromodulation in connection with central-nervous and peripheral nerve lesions and the functional neurosurgical treatment of therapy-resistant spasticity in connection with pain therapy are becoming more and more integral part of neurorehabilitation.

Particular emphasis here is attached to the implantation of neuronal networks and stimulation systems (e.g., Stand Up And Walk – a project by Pierre Rabischong and co-workers to enable walking in spinal cord transsection D10). However, in respect to the high frequency of complications during the early phase, it is still more important to eliminate secondary and tertiary complications such as CSF fistulae, hydrocephalus, cranioplasty, and plastic-reconstructive interventions.

Both conceptually and structurally, early rehabilitation measures should accompany acute therapy from very early on in the care of the patient in the ICU once the vegetative functions have been stabilized and the intracranial pressure has normalized. In this regard there are a number of models undergoing clinical tests for adults and children. In a responsible and integrated manner, the neurosurgeon leads the interdisciplinary rehabilitation team, coordinates the multidisciplinary conciliatory treatment of other medical departments and directly assists in the transdisciplinary implementation of the complex rehabilitation concept that has been established for the individual patient right up to the time that he or she is transferred to community rehabilitation. In this late phase of rehabilitation, the neurosurgeon should play an active role. In the *neurorehabilitation spectrum*, the neurosurgeon today plays an ever more important role, including the establishment and management of the corresponding medical departments and clinics for neurorehabilitation.

Perspectives

While continuing our efforts in the area of brain trauma research at the end of the "Decade of the Brain," we must still rely on the classical strategies of neurological rehabilitation in the form of prevention, diagnosis and treatment of secondary and tertiary damage, as well as for other complications or sequelae. There is much need for an evidence-based, post-traumatic rehabilitation strategy that is reliable, validated, and culturally sensitive. We believe that the spectrum of neurorehabilitation is a challenge for every neurosurgeon and neurologist who is interested in plasticity, regeneration and restoration after brain and spinal cord damage in order to reduce the handicap and to enable patients to go back to their family and friends with as independent a social and vocational life as possible.

Concluding remarks

This brief synopsis makes it clear why guidelines for a standardized neurotraumatological rehabilitation concept in patients with head injury are needed. However, recent results are promising for continuing with carefully designed, prospective and randomized controlled clinical studies to fulfill the criteria of evidence-based medicine in the future. This will be a challenging task for both the neurotraumatology committee and the WFNS novel committee on neurorehabilitation at the beginning of this millennium.

References

1. American Association of Neurological Surgeons and Brain Trauma Foundation (1995). *Guidelines for the management of severe head injury.* New York: Brain Trauma Foundation.
2. Teasdale, G., & Jennett, B. (1974). Assessment of coma and impaired consciousness. A practical scale. *Lancet, 2*, 81–85.
3. Jennett, B., & Bond, M. (1975). Assessment of outcome after severe head injury. *Lancet, 1*, 480–484.
4. Murray, G. D., et al. (1999). The European brain injury consortium survey of head injuries. *Acta Neurochir. (Wien), 141*, 223–236.
5. Narayan, R. K., Wilberger, J. E. Jr, & Povlishock, J. T. (1996). *Neurotrauma.* New York: McGraw-Hill.
6. Freund, H. J., Sabel, B. A., & Witte, O. W. (. . .). Brain plasticity. *Adv. Neurol., 73*, 1–1408.
7. Stein, D. G., Brailowsky, S., & Will, B. (1995). *Brain repair.* New York: Oxford University Press.
8. Stein, D. G. (1993). Brain injury and theories of recovery. In L. B. Goldstein (Ed.), *Restorative neurology: Advances in pharmacotherapy of recovery after stroke* (pp. 1–34). Armong, NY: Futura.
9. von Wild, K., & Janzik, H. H. (Eds.) (1990). *Neurologische Frührehabilitation.* München, Bern, Wien, San Francisco, CA: Zuckschwerdt-Verlag.
10. Voss, A., von Wild, K., Ortega-Suhrkamp, E., & the German Task Force on Early Neurorehabilitation (1993). Standards der neurologisch–neurochirurgischen Frührehabilitation. Ein Konzept der Arbeitsgemeinschaft Neurologische–Neurochirurgische Frührehabilitation. In K. von Wild (Ed.), *Spektrum Neuro-rehabilitatation* (pp. 112–120). München, Bern, Wien, New York: W. Zuckschwerdt-Verlag.
11. Voss, A., von Wild, K. R. H., & Prosiegel M. (Eds.) (1999). *Qualitätsmanagement in neurologischer und neurochirurgischer Frührehabilitation.* München, Bern, Wien, New York: Zuckschwerdt-Verlag.
12. Chesnut, M. R. (1997). Guidelines for the management of severe head injury: what we know and what we think we know. *J. Trauma, 5*, 19.
13. von Wild, K. (Ed.) (1993). *Spektrum der Neurorehabilitation.* München, Bern, Wien, New York: W. Zuckschwerdt-Verlag.
14. Kemper, B., & von Wild, K. R. H. (1999). Neuropsychologische Aspekte in der Frührehabilitation schädelhirnverletzter Patienten. In P. Frommelt and H. Grötzbach (Eds.), *Neurorehabilitation* (pp. 434–439). Berlin, Wien: Blackwell Wissenschaftsverlag.

15. Walshe, T. M. (1997). Neurological concepts in archaic Greece: what did Homer know? *J. Hist. Neurosci., 6*, 72–81.
16. Goldstein, K. (1919). *Die Behandlung, Fürsorge und Begutachtung der Hirnverletzten* (p. 82). Leipzig: F. C. W. Vogel.
17. Tönnis, W. (1942). *Richtlinien für die Behandlung der Schussverletzungen des Gehirns und die Beurteilung ihrer Folgezustände.* München: J. F. Lehmanns.
18. Bothe, H. W., & Engel, M. (1998). *Neurobionik: Medizin mit mikroelektronischen Implanten.* Frankfurt: Umschan.
19. Foerster, O. (1916). Therapie der Motilitätsstörungen bei den Erkrankungen des zentralen Nervensystems. In H. Vogt (Ed.), *Handbuch der Therapie der Nervenkrankheiten (vol. 2), Symptomatische Therapie und Therapie der Organneurosen. Krankheitsbilder und deren Behandlung* (pp. 860–940). Jena: Fischer.
20. Foerster, O. (1936). Übungstherapie. In O. Bumke and O. Foerster (Eds.), *Handbuch der Neurologie* (vol. 8, pp. 316–414). Berlin: Springer.
21. Luria, A. R. (1963). *Restoration of function after brain injury.* Oxford: Pergamon.
22. Luria, A. R. (1980). *Higher cortical functions in man* (2nd ed.). New York: Basic Books.
23. Christensen, A. L. (1984). *Luria's neuropsychological investigation.* Copenhagen: Munsgaard.
24. Christensen, A. L. (1996). Is there a need for psychological interventions in primary care? In H. E. Diemath, J. Sommerauer and K. R. H. von Wild (Eds.), *Brain protection in severe head injury* (pp. 160–161). München, Bern, Wien, New York: Zuckswerdt-Verlag.
25. Christensen, A. L., & Caetono, C. (1996). Alexandr Romanovich Luria (1902–1907): Contributions to neuropsychological rehabilitation. *Neuropsychol. Rehab., 6*, 279–303.
26. Christensen, A. L., & Uzzel, B. P. (Eds.). (2000). *International handbook of neuropsychological rehabilitation.* New York, Boston, Dordrecht, London, Moscow: Kluwer Academic/Plenum.
27. Goldstein, K. (1934). *Der Aufbau des Organismus.* Den Haag: Nijhoff.
28. Goldstein, K. (1942). *After-effects of brain injury in war.* London: Heinemann.
29. von Wild, K., & Janzik, H. H. (1993). Zur Begriffsbestimmung: Neurologisch–neurochirurgische Frührehabilitation. In K. von Wild (Ed.), *Spektrum der Neurorehabilitation.* München, Bern, Wien, San Francisco: Zuckschwerdt-Verlag.
30. Greenspan L. B., McLellan A., & Greig H. (1985). Abbreviated injury scale and injury severity score: a scoring chart. *J. Trauma, 25*(1), 60–64.
31. Baker, S. P., O'Neill, B., Haddon, W., et al. (1974). The injury severity score. a method for describing patients with multiple injuries and evaluating emergency care. *J. Trauma, 14*, 187–196.
32. Baker, S. P., O'Neill, P., Haddon, W., et al. (1994). The Injury Severity Score: a method of describing patients with multiple injuries and evaluating emergency care. *J. Trauma, 15*, 187.
33. Champion, H. R., Sacco, W. J., Copes, W. S., et al. (1989). A revision of trauma score. *J. Trauma, 29*, 632.
34. Regel, G., Pape, H. C., Pohlemann, T., et al. (1994). Score systems – an instrument of decision making in trauma care. *Unfallchirurgie, 97*, 211.
35. Oestern, H. J., & Kabus, K. (1997). Comparison of different trauma scoring systems. A review. *Unfallchirurgie, 97*, 177.
36. Janzik, H. H., von Wild, K., & Hömberg, V. (December 1992) (. . .) Gutachten zur

Versorgung von Patienten mit schweren Schädel-Hirn-Verletzungen in Nordrhein-Westfälischen Krankenhäusern. Gutachten zu den Standards der neurologischen Rehabilitation unter besonderer Berücksichtigung der Frührehabilitation und der Nachsorge und Verwirklichungsmöglichkeiten im bestehenden Versicherungssystem Ministerium für Arbeit, Gesundheit und Soziales des Landes Nordrhein-Westfalen Ahlen: Partner Druck.

37. Mayer, K., & Wiechers, R. (1993). Zur Epidemiologie der Hirnverletzungen und Hirngefässerkrankungen. In K. von Wild (Ed.). *Sprektrum der Neurorehabilitation* (pp. 87–93). München, Bern, Wien, New York: W. Zuckschwerdt-Verlag.

38. Durkin, M. S., Olsen, S., Barlow, B., et al. (1998). The epidemiology of urban pediatric neurological trauma: evaluation of, and implications for, injury prevention programs. *Neurosurgery, 42*, 300–310.

39. Bouillon, B., Raum, M., Fach, H., et al. (1999). The incidence and outcome of severe brain trauma. Design and first results of an epidemiological study in an urban area. *Restor. Neurol. Neurosci., 14*, 85–89.

40. Kwasny, O., Kemtzhofer, P., Fialka, C., & Nau, T. (1999). Guidelines of prehospital care of patients with severe head injury. *Acta Chir. Austriaca, 31*, 27.

41. Granger, C., Hamilton, B., Sherwin, F. (1986). Guide for use of uniform data set for medical rehabilitation. Buffalo, NY: Buffalo General Hospital.

42. Zasler, N. D., & Horn, L. J., (Eds.). (1995). *Medical rehabilitation of traumatic brain injury*. Philadelphia, PA: Hanley Belfus.

43. Schönle, P. (1996). Frühe Phasen der neurologischen Rehabilitation: Differentielle Schweregradbeurteilung bei Patienten in der Phase B (Frührehabilitation) und in der Phase C (Frühmobilisation/Postprimäre Rehabilitation) mit Hilfe des Frühreha-Barthel-Index (FRB). *Neurol. Rehabil., 1*, 21–25.

44. Berger, E., Leven, F., Pirente, N., et al. (1999). Quality of life after traumatic brain injury: a systematic review of the literature. *Restor. Neurol. Neurosci., 14*, 93–102.

45. von Wild, K. R. H., & Diemath H. E. Euroacademy of Multidisciplinary Neurotraumatology (EMN) – A better chance for head injured patients in the third millennium. *Acta Chir. Austriaca, 31*, 5.

5   Electrical treatment of coma

Experience in the eastern USA and central Japan

Edwin Cooper and Tetsuo Kanno

Introduction

In the third millennium, the useful applications of electricity abound. So accustomed are we to multitasking that we talk on a cell phone while reading e-mail for the few minutes a frozen steak is thawing in a microwave, all interrupted by a beeper . . . The electronic extensions of our brain and body have stretched our abilities which are driven by internal electrochemical reactions. The complicated but finite digital real world processing of information has retrained our infinite minds. No longer do we plan and work in a linear sequence. The cerebrum mimics computer brains. We think in parallel circuits while racing forward and backward to amplify the truth that emerges. But just as sophisticated modern computers can crash and lose data, the human brain can be seriously injured, electrically and structurally, by trauma. Brain trauma in the third millennium comes in two species: (1) blunt head injury from motor vehicle collisions; (2) penetrating trauma from civilian gunshot wounds.

Neurological salvage is more predictable and more successful in diffuse brain injury resulting from a collision. Usually there is more structural damage when the injury is caused by the violent penetration of a missile.

Just as electricity has been our servant and instructor in the daily world, electrical stimulation can be our rescuer in the post-traumatic coma world.

There exists a certain pessimism regarding the treatment of severe closed head injuries. Physicians are reluctant to offer much hope to the families of the acutely comatose brain injured victim. The patients are often teenagers, inexperienced drivers involved in high speed collisions. Usually there are multisystem injuries that add to the seriousness of the condition.

But deep coma, with sluggish pupils, and abnormal motor responses governed by the brainstem, does not universally indicate a poor outcome. Clinical and computerized tomography (CT) findings have been used to predict outcome. With the advent of intracranial pressure monitoring, and regulation of the elevated pressure by diuresis and chemically induced coma, serial Glasgow Coma Scale (GCS) scores may not be reliable prognosticators in the first few days of coma. In the absence of severe anatomical damage on the initial and follow-up CT scans, but in the presence of cerebral edema, a favorable recovery may still be possible for the patient.

This chapter will present traditional measures of prognosis and standard treatments for closed head injury and a discussion of the anticipated outcomes. This will be followed by a presentation of a novel treatment of coma, electrical stimulation.

Implanted electrical stimulation of the dorsal column cervical spinal cord has been used for over a decade, mainly in Japan, to treat the persistent vegetative state. In the USA superficial electrical stimulation of the right median nerve has been used for the treatment of acute post-traumatic coma since the early 1990s.[1]

History of electrical stimulation

Electricity's potent physiological effects have been recognized for most of recorded history. Almost 2000 years ago, 40–100 AD, the Romans and Greeks adopted electric therapy. The torpedo fish, an electric ray, was applied to patients complaining of headache, hemorrhoids, gout, depression, and epilepsy.[2] In the mid-1800s, an English surgeon, John Birch, reported the use of electrical stimulation to treat a patient with a hand injury for the purpose of restoring function and decreasing pain.[3]

The medical advent of neurostimulation in pain control can be attributed to the work of Melzack and Wall in 1965.[4] Stimulation as a means of muscular control and improving function has been researched through the past three decades by Cooper, Hildebrandt, Keith, Kralj, Marsolais, Mortimer, Peckham, Petrofsky, Salmons and Verbova, Vdovink, and others. Most of the research has focused on the clinical and functional applications of electrical stimulation for the control of the paralyzed muscles of persons who are quadriplegic or paraplegic, and stroke victims.

Functional electrical stimulation has been used to assist paraplegic patients in walking.[5] Much research has been devoted to restoring basic functions to the quadriplegic hand. Grasping objects under computer control has been developed by Peckham, Mortimer, Marsolais, Cooper, McElhaney, and Han.[6] In the treatment of motor neuron deficits, electrical stimulation is used to mimic cerebral control of muscle fibers.

Implanted or transcutaneous electrodes transfer current to local tissues that is communicated through the axons of nerves. The action potential begins when the plasma membrane of the axon allows passage of certain ions. The ions diffuse along concentration gradients, electrically induced currents flow in complete circuits, and a capacitive current is established.[7] Once a capacitive current is established in the axon of a nerve, an action potential indifferentiable from those initiated by physiological mechanisms is propagated.[8] The resultant potential travels down the axon independent of the electrical stimulation.

When the action potential reaches the neuromuscular junction, acetylcholine streams across the cleft interacting with receptors on the muscle end-plate. The signal is transduced into the muscle fibers through the T-tubules, Ca^{2+} is sequestered from the sarcoplasmic reticulum, the actin/troponin/tropomyosin complex is activated, and the muscle contracts. The amplitude and pulse width of the current must be sufficient to exceed the threshold of excitability.[9]

Electrical stimulation induces changes in levels of neurotransmitters, some neural hormones, and cerebral blood flow. Direct stimulation of the nucleus raphe dorsalis was shown to reduce nociception through increased release of serotonin.[10] Pain reducing stimulation often involves chronic stimulation of the spinal cord in conjunction with narcotic treatment. Stimulation of the thalamus, periventricular gray, and the nucleus raphe dorsalis of the brain have been shown to successfully produce results in pain management.[10]

An increase in neurotransmitter release has been hypothesized to mitigate the improvement of patients with Alzheimer's type dementia undergoing transcutaneous electrical stimulation.[11]

Significant increases in norepinephrine and dopamine in the cerebrospinal fluid and increases in cerebral blood flow have been observed in comatose individuals receiving dorsal column electrical stimulation.[12]

Electrical stimulation techniques

Two contraindications to the use of transcutaneous electrical stimulation have been stated by the Federal Food and Drug Administration.[13] Transcutaneous electrical nerve stimulation (TENS) should not be used for patients with a demand cardiac pacemaker, nor should it be applied over the carotid sinus. Special precaution should be taken with patients and young children with cognitive dysfunction.[7]

Possible adverse reactions to transcutaneous stimulation are infrequent but could include skin irritation from the electrical reaction or allergic reactions to the electrodes, the lubricant, the tape, or the mechanical irritation of the electrodes. Close monitoring is needed for the skin and denervated areas where the patient would not feel the electrical stimulation. Burns could occur if the current density is too high under the electrode.[8] Electrical stimulation over an electrical implant including pacemakers and defibrillators could interfere with the function of those devices. However, electrical stimulation at an area away from the implant could be done safely.[14]

The safety of TENS during pregnancy has not been established. It was stated by Nelson et al.: "Effects on patients with cerebral vascular accidents, transit ischemic attacks, epilepsy, and seizure disorders, or stimulation on the head or upper cervical regions, are not well established thus close monitoring is required."[14]

The manual for the Focus® electrical stimulator (Empi, Inc., St. Paul, Minnesota) stated that neuromuscular electrical stimulation (NMES) is contraindicated for use in patients with implanted demand-type cardiac pacemakers or defibrillators.[15] They also suggest caution when stimulating patients with a history of heart disease or epilepsy. NMES should be applied with caution to patients with cardiac conditions such as arrhythmia or conduction disturbances.[7] Empi also listed contraindicated locations as placement over the carotid sinus region of the neck, transcerebral placement and transthoracic locations.

Electrotherapy for enhancing neuromuscular performance has greatly increased over the past 20 years in the USA.[14] Prior to the mid-1970s electrical stimulation was used mainly to treat atrophy in skeletal muscles. NMES on the skin over a motor point of the muscle produces active potential in the muscle or nerve fiber identical to the potential generated by a nerve. The evoked potential travels in both directions along the nerve fiber from the site. NMES involves stimulating peripheral nerves with a mixture of motor and sensory fibers.

For patients who were unable to contract a specific muscle, NMES activates the muscle and may help with muscle re-education. However, motor units must be intact for this to be useful. Spasticity may be reduced by applying the NMES alternately to the spastic agonist muscle and the antagonist and the combined effect may give reciprocal inhibition, muscle fatigue, and therefore help reduce the spasticity. However, the effectiveness of NMES in the treatment of spasticity is unpredictable.[14,16]

NMES has been approved by the FDA as safe and effective for treatment of disuse atrophy, increasing the maintenance of range of motion and muscle re-education and facilitation.[7,17] Other areas of use include spasticity reduction or orthotic substitution and augmentation of motor recruitment.[7]

The asymmetrical biphasic square waves are suitable for smaller muscles. The symmetric biphasic pulse is for large muscle groups. The duration of 0.3 milliseconds (ms) (300 microseconds, μs) is for muscle stimulation.[7] The frequency in the range of 10–20 pulses/s causes a sensation of vibration or incomplete tetany. Above 30 pulses/s, the muscle contractions become fused (tetanic) so that a smooth contraction is produced.[7]

The amount of resistance (impedance) for dry skin is in the range of 500,000 ohms (Ω) and 1000 Ω for wet skin. For our projects we have considered the resistance of the skin under the lubricated electrodes to have an impedance of 1000 Ω.[1]

Various duty cycles are used for balancing the on time and the off time to prevent fatigue. A 1:5 ratio of on:off is recommended for the initiation of an NMES program.[7] For nerve stimulation of coma patients a 1:2 cycle of 20 s on:40 or 50 s off has proved useful for the last decade.[1,18] Up to 100 milliamps (mA) of surface stimulation have been used for stimulation of the quadriceps in paraplegics.[8] Much lower levels are used when the stimulation is over the skin at the wrist.

For median nerve stimulation, the range of 10–20 mA has been used as tolerated in the University of Virginia and East Carolina University studies.[1,18] The delivered dose to the nerve would be measured in μA. In working with stroke patients, with shoulder subluxation, amplitudes of 30–35 mA have been used for muscle strengthening.[7]

Electrical current that is transported through a biological conductive medium causes three effects: electrochemical, electrophysical, and electro-thermal. The electrophysical effect could also be termed electrokinetic.[14] Sodium and potassium ions move across the semipermeable cell membrane (of the muscle) producing the action potential which results in the contraction of the skeletal muscle. With peripheral nerve stimulation, afferent stimulation of the sensory nerves to the spinal cord, brainstem, thalamus and cerebrum occurs.

Surface, as opposed to implanted, electrodes are used for the acute coma stimulation for the ease of application, economy, and noninvasive features. Higher currents are required from the stimulator for transcutaneous stimulation than for implanted devices.

Smaller width, smaller duration pulses can be tolerated at relatively higher amplitudes than longer-duration pulses.[14] At the 200 μs width of pulse, sensation is noted around 10 mA, motor function at 20 mA or less, and pain at 30–40 mA.[1,14]

Neural excitability comes from voltage-gated ionic channels within the semipermeable membranes. At the resting threshold of −40 to −60 millivolts (mV), the channels open to allow a quick flow of sodium ions inward thus reversing the membrane potential to +20 to +30 mV. There is also an outflow of potassium ions after that restoring the potential back to the resting level. This rapid sequence is called the action potential and is propagated along the neural membrane.

Monophasic pulses are preferred when the responses need to be accurately quantified. These pulses can be electrically differentiated to retard fatigue. Most physiological studies are done with constant-current electrical stimulators that supply a pulse of constant intensity.[14] This is important as the impedance of the skin may vary, depending on sweating and the amount of lubrication.

Incidence of traumatic brain injury

Traumatic brain injury (TBI) is caused by vehicular crashes, falls, violence, and sports injuries. TBI is twice as frequent in males than in females. The estimated incidence is 100/1000 persons, with 52,000 annual deaths.[19] The highest incidence is among persons aged 15–24 years. There are also peaks in the very young and the elderly. TBI may result in lifelong impairment of physical, cognitive, and psychosocial functions. The prevalence in the USA is estimated to be 2.5 million to 6.5 million individuals.

About 2 million persons/year have a traumatic brain injury. The number of survivors has increased significantly in recent years secondary to fast and more effective emergency care, more rapid transportation to specialized treatment centers and advances in acute management. But up to 90,000 persons incur a TBI resulting in lifelong impairments: reduced physical, cognitive, and emotional functions. TBI may result in physical impairment. But the more serious consequences involve the person's cognition, emotional function and behavior.[19]

The evolution of electrical stimulation for TBI

In Japan and in the USA in the 1980s, parallel observations were made by unrelated observers, Tetsuo Kanno and Ed Cooper. These revelations led to the concept of electrical stimulation for the treatment of comatose states, chronic and acute.

Kanno was using dorsal column stimulation (DCS) for the relief of spasticity.[12] Near the same time, Cooper was using right forearm stimulation (involving the median nerve and the flexor muscles) to try to decrease right arm spasticity in a young man with spastic quadriplegia. The man was residing at Caswell Center in Kinston, North Carolina's largest facility for persons with mental/motor delays. Both Kanno and Cooper separately observed increased levels of consciousness in their patients who were given electrical stimulation for the purpose of decreasing spasticity.[12,20] Almost two decades ago, this important observation led both physicians to research electrical stimulation for the purpose of central nervous system arousal.

A second parallel observation was made by researchers in the USA and Japan: brief periods of median nerve stimulation led to temporary although slight increases in awareness of comatose patients. This was noted in both countries during median nerve stimulation for sensory evoked potentials.[21,22]

Cooper also noted gradual improvement in mental function in a semi-vegetative 52-year-old male physician who had suffered a brain injury and stroke as a result of head trauma in 1987. After treatment, he was noted to have no rehabilitation potential. This patient was transferred to Duke University Medical Center (Durham, NC) nine months after the onset of severe coma followed by a semi-vegetative state. At Duke, with control of pain and electrical stimulation of his right forearm and both quadriceps, he gradually regained the abilities to walk, talk, and operate his computer and to live at home with his wife.

Experience in Japan with electrical stimulation for coma

In Japan, Kanno's keen observations led him to become the world pioneer for dorsal column stimulation for patients in the persistent vegetative state after head injury, stroke, hypoxia, and other neurologic etiologies.[23] Cooper et al.'s observations in the USA of increased awareness after peripheral nerve stimulation evolved into the coma stimulation projects at East Carolina University in (Greenville, NC, 1992 through the present) and the University of Virginia (Charlottesville VA, 1994–1995, 1998–1999).[1,18] This chapter will describe the goals, methods and theories of the techniques of dorsal column stimulation

(DCS) for persistent vegetative state (PVS) and right median nerve electrical stimulation (RMNS) for treatment of acute coma.

Kanno et al. in Japan observed that it is clear that neurosurgeons must be familiar with the morbid conditions and therapeutic modalities related to prolonged coma: the persistent vegetative state.[23] He observed that although diagnostic instruments and methods of treatment have improved, patients with prolonged coma are still found in most hospital wards. Unfortunately, no special modality of treatment has yet been established, and the condition is being left to follow a natural course. On the other hand, the social climate is increasingly focused on the importance of quality of life, which is naturally problematic in patients with prolonged coma, who are confined to bed without effective treatment.[23]

Dorsal column stimulation for the persistent vegetative state

At the first annual meeting of the Society for Treatment of Coma (held in Kyoto in 1992) Kanno, Kamei and Yokoyama at the Department of Neurosurgery, Fujita Health University, School of Medicine, Toyoake, Japan, reported on their experience for the previous 8 years with dorsal column stimulation. Of 42 cases treated, 18 (42.9%) showed clinical improvement. This was much higher than expected in the incidence of natural recovery.[23]

Previously, dorsal column stimulation was known to be effective for treatment of pain and spasticity. Improvement in the level of activity and also improvement on the electroencephalogram (EEG) was observed in some patients who were treated with DCS for spasticity and cerebral vascular diseases. This led to the use of DCS for treatment of the persistent vegetative state (PVS). Of the 42 patients, 23 were cases of PVS secondary to trauma, 11 were due to cerebrovascular disease, seven to hypoxia and one was a complication of surgery for a brain tumor. Twenty-five patients (60%) were under the age of 30.[23]

The clinical conditions that satisfied the definition of the vegetative state include inability to recognize and/or communicate, inability to move or eat, and loss of bowel and bladder control for a minimum period of 3 months. In their study, the patients had been in a morbid condition for 3–78 months (an average of 19.2 months) before DCS therapy was commenced. Before and during DCS therapy, 37 patients were studied for changes in rCBF (regional cerebral blood flow) using SPECT (single photon emission computerized tomography), and electroencephalography (EEG) in all 42 cases.

The rCBF was increased by DCS therapy in 22/37 cases. The EEG improved in 23/42 cases. They found that the original disease in the improved group was head trauma in 72.2% of the cases. PVS due to vascular or hypoxic injury rarely improved with DCS. On average, 89.9% of the improved patients were under the age of 30, but patients over the age of 50 did not show any improvement by DCS therapy.

These data show a general trend that computerized tomography (CT) in the improved cases shows no marked cerebral atrophy, no large low density area and no involvement of thalamus.

There was good clinical improvement in 18/42 cases. None of the patients showed a return to normal functioning such as being able to walk, but the patients with a good outcome were able to have some communication with the outside world and/or express some emotion. The interval from the start of DCS therapy to the first sign of improvement is variable (6 months to 5 years). Therefore, the effectiveness of therapy may not be able to be evaluated for some time. Based on their results, the indications for DCS therapy for patients in a vegetative state are as follows:

1   Young age.
2   Head trauma.
3   Coma for over 3 months, without improvement by medical treatment.
4   Head CT does not show signs of severe damage.

After marked cerebral atrophy has occurred, it appears that DCS therapy is not effective.

The mechanism of action of DCS is not clear but, as already reported: DCS increases rCBF, enhances catecholamine metabolism, and improves EEG. The increase in rCBF appears in all parts of the brain. The rCBF in the cerebral cortex and brainstem in cases of vegetative coma is usually 10–25 ml/min/100 gm, which is markedly low compared with controls. After DCS therapy, rCBF increases by 10–20% in most areas. The same phenomenon was also observed in the experimental model. It appears that DCS enhances the metabolism of catecholamine in the central nervous system.[23]

The improvement in the EEG tracing was usually bilateral, dominant on the unaffected side, and characterized by alpha-waves tending to increase. However, improvement in the EEG probably was followed by improvement of the clinical status. DCS enhances catecholamine metabolism and increases rCBF. This resulted in EEG and clinical improvement.[23]

By July 2000, Kanno's group had treated 131 dorsal column stimulation cases (65 in coma from trauma, 28 from hypoxic cerebropathy, 25 from cerebrovascular accidents, 3 from brain tumors; other causes, 10 cases). The mean age was 33 years. The percentage of favorable outcome was the same 43% as had been observed earlier. In cases that were under 35 years of age, there was clinical improvement in 58% of the cases.

Kanno at the University of Virginia

In June 1995, Tetsuo Kanno was the visiting professor at John Jane's Department of Neurosurgery at the University of Virginia in Charlottesville. Kanno gave a lecture on an expanded series of patients in the persistent vegetative state that had been treated by dorsal column stimulation. He explained in detail the physiological mechanisms of the electrical stimulation.

In the discussion, John Jane asked if the targets in the thalamus reached by dorsal column stimulation and by peripheral nerve stimulation were the same. Kanno concluded that they were the same.[24]

University of Virginia series presented in Japan

One year later in Sendai, Japan, at the Fifth Annual Meeting for the Society for Treatment of Coma (August 1996), Cooper presented the results of the first series of six acutely comatose patients treated at the University of Virginia (1994–1995). Kanno stated: "This was the very first lecture regarding median nerve stimulation in Japan."

In that UVa series, three patients were treated with right median nerve electrical stimulation and three were given sham stimulation.[25] All patients were in coma after acute closed head injury. All acute brain injury patients were screened by the neuroclinical nurses. Admission criteria included acute traumatic brain injury and Glasgow Coma Scale (GCS) 4–8 after resuscitation. Patients with severe cardiac arrhythmia, pacemakers, implanted defibrillators, uncontrolled seizures, cerebral palsy, mental retardation, or pregnancy were excluded. The neurological exclusions were spinal cord, brachial plexus or right median nerve injury. Patients were randomly assigned to the electrical stimulation or the sham stimulation group.

Battery powered Respond Select® (Empi) electrical neuromuscular stimulators were connected by lead wires to a pair of 2.5 × 2.5 cm rubber electrodes in a plastic orthosis cuff applied onto the right wrist over the median nerve. Electrical stimulation was performed at 40 pulses/s (300 μs duration) at approximately 20 mA, 20 s on and 40 s off for 8 h/day for a period of 2 weeks. Stimulation was discontinued if the patient awoke during that time. There were no complications from the stimulation.

Intracranial pressure monitoring was done. No patients had prolonged elevations of the pressure above 20 mmHg during the first 5 days after injury. CT scans were noted for the presence of cisterns, midline shift, subarachnoid blood, and cerebral edema. Patients were also evaluated regarding their multisystem injuries. In all cases the brain injury was the most significant injury. The afferent pathway of the right median nerve was chosen in this study because the cortical representation of the hand resides in close proximity to the motor speech planning center. Increases in release of neurotransmitters in areas of the brain may facilitate the progression of individuals from a vegetative or comatose condition to a conscious and more functional state.[25] The results of the coma treatment are presented in Table 5.1.

In this small one-and-a-half-year pilot study, only six patients met the criteria including informed consents from the families. There were two males and four females, range age 13–42 years. The GCS for both groups was in the range of 7. The average age of the treated group (32 years) was moderately higher than the control group (24 years). The severity of the multisystem injuries was mildly less in the treated group than the control group (Injury

Table 5.1 Initial Glasgow Coma Scale (GCS) ratings

Patient's name	Age	GCS
Treated group		
SI	16	7
DS	37	8
AC	42	7
Mean	32	7.3
Control group		
RB	13	7
WM	42	7
JB	18	7
Mean	24	7

Table 5.2 Follow-up

Patient's name	7 day Glasgow Coma Scale	14 day Glasgow Coma Scale
Treated group		
SI	10	14
DS	11	14
AC	13	13
Mean	11.3	13.7
Control group		
RB	9	9
WM	7	5
JB	7	11
Mean	7.7	8.3

Severity Scores: treated group mean of 28.3, control group mean of 34.3). The follow-up results after one and two weeks of stimulation are presented in Table 5.2.

After 1 week of stimulation, the treated group average GCS had risen to 11.3 while the control group was at a level of 7.7. At 2 weeks the treated group had risen to 13.7 GCS and the control group was at 8.3. The comparison of the pre-stimulation and post-stimulation status was dramatic in the treated group contrasted to the controlled group (Table 5.3).

Therefore, the mean increase in the GCS for the treated group over a 2 week period was 6.3 compared to 0.8 in the control group.

At 1 month all of the treated patients were at a Glasgow Outcome Score (GOS) of III with severe disability. The three patients in the control group had a score of II, the persistent vegetative state (Table 5.4).

Frequent assessments of both groups were done daily by the nurses and once daily by a physical therapist. The physicians, nurses, and evaluators

Table 5.3 Change over 14 days

Patient	Group	Change
SI	Treated	+7
DS	Treated	+6
AC	Treated	+6
RB	Control	+2
WM	Control	−2
JB	Control	+4

Table 5.4 Glasgow Outcome Scale (GOS) 1 month post-injury

Patient	Group	GOS	Score
SI	Treated	Severe disability	III
DS	Treated	Severe disability	III
AC	Treated	Severe disability	III
RB	Control	Persistent vegetative state	II
WM	Control	Persistent vegetative state	II
JB	Control	Persistent vegetative state	II

Table 5.5 Days in intensive care unit

Patient	Group	Days
SI	Treated	6
DS	Treated	9
AC	Treated	8
RB	Control	8
WM	Control	28
JB	Control	15

were blinded as to which patients were receiving real or sham electrical stimulation. An interesting difference in length of stay in the ICU was noted (Table 5.5).

When the data were encapsulated in summary form the differences between the treated and sham treatment group were striking (Table 5.6).

In recent years in the USA, there has been much interest in the economics of medical care. We looked at the length of stay in the intensive care unit for the two groups and there was a significant difference there also. The treated group stayed an average of 7.7 days and the control group 17 days. The decrease in the bed days of the treated group was driven by the significant improvement in the GCS during the first week. The treated group mean GCS increased by 4 points, the control group by 0.7 points. We concluded that early right median nerve stimulation could be an effective treatment for acutely comatose patients.[25]

Table 5.6 Glasgow Coma Scale change and intensive care days

Group	Positive change	
	GCS	Bed days
Treated	6.3	7.7
Control	0.8	17.0

The use of right median nerve stimulation in Japan

Society for treatment of coma meeting, 1996

At the same 1996 meeting in Japan, Yokoyama reported on work that he, Kamei and Kanno had done using the right median nerve stimulation technique for comatose patients.[26] They selected two unconscious patients: a 59-year-old female with hypoxic brain damage, and a 40-year-old male with severe head trauma. Both of these patients showed increased level of consciousness after two weeks of electrical nerve stimulation.

The 59-year-old woman (KJ) was suspected of having a right cerebellopontine angle tumor at another hospital. She was admitted for detailed examination. There were no distinct neurological abnormalities other than numbness of the right upper and lower extremities. Cerebral angiography was performed. The following day the patient had systemic convulsions that deteriorated to respiratory arrest. Despite emergency resuscitation, the patient sustained prolonged consciousness disturbance since the ictus.

Three weeks after the onset, the patient showed a Glasgow Coma Scale (GCS) score of 1.T.3, and median nerve stimulation was initiated. The patient's condition changed from a comatose state to one of arousal within approximately 2 weeks after the start of stimulation. The patient became more oriented, involving both eyes in response to the electrical stimulation.[26]

Society for treatment of coma meeting, 1997

Yamamoto and colleagues from the Department of Neurosurgery at Kurume University School of Medicine in Japan reported on "A case of persistent vegetative state treated with median nerve stimulation."[27] They used this technique for an 18 year-old woman who was in a vegetative state after a brain contusion and open head injury from a traffic accident with admission GCS of 4 with decerebrate rigidity and unequal pupils.

The right median nerve stimulation (RMNS) was started three months after the injury when she was in a persistent vegetative state (PVS). The Focus electrical stimulator was set at 20 mA and pulses at 40 Hz. There was no change in the level of consciousness (GSC 7) before and after the 1 month period of stimulation 12 h/day. There were no marked changes on the EEG, nor were there increases in the cerebral blood flow to the left hemisphere (measured by single photon emission computed tomography, SPECT). There were no changes in adrenalin or serotonin in the spinal fluid but GABA and dopamine each almost doubled. These findings suggested one possible mechanism for the therapeutic effects of RMNS.[27]

At the same meeting, Hayashi from Nihon University in Tokyo, reported on "Prevention of vegetation after severe head injury and stroke by combination therapy of cerebral hypothermia and activation of immune-dopaminergic nervous system."[28] It has been their practice to use cerebral hypothermia for 1–2 weeks in the treatment of severely brain injured patients with GCS scores of less than 6 with a high incidence of good recovery (54%). Similar treatments were also used after cerebrovascular accidents.

In this study they treated (RMNS) five cases of vegetation after cerebral hypothermia treatment. All of these persons had suffered cardiac arrest following trauma or a stroke. The RMNS therapy was done to increase cerebral dopamine. Hayashi stated: "Our preliminary clinical trials of these combination therapy have revealed very useful effects for the neuronal recovery."[28] One case returned to an ordinary lifestyle while others retained neurological deficits.

Society for treatment of coma meeting, 1998

Moriya et al. reported on median nerve stimulation for unconscious patients: "New therapeutic strategies for patients with unconsciousness and neurological deficits in acute stage with median nerve stimulation."[29] They used 2 weeks of median nerve stimulation (MNS) to treat 17 intensive care patients. Seven had severe head injury, four cerebrovascular disease, four with encephalopathy following cardiopulmonary resuscitation, two with hypoxic encephalopathy due to chronic obstructive pulmonary disease.

Nine (53%) showed improved clinical status within 2 weeks. They noted significant rises of the dopamine in the spinal fluid within 1 h after the stimulation. There were no complications induced by the MNS. Hayashi and Moriya concluded that the MNS may be useful for patients in coma with neurological deficits in the acute stage. This treatment may be a therapeutic strategy for comatose patients and could result in lower hospital costs and shorter hospitalizations.[29]

Society for treatment of coma meeting, 1999

Moriya and colleagues at the Department of Emergency and Critical Care Medicine at Nihon University observed the change of clinical symptoms caused by median nerve stimulation.[30] Their protocol was 6 h a day of RMNS, 20 s on and 50 s off. Clinical symptoms improved in 17/37 cases of severe brain damage. The average admission GCS was in the 3.3–5.6 range and the average was 44 years.

The etiology of the brain damage in the 17 improved cases was trauma (nine cases) encephalopathy after cardiopulmonary resuscitation (four cases) and two cases each of severe subarachnoid bleeding and hypoxic encephalopathy. RMNS was started an average of three weeks after admission. In the improved cases, changes in the muscles of facial expression occurred after 3 days of electrical stimulation. They also noted improvements in phonation.

They concluded that median nerve stimulation improved the arousal response. Effectiveness could be expected in cases where increases in spontaneous movement of the extremities and changes of facial expression were observed.[30]

Society for treatment of coma meeting, 2000

Tetsuo Kanno in a special lecture on surgical neurorehabilitation concluded:

> The treatment for severe trauma and vascular diseases at acute stage is carried out very enthusiastically by neurosurgeons, while the treatment at chronic stage is done well by the rehabilitation people. However, at subacute stage, the patients do not have any special treatment. But at this time, the brain atrophy is in progress. Some new treatments must develop to awake the patient and inhibit the progress of the brain atrophy. The author considers that DCS, MNS (median nerve stimulation), and deep brain stimulation could be the modalities for the new treatment. Surgical neurorehabilitation will play an important role in the very near future.[31]

Hirata and Ushio reported on a new application of median nerve stimulation for consciousness disturbance in the chronic phase following subarachnoid hemorrhage in an elderly female. She had already had a ventricular atrial shunt inserted but still had a severe eating disorder taking 2 hours to finish a meal with help. Xenon-CT scanning revealed decreased cerebral blood flow. However, after right median nerve stimulation was started blood flow increased by 40–75% in both cerebral hemispheres. The therapy was given three times daily before each meal for 30 min each. In 2 weeks the patient was able to finish ordinary meals in a half-hour with help. More importantly, her phonation and level of intelligence improved. Months later she was able to walk between parallel bars. They concluded: "Above all, MNS (median nerve stimulation) therapy is characterized by non-invasiveness, simple procedures, and no complications, and is believed to be more suitable than SCS therapy as the first-choice for elderly patients with complications."[32]

The final paper of that meeting pertaining to the nerve stimulation was presented by Moriya and colleagues from Nihon University School of Medicine in Toyoko. He noted the correlation between the median nerve stimulation and changes in the cerebral spinal fluid dopamine in patients with severe traumatic brain injury who responded to the treatment. In those patients whose level of dopamine was low before the startup of the electrical therapy, there was increase in the spinal fluid dopamine concentration and clinical improvement regarding consciousness and motor control. They concluded: "Since dopamine is involved in vigilance and motor control via the A-10 nervous system, which centers on the limbic system, consistency with the improvement of clinical symptoms after MNS is believed to be significant when associated with cerebral changes caused by dopamine."[33]

Society for treatment of coma, 2001

At this meeting Isao Okuma gave a lecture and mentioned that both median nerve stimulation and dorsal column stimulation were performed at Fujita Health University in Toyoake City. These electrical therapies were used for patients with prolonged consciousness disturbance.[34]

Society for treatment of coma, 2002

During this meeting at Tokyo Bay there were two lectures presenting clinical results of acute coma patients treated by right median nerve stimulation. Ed Cooper gave a six-year follow-up of young coma patients treated with RMNS that had been previously presented by him at the 1996 Society for Treatment of Coma meeting. Better than expected results have been obtained in half of the GCS four coma patients treated with RMNS within the first 2 weeks after their closed head injuries. Three young patients were presented by videotape. These patients are discussed later in this chapter.

Jun-Tung Liu from Taiwan, ROC (China Medical College Hospital) presented a recent series of six patients aged 1.5–66 years treated with RMNS in the subacute phase. Cerebral profusion rose in all cases. Neurotransmitter amounts increased in the spinal fluid in five of the six cases.

The details of these and other lectures at Tokyo Bay, July 2002, are published in a supplement of *Acta Neurochirurgica*.

Observations of the central nervous system effect of peripheral nerve stimulation

Neuroimaging in Europe

The central nervous system effect of median nerve electrical stimulation has been demonstrated in several ways. In an article from Mainz, Germany, this effect was noted by using functional magnetic resonance imaging (fMRI).[35] Increased signals in the contralateral somatosensory cortex were noted during median nerve stimulation at a rate of 30–50 Hz (similar to what was used in the University of Virginia and East Carolina University studies). The stimulation was 200 microseconds and the intensity was at motor threshold. In seven out of nine normal subjects, there was significant activity in the hand area on the side opposite to the median nerve stimulation involving the sensory and the motor strips (see Figure 5.1).

In Austria it was also noted with functional MRI that there was an increase in the signal in the primary and secondary motor and somatosensory areas after mesh-glove electrical stimulation of the hand of normal subjects.[36] The pulse frequency was 50 Hz with a pulse width of 300 microseconds. In this study variable amounts of ipsilateral and contralateral hemisphere uptake were noted. Based on this information, it was hypothesized that the stimulation triggered input to the posterior column nuclei of the spinal cord, then to the thalamus and to the cortex of the brain.[36]

In Munich, Germany functional MRI was used to identify cortical areas dedicated to motor hand function prior to removal of space occupying lesions.[37] At the time of brain surgery, electrical stimulation at 50 Hz was

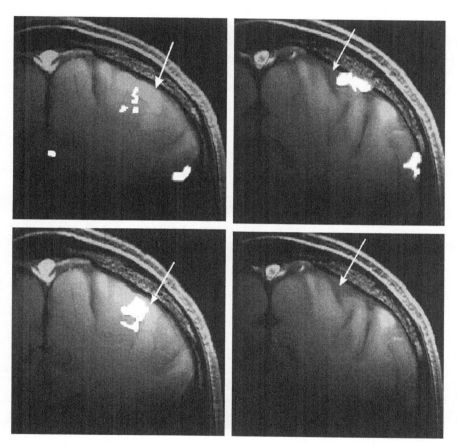

Figure 5.1 Close-up of functional MRI, left hemisphere, showing the uptake in the sensory strip during right median nerve electrical stimulation. Reproduced by permission from Spiegel et al.[35]

done to identify the hand areas. The movements of the contralateral limbs were observed as well as measuring compound muscle action potentials from the contralateral hand (thenar and hypothenar muscles). The motor hand area was located in each case in the precentral gyrus. By doing this open stimulation technique, the pathways were again stimulated.[37]

Observations in rats

In Minnesota, electrical stimulation of the forepaw of ten male rats produced increases in cerebral blood flow (CBF) in the somatosensory cortex.[38] This animal model gives further credence to the theory that peripheral nerve stimulation causes measurable central nervous system effects which might lead toward clinical changes.

Review of prognosis and outcomes in the literature

The following section is a review of articles over the last quarter of the twentieth century. This chronological progression will show the evolution of the treatment and prognosis of severe brain injury. The original Glasgow Coma Scale was described in a 1974 article by Teasdale and Jennett "Assessment of Coma and Impaired Consciousness".[39]

Twenty-five years ago in Italy there was a report of 282 comatose patients; there were 140 fatalities (49%). Age was an important factor in recovery from brain injury. Age 20 was the positive limit for complete recovery and age 40 represented the positive limit for survival. After age 60 the probability of dying was greater than that of surviving.[40]

Twenty years ago a study was done at the Medical College of Virginia in Richmond doing a competitive analysis with the clinical examination evoked potentials, CT scanning, and measurement of intracranial pressure.[41] Age was also an important factor. The proportion of good versus poor outcomes changed at age 40. In their review they used the Glasgow Outcome Scale of Good, Moderately Disabled (that prevents normal function but allows self-care), Severely Disabled (marked deficits that prevent self-care), Vegetative (no higher mental function), and Dead.

The proportion of Good/Moderate Disability versus Severe Disability/Vegetative/Dead outcomes reversed after the age of 40. In patients over the age 60, 78% had a Severe Disability/Vegetative/Dead outcome. Under the age 20, 72% of patients had a Good/Moderate Disability outcome. Only 30% of patients with abnormal pupillary functions had good outcome contrasted to 76% of those with normal pupil responses.

A higher proportion (83%) of Good/Moderate Disability outcomes was observed in patients with normal computerized tomography (CT) scans on admission. Elevated intracranial pressure (ICP) was predictive of a poor prognosis. If ICPs remained elevated throughout then there was only an 11% Good/Moderate Disability outcome.

With the combination of age, Glasgow Coma Scale, pupillary reaction, presence or absence of a surgical mass lesion, eye movements, and motor responses, the prognosis of severe head injury could be estimated with 82% accuracy. This study of 133 patients was in the period 1976–1979.[41]

John Jane presented a description of the outcome following head injury based on material from the University of Virginia Head Injury Service and the National Coma Data Bank.[42] This report from 25 years ago presents the predictive value of the Glasgow Coma Scale motor score alone. Of the three scales, the motor score was the most significant as the patient in deep coma would usually have the eyes closed and would be intubated.

The lower Glasgow Coma Scales of 3, 4 and 5 yielded high mortalities (over 60%). The outcome of patients with GCS less than 8 depended largely on three preventable or treatable factors of hypoxia, shock, and increased intracranial pressure.[42]

Five hundred and eighty-one patients with severe brain injury (nonpenetrating) with GSC score of 8 or less following resuscitation were described in the follow-up phase of the National Traumatic Coma Data Bank in the *Journal of Neurosurgery* in 1983.[43] Experience was gathered from the four participating hospitals: University of Virginia, University of Texas at Galveston, Medical College of Virginia, and University of California at San Diego. In the second year of the study two other centers were added: Albert Einstein College of Medicine in New York and Baylor University in Houston.

The data was stored at Stanford University (Palo Alto, CA). The data was collected between 1980 and 1982. The largest group of patients (28%) were white males aged 19–29 with head injury resulting from a motor vehicle accident. This effort served as a model for further multiple center studies of complex neurosurgical problems.

The appearance of the basal cisterns on the initial CT scan was assessed in 218 severely head injured patients (University of California Medical Center, San Diego) in the early 1980s.[44] When the cisterns were normal the mortality rate was 22%, if they were compressed the death rate was 39% and if the cisterns were absent mortality was 77%. In 25/34 patients (74%) in which the ICPs were monitored and the cisterns were absent, there was severe intracranial hypertension exceeding 30 mmHg.

An important article from 1987 about the outcome after severe head injury reported a series of 330 severely head injured patients at the Medical College of Virginia.[45] The pediatric patients had a higher percentage of good outcome (43%) than the adult patients (28%). The mortality rate for the children was 24% and for the adults 45%. At 1 year post-injury 55% of the pediatric patients had a good outcome overall compared to only 21% of the adults. The overall percentage of good outcome for all patients in the series was 32% with mortality of 38%. Moderate disability combined with good outcome yielded a 52% favorable result.

For patients in whom ICP was elevated above 20 mmHg and the pressure did not come down with treatment (pharmacological paralysis, morphine sedation, hyperventilation, CFS drainage, Mannitol, barbiturate coma), there was only 8% good outcome in the pediatric group and 0% good outcome in the adult group. Mortality rates were 92% and 95% respectively. If the patient had treatable intracranial hypertension, the good outcome was still low, only 27%. It was concluded that "by the time a severe injury had manifested itself with an increased ICP, it may already be too late to effect an improved outcome." It appeared that the children and the adults both fared badly with increased ICP.[45]

In an article by Marshall in 1988, the role of aggressive therapy was discussed.[46] Aggressive management of intracranial hypertension is important. However, some brain injuries are so severe at the beginning that the outcome is inevitable. Outcome studies elsewhere had indicated a mortality of approximately 35–40%. Of the patients who reached the hospital alive, the neurosurgeon could only influence the outcome in a group no greater than 50%, Marshall estimated. He concluded: "Further refinements in head injury care await a better understanding of the neurobiology of such injuries and the imaginative application of therapies by young investigators."[46]

A five-center study of 73 patients was done to investigate the role of high-dose barbiturate control of elevated intracranial pressure in patients with severe head injury.[47] Eisenberg noted that when ICP control using other protocols failed, high-dose barbiturates can be effective. Their study confirmed the findings of others: a strong association between controlled ICP and mortality from TBI.[47]

From four hospitals in Barcelona, Spain, a paper emerged on "Diffuse axonal injury [DAI] after severe head trauma" published in 1989.[48] DAI is considered to be the cases rendered unconscious at the moment of impact in which the CT scan does not show mass lesions, but there is diffuse axonal damage with rotational acceleration producing shear and tensile injuries. The shear injuries of the brain could explain the poor outcome in certain patients in spite of rapid surgical treatment and control of intracranial pressure. The initial CT scan is important in predicting the clinical evolution and outcome. Those with intracerebral hemorrhages have a worse outcome than those who do not. The most severe forms show lesions in the corpus callosum and/or the dorsolateral rostral brainstem.[48]

In 1990, a multicenter study from the Neurosurgery Departments of the University of Texas, University of Virginia, Medical College of Virginia, University of California (San Diego) and the National Institute of Neurological Diseases and Stroke was reported. This prospective study looked at the initial CT scans of 753 patients with severe head injury.[49] It was found that the risk of dying in severe head injured patients is increased twofold if the mesencephalic cisterns are obliterated or compressed. In general, if the initial CT scan is normal, then the patient does not develop intracranial hypertension.[49]

In another study from the same multiple centers, neurobehavioral outcome was evaluated one year after severe head injury.[50] The lowest post resuscitation Glasgow Coma Scale score and the pupillary reactivity were predictive of the 1 year Glasgow Outcome Scale score and the neurophysiological performance. Patients with the lowest score below 4 all ended up in a vegetative state. Those with scores between 4 and 6 were more likely to end up with severe than moderate disability and only those with scores of 6 and above had a good outcome. One year after injury, memory for new information was impaired. It was concluded that the 24 h GCS score was more predictive of neurobehavioral outcome than the GCS score obtained on admission.[50]

From the same centers, a new classification of head injury was based primarily on information from the first computerized tomography scan.[51] In category III, where the cisterns were compressed or absent, or there was a midline shift of 0–5 mm, but no high or mixed density lesions greater than 25 ml, only 16% made a satisfactory recovery. There was an unsatisfactory result in 50% of these patients and 34% expired for a total of 100%.

It was noted that the CT classification appeared to have significant application to the critical care head injury patients. There was a strong relationship between the CT scan, mortality and elevated intracranial pressure. The authors stated, however: "In patients with less substantial biomechanical injuries, it appears likely that early intervention might prevent the development of other insults and improve both mortality and the overall quality of life."[51] They concluded that the frequency of diffuse head injury with midline shift was relatively low. But the very high mortality rates suggest that these severely injured patients represent a target group in which innovative therapies might first be tested.[51]

In Waxman et al.'s 1991 article "Is early prediction of outcome in severe head injury possible?" he noted a poor correlation between the initial Glasgow Coma Scale score at patient arrival and eventual outcome.[52] But scores 6 h after presentation correlated better with the outcome. In patients even as low as GCS 3 there could be a good neurological outcome.

Several factors affect survival including the age, other injuries, blood pressure, mechanism of injury, presence of spontaneous ventilation, CT scan findings. He reasoned that the initial therapy should be aggressive for patients with severe TBI. Regardless of the initial neurologic status, accurate prediction of outcome within 6 h of presentation is not possible. This included a review of patient records between 1985 and 1987 at the University of California Irvine Medical Center. Of patients with initial blood pressure of less than 60 mmHg, 96% died, and the one survivor was in a vegetative state.

In patients in the 13–20 year-old group (74 patients), the initial Glasgow Coma Scale score was 5.9. Of this group 32% died, 7% went into a vegetative state, 26% had severe disability, 14% had moderate disability, and 20% a good outcome. The improved correlation using scores 6 h after admission was due in part to the natural history of the brain injury: some patients had already died by that time. The effects of drugs and alcohol diminished and there was time for the treatment of associated injuries.[52] The conclusion by the authors deserves quoting:

> To provide appropriate care for patients with potential for good outcome, we conclude that initial therapy should be aggressive, regardless of the initial GCS score . . . the risk of withholding therapy must be considered, namely, that salvageable patient may die or suffer unnecessary disability. We believe this risk offsets any cost savings . . . prolonged hospitalization need not precede death.[52]

The same multiple centers published an article in 1991: "The outcome of severe closed head injury".[53] They studied patients enrolled in the Traumatic Coma Data Bank prospectively from January 1984 through September 1987 and this included 1030 consecutive patients admitted with severe head injury who had GCS of 8 or less after resuscitation.

Of these, 284 were brain dead or had a gunshot wound to the brain so those groups were excluded, leaving 746 patients. The overall mortality for this group was 36% by 6 months post-injury. The highest mortality group were the GCS 3 patients (76%) but only 18% for patients of 6, 7, or 8. Among patients with nonsurgical lesions overall mortality rate was 31%. At the time of hospital discharge 33% of patients had died, 14% were vegetative and only 7% were showing a good outcome at that point. Higher proportions of patients with Diffuse Injury III and IV (swelling and shift) were vegetative. Only the Diffuse Injury I (no visible CT scan pathology) had a high proportion of good outcomes of 27%.

For Diffuse Injury II group patients, 15% of those under 40 years of age had a good recovery, 44% moderate disability for a total of 59% satisfactory. If they were over 40 years old then there were no good category survivors and 8.3% moderate disability.[53]

Dacey et al. analyzed a series of 242 consecutive surviving head injured patients and 132 general trauma patients.[54] The neuropsychological outcome was related to the brain injury and the injury severity though it is not independently related to other system injuries. The psychosocial outcome was related to both the brain and non-brain injuries independently. Therefore, both sets of injuries should be considered.

The severity of the brain injury was the dominant factor in determining mortality in patients with multisystem injuries. The mortality was about 30% from patients with major blunt trauma and severe brain injury. When there is major trauma alone the mortality is very low. Cognitive outcome was mainly related to the severity of the brain injury. The psychosocial outcome was affected by both the brain injury and the multisystem injuries.[54]

The usefulness of CT scan in predicting the outcome of TBI patients was discussed by Kido et al. at Rochester Medical Center in New York.[55] Patients with normal CT scans were more likely to have mild neurological dysfunction or normal recovery than patients with an abnormal CT scan. Norepinephrine levels were higher in patients with severe brain injury and this was associated with the outcome. However, even with a normal CT scan, 41% remained moderately severely disabled. The lesion size was most critical for intracranial hematomas. Prognosis was poor for patients with a lesion larger than 4100 mm^3.[55]

In 1992 Levin et al. investigated the outcome at six months and at one year of children (0–15 years old) who had suffered severe head injuries.[56] The children in the 0–4 year-old group had a high mortality (62% by 1 year). Only one in five obtained a favorable outcome. In the 5–10 year-old group three-quarters had a favorable outcome. In terms of the CT scans, the most common finding was bilateral swelling (36% of the patients). Mass lesions of at least 15 ml and bilateral swelling were associated with elevated ICP and poor outcome. Children with diffuse axonal injury but without diffuse brain swelling usually did not have increased ICP. More than two-thirds of these children obtained a favorable outcome.[56]

Choi and Barnes noted that extremely good or poor outcomes could be predicted with confidence.[57] Intermediate outcomes are more difficult to predict. They reviewed 786 patients with severe head injury treated between 1976 and 1991 at the Medical College of Virginia. Comparing GCS scores and age relative to favorable or unfavorable outcome, there was a "J" shaped curve. The turning point was at age 30–40 years in terms of more unfavorable outcomes. Above age 40 all patients with a GCS of 5 or less had an unfavorable outcome.[57]

Gruen reported in 1996 on the management of complicated neurologic injuries.[58] An injury was called complicated if associated with an injury of any other organ system which jeopardizes the neurologic outcome. It was noted that of the 60,000 patients each year in the USA with severe head injury who were alive for transfer to the hospital, 50% had intracranial pressure elevation.

Cerebral oxygen delivery can be measured and may be a better indicator of ischemia. Refractory intracranial hypertension with increases in ICP led to neurologic deterioration and death. Gruen noted that all neural tissue is very dependent on an uninterrupted supply of oxygen and glucose, the fuels for sustaining the metabolic machinery.[58]

Baltas and others reported on the outcome in severely head injured patients with and without multiple trauma.[59] They concluded that the non-shock severely head injured patients with multiple trauma had similar mortality to those without multiple trauma. Mortality was dependent on the severity of the intracranial pathology.

The Guidelines for the Management of Severe Head Injury, published in 1996 by the Brain Trauma Foundation and the American Association of Neurological Surgeons gave standards that could improve the outcome.[60] The understanding of events that determine the functional outcome depends on: (1) primary brain injury; (2) secondary brain injury; (3) inflammation: the cellular inflammatory response adds to the damage begun by the oxygen-free radicals and other toxic chemicals; (4) repair/regeneration – this is the area that is least known. Future advances will include neuronal regeneration, axonal guidance and central nervous system transplantation. The incidence of gunshot wound to the head has steadily risen during the past 10–20 years as the most common cause of fatal head injury.[60,61]

Letarte at Loyola University Medical School wrote the article "Neurotrauma care in the new millennium."[62] He observed:

> The dawn of the new millennium occurs as the paradigm for the treatment of patients with head injuries is changing. The treatment of patients with head injuries started in the 1900s as a surgical disease; craniotomy for evacuation of hematoma was the only modality available for the reduction of intracranial pressure (ICP) and the maintenance of cerebral profusion pressure (CPP). Over the past 50 years there has been the introduction of surgical modalities for treatment of patients' traumatic brain injury (TBI). As the new millennium dawns, surgery is becoming but one modality in what is now seen as the resuscitation of the injured brain. . . .[62]

In *Neurology and Trauma* by Evans, chapter 12 entitled "Neurobehavioral Outcome of Head Trauma", the Glasgow Coma Scale and Glasgow Outcome Scale were explained. Age is important: in adults 50 years or older age is a poor prognostic factor, partly because of the higher incidence of intracranial hematoma in older patients. Older patients have other medical complications that could contribute to a poor outcome.[63]

In those patients with nonreactive pupils in the first 24 h of coma, 95% will die or become vegetative. Only 4% will have a moderate disability or good recovery. If the pupils are reactive, there is a 50% rate of moderate or good recovery.

Cognitive impairments are the most disabling results of head injury. In the recovery from moderate to severe closed head injury, there is a period of post-traumatic amnesia (PTA) that is often accompanied by a reduced level of consciousness or agitation. Initial severity of trauma, age and length of PTA are some of the variables predictive of outcome.[63]

In the textbook *Neurosurgery* by Wilkins and Rengachary (1996), Marshall observed that prediction after severe head injury continues to be an area of intense interest because of the natural curiosity of neurosurgeons and society's attention to resource allocation. The ability to predict outcome becomes very important to the targeting of resources.[64]

Right median nerve electrical stimulation (RMNS)

The median nerve serves as a peripheral gateway to the central nervous system. The sensory distribution of the hand exhibits disproportionately large cortical representation. Within the brainstem, the ascending reticular activating system (ARAS) maintains wakefulness. The spinoreticular component of the median nerve synapses with neurons of the ARAS. The nearby locus coeruleus releases norepinephrine causing a monoaminergic arousal of the cortex directed to cortical layer 1.[65] The intralaminar nuclei of the thalamus are activated by acetylcholinergic input from the ARAS. These intralaminar thalamic nuclei provide nonspecific excitatory input to the cortical layer 1 leading to the initiation of awakening. The excited ARAS also stimulates the forebrain basal nucleus of Meynert which delivers diffusely spread acetylcholine to the cerebral cortex.[66]

The right median nerve was chosen as a portal to stimulate the brainstem and cerebrum because increased alertness and better speech have been observed after RMNS.[1,18] Broca's motor speech planning area in the left frontotemporal region has been shown in positron emission tomography (PET) to become more active when a subject moves, or even contemplates moving his or her hand.[67] This process is mimicked in RMNS.

The author's interest in stimulation began 30 years ago with a study involving a paraplegic individual at University of Virginia (UVa) in Charlottesville, Virginia. Radio-linked, implanted electrodes strengthened muscles and allowed crude ambulation.[5] From 1987 to 1989 individuals suffering from quadriplegia were helped to use their forearm muscles through voice-activated electrical stimulation to produce hand opening and closing at the Department of Biomedical Engineering at Duke University in Durham, North Carolina. Significant improvement was noted in distal motor abilities in response to electrical stimulation in this and previous studies by Cooper and associates.[5,6,68] Proximal voluntary and contralateral arm increases in performance were also noted during strength testing.[6]

Similar computerized electrical stimulation was applied to adult individuals with severe mental/motor delays at Caswell Center in Kinston, North Carolina, in hopes of improving function and awareness.[69] While viewing serial videos of patients in the treated group, progressive augmentation of mental awareness was noted. The observed cross-over effect in the quadriplegic population, along with the central arousal of the mentally challenged population, led to the postulation that stimulation of the median nerve causes significant central nervous system activation.[1,18,69]

The electrical stimulators, Respond Select at the University of Virginia project and Respond II® (Empi) at the East Carolina University project were battery-powered units. They supplied trains of asymmetric biphasic pulses at an amplitude of 15–20 milliamps (mA) as tolerated with a pulse width of 300 μs at 40 Hz for 20 s/min. The treatment was done for 12 h daily at ECU and 8 h/day at UVa for 2 weeks. The trains of pulses were delivered to the volar aspect of the right distal forearm over the median nerve via lubricated surface rubber electrodes measuring 2.5 × 2.5 cm. The electrodes were embedded 2 cm apart in the midline of plastic cuffs (Carolina Ortho Prosthetics, Greenville, NC; see Figure 5.2).

In our UVa and ECU coma projects, electrical treatment was usually started in the first week post traumatic brain injury (TBI).[1,18] Stimulation was not done in the first 2 days to allow time for clearing of any intoxicants and also for emergency surgery.

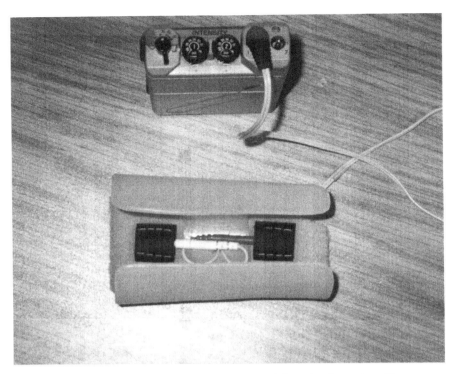

Figure 5.2 An electrical stimulator connected to a right wrist electrode cuff.

If there is concern about the dopamine rush in the first week after severe TBI with neuronal cell death, then the coma stimulation may be delayed as needed. However, with advancing time post-injury, there may be a slower response to the electrical treatment and diminishing returns for the final neurological outcome.

For children and small adults, a setting of up to 15 mA is recommended and also for those adults with agitation at the 20 mA setting. For safety purposes, a plastic cap or clear tape should be applied over the external power dial on the electrical stimulator to prevent inadvertent overstimulation.

Peripheral nerve electrical stimulation (FDA approved stimulators) was cleared by the institutional review boards of UVa and ECU for the coma projects. Informed consents for the participation of the comatose patients were obtained from the families.

The right median nerve motor stimulation was done at approximately 1.5 times the motor threshold. This usually produced strong right thenar abduction and flexion of the index and middle fingers plus some wrist flexion. In conscious volunteers, obvious tingling (but not painful) was felt in a median nerve distribution in the right hand. Depending on the depth of coma of the TBI patients, RMNS may elicit withdrawal of the right forearm, head turning and partial opening of the eyes. Temporary mild elevation of the vital signs is not unusual, but intracranial pressures usually remain stable. The motor responses gradually diminish during the 8–12 h treatment sessions. If the coma patient has been chemically paralyzed, hand movements during the "on" cycles may be absent, but the therapeutic afferent stimulation should continue to be effective.

In the first few days of treatment, mirror movements of the unstimulated left hand may occur. This cross-over effect was first discovered in the Duke quadriplegic hand stimulation study as evidenced by the strength gains in bilateral proximal arm muscles. The effect was noted in the Caswell computerized electrical stimulation projects as evidenced by the generalized motor and emotional improvements.[6]

This dynamic cross-over effect heralds the reactivation of the cerebral hemispheres in the electrically stimulated comatose patient. First the left hemisphere, then the right, is reanimated via the corpus callosum.[70] Usually the first simple command ("touch your thumb to your finger") to which the patient will respond after one or two weeks of RMNS is a sluggish opposition of the right thumb and index finger. *This unique "O sign" is the earliest signal of the progressive emergence from deep coma.*

In computer parlance, this voluntary hand response while the TBI patient still appears to be semi-comatose, demonstrates that the 5 million electrical pulses delivered to the nervous system in the first 10 days of treatment have been copied and stored in the hard drive of the brain. The message can be retrieved on command: purposeful hand movement, a very human and not a vegetative function. It is the outward and physical sign of internal electro-chemical partial healing.[1]

As reported earlier in this chapter, in the UVa study at 1 week, the treated group had improved by an average of 4.0 on the GCS and the control group had improved by an average of 0.7 on the GCS. By 2 weeks, the treated group had improved by an average of 6.4 on the GCS and the control group had improved by an average of 1.3 on the GCS (refer to Tables 5.1 and 5.2). The treated group stayed in the intensive care unit for an average of 7.7 days and the control group stayed in the ICU for an average of 17.0 days (refer to Table 5.6).

In a more recent study (1998–1999) with similar methods and similar comatose patients, Cristian Peri noted that the electrically treated group required a shorter period of endotracheal intubation/respirator than the sham treatment group.[18] Although the statistical significance has not been determined, it appears that the difference in intubation time is an even more refined measure of brainstem function than the previously observed total days in the ICU for the two groups.[25]

Right median nerve stimulation (RMNS) by way of the afferent pathways through the spinal cord and brainstem probably activates the cells of the medullary "respiratory centers".[71] Injuries to the brainstem particularly in the medulla may result in ataxic or irregular respiration or a cessation of respiration.[72]

History of RMNS in the eastern USA

Four selected American cases

The following four young patients with severe TBI from motor vehicle collisions were treated with right median nerve electrical stimulation (RMNS) at two university medical centers in North Carolina within the last few years. These cases are presented to show the possibility of functional recovery with RMNS in situations where the initial prognosis was very grim.

1   CP, a 16-year-old female, was involved in an motor vehicle crash (MVC 1993) and sustained a severe closed head injury. She had a mandibular fracture and an intracranial pressure of 18. After resuscitation she continued with decerebrate posturing. Her initial head CT scan was normal. She was dependent on a respirator and had a brief cardiac arrest. One week later she remained comatose and RMNS was commenced. After 1 week of stimulation her GCS had improved to 9. After a total of 2 weeks of stimulation she scored 14 on the GCS, an improvement of 9 and near the fully alert state. Within 1 month of her injury, CP could speak, eat, and walk with assistance. CP was discharged to home within 2 months of her trauma. She made a full recovery by one year. She has had held a full-time job as a cashier and has been promoted to the administrative office.

2   AT, a 14-year-old female, was involved in an MVC (1995) and sustained a severe closed head injury. She had a hemothorax and a pulmonary contusion. Her right mandibular condyle penetrated the base of her skull through the temporal bone into the middle cranial fossa. CT scan showed hemorrhagic foci in the left cerebral hemisphere. She exhibited alternating decerebrate and decorticate posturing and received a GCS of 4. Within the first week of stimulation she began gripping spontaneously. After 1 week of stimulation her GCS was 6. After 2 weeks of stimulation she began to open her eyes spontaneously and received a GCS of 8. At 2 months post-injury she was eating well and speaking. Within 5 months she was playing volleyball and doing well in school. She recently graduated from college ("B" average) and is now married.

3   CI, a 16-year-old female, was involved in an MVC (1994) and sustained severe closed head injury. She suffered a basilar skull fracture, cerebrospinal fluid otorrhea, left facial fracture, and left pelvic fracture. CT scan revealed left internal capsule contusion, right cerebellar subarachnoid hemorrhage, and blood in the fourth ventricle. Decerebrate posturing was observed and she received a GCS of 4. She was briefly given electrical stimulation but intracranial pressures continued to rise. With her extremely poor prognosis, she was expected to die and was extubated. She breathed spontaneously and electrical stimulation was resumed to the right median nerve. Within 1 week of stimulation, she exhibited semi-purposeful movement of her right arm and leg and scored 7 on the GCS.

After a total of 2 weeks of stimulation, she scored 10 on the GCS. This increase of 6 was consistent with the UVa pilot project observation.[1,25] One month after the injury, CI followed simple commands. At 2 months post-injury CI could walk with assistance and read aloud. Two years later CI talked and walked well. She resumed dancing and driving. She completed high school and college with a "B" average. Now she is the recreation/activities director at a rest home.

4   In March of 2000, a 12-year-old boy, KF, was struck by a van and had severe brain and intra-abdominal injuries plus multiple extremity fractures including compound fractures of the pelvis. On his initial CT scan there was left frontal contusion, a small amount of subarachnoid hemorrhage in the interpeduncular cistern and a non-depressed skull fracture of the left parietal bone. There was also a fracture of the left temporal bone. On the follow-up scan two days later, a right frontal ventricular catheter was noted. There were several contusions (right frontal and left temporal), increased edema with marked effacement of the cortical sulci, and intraventricular hemorrhage. On the scan 1 week post-injury there was diffuse brain swelling and multiple hemorrhagic shearing injuries and hemorrhagic contusions of the left frontal lobe extending into the temporal lobe. He underwent multiple abdominal and orthopaedic operations. He remained comatose with elevated intracranial pressures (over 70 mmHg) in spite of two courses of barbiturate therapy. Pupils remained unequal. Survival was very questionable. Surface electrical stimulation in the 15 mA range to the left median nerve was commenced 2 weeks post-injury. The right forearm was in a cast. After 2 weeks of daily stimulation, he began to emerge from the coma. He progressively improved and regained his ability to speak. He could use his hands in spite of a right hemiparesis. Two months post-injury, he was transferred to a rehabilitation center. Electrical stimulation was resumed, but switched to the right median nerve to help reduce the right hemiparesis. He continued to improve and was discharged to home 6 weeks later. He started home schooling and made good grades. On his final neurosurgical evaluation 4 months post-injury KF was noted to have made a very good recovery. On a home visit 8 months post-injury, his speech was almost normal. His right hemiparesis was very mild, walking with only a slight limp. Two years post-injury in the spring of 2002 his junior high school grade average was a "B". He returned to some athletic activities.

Analysis of GCS-4 decerebrate patients

At the heart of the controversy regarding electrical stimulation for coma lies the stark question, *Does early electrical stimulation improve the outcome of severely comatose patients?*

To best answer this question a series of 100 comatose patients from acute brain injury would be needed. They would be randomized so that approximately 50 would be in a treated group and 50 in a control group with sham electrical stimulation, double blinded. With the large number of patients, variations in the severity and types of injuries would balance out.[73] To accomplish such a study, a multicenter effort in the USA, Asia and Europe would be needed. This work needs to be done in the near future. To provide a quick answer to the efficacy of early stimulation, looking at a group of patients with an extremely poor prognosis when treated by conventional methods would be helpful.

Within our series of 22 comatose patients treated with electrical stimulation at the medical center at East Carolina University from 1993 through 1999, 12 of the patients were in the Glasgow Coma Scale 4 category. They exhibited decerebrate posturing. These patients were in deep coma for more than a week. It is known that GCS 4 patients have a very poor prognosis.[41–46,48–57]

In the textbook by Wilkins and Rengachary, *Neurosurgery*, 1996, there is a chapter written by Marshall and Marshall on "Outcome prediction in severe head injury". The outcome at the last contact was discussed by categories of the post-resuscitation Glasgow Coma Scale scores.[64] Out of 111 patients in the GCS 4 category, 62 expired. This left 49 patients for comparison to our 12 GCS 4 patients who survived. Of their 49 patients, 7 had a Good outcome (14%), 9 had Moderate Disability (18%) for a total of 32% favorable outcome of the GCS 4 patients who survived. Other survivors included 21 with Severe Disability (43%) and 12 Vegetative patients (25%) for a total of 100% for the surviving group of 49 patients.

Using the Glasgow Outcome Scale, Good recovery is characterized as "resumption of normal life even though there may be minor neurologic and pathologic deficits".[74,75] A patient in the category of Moderate Disability is "Disabled but independent". The person could work in a sheltered environment and travel by public transport. However, various degrees of neurological deficit and also intellectual and memory deficits and personality change would remain. Those in the Severe Disability category are dependent for daily support, usually with a combination of mental and physical disabilities.

In our small uncontrolled series at East Carolina University, the comatose patients were treated with RMNS as described in the protocol plus traditional neurosurgical aggressive management with intracranial monitoring.[1,18] The right median nerve electrical stimulation was usually started at 1 week post-injury and continued for 2–3 weeks. The outcome of the surviving GCS 4 subset of patients (12) is shown in Tables 5.7 and 5.8.

In summary, a satisfactory result (Good plus Moderate) was reached by 1 year in 58% of the GCS 4 patients treated with right median nerve electrical stimulation.[25]

In the chapter by Marshall, the outcome scoring was done at "last contact".[64] The outcomes in our series as noted in Tables 5.7 and 5.8 were at 1 year or less. In the Severe cases (42%), the outcome was judged much earlier, usually several months post injury when the patient was transferred from the rehabilitation center to a long-term facility elsewhere. It is not known

Table 5.7 Twelve GCS-4 survivor patients treated with early RMNS at ECU

Initials	Age	Sex	Injury year	Outcome at ≤ 1 year
1. CP	16	F	1993	Good recovery
2. PW	21	M	1994	Severe disability
3. MS	22	M	1994	Severe disability
4. CI	16	F	1994	Moderate disability
5. AT	15	F	1995	Good recovery
6. AP	17	F	1995	Good recovery
7. MC	26	F	1996	Moderate disability
8. KB	19	F	1996	Good recovery
9. KB	7	M	1997	Severe disability
10. RR	14	M	1997	Severe disability
11. DV	21	M	1997	Severe disability
12. EW	15	F	1999	Moderate disability

Table 5.8 Outcome at 1 year or less

Outcome	(n)	Proportion
Good	4	33%
Moderate disability	3	25%
Severe disability	5	42%
Vegetative	0	–
Dead	Not included	–
Total	12	100%

whether some of the patients in the Severe category might have progressed to the Moderate category by 1 year.

As demonstrated by one of the Severe category patients (PW, age 21), by last report a little over 1 year post-injury he was making progress toward Moderate Disability. He was living in an apartment, receiving physical therapy, having difficulty walking because of heterotopic ossification in his hips, but he was able to talk.

There were three patients in the Moderate outcome category (25%). In the Good recovery group at 1 year there were four patients (33%). One of the teenage patients (CI) in the Moderate category progressed to the Good outcome group by 3 years post-injury.

EW (Moderate Disability) is now almost 2 years post-severe brain injury, making As and Bs in high school, playing basketball, but has short-term memory deficits. Based on her rate of progress, she too will probably be in the Good outcome category by 3 years post-injury.

The time required to reach the Good category in our patients corresponded inversely to the severity of the findings on the early CT scans.[1,25] This relationship between the early CT scans and the final outcome has been well reported in the literature.[49,55,76] The Good outcomes were judged on the basis of physical and speaking abilities, resuming driving an automobile and making good grades in school. Most of these Good outcome patients went on to be fully employed.

There was a satisfactory outcome (Good plus Moderate) in 58% of the GCS-4 patients treated with right median nerve electrical stimulation. Three of our Good outcome patients had excellent outcomes, virtually normal according to the families.

While the number of treated patients was quite small and not randomized, there was a definite trend toward Good recovery. This would suggest a significant treatment effect by the early electrical stimulation.[1,25]

Discussion

Electrical stimulation of the right median nerve may help acutely brain-injured persons to recover from coma more rapidly (Figure 5.3). The patients receiving RMNS suffered no ill consequences.[1,25,77] Many have recovered more quickly than was anticipated.

Through maintenance of existing neuronal circuitry, earlier awakening from coma may lead to a higher final level of function. Increased cerebral activity, as observed in RMNS, may also facilitate synaptogenesis in damaged cerebral cortex.[78,79,80] The clinical observations indicate that RMNS has a beneficial effect on the resumption of language capabilities, possibly through stimulation of Broca's motor speech area.[1,25]

The pilot project at the University of Virginia reflects the observations at ECU: treated patients' Glasgow Coma Scale scores rose more quickly than those in the control group.[1,25] But the burden of proof in establishing a cause and effect relationship in the comatose population is immense. Both the treated group in the UVa pilot project and the three cases presented from the ECU series showed a mean improvement of 6.4 on the GCS after 2 weeks of treatment. This suggests that the treatment may show dose-dependent efficacy.[1] Future clinical trials at the University of Virginia and other medical centers in the USA and Japan should produce more substantial results.

Conclusion

Electrical stimulation is not a panacea for all severe head injuries. Those patients with extensive cerebral structural damage and/or intractable intracranial hypertension may not respond to the electrical stimulation. Those patients with mild and moderate brain injury can be expected to respond to standard neurosurgical protocols. But there is a subset of severe TBI patients, usually in the Glasgow Coma Scale post-resuscitation range of 4 and 5 with a mixture of decerebrate and decorticate movements. They may benefit from early electrical stimulation. Especially in comatose teenagers with CT scans that do not show excessive structural damage, electrical stimulation may yield a better than expected outcome.

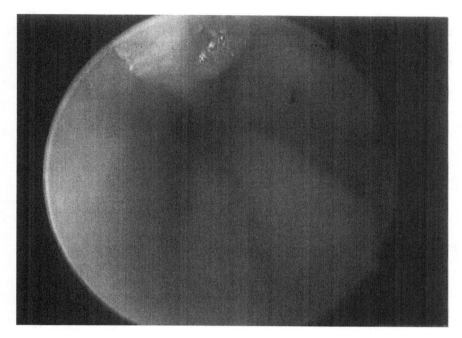

Figure 5.3 Endoscopic photo of the right median nerve.

Anecdotally, our patients' history show a tendency toward better recovery than expected in the literature. The strong message gained from the last 10 years of clinical research is that there is a subset of young patients who appear at first to have a hopeless neurological injury. With the proper treatment, the majority of persons who survive their brain injuries may make a semi-functional recovery. About half of the patients could make a good recovery, a few excellent.

For patients with severe traumatic brain injury, electrical stimulation can be a therapeutic adjunct to the standard neurosurgical treatment. Through peripheral nerve stimulation, cerebral blood flow may be increased, catecholamine output enhanced, and maintenance of neuronal circuitry in spite of massive blunt trauma to the brain.

The reawakening and partial healing of the non-fatally injured brain can be driven from below.[78,79,80] The median nerve is an available portal to the brainstem and cerebral cortex.[81] Electrical stimulation provides a strong force to unmask a subset of salvageable patients whose grim clinical picture exceeds the amount of anatomical brain damage. Right median nerve stimulation, by avoiding disuse atrophy, may allow patients to begin rehabilitation with fewer deficits.

These patients may obtain a better outcome as a result of the stimulation. The observations gained from the treated series of patients at ECU, Fujita

Health University, and the pilot projects at UVa suggest that RMNS may have a positive effect on brain-injured comatose individuals. Non-invasive RMNS is easily employed with little risk and is cost effective. This new technique *can* improve neurological outcomes. In the words of Shakespeare:

> Diseases desperate grown
> By desperate appliance are relieved,
> Or not at all.
> (*Hamlet*, Act IV, scene iii)[82]

To empower brains that have crashed, median nerve stimulation will be an easy, safe, and economical adjunctive treatment for severe brain injury.

References

1. Cooper, J., Jane, J., Alves, W., & Cooper, E. (1999). Right median nerve electrical stimulation to hasten awakening from coma. *Brain Injury, 13*, 261–267.
2. Devinsky, O. (1993). Electrical and magnetic stimulation of the central nervous system, historical overview. In O. Devinsky, A. Beric and M. Dogali (Eds.), *Electrical and magnetic stimulation of the brain and spinal cord*. New York: Raven.
3. Soric, R., & Devlin, M. (1985). Transcutaneous electrical nerve stimulation. *Postgrad. Med. 78*, 101–107.
4. Mullet, K. (1985). Implanted versus transcutaneous neurostimulation devices in pain management. In Y. Azaorthes and A. Upton (Eds.), *Neurostimulation: An overview* (pp. 61–65). Mt. Kisco, NY: Futura
5. Cooper, E., Bunch, W., & Campa, J. (1973). Effects of chronic human neuromuscular stimulation. *Surg. Forum, 24*, 477–479.
6. Cooper, E., Han, D., & McElhaney, J. (1988). *A voice-controlled computer system for restoring limited hand functions in quadriplegics, Proceedings of the American Input Output Systems Applications Conference*. San Francisco, CA; 1988.
7. Gersh, M. (1992). *Electrotherapy in rehabilitation*. Philadelphia, PA: F. A. Davis.
8. Mortimer, J. (1981). Motor prostheses. In V. Brooks (Ed.), *Handbook of physiology: The nervous system, II* (pp. 155–187). Bethesda, MD: American Physiological Society.
9. Benton, L. (1981). *Functional electrical stimulation – A practical clinical guide* (2nd ed.). Rancho Los Amigos, Downey, CA: The Professional Staff Association of the Rancho Los Amigos Hospital, Inc.
10. Scherder, E., & Bouma, A. (1993). Possible role of the nucleus raphe dorsalis in analgesia by peripheral stimulation: theoretical considerations. *Int. J. Acupunct. Electrother. Res. 18*, 195–205.
11. Scherder, E., Bouma, A., & Steen, L. (1992). Influence of transcutaneous electrical nerve stimulation on memory in patients with dementia of the Alzheimer type. *J. Clin. Exp. Neuropsychol. 14*, 951–960.
12. Kanno, T., Karmel, Y., & Yokoyama, T. (1989). Effects of dorsal spinal cord stimulation (DCS) on reversibility of neuronal function – experience of treatment for vegetative states. *Pace 12*, 733–738.
13. FDA (1975). *Food and Drug Administration guidelines for electromedical devices*. Washington, DC: FDA.

14. Nelson, R., Hayes, K. & Currier, D. (Eds.) (1999). *Clinical electrotherapy.* Stamford, CT: Appleton & Lange.
15. Focus (1999). *Focus instruction manual.* St. Paul, MN: Empi, Inc.
16. Robinson, C., Kett, N., & Bolam, J. (1988). Spasticity in spinal cord injured patients: 1. Short-term effects of surface electrical stimulation. *Arch. Phys. Med. Rehab. 69,* 598–604.
17. FDA (1982). *Food and Drug Administration compliance policy guidelines.* Guide No. 7124.26. Washington, DC: FDA.
18. Peri, C., Shaffrey, M., Farace, E., Cooper, E., Cooper, B., & Jane, J. (2001). Pilot study of electrical stimulation on median nerve in comatose severe brain injured patients: 3-month outcome. *Brain Inj., 15,* 903–910.
19. NIH (1998). Rehabilitation of persons with traumatic brain injury. *NIH Consensus Statement, 16,* 1–29.
20. Alfieri, V. (1982). Electrical treatment of spasticity. *Scand. J. Rehab. Med. 14,* 177–182.
21. Greenberg, R., Newton, P., Hyatt, M., Narayan, R., & Becker, D. (1981). Prognostic implications of early multimodality evoked potentials in severely head-injured patients. *J. Neurosurg., 55,* 227–236.
22. Pfurtscheller, G., Schwarz, G., & List, W. (1986). Long-lasting EEG reactions in comatose patients after repetitive stimulation. *Electroencephalog. Clin. Neurophysiol. 64,* 402–410.
23. Kanno, T., Kamei, Y., & Yokoyama, T. (1992). Treating the vegetative state with dorsal column stimulation. *Soc. Treatm. Coma, 1,* 67–75.
24. Kanno, T. (1995). Dorsal column stimulation for the persistent vegetative state. University of Virginia neurosurgery lecture (unpublished).
25. Cooper, E., Cooper, J., Alves, W., & Jane, J. (1996). Right median nerve electrical stimulation of comatose patients. *Society for Treatment of Coma, 5,* (unpublished Keynote address).
26. Yokoyama, T., Kamei, T., & Kanno, T. (1996). Right median nerve stimulation for comatose patients. *Soc. Treatm. Coma, 5,* 117–125.
27. Yamamoto, K., Sugita, S., Ishikowa, K., Morimitsu, H., Shimamoto, H., & Shigemori, M. (1997). A case of persistent vegetative state treated with median nerve stimulation. *Soc. Treatm. Coma, 6,* 117–121.
28. Hayashi, N. (1997). Prevention of vegetation after severe head trauma and stroke by combination therapy of cerebral hypothermia and activation of immune-dopaminergic nervous system. *Soc. Treatm. Coma, 6,* 133–147.
29. Moriya, T., Hayashi, N., Sakurai, A., et al. (1998). New therapeutic strategies for patients with unconscious and neurological deficits in acute stage with median nerve stimulation. *Soc. Treatm. Coma, 7,* 65–67.
30. Moriya, T., Hayashi, N., Utagawa, A., et al. (1999). Median nerve stimulation method for severe brain damage, with its clinical improvement. *Soc. Treatm. Coma, 8,* 111–114.
31. Kanno, T. (2000). Development of surgical neurorehabilitation. *Soc. Treatm. Coma, 9,* 23–24.
32. Hirata, Y., & Ushio, U. (2000). A case of successful treatment by median nerve stimulation for prolonged moderate consciousness disturbance in the chronic phase following subarachnoid hemorrhage. *Soc. Treatm. Coma, 9,* 85–89.
33. Moriya, T., Hayashi, N., Sakurai, A., Utagawa, A., Kobayashi, Y., Yajima, K.,

et al. (2000). Usefulness of median nerve stimulation in patients with severe traumatic brain injury determined on the basis of changes in cerebrospinal fluid dopamine. *Soc. Treatm. Coma, 9*, 159–161.

34. Okuma, I., Kaitou, T., Hayashi, J., Funahashi, M., & Kanno, T. (2001). Electrical stimulation therapy for prolonged consciousness disturbance. *Soc. Treatm. Coma, 10*, 67–71.

35. Spiegel, J., Tintera, J., Gawehn, J., Stoeter, P., & Treede, R. (1999). Functional MRI of human primary somatosensory and motor cortex during median nerve stimulation. *Clin. Neurophysiol. 110*, 47–52.

36. Golaszewski, S., Kremser, C., Wagner, M., Felber, S., Aichner, F., & Dimitrijevic, M. (1998). Functional magnetic resonance imaging of the human motor cortex before and after whole-hand afferent electrical stimulation. *Scand. J. Rehab. Med. 31*, 165–173.

37. Yousry, T., Schmid, U., Jassoy, A., et al. (1995). Topography of the cortical motor hand area: prospective study with functional MR imaging and direct motor mapping at surgery. *Radiology, 195*, 23–29.

38. Silva, A., Lee, S., Iadecola, C., Kim, S., et al. (2000). Early temporal characteristics of cerebral blood flow and deoxyhemoglobin changes during somatosensory stimulation. *J. Cerebr. Blood Flow Metab. 20*, 201–206.

39. Teasdale, G., & Jennett, B. (1974). Assessment of coma and impaired consciousness, a practice scale. *Lancet, 2*, 81–84.

40. Pazzaglia, P., Frank, G., Frank, F., Gaist, G., et al. (1975). Clinical course and prognosis of acute post-traumatic coma. *J. Neurol. Neurosurg. Psychiat. 38*, 149–154.

41. Narayan, R., Greenberg, R., Miller, J., et al. (1981). Improved confidence of outcome prediction in severe head injury. *J. Neurosurg. 54*, 751–762.

42. Jane, J., & Rimel, R. (1982). Prognosis in head injury. *Clin. Neurosurg., 29*, 346–352.

43. Marshall, L., Becker, D., Bowers, S., et al. (1983). The National Traumatic Coma Data Bank – design, purpose, goals, and results. *J. Neurosurg., 59*, 276–284.

44. Toutant, S., Klauber, M., Marshall, L., et al. (1984). Absent or compressed basal cisterns on first CT scan: ominous predictors of outcome in severe head injury. *J. Neurosurg., 61*, 691–694.

45. Alberico, A. (1987). Outcome after severe head injury. *J. Neurosurg., 67*, 648–656.

46. Marshall, L. (1988). The role of aggressive therapy for head injury: does it matter? *Clin. Neurosurg., 34*, 549–559.

47. Eisenberg, H., Frankowski, R., Contant, C., et al. (1988). High-dose barbiturate control of elevated intracranial pressure in patients with severe head injury. *J. Neurosurg., 69*, 15–23.

48. Sahuguillo, J., Vilalta, J., Lamarca, J., Rubio, E., Rodriquez-Pazos, M., & Salva, J. (1989). Diffuse axonal injury after severe head trauma. *Acta Neurochirurg. 101*, 149–158.

49. Eisenberg, H., Jane, J., Marmarou, A., et al. (1990). Initial CT findings in 753 patients with severe head injury. NIH Traumatic Coma Data Bank Report. *J. Neurosurg., 73*, 688–698.

50. Levin, H., Eisenberg, H., Jane, J., et al. (1990). Neurobehavioral outcome 1 year after severe head injury. *J. Neurosurg., 73*, 699–709.

51. Marshall, L., Eisenberg, H., Jane, J., et al. (1991). A new classification of head injury based on computerized tomography. *J. Neurosurg., 75*, S14–S20.
52. Waxman, K., Sundine, M., & Young, R. (1991). Is early prediction of outcome in severe head injury possible? *Arch. Surg. 126*, 1237–1242.
53. Marshall, L., Gautille, T., Klauber, M., et al. (1991). The outcome of severe closed head injury. *J. Neurosurg., 75*, S28–S36.
54. Dacey, R., Dikmen, S., Temkin, N., McLean, A., Armsden, G., & Winn, H. (1991). Relative effects of brain and non-brain injuries on neuropsychological and psychosocial outcome. *J. Trauma, 31*, 217–222.
55. Kido, D., Cox, C., Hamill, R., Rothenberg, B., & Woolf, P. (1992). Traumatic brain injuries: predictive usefulness of CT. *Radiology, 182*, 777–781.
56. Levin, H., Jane, J., Marmarou, A., et al. (1992). Severe head injury in children: Experience of the Traumatic Coma Data Bank. *Neurosurgery, 31*, 435–444.
57. Choi, S., & Barnes, T. (1996). Predicting outcome in the head-injured patient. In R. K. Narayan, J. E. Wilberger, and J. T. Povlishock (Eds.), *Neurotrauma* (pp. 779–792). New York: McGraw-Hill.
58. Gruen, J., & Weiss, M. (1996). Management of complicated neurologic injuries. *Surg. Clin. N. Am., 76*, 905–922.
59. Baltas, I., Gerogiannis, N., Sakellariou, P., Matamis, D., Prassas, A., & Fylaktakis, M. (1998). Outcome in severely head injured patients with and without multiple trauma. *J. Neurosurg. Sci. 42*, 85–88.
60. Bullock, R., Chesnut, R., Clifton, G., et al. (1996). Guidelines for the management of severe head injury. *J. Neurotrauma, 13*, 639–734.
61. Marion, D. (1999). Management of traumatic brain injury: past, present and future. *Clin. Neurosurg., 45*, 184–191.
62. Letarte, P. (1999). Neurotrauma care in the new millennium. *Surg. Clin. N. Am., 79*, 1449–1470.
63. Capruso, D., & Levin, S. (1996). Neurobehavioral outcome of head trauma. In R. Evans (Ed.), *Neurology and trauma* (pp. 201–221). Philadelphia, PA: W. B. Saunders.
64. Marshall, F., & Marshall, S. (1996). Outcome prediction in severe head injury. In R. Wilkins and S. Rengachary (Eds.), *Neurosurgery* (pp. 2717–2722). New York: McGraw-Hill.
65. Parent, A. (1996). Pons. In *Carpenter's Human Neuroanatomy* (pp. 469–526). Media, PA: Williams & Wilkins.
66. Parent, A. (1996). Limbic system. In *Carpenter's Human Neuroanatomy* (pp. 744–794). Media, PA: Williams & Wilkins.
67. Montgomery, G. (1989). The mind in motion. *Discover, 10*, 58–68.
68. Hamilton, G., & Cooper, E. (1987). *Functional electrical stimulation (FES) in paralytic hand musculature.* Proceedings of the Tenth International World Confederation of Physical Therapy.
69. Han, D. (1992). The voice operated electrical stimulation system. *The Proceedings of the Johns Hopkins National Search for Computing Applications to Assist Persons with Disabilities.* Baltimore, MD: Johns Hopkins.
70. Haines, D. (2000). *Neuroanatomy: An atlas of structures, sections, and systems* (5th ed.). Philadelphia, PA: Lippincott, Williams & Wilkins.
71. Parent, A. (1996). Medulla. In *Carpenter's human neuroanatomy* (pp. 421–468). Media, PA: Williams & Wilkins.
72. Turner, D. (1996). Neurological evaluation of a patient with head trauma: coma

scales. In R. Wilkins and S. Rengachary (Eds.), *Neurosurgery* (pp. 2667–2674). New York: McGraw-Hill.

73. Kaye, A. (1991). *Essential neurosurgery*. New York: Churchill Livingstone.
74. Jennett, B., & Bond, M. (1975). Assessment of outcome after severe brain damage. *Lancet, 1*, 480–484.
75. Whyte, J., & Rosenthal, M. (1999). Rehabilitation of the patient with traumatic brain injury. In J. DeLisa (Ed.), *Rehabilitation medicine*. Philadelphia, PA: Lippincott.
76. Servadei, F., Murray, G., Penny, K., et al. (2000). The value of the "worst" computed tomographic scan in clinical studies of moderate and severe head injury. European Brain Injury Consortium. *Neurosurgery, 46*, 70–75.
77. Cooper, I., Amin, I., Upton, A., et al. (1977). Safety and efficacy of chronic stimulation. *Neurosurgery, 2*, 203–205.
78. Robertson, I., & Murre, J. (1999). Rehabilitation of brain damage: brain plasticity and principles of guided recovery. *APA Psychol. Bull., 125*, 544–575.
79. Seitz, R., Huang, Y., Knorr, U., Tellmann, L., Herzog, H., & Freund, H. (1955). Large-scale plasticity of the human motor cortex. *Clin. Neurosci. Neuropathol. 6*, 742–744.
80. Grady, M., Jane, J., & Steward, O. (1989). Synaptic reorganization within the human central nervous system following injury. *J. Neurosurg., 71*, 534–537.
81. Walser, H. (1986). Somatosensory evoked potentials in comatose patients: correlation with outcome and neuropathological findings. *J. Neurol., 233*, 34.
82. Shakespeare, W. (1980). *The complete works of William Shakespeare*. London: Cambridge University Press.

6   Low-level responsive states

José León-Carrión, María del Rosario Domínguez-Morales, and José María Domínguez-Roldán

Coma

The term coma is used to refer to patients whose eyes are permanently closed and who cannot be awakened nor are in a functioning state.[1] According to Zasler,[2] coma is a state in which there is no meaningful response. Comatose patients normally maintain their eyes closed without evidence of opening spontaneously or to external stimuli, do not follow instructions, do not show goal-directed or voluntary conduct, do not speak and cannot sustain looking or tracking movements of more than a 45° angle. Excluded are secondary neurobehavioral signs and symptoms in coma that have been treated pharmacologically with sedatives. The definition of coma in terms of cerebral functioning refers to a state of acute brain failure not strictly related to any particular cerebral substratum or specific anatomical level of lesion. Coma normally occurs when broad areas in the upper and lower brain stems, or cerebral hemispheres, or simultaneously in the cerebral hemispheres and brain stem are damaged. The most frequent causes of coma are diffuse axonal pathology, hypoxia and secondary lesions which affect the brainstem (Figures 6.1, 6.2, 6.3, 6.4).

A special situation is deep coma induced by barbituates or iatrogenically induced which can happen during an intent to protect the brain from secondary injury while the patient is in an intensive care unit. In such cases, doctors cannot evaluate the neurological integrity of the patient with the usual techniques and methods because the brainstem reflexes disappear and the EEG is isoelectric. Thus therapy decisions are based on changes produced when monitoring intercranial pressure. A study by Schalén et al.[3] reported the clinical outcome of 38 patients with severe head trauma (post-traumatic coma for 6 hours or more) treated with barbiturate coma because of intracranial hypertension. Eighteen patients died, four patients remained in a severely disabled or chronic vegetative state, and sixteen patients reached levels of good recovery/moderate disability. Six of these patients returned to work or school full-time, four half-time and three were in a rehabilitation program. Fourteen patients were assessed by neuropsychologists: all patients except one exhibited varying degrees of cognitive dysfunction and six patients

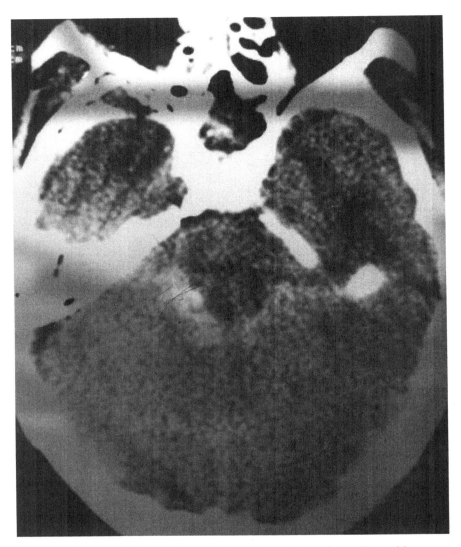

Figure 6.1 Computerized axial tomography at admission of a patient with severe traumatic brain injury showing an intense subarachnoid hemorrhage in the quadrigeminal cistern with the focal point of bleeding found in the posterior mesencephalon. These lesions are compatible with a severe diffuse axonal lesion.

had signs of personality changes. The quality of life for the majority of the surviving patients was relatively good. The author also found that the effects of barbiturate coma therapy in the age groups over 40 appeared to be limited.

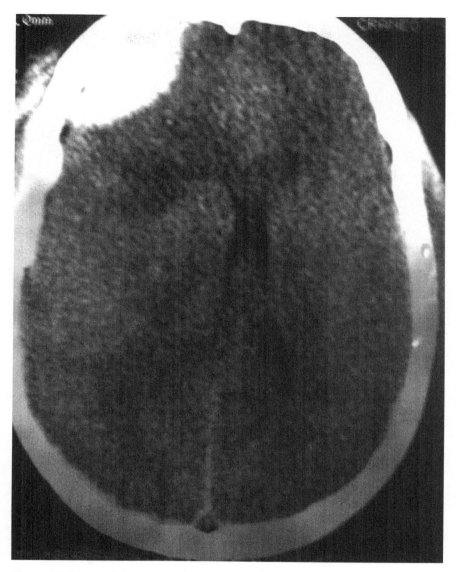

Figure 6.2 Image of the same patient in whom a frontal epidural hematoma, which was surgically evacuated, also has a lesion in the right putamen. These lesions are compatible with a severe diffuse axonal lesion.

Clinical evaluation of the integrity of the motor and sensory systems of comatose patients is a difficult task and, at times, the diagnostic value of techniques which evaluate brain injury is relative. There are times when we cannot find any morphological substratum which is clearly responsible for the

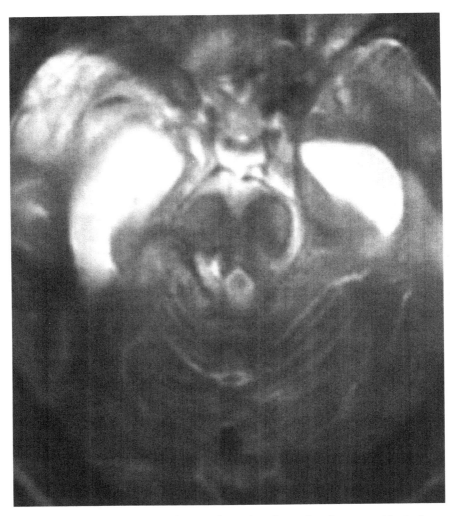

Figure 6.3 Magnetic resonance image of a patient 2 months after an accident, showing an image in T2 of the right side of the mesencephalon, compatible with
a diffuse axonal lesion.

state of coma. We can even observe deterioration or improvement without
there being any apparent structural cerebral changes. The Glasgow Coma
Scale (GCS) is the most widely accepted clinical instrument for evaluating
the depth of coma in an acute post-critical state, although it is not useful
in prolonged coma or in the vegetative state. According to Jennett and
Dyer,[4] diagnosing coma depends a great deal on the skill and expertise of
the specialist in his or her observations since current neuroimaging
methods, as well as computerized tomography, magnetic resonance imaging,

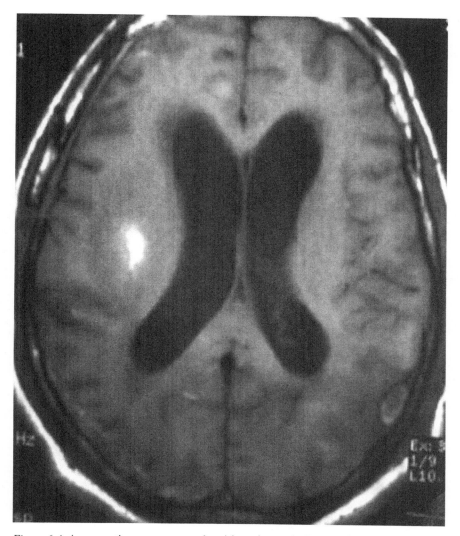

Figure 6.4 A magnetic resonance study with an image in T1 showing the right putamen compatible with a severe diffuse axonal lesion. The patient was in a
low-level response state 1 year after the accident.

electroencephalography, etc., which are normally of help, do not work in
some cases. In Table 6.1 we can observe the items making up this scale.

The Glasgow Coma Scale[5,6] allows precise, objective evaluation of patterns of conduct in three categories of response: stimulation required to bring
about opening of the eyes, quality and type of verbal response and obtaining
the best motor response. The scoring of a patient can vary from 3 to 15
points. The lower the score, the more profound the coma. A score below 9 is

Table 6.1 Glasgow Coma Scale (GCS) after age 4

	Points
Eye opening	
Spontaneously	4
Verbal commands	3
From pain	2
No response	1
Better motor response	
Obeys verbal commands	6
Locates pain	5
Withdrawn	4
Abnormal flexion	3
Pronation/extension	2
No response	1
Better verbal response	
Oriented response	5
Disoriented response	4
Inappropriate words	3
Uncomprehensible sounds	2
No response	1
Total GCS	3–15

Table 6.2 Glasgow Coma Scale and percentage of survival in each interval of points. Percentages have been noted and averaged by Nagib et al.[10] and Aldrich et al.[11]

GCS scoring	3–5	6–8	9–12	13–15
Survival (%)	4	51	84	87

considered severe brain injury; between 3 and 5 is very severe and profound coma. A score between 9 and 13 is considered moderate brain injury without being in coma; 14 or 15 is mild brain injury. To determine if a patient has come out of coma, the scale should be administered at different times to see the variety in the scores. When the person recovers consciousness, the Glasgow Coma Scale should be discontinued. A few considerations should be taken into account when interpreting some patients' scores obtained from the Glascow Coma Scale, especially when predicting evolution after cardio-respiratory arrest with ischemic-anoxic encephalopathy. Mullie and colleagues[7] recommend certain precautions with patients who are under the effects of strong sedation and/or who have metabolic encephalopathy.

Intensive care units equipped with the most modern techniques, although rather invasive, facilitate survival for the majority of patients with traumatic brain injury (see Table 6.2). The probability of death varies between 9% and 35% while a patient is in the ICU, depending on the pathology. The death rate in the ICU has fallen considerably in the past decades. This achievement, which still holds true at present, poses new challenges not only from the scientific point of view but the attention to, and care of, patients as well. Survivors of traumatic brain injury who emerge from a state of coma often have marked neurocognitive, behavioral, affective and social deficits.[8] Many of them remain in coma for an undetermined length of time. All of them need specialized care. The Traumatic Coma Data Bank showed a 5% incidence of persistent vegetative state after brain trauma due to severe brain injury after 6 months.[9] There is a notable variety of outcomes for these patients, but few of them manage to gain more independence.[1]

The most frequently asked questions to professionals in the field of traumatic brain injury are those to do with outcome of the survivor. The questions refer to the patient's recovery. The answer is not totally clear, but we can provide some considerations. Some studies suggest that outcome is closely related to the type of lesion the patient has. Recovery of consciousness after a prolonged period of coma is strange, although some cases have been reported in the scientific literature. Tanhenco and Kaplan.[12] reported a head trauma patient, comatose for 6 years in a nursing home, who began to respond to her environment and to the rehabilitation program she underwent after regaining conciousness. Speech and psychological functions improved considerably after 9 months of training and, after 14 months of intensive rehabilitation and family teaching, the patient was able to live at home with her family.

Outcome in a group of 31 patients who were comatose for more than 24 hours after cardiopulmonary arrest was studied by Groswasser et al.[13] They found that 17 regained functional ambulation, 20 regained oral communication and 13 regained full independence in activities of daily living. Two regained their approximate previous cognitive level, and one regained his previous level of employment. These results demonstrate that these outcomes are strikingly inferior to those of patients with prolonged coma after traumatic brain injury who were hospitalized in the same center during the same period. Both age and coma duration were correlated with outcome. The relatively better outcomes were seen in patients who were 25 years old or younger at the time of anoxic injury, and whose coma lasted less than 24 hours. In Table 6.3, some considerations about outcome are shown in regard to anoxic brain injury.

A retrospective study of 134 patients in prolonged coma (coma > 1 month) as a consequence of brain injury was carried out by Sazbon and Groswasser.[14]

Table 6.3 Outcome for lesions produced by cerebral anoxia

- High probability of persistent vegetative state if it lasts more than 3 months
- Relatively better outcome if the patient is under age 40 years
- High rate of survival
- Very poor outcome if there is absence of photomotor reflex 6–24 h after onset of coma
- Poor outcome if there is hypoglycemia at admission

Outcome values were established at simple baseline parameters: signs of damage to the hypothalamus, abnormal motor reactivity, manifestations of general character, epilepsy and hydrocephaly (Table 6.4).

For Bates[15] it is certain that clinical signs, especially brainstem response and motor and verbal response, are the most useful and valid predictors. However, even the most exact clinical predictors are not sufficient for avoiding 5% false positives and, therefore, although exam results are valid for informing professionals and family members about the patients, they should not be used without therapy when making decisions. In the future, identification of patients for whom it would be reasonable to consider using neurorestorative medicine and therapy could be useful, but at present they cannot be considered criteria for removing the supports that sustain a patient's life.

Table 6.4 Parameters of poor prognosis in patients in prolonged state of coma (Sazbon & Groswasser, 1990)

Characteristics	n	Group with recovery		Group without recovery		Significance
		n	%	n	%	
No. of cases	72					
Acute phase						
Signs of hypothalamic damage						
Fever of central origin	28	16/54	29.6	12/21	57.1	$p < 0.03$
Diffuse body perspiration	14	7/44	15.9	7/13	53.8	$p < 0.005$
Abnormal secretion of ADH	16	5/72	6.9	11/58	18.9	$p < 0.04$
Motor reactivity						
Normal motor reactivity	4	–	–	4/4	100.0	
Abnormal motor reactivity	95					$p < 0.002$
No answer	13	1/13	7.7	12/13	92.3	
Decerebrate	67	33/67	49.3	34/67	50.7	
Decorticate	15	11/15	73.3	4/15	26.7	
General manifestations						
Respiratory disorders	76	38/70	54.3	38/55	69.1	$p < 0.04$
Associated damage	79	36/72	50.0	43/62	69.4	$p < 0.03$
Late phase						
Epilepsy	40	12/66	18.2	28/57	49.1	$p < 0.001$
Hydrocephalus	54	17/62	27.4	37/43	86.1	$p < 0.001$

ADH, antidiuretic hormone. The significance was measured by the χ^2 test.

Coma stimulation programs

In the 1980s, the use of sensory stimulation for coma was popular but there were many discrepancies among professionals about its efficacy. Recently, Lombardi et al.[16] searched the Injuries Group specialized register, the Cochrane Controlled Trials Register, from 1966 to January 2002. They compared sensory stimulation programs with standard rehabilitation in patients in coma or vegetative states. Their systematic review indicated that there is not reliable evidence to support, or rule out, the effectiveness of multisensory programmes in patients in coma or vegetative states. The same conclusion was reached by Pierce et al.[17] They were unable to find any evidence that coma arousal, for all its arduous patient contact, had a markedly better outcome compared to conventional treatment.

However, Wood et al.[18] made a controlled pilot study based on a sensory regulation model. The study contrasted the outcome of four patients treated in a sensory-regulated environment with four who were exposed to sensory stimulation of an unregulated kind. The results obtained are, for the authors, quite encouraging in favor of a sensory regulation approach. In the same way, Mitchell and colleagues[19] report on the efficacy of a "coma arousal procedure". The procedure involved a program of vigorous sensory stimulation administered to comatose patients by relatives using Comakits. The coma arousal procedure was applied to an experimental group of patients with severe brain injury and results were compared to those obtained by a matched control group who did not receive the procedure. Total duration of coma and weekly Glasgow Coma Scores were recorded for the two groups. Their results indicate that the total duration of coma was significantly shorter and that coma lightened more rapidly for the group receiving the procedure. Other authors[20] recommend that coma stimulation programs should be individualized and that families should be encouraged to participate even while the patient is in the intensive care unit. Helwick said that "recovery from coma is often long and tedious, but with the use of a coma stimulation program, there is hope for recovery from coma".[20]

An interesting study was carried out by Mazaux et al.[21] They reviewed some aspects of early rehabilitation and illustrated their discussion with data from 876 French TBI patients admitted over the course of 1 year at 18 rehabilitation units. They found that preservation of vital functions follows standardized protocols, but rehabilitation is more controversial. Few controlled trials are available. There is agreement among clinicians about the prevention of orthopedic complications and treatment of spasticity. However, there is not much consensus about treatment of non-pyramidal hypertonia and spasms or about procedures that can be undertaken to improve arousal from a coma or vegetative state. Bernard et al.[22] studied 77 patients with cardiac arrest who were randomly assigned to treatment with hypothermia: core body temperature reduced to 33 °C within 2 h after the return of spontaneous circulation and maintained at that temperature for 12 h, or normothermia. They concluded that treatment with moderate hypothermia appears to improve outcomes in patients with coma after resuscitation from out-of-hospital cardiac arrest.

The changes of vegetative parameters and behavioral assessment in comatose patients after severe brain injury were evaluated by Lippert-Grüner et al.[23] during the Multimodal-Early-Onset-Stimulation (MEOS) early rehabilitation. They found two significant vegetative parameter changes: heart and respiratory frequencies. Stimulation of tactile and acustic senses resulted mainly in mimical head and eye movements. When they followed up 14 patients, they found that one remained in a vegetative state, two exhibited severe neurological/neuropsychological deficits, depending on care, six sustained major functional deficits, three were able to perform the tasks of daily life, and two returned to their former jobs. The authors concluded by indicating that stimulation therapy should be based on close observation of behavior patterns and, at least in deep coma stages, involve the registration of vegetative parameters. It may be sensitive to identify parameters predicting a favorable or unfavorable outcome. They suggest that the absence of any response to external stimuli is indicative of unfavorable outcome.

Sequelae after coma

Normally, patients who emerge from coma suffer cognitive and motor dysfunctions[24] such as aphasia, executive dysfunction, memory disorders, attentional deficits, orientation problems, etc. This situation interferes with the normal course of treatment. The most serious physical problems patients may have are fractures, flaccidity or spasticity, heterotopic ossification, etc. The severity of the clinical picture depends on various factors: place and quantity of the lesioned area, duration of coma, depth of coma and duration of post-traumatic amnesia (PTA). Having been in prolonged comas does not mean that patients cannot or should not be given rehabilitation treatment as soon as possible or that they are not going to improve. Different studies show good rehabilitation outcome in patients awakened from prolonged coma when comprehensive, holistic, intensive, and multidisciplinary programs are performed.[25,26] Cohadon and Richer[27] found that functional outcome is not related to the depth of initial coma but rather to the length of the comatose period. A study by Johnstone and Bouman[28] report a case of near-drowning (5–15 min of anoxia) followed by 15 h of coma. After regaining consciousness, the patient had an absence of neuropsychological and neurological deficits 3.5 months post-injury. The authors suggest that anoxic encephalopathy does not automatically result in neurological or cognitive impairment.

The early clinical stages of recovery of consciousness after coma were studied in 48 selected patients by Van de Kelft et al.[29] They confirm the classical clinical sequence of arousal and recovery of consciousness characterized by consecutive appearance of stimulated opening of the eyes, the blink reflex, opening of the eyes, localizing pain, and obeying commands. When the appearance of stimulated eye opening and blink reflex are considered separately, they found a significant difference, suggesting different structural and functional brain recovery processes.

A study carried out by Ross et al.[30] indicated that both coma length and the presence of focal abnormalities on computer tomography scans contribute independently to neuropsychological outcome. They found that the effects of coma length are stronger than the effects of focal abnormalities evident in CT scans and continue to exert a stronger influence on neuropsychological outcome over the year post-injury. These results suggest to the author that the extent of diffuse pathology may be a more important determinant of long-term behavioral outcome than the presence of focal lesions. In predicting the recovery of equilibrium and protective reactions both at 3 and 6 months post-injury, Macpherson et al.[31] found that coma duration followed by age contributed significantly to the predictive capability. In another study by Stover and Zeiger,[32] residual impairments and mortality were assessed in 48 patients under 20 years of age at least 2 years after a severe traumatic brain injury had caused coma lasting more than 7 days. They concluded that the prognosis for recovery in this age group is much better than expected after severe brain injury and that rehabilitation medicine needs to be involved in patient care during the period of coma to prevent contractures and other complications which often interfere with and delay later rehabilitation.

Persistent vegetative state

In Europe, the term "coma vigile" as a synonym for vegetative state has been used for many years as a diagnostic term referring to patients whose eyes are open but do not respond to any kind of stimulation, nor exhibit any type of spontaneous behavior after a certain time in coma.[33] According to Jennett,[34] it is an old French term describing some patients with typhoid fever or severe typhus, but this author suggests that the term does not adequately describe the vegetative state. In order to diagnose persistent vegetative state (see Table 6.5), it is necessary for the patient to have been at least 12 months in coma after first opening his or her eyes. The vegetative state is a term proposed by Jennett and Plum in 1972[24] which describes patients who return to wakefulness with a total lack of cognitive functioning after severe brain injury. These patients open their eyes in response to sounds, they maintain respiration and normal cardiocirculatory activity as well as autonomous or preserved vegetative functions. The majority of these patients have normal brainstem functions (pupillary activity, ocular response, chewing, swallowing, breathing and control of circulation), although EEG studies reveal diverse patterns from isoelectric EEGs to distinct models of rhythm and extent. In a study made by Zeithofer and colleagues,[35] no correlations were found between results of evoked potentials and clinical state. Evoked potential measurements of vegetative patients allowed no prognosis. Authors said

Table 6.5 Criteria for vegetative state of the American Neurological Association Committee on Ethical Affairs (1993)

- Reflex or spontaneous eye opening. No evidence of awareness of self or surroundings
- Not the slightest communication between examiner and patient. No following of visual stimuli, although visual tracking can occasionally occur. No emotional response
- No comprehensive speech or mouthing of words
- Smiling, frowning, and crying may inconsistently appear
- There are sleep–wake cycles
- Brainstem and spinal reflex activity are variable. Primitive reflexes (sucking, rooting, chewing and swallowing) may be preserved. Pupillary reactivity to light, oculocephalic reflexes, grasp reflexes and tendon reflexes may also be present
- The presence of voluntary movements and behavior, no matter how rudimentary, is a sign of cognition and is not compatible with the diagnosis of persistent vegetative state. There is no motor activity suggesting learned behavior and no mimicry. Rudimentary movements (such as withdrawal or posturing) may be seen with noxious or disagreeable stimuli
- Blood pressure control and cardiorespiratory functions usually are intact. Incontinence of bladder and bowel

that evoked potentials are an important prognostic factor after severe brain injury, but have no value for the prognosis of vegetative or apallic patients.

The apallic syndrome, an old term describing consequences of diffuse bilateral degeneration of the brain cortex, has been identified on occasion as a synonym for vegetative state since the concept includes patients with absence of neocortical function but that have brainstem functions relatively intact. It was initially described in patients with ischemic-anoxic encephalopathy and encephalitis.

According to Andrews,[36] physicians facing long-term care of patients in vegetative state are confronted with various problems. They have to decide if withdrawal of tube feeding is an appropriate form of management, what the clinical advantages are, at what level of awareness can a patient be said to have a quality of life, and who should determine a patient's right to die. They conclude that these problems are determined more by social, legal, emotional, cultural, religious, and economic forces than by clinical facts. Jennett[37] wrote:

It is clear that the majority of those questioned support the withdrawal of life-prolonging treatment from permanently vegetative patients, and indeed this has been sanctioned by many institutional statements and supported by many courts of law, as well as by most comments in the media. Certainly most people in several countries appear to consider that indefinite survival in the vegetative state is worse than death.

Medication of patients in vegetative states

Some studies have reported that medication can help vegetative patients recover consciousness. The effects of multidisciplinary rehabilitation interventions and use of *bromocriptine* on outcome in patients with traumatic brain injury-vegetative state (TBI-VS) was studied by Passler and Riggs[38] in a retrospective review of clinical cases. They found that bromocriptine administration, systematic neuropsychological testing, sensory stimulation, a comprehensive rehabilitation program or a combination of these treatments may enhance functional recovery in the TBI-VS patient group. Kaelin et al.[39] found that the use of *methylphenidate* in acutely brain-injured adults is well tolerated and they demonstrated that there was a significant improvement in attention compared to natural recovery in a rehabilitation setting. Methylphenidate also correlates with faster functional recovery as measured by the Disability Rating Scale, although the improvement did not achieve statistical significance. The use of *Sinemet* has also been attempted but results are not yet clear.[40] However, Haig and Ruess[41] recommended the use of Sinemet because of the relative small risk of side-effects. They presented a case of a 24-year-old man with TBI who remained unresponsive to commands and unchanged for 6 months despite periodic aggressive therapy. Within days of beginning Sinemet, the patient became conversant and responsive. They argued that the reported low likelihood of spontaneous recovery of cognition in patients who are vegetative for 6 months suggests that Sinemet was responsible for this patient's recovery. Meythaler et al.,[42] using amantadine 200 mg, studied 35 subjects sustaining TBI who were initially seen with a Glasgow Coma Scale score of 10 or less within the first 24 h after admission in a randomly double-blind, placebo-controlled, crossover design trial. They found that there was a consistent trend toward a more rapid functional improvement regardless of when a patient with diffuse axonal injury-associated TBI was started on amantadine in the first 3 months after injury. The toxic effect of amantadine (coma, psychosis, death, cardivascular problems) is a particular problem in patients with renal insufficiency because 90% of an oral dose is excreted unchanged in the urine.[43] No significant difference for amantadine versus placebo was found by Schneider et al.[44] in 10 TBI adult patients in an acute brain injury rehabilitation unit.

Prognosis of vegetative states

Coma and vegetative state follow traumatic brain injury in about 1/8 patients, and the prognosis is worse in patients with non-traumatic brain injury. The most frequent causes of persistent vegetative state are brain trauma, cerebrovascular disorders, brain tumors, ischemic-anoxic encephalitis and other disorders. In general, the patients who remain in a persistent vegetative state for more than 1 year survive many more. Minderhound and Braakman[45] found that 58% survive more than 3 years, 34% more than 6 years, and 22%

more than 8 years. Normally, those who survive a long time and are able to improve their level of consciousness usually remain severely incapacitated.[1] Approximately 10% of the patients who have had severe brain trauma (TBI) are released from hospital in a vegetative state characterized by the total absence of cognitive interaction with the environment. Zasler[2] wrote:

> In general, it has been my philosophy to endorse a time frame of 1 year for traumatic and 3 months for hypoxic-ischemic brain injury for prognostic purposes relative to determining that emergence from vegetative state is statistically highly unlikely. Such a determination should only occur after an adequate period of extended patient observation and sufficient neuromedical assessment to rule out treatable conditions potentially affecting ongoing neural and functional recovery.

A retrospective review of 43 cases of patients with PVS was made by Andrews.[46] He found that 11 of these patients regained awareness 4 months or more after suffering brain injury. First report of eye tracking was between 4 months and 3 years, and the first response to command was between 4 and 12 months. Only one patient was eventually unable to communicate, six used non-verbal methods for communicating at least yes or no, and four patients were able to speak. Six patients remained totally dependent for daily living activities and two became independent. For feeding, four became independent, three required help and four remained on gastrostomy feeding. The author concluded that some patients can regain awareness after more than 4 months in a vegetative state and, although few reach full independence, most can achieve an improved quality of life within the limitations of their disabilities. The recovery period is prolonged and may continue for several years. He recommends that even patients with profound brain damage should have the opportunity of a specialized rehabilitation program. Regarding communication, Najeson and colleagues[47] found that communicative recovery began as late as 5.7 months after injury, and roughly paralleled recovery in locomotion and activities of daily living. Restlessness and sweating were favorable prognostic factors: excessive salivation, snout reflex, corneomandibular reflex, retractory nistagmus, and stereotypic movements were unfavorable.

Another interesting study was carried out by Heindl and Laub.[48] They studied the outcome of 127 children and adolescents who were in PVS more than 30 days after a traumatic ($n = 82$) or hypoxic ($n = 45$) brain injury. They followed up the patients for 19 months. At that time, they found that 84% of the patients with TBI and only 55% of the patients with hypoxia had left persistent vegetative state ($p < 0.001$). The patients with TBI regained consciousness earlier. If it was later than 9 months post-trauma, less than 5% of the patients in both groups left PVS. Patients sustaining hypoxic brain injury had a higher incidence of seizures ($p < 0.01$) and a higher seizure frequency, and also had significantly more complications (pneumonia, gastrointestinal disturbances, heterotopic ossification). Post-traumatic hyperthermia and autonomic dysfunction correlated with worse outcome in the TBI group, but not in the anoxic group. Of patients with TBI, 16% became independent in everyday life versus only 4% with anoxia. Authors concluded by underlining the important contribution of hypoxia in severe and permanent brain impairment and in establishing a prognosis for people in PVS.

The quality of life of patients in a vegetative state depends on the care that is given to them since most are sent home where they should continue to be cared for normally by family members. Not all families have the capacity to assist a patient with these characteristics. On the other hand, the cost of attention to these patients at home is elevated and not all families have such economic resources, have received compensation in accord with new necessities, or have had costs of care giving taken care of by insurance. In general, an additional 25% of patients hospitalized with severe TBI recover consciousness with sequelae that make them dependent on others for daily activities. Taken as a whole, approximately one-third of the patients who have survived severe TBI live in precarious conditions. It seems that 10% of these patients are able to recover consciousness within 5 years of the trauma, 25% survive more than 5 years, and over 48% more than 10 years. The main causes of death in patients in persistent vegetative states are respiratory infections (around 50%) and heart failure (30%). Although, according to Zasler:[2]

> Any cases of late emergence from the vegetative state, that is more than one year following trauma or 3 months following hypoxic-ischemic insult, from vegetative state should without a doubt be reported in peer-reviewed scientific literature.

The course and outcome of patients in vegetative state of non-traumatic etiology have been studied by Sazbon et al.[49] They studied 100 consecutive unconscious patients admitted to an intensive care coma facility with a history of 30 days or more of unconciousness due to a non-traumatic cause: 20 recovered consciousness within 5 months after injury; 31 of the remaining patients died within 6 months of injury; 49 remained unconscious until death with a mean life expectancy of 26–34 months. All 20 patients who recovered awareness suffered severe sequelae. The prognosis for life or death and for recovery or not of consciousness was not significantly correlated with age or etiology of the vegetative state. Young patients who recovered consciousness showed somewhat better results in three parameters of functions: locomotion, activities of daily living, and day placement, but not in cognition, behavior or speech accuracy and fluency. Authors concluded that the overall results for these non-traumatic patients with post-comatose unawareness are clearly worse than those for patients with a similar period of unconsciousness following brain injury.

It should be remembered that persistent vegetative state should not be diagnosed until 12 months after the patient has emerged from coma and opened his or her eyes and, after that time, remained in that state in traumatic brain injury patients. We conclude this section by quoting from the epilogue in the last book by Professor Bryant Jennett.

> In the 30 years since the vegetative state was defined and named there has been a gradual evolution of medical knowledge about its diagnosis, prognosis, and pathology. However, there remains much that we do not yet know – especially about the nature of conciousness and about how even partial recovery can occur after many months. Diagnosis and prognosis remain matters of probability rather than of certainty. This makes the condition no different from many others in medicine that require decisions to be made about management in order to provide compassionate care . . . but there is also the question of the equitable use of scarce medical resources when it comes to indefinite life support for permanently vegetative patients. This is particularly difficult to justify when there is such a broad consensus among doctors, ethicists and lawyers that prolonging survival in this condition brings no benefit to the patient.[37]

Locked-in syndrome (LIS)

The Locked-in syndrome (LIS) is a state characterized by quadriplegia involving cranial nerve pairs, with lateral gaze palsy and paralytic mutism. The patient is normally fully conscious and aware of his or her environment. Generally, vertical eye movement and blinking are preserved, this ability usually being the only means of communication with the surrounding world. LIS is a consequence of a brainstem lesion, normally in the ventral zone of the pons with an implication of the cortico-spinal tract which produces acute tetraplegia (quadriplegia). This pontine lesion affects the long pathways running through the brainstem as well as cranial nerves III and XII (interruption of the cortico-bulbar tract); normally the reticular formation is preserved. Most patients with LIS suffer from decerebrate posturing, the rigid extension of both the upper and lower limbs. This posturing can be either spontaneous or caused by painful stimuli. In addition, patients with LIS present respiratory problems, associated with breathing insufficiency. The lesions to the last pair of cranial nerves produce a facial, tongue and pharyngeal diplegia with anarthria causing severe difficulties in swallowing and producing sounds. While awake, patients can open their eyes, blink and make voluntary conjugated vertical movements of the eyeballs. According to Plum and Posner,[50] this is due to the fact that "the supranuclear ocular motor pathways travel caudally in the brainstem via Dejarine's bundle, which lies dorsal to the main destructive lesion and remains unscathed". These movements are possible because of the partial preservation of cranial nerve XI and the mesencephalic reticular substance. Abnormal eye movements can be present, with so-called "eye bobbing" (a brisk deviation of the eyes in a downwards direction followed by a slow movement upward toward the resting position) being the most typical. The pupils are generally small but do react to light.

León-Carrión and colleagues[51] have done a survey of 44 people diagnosed with LIS, all of them belonging to the Association for Locked-in Syndrome (ALIS) of France. Results of the survey showed that LIS was equally frequent in men and women (51.2% vs. 48.1%) and had occurred at any age between 22 and 77 years of age (normally between 41 and 52 years, the mean age being 46.79 years). The average time that transpired post-insult was 71.35 months. The principal cause of LIS was stroke (86.4%), with traumatic brain injury (TBI) being a distant second cause with an incidence of only 13.6%. The diagnosis of LIS was usually made around the middle of the second month after onset (mean of 78.76 days). The principal treatments, when present, were pharmacological and physiotherapy. However, 47.1% of the patients were not receiving treatment of any kind at the time of the survey. Neuropsychologically, 86% had a good attentional level, 97.6% were temporally oriented, and 76.7% could read. Memory problems were reported by 18.6%, and 24% showed visual deficit (found mainly in patients with LIS originated by TBI). Also 47.5% of patients reported a good mood state, and 12.5% reported feeling depressed; 61.1% reported having sexual desire, but only 30% maintained sexual relations; 78% of patients were capable of emitting sounds, and 65.8% could communicate without technical aid. In addition 73.2% enjoyed going out, and 81% met with friends at least twice a month. Only 14.3% participated in social activities and 23.8% watched television regularly. Nearly 100% of the patients reported being sensitive to touch to any part of their bodies. The authors suggest diagnostics and rehabilitation procedures.

Diagnosis of patients with LIS

From the point of view of its classic diagnosis, three categories of Locked-in syndrome can be found. The first category would be *Complete LIS*, caused by a primary massive lesion to the brainstem (ventral pons), of either vascular or traumatic origin, in which the patient suffers total immobility (with the exception of vertical eye movements and blinking) and shows signs of normal cortical function in the EEG. Second would be *Incomplete LIS*, also caused by a primary lesion to the brainstem, but in which a partial recovery of the injured zone is produced during the first few weeks following the event, allowing the patient to be able to make certain movements. The third category that we find is *Pseudo-LIS*, occurring when a cortical lesion to the cerebellum causes secondary damage to the brainstem. Clinically, patients with pseudo-LIS present the profile of LIS. This is generally accompanied by other disorders, as when the original supratentorial lesions produce language, memory, and reasoning disorders.[52] Given that not all basilar strokes are the same, a clinico-radiological study may be useful in establishing a diagnosis and prognosis.

In a 1993 study, Thajeb and co-workers[53] conclude that, although initial CT scanning may sometimes be unrevealing, serial and follow-up CT scanning have proven their usefulness in the majority of cases as a non-invasive tool – in contrast to cerebral angiography – for predicting the short-term prognosis of basilar artery (BA) syndrome. This conclusion is based on research done on 22 patients with ischemic stroke, as a single event, in the territory of basilar artery (BA) using computerized tomography (CT) and clinico-radiological features. The authors found that the basilar artery syndrome may be divided into five subtypes:

- Type 1, incompatible with life, is the complete type and is characterized by infarctions in the whole territory of the BA.
- Type 2 involves extensive brainstem infarct and may result in LIS.
- Type 3 involves infarction in part of the BA territory (incomplete form or partial syndrome) and may have a more variable clinical outcome.
- Type 4, characterized by "top of the BA" syndrome, is often more benign.
- Type 5, with negative CT BA syndrome (angiographically verified) is often more benign.

These patients generally have their ocular vertical movements preserved, movements of the eyelids (blinking) being the only form of communicating with the outside world. These patients are in a dramatic state as they can be conscious of everything that is happening around them but are incapable of communicating with the outside world. Days and months can pass before someone notices that they are conscious yet unable to communicate.

Due to the difficulties in diagnosing LIS, greater care must be taken at the time of diagnosis and more widespread use of available diagnostic equipment must be made. The use of modern diagnostic technology and complementary testing should be made routine and included in the protocols in order to establish a differential diagnosis between patients in vegetative state, in minimally conscious state, with akinetic mutism and with LIS. Giacino et al.[54] proposed a differential diagnosis between vegetative and minimally conscious states that could also be applied to an extent to LIS patients. They proposed that one or more of the following clinical features should be present to diagnose minimally conscious states (MCS): following simple commands; manipulation of objects; gestural or verbal "yes/no" responses; intelligible verbalization; stereotypical movements (blinking, smiling) that occur in a meaningful relationship to the eliciting stimulus and are not attributable to reflexive activity. The authors also maintain that all of these responses must occur on a sustained basis before the diagnosis of MCS can be applied. In another paper, Giacino and Kalmar[55] found that patients diagnosed with MCS on admission to rehabilitation had significantly more favorable outcomes in the first year post-injury, in contrast to patients diagnosed with vegetative state.

In addition, they suggest:

Routine bedside examination is often inadequate for conducting diagnostic and prognostic assessment. Specialized assessment procedures, designed specifically for use with this population, should be utilized for evaluation and monitoring purposes, since these techniques appear to be superior to traditional assessment methods. Individualized as well as standardized approaches are available and can be used alone or in combination.

Although we agree that diagnostic tools should play an important part in diagnosis, the role of bedside examination in diagnosing LIS cannot be discounted. This is demonstrated by the fact that it is normally a family member who, without the use of diagnostic equipment, first discovers that a patient with LIS is aware. We recommend the use of bedside diagnosis of LIS in conjunction with the use of valid sophisticated technology.

One of the most difficult differential diagnoses is between LIS and akinetic mutism given that they share certain clinical similarities Akinetic mutism is associated with bilateral mesodiencephalic or frontal lesions of various etiologies. Ackerman and Ziegler[56] distinguish at least two pathomechanisms: first, a reduced arousal of cortical functions due to lesions at or rostral to the mesodiencephalic junction; second, impaired activation of the motor system following bilateral damage to the frontal lobes. For Hazouard and co-workers,[57] the accountable lesions producing akinetic mutism are always bilateral, and the injured structures include the frontal gyri, the thalami or the mesencephalic areas. A bilateral frontal hypoactivity was observed in the SPECT of their patient. An anatomical correspondence between the mesolimbocortical dopaminergic system and the circumscribed bilateral lesion of the medial prefrontal cortex are suggested by Nemeth and co-workers.[58] The pathological features common to their patients were bilateral lesions of the rostral part of the anterior cingulated gyri which overlapped onto the neighboring supplementary motor area. They found that damage of the mesolimbocortical dopaminergic terminal fields in the anteromedial frontal cortex is essential for a type of akinetic mutism characterized by almost absolute mutism, immobility, and inability to communicate in any way. These same authors studied the functional-anatomical basis for the differentiation of akinetic mutism and LIS. The results of their review lead them to argue that mesocoeruleo, diencephalospinal and/or mesocorticolimbic dopaminergic systems are selectively damaged in akinetic mutism but preserved in LIS.

Prognosis and therapeutic interventions in patients with LIS

The prognosis of patients with LIS may be directly related to the long-term treatment they receive and, based on our clinical experience, to the individual family's ability to access and make use of medical and paramedical resources. Families who unquestioningly accepted a bad prognosis denied the patient with LIS any possibility of obtaining even a minimum recovery.

Criteria concerning the most adequate protocol to be followed with LIS patients are varied and as yet there is no general agreement as to how to proceed. Interesting are the responses obtained in a written survey of physicians on neurological intensive care units in Germany regarding the treatment of patients with basilar artery thrombosis and LIS. Out of 93 physicians, 52% advocated not treating severe infections with antibiotics, and 38% were in favor of stopping intensive care. Nonetheless, intubating the patient when swallowing disturbances were present as well in the presence of imminent aspiration was recommended by 55% of the physicians. Discussing these problems with relatives was advocated by 87%, with 58% favoring discussing them in detail with the patient. Of these physicians 97% recommended the use of opiates and benzodiazepines. Part of the reason for this lack of a general agreement, as well as the lack of adequate therapeutic measures to be taken for these patients, is owing to the firm belief that whatever is done, these patients will not get better. This belief, however, has no scientific basis. It is based on the observation that, as time passes, LIS patients remain in the same state, often for years. The situation is exacerbated when therapy is discontinued after 2–3 years due to poor observable results. At this point any possibility of further recovery is lost, and the belief that no recovery is possible is once again reinforced. We found very little in the literature regarding continued therapeutic action. Nonetheless, some cases show thought-provoking results.[51,52]

Most patients with LIS, even those receiving only maintenance care after hospital discharge, may live for quite a long time, possibly more than 20 years. This is particularly true for patients with onset at an early age. The pessimistic outlook with which LIS treatment is commonly viewed needs to be dismissed. It must be assumed that the treatment of LIS is very long term and should be undertaken in a positive manner. We recommend early intervention during the acute phase, and, circumstances allowing, within the first 12 h. For the post-acute phase we recommend a long-term, intensive, holistic and multidisciplinary rehabilitation program. Short-term programs or isolated rehabilitation measures should be avoided as a treatment. More imagination should be used to seek creative measures, and further research in rehabilitation for LIS needs to be carried out.

We recommend that long-term holistic, intensive and multidisciplinary treatment be commenced as soon as these patients are available. Protocols must be developed to make the ongoing results evident to scientific and professional communities. Facilitating breathing, swallowing, and speech are key targets when caring for and treating patients with LIS. More research on different physiotherapeutic treatment is needed, including the effect of medication on physical and motor problems. Precautions need to be taken with regard to the manipulation of the cervical spine of patients with vascular disorders. Without exclusion of speech therapy, active communication with patients with LIS by whatever methods is encouraged. The role of the family and the social environment have to be taken into account when designing long-term treatment or long-term care. A more positive outlook on the part of the different professionals involved in the treatment, care and therapy of patients, as well as more imaginative research will facilitate positive new treatment strategies for LIS.[51,52]

From the legal point of view, these patients' cases should be considered as probably some of the hardest conditions that can affect an individual during their lifetime: being unable to communicate, only with a vertical movement of the eyes and blinking, yet conscious and aware of everything occurring around them. The costs of treatment should be considered very high.

Minimally responsive state

An emerging term is that of minimally responsive state (MCS). This term is used to describe a subgroup of patients with severe disturbances of consciousness that do not fulfill diagnostic criteria for coma or vegetative state. The main characteristic is that evidence of awareness is inconsistently discernible, that is to say, not always. The distinction between coma and MCS is very important from the point of view of treatment planning and results obtained since outcome is more favorable for patients in MCS than those in prolonged coma or persistent vegetative state. An attempt to find consensus in the definition of this state was carried out by Giacino et al.[54] For them, the minimally responsive state is defined by clear evidence of behavioral awareness, even though inconsistent, and it can be differentiated from coma and persistent vegetative state because behavioral response is not found in patients in the other two states. Patients in coma can evolve towards MCS or a vegetative state after 1 year following acute brain injury. MCS can also be the result of degenerative or cognitive disorders of the central nervous system. The minimally responsive state is often transitory, but can also be permanent. Legally, they should be considered patients in a vegetative state, however, neuropsychological, multidisciplinary and intensive rehabilitation treatment should be attempted with these patients as there is hope that important steps towards functional recovery can be achieved.

Inconsistent but *clearly discernible* behavioral evidence of consciousness on a reproducible or sustained basis is documented by one of more of the behaviors listed in Table 6.6.

Canedo et al.[59] observed that that there is a subgroup of minimally responsive patients who, when given sensory stimulation, show an increase in responding not always detected through usual instruments of assessment. These are subtle changes in responding that are not always reported and, therefore, no rehabilitation measures are taken to improve this response. These clinical observations are better made by a clinician with experience with these patients. The authors' observations suggest that clinical findings do not correlate with assessment scores. Authors also suggest that these provisory

Table 6.6 The minimally conscious state diagnostic criteria, Giacino et al.[54]

1. The patient is able to follow simple commands.
2. Independent of accuracy, patient is able to respond *yes* or *no*.
3. Some intelligible verbalization.
4. Patient shows purposeful or intentional behavior through movement, affective reactions in contingent relation to a relevant stimuli, e.g.:
   - smiling or crying to relevant visual or verbal stimuli
   - response to verbal question by vocalization or gesture
   - trying to reach objects
   - touching or holding objects adjusting to size and shape
   - sustaining tracking and visual fixation

observations indicate that there is a need to develop methodologically sound tools that will accurately monitor individuals throughout rehabilitative processes.

Akinetic mutism

The term akinetic mutism was introduced by Cairns et al.[60] to describe the behavior of a young woman with a third ventricle cystic tumor. The most important neurobehavioral observations were the marked lack of movement and speech in a patient that was otherwise alert and visually tracking. Akinetic mutism is usually used to describe those patients who are totally immobile but not completely paralyzed who can maintain their eyes open as if they were aware of something near them or something said in a given moment, but are incapable of communicating although, in general, lie with their eyes closed, maintain cycles of alert and give the impression that they are alert. These patients make few muscular movements and, in general, they would be basic movements following nociceptive stimulation. Sometimes they emit a word or signs of communication. The associated anatomical lesions are frontal-basal (sella Turca) areas and posterior region of the midbrain.[61] Although some authors have at times identified akinetic mutism as vegetative state, it should not be assumed.

Legal aspects

When a patient has been in coma or persistent vegetative state for a long time, the family, professionals, and even judges debate the possibility of ending the life support system which has been sustaining the patient's life. In the last few years, some judges have approved decisions like these. Normally, the family resists making such a decision since there is always hope of recovery, that a miracle could occur or that new technological advances might discover something that would help their loved one. At the same time, they ask themselves if this is what the patient would want if they could make the decision on their own. Professionals agree that patients in a persistent vegetative state do not generally recover and that, at any moment, a medical complication (normally respiratory) will end the patient's life. In the end, doctors, neuropsychologists and neuroscientists are the only ones who can legally determine when cerebral functions are completely lost and unable to be recovered, and they help the family to make the decision. Finally, for judges:

> The suggestion that finalizing a patient's treatment in these circumstances is a form of criminal homicide has been firmly rejected. However, when judges or others dissent, the issues are put on the table as to whether the particular decision is correct, if they have challenged logic by denying a casual relationship between ending treatment and inducing death, and preoccupations about the kind of person whose death has been hastened being applied beyond morally-tolerable limits once society begins to permit permanently unconscious persons to die. (Council of Scientific Issues and Council of Ethical and Judicial Issues, 1990)[62]

Doctors and other professionals confront the problem of having to advise family members of patients in coma or persistent vegetative state. Before offering a reply, they should reflect upon certain aspects of the issue, as suggested by the Council of Scientific Issues and Council of Ethical and Judicial Issues without forgetting different legal perspectives existing in different states on whether treatment should be maintained or discontinued.

First of all, the desires of a patient when he or she is conscious should be clearly known. Judges have no problem in accepting this. However, a patient's desires are not so clear or convincing since doubt exists as to what someone comments are his or her desires when he or she was young and healthy, never imagining that he or she could find themselves in these circumstances. The Supreme Court of New York proposes that sustaining life artificially should not be done unless a patient has clearly and explicitly solicited it. Other justice departments and states have suggested certain conditions for deciding when it is appropriate to end treatment while others reject any methods which facilitate death.

Second, the diagnosis of prolonged coma or persistent vegetative state should be as well defined and clear as possible. In many situations, diagnosis of persistent vegetative state is unclear or mistakenly pronounced by doctors and professionals since it is made only because they cannot find a way to communicate with the patient. The correct thing to do, especially from a legal point of view, would be to contrast the diagnosis with a second or third opinion by other specialized doctors and neuropsychologists in order to confirm the diagnosis.

Third, when there are discrepancies among different diagnoses of doctors and doctors consulted, or when there are disputes between family members over different points of view, it is advisable to consult an ethical group to help the family make a decision.

There is no doubt that these options should be contemplated within the strictest legal framework in force in the respective country.

Conclusions

Evaluation and assessment of catastrophic brain injury should be carried out with maximum rigor in accordance with time of evolution and mechanisms of causes, and, at the same time, using the latest state-of-the-art technology possible. Research about and clinical intervention in patients with a low level of response is a challenge for all those professionals who have to demonstrate their ability and efficacy. It is a multidisciplinary matter and all diverse professionals working on a team have to combine their knowledge, clinical abilities, and capacity of integration in order to obtain better results in the treatment of these patients. Imagination is needed to seek more creative measures for rehabilitation. Most of the patients are going to need special care while they are alive, or constant supervision, by a third person. It is very important for these patients to be involved in specialized programs of stimulation and rehabilitation. A more positive outlook on the part of different professionals involved in the treatments will facilitate positive new treatment strategies for low-level responsive patients.

References

1. Jennett, B. (1993). Mental incapacity and medical treatment. *Lancet, 3*(342), 8862.
2. Zasler, N. D. (1993). Some aspects of the humoral and neutrophil functions in post-comatose unawareness patient. *Brain Injury, 7*, 379–381.
3. Schalén, W., Sonenson, B., Messeter, K., Norstrom, G., & Nordstrom, C. H. (1992). Clinical outcome and cognitive impairment in patients with severe head injuries treated with barbiturate coma. *Acta Neurochir., 117*, 153–159.
4. Jennett, B., & Dyer, C. (1991). Persistent vegetative state and the right to die: the United States and Britain. *Br. Med. J., 302*, 1256–1258.
5. Teasdale, G., & Jennett, B. (1974). Assessment of coma and impaired consciousness. A practical scale. *Lancet, 13*(2), 81–84.
6. Teasdale, G., & Jennett, B. (1976). Assessment and prognosis of coma after head injury. *Acta Neurochir., 34*(1–4), 45–55.
7. Mullie, A., Verstringe, P., Buylaert, W., et al. (1988). Predictive value of Glasgow coma score for awakening after out-of-hospital cardiac arrest. Cerebral Resuscitation Study Group of the Belgian Society for Intensive Care. *Lancet, 23*(1), 137–140.
8. León-Carrión, J. (1994). *Brain injury: Guide for family members and caretakers.* Madrid: Siglo XXI.
9. Marshall, L. F. (1991). Evoked potentials: a decade later. *Crit. Care. Med., 19*(11), 1337.
10. Nagib, M. G., Rockswold, G. L., Sherman, R. S., & Lagaard, M. W. (1986). Civilian gunshot wounds to the brain: prognosis and management. *Neurosurgery, 18*(5), 533–537.

11. Aldrich, E. F., Eisenberg, H. M., Saydjari, C., et al. (1992). Predictors of mortality in severely head-injured patients with civilian gunshot wounds: a report from the NIH Traumatic Coma Data Bank. *Surg. Neurol., 38*(6), 418–423.
12. Tanhenco, J., & Kaplan, P. E. (1982). Physical and surgical examination of patient after 6-year coma. *Arch. Phys. Med. Rehabil., 63*, 36–38.
13. Groswasser, Z., Cohen, M., & Costeff, H. (1989). Rehabilitation outcome after anoxic brain damage. *Arch. Phys. Med. Rehabil., 70*, 186–188.
14. Sazbon, L., & Groswasser, Z. (1990). Outcome in 134 patients with prolonged posttraumatic unawareness. Part 1: Parameters determining late recovery of consciousness. *J. Neurosurg., 72*(1), 75–80.
15. Bates, D. (1991). Defining prognosis in medical coma. *J. Neurol. Neurosurg. Psychiatry., 54*(7), 569–571.
16. Lombardi, F., Taricco, M., De Tanti, A., Telaro, E., & Liberati, A. (2002). Sensory stimulation for brain injured individuals in coma or vegetative state. *Cochrane Database Syst. Rev., CD001427*, 8.
17. Pierce, J. P., Lyle, D. M., Quine, S., Evans, N. J., Morris, J., & Fearnside, M. R. (1990). The effectiveness of coma arousal intervention. *Brain Inj., 4*, 191–197.
18. Wood, R. L., Winkowski, T. B., Miller, J. L., Tierney, L., & Goldman, L. (1992). Evaluating sensory regulation as a method to improve awareness patients with altered states of consciousness: a pilot study. *Brain. Inj., 6*, 411–418.
19. Mitchell, S., Bradley, V. A., Welch, J. L., & Britton, P. G. (1990). Coma arousal procedure: a therapeutic intervention in the treatment of head injury. *Brain. Inj., 4*, 273–279.
20. Helwick, L. D. (1994). Stimulation programs for coma patients. *Crit. Care Nurs., 14*, 47–52.
21. Mazaux, J. M., De Sèze, M., Joseph, P. A., & Barat, M. (2001). Early rehabilitation after severe brain injury: a French perspective. *J. Rehabil. Med., 33*, 99–109.
22. Bernard, S. A., Gray, T. W., Buist, M. D., et al. (2002). Treatment of comatose survivors of out-of-hospital cardiac arrest with induced hypothermia. *N. Engl. J. Med., 346*, 557–563.
23. Lippert-Grüner, M., Wedekind, C., Ernestus, R. I., & Klug, N. (2002). Early rehabilitative concepts in therapy of the comatose brain injured patients. *Acta Neurochir. Suppl., 79*, 21–23.
24. Jennett, B., & Plum, F. (1972). The persistent vegetative state: a syndrome in search of a name. *Lancet, 1*, 734–737.
25. Domínguez-Morales, M. R., & León-Carrión, J. (2001). Impact of treatments in the economical compensation of brain injury patients. *Revist. Española Neuropsicol., 3*(1–2), 77–84.
26. Talar, J. (2002). Rehabilitation outcome in a patient awakened from prolonged coma. *Med. Sci. Monit., 8*, CS31–CS38.
27. Cohadon, F., & Richer, E. (1983). Course and outcome of severe traumatic coma. *Neurochirurgie, 29*, 303–325.
28. Johnstone, B., & Bouman, D. E. (1992). Anoxic encephalopathy: a case study of an eight-year-old male with no residual cognitive deficits. *Int. J. Neurosci., 62*, 207–213.
29. Van de Kelft, E., Candon, E., Couchet, P., Frèrebeau, P., & Daures, J. P. (1995). Early restructuration of consciousness after traumatic coma. *Acta Neurol. Belg., 95*, 88–91.
30. Ross, B. L., Temkim, N. R., Newell, D., & Dikmen, S. S. (1994). Neuro-

psychological outcome in relation to head injury severity. Contributions of coma length and focal abnormalities. *Am. J. Phys. Med. Rehabil., 73*, 341–347.

31. Macpherson, V., Sullivan, S. J., & Lambert, J. (1992). Prediction of motor status 3 and 6 months post severe traumatic brain injury: a preliminary study. *Brain Inj., 6*, 489–498.

32. Stover, S. L., & Zeiger, H. E. (1976). Head injury in children and teenagers; functional recovery correlated with the duration of coma. *Arch. Phys. Med. Rehabil., 57*, 201–205.

33. Wade, D. T., & Johnston, C. (1999). The permanent vegetative state: practical guidance on diagnosis and management. *Br. Med. J., 25*(319), 841–844.

34. Jennett, B. (1996). Epidemiology of head injury. *J. Neurol. Neurosurg. Psychiat., 60*(4), 362–369.

35. Zeithofer, O., Steiner, M., Oder, W., Obergottsberger, S., Mayr, N., & Deecke, L. (1991). The prognostic value of evoked potentials in early neurologic rehabilitation of patients with the apallic syndrome. *EEG EMG Z Elektroenzephalogr Elektromyogr Verwandte Geb., 22*, 10–14.

36. Andrews, K. (1993). Patients in the persistent vegetative state: problems in their long-term management. *Br. Med. J., 306*, 6892.

37. Jennett, B. (2002). *The vegetative state*. Cambridge: Cambridge University Press.

38. Passler, M. A., & Riggs, R. V. (2001). Positive outcomes in traumatic brain injury-vegetative state: patients treated with bromocriptine. *Arch. Phys. Med. Rehabil., 82*, 311–315.

39. Kaelin, D. L., Cifu, D. X., & Matthies, B. (1996). Methylphenidate effect on attention deficit in the acutely brain-injured adult. *Arch. Phys. Med. Rehabil., 77*, 6–9.

40. Wolf, A. P., & Gleckman, A. D. (1995). Sinemet and brain injury: functional versus statistical change and suggestions for future research designs. *Brain Inj., 9*, 487–493.

41. Haig, A. J., & Ruess, J. M. (1990). Recovery from vegetative state of six months' duration associated with Sinemet (levadopa/carbidopa). *Arch. Phys. Med. Rehabil., 71*, 1081–1083.

42. Meythaler, J. M., Brunner, R. C., Johnson, A., & Novack, T. A. (2002). Amantadine to improve neurorecovery in traumatic brain injury-associated diffuse axonal injury: a pilot double-blind randomized trial. *J. Head Trauma Rehabil., 17*, 300–313.

43. Macchio, G. J., Ito, V., & Sahgal, V. (1993). Amantadine-induced coma. *Arch. Phys. Med. Rehabil., 74*, 1119–1120.

44. Schneider, W. N., Drew-Cates, J., Wong, T. M., & Dombovy, M. L. (1999). Cognitive and behavioral efficacy of amantadine in acute traumatic brain injury: an initial double-blind placebo-controlled study. *Brain Inj., 13*, 863–872.

45. Minderhound, J. M., & Braakman, R. (1985). Het vegeterende bestaan. *Nederlandes Tijdsch. Geneeskunde, 129*, 2385–2388.

46. Andrews, K. (1993). Recovery of patients after four months or more in the persistent vegetative state. *Br. Med. J. 306*, 1597–1600.

47. Najeson, T., Sazbon, L., Fiselzon, J., Becker, E., & Schechter, I. (1978). Recovery of communicative functions after prolonged traumatic coma. *Scand. J. Rehabil. Med., 10*, 15–21.

48. Heindl, U. T., & Laub, M. C. (1996). Outcome of persistent vegetative state following hypoxic or traumatic brain injury in children and adolescents. *Neuropediatrics, 27*, 94–100.

49. Sazbon, L., Zagreba, F., Ronen, J., Solzi, P., & Costeff, H. (1993). Course and outcome of patients in vegetative state of nontraumatic aetiology. *J. Neurol. Neurosurg. Psychiatry., 56*, 407–409.

50. Plum, F., & Posner, J. B. (1972). Diagnosis of stupor and of coma. *Contemp. Neurol. Ser., 10* 1–286.

51. León-Carrión, J., Van Eeckaout, P., Pérez-Santamaría, F. J., & Domínguez-Morales, M. R. (2002). The locked-in syndrome: a syndrome looking for a therapy. Review of subjects. *Brain Inj., 15*(5), 60–72.

52. León-Carrión, J., Van Eeckaout, P., & Domínguez-Morales, M. R. (2002). The locked-in syndrome: a syndrome looking for a therapy survey. *Brain Inj., 15*(5), 1–12.

53. Thajeb, P., Lie, L. K., & Chang, T. R. (1993). Types of basilar artery syndrome: clinicoradiologic correlation. *Angiology, 44*, 368–375.

54. Giacino, J. T., Ashwal, S., Childs, N., et al. (2002). The minimally conscious state: definition and diagnostic criteria. *Neurology, 58*(3), 349–353.

55. Giacino, J. T., & Kalmar, K. (1997). The vegetative and minimally conscious states: a comparison of clinical features and functional outcomes. *J. Head Trauma Rehab., 12*(4), 36–51.

56. Ackerman, H., & Ziegler, W. (1995). Akinetic mutism – a review of the literature. *Fortschr. Neurol. Psychiat., 63*(2), 59–67.

57. Hazouard, E., Legras, A., Corcia, P., et al. (1998). Significance of single photon emission computed tomography and akinetic mutism. *Rev. Neurol., 154*(12), 856–858.

58. Nemeth, G., Hegedus, K., & Molnar, L. (1986). Akinetic mutism associated with bicingular lesions: clinicopathological and functional anatomical correlates. *Eur. Arch. Psychiat. Neurol. Sci., 237*, 218–222.

59. Canedo, A., Grix, M. C., & Nicoletti, J. (2002). An analysis of assessment instruments for the minimally responsive patient (MRP): clinical observations. *Brain Inj., 16*, 453–461.

60. Cairns, H., Olfield, R. C., Pennybacker, J. B., & Whitteridge, D. (1941). Akinetic mutism with an epidermoid cyst of the 3rd ventricle. *Brain, 64*, 273–280.

61. Berrol, C. (1990). Dance/movement therapy in head injury rehabilitation. *Brain Inj., 4*(3), 257–265.

62. Council on Ethical and Judicial Affairs. (1990). Persistent Vegetive State and the Decision to Withdraw or Withhold Life Support, *JAMA 263*, (3): 426–30.

7   Diagnosing and treating affective disorders after brain injury

Dale F. Thomas and José León-Carrión

Introduction

The affective and emotional problems that occur as the result of a brain injury tend to be among the more common sequelae likely to affect interpersonal, family, and work relations. Affective disturbances, in some instances, may be even more debilitating than cognitive or physical changes.[1] The reasons that affective disturbances occur following brain injury are complex and may be a direct result of damage to the cortical systems involved with regulation of emotion, initiation of activities, self-awareness, and impulse control. Affective disturbances may also result from a host of other related variables such as adjustment to disability or grieving the losses that accompanied the brain injury.[2] Family and social adjustment issues resulting from changes in family dynamics, income, work, or the social isolation often experienced, may be the cause of or may interact with emotional or behavioral stressors resulting in affective disturbances.

The clinician involved in the evaluation and treatment of people with a brain injury must be thoroughly prepared from an educational and training perspective in order to be an effective part of a treatment team. When developing assessment and treatment strategies, clinicians must be acutely aware of the nature of the brain injury that the person sustained, their pre-morbid personality characteristics, and present personality features. A thorough knowledge of brain behavior relationships and the effects that various types of neurotrauma injuries may have on behavior and cognition is an essential prerequisite. Some authors, for example, suggest that a brain injury may produce exaggerations in previous underlying personality characteristics in clinical populations.[3–5] Individuals who previously had been somewhat impulsive, prone to angry outbursts, or had obsessive and compulsive traits may show exaggeration of these pre-morbid personality characteristics after the brain injury.[6] Changes from pre-morbid personality features may be a dramatic change from the person's pre-morbid personality, but they are often quite subtle.

Other sequelae of a brain injury are also important to understand, such as the effect of a neurotrauma injury on initiating behavior and following through on tasks, awareness of self, and ability to regulate emotions and affective expression. Cultural differences among different populations is yet another important factor to consider. Prigatano,[7] for example, stresses the importance of understanding individual and cultural differences in assessment procedures, since a person's willingness to acknowledge how a brain injury has affected their life, how family members may not be candid in describing relationship changes, and how the outward directedness of many cultures may affect ability to disclose personal information or provide an adequate self-appraisal or appraisal of family members.

León-Carrión[8] reports that in the majority of patients who have suffered a brain injury, changes in the manner of expressing their emotions or feelings can readily be observed. He stresses the importance of neuropsychological rehabilitation designed to approach not only the cognitive deficits, but also the emotional and affective aspects of a person's functioning in order for a program to be effective. Holistic neuropsychological rehabilitation programs have been identified as being among the most effective in treating individuals with brain injury when compared to other methods.[8,9] In a meta-analysis of reported outcomes from holistic neuropsychological rehabilitation programs Malec and Basford[9] site the importance of a thorough and comprehensive evaluation, family involvement, treatment in a program milieu, as well as involvement in group and individual psychotherapy and family treatment sessions as being critically important components of brain injury rehabilitation programs. When such holistic and comprehensive neuropsychological rehabilitation programs are not available due to financial constraints, distance to treatment programs, or lack of qualified professionals, clinicians must assume a greater role for coordinating all available resources and working with family members and community support systems in the most effective manner possible.[10]

This chapter will focus upon the fundamental issues relative to the diagnosis of affective changes resulting from an acquired brain injury, the role and effectiveness of various intervention strategies, and the incidents and reported success rates of various types of pharmacological, behavioral, and psychotherapeutic interventions. Contemporary issues and theories as to why affective disturbances occur following brain injury will be presented, followed by a discussion of assessment and intervention strategies.

Epidemiological data

Numerous studies have been published that identified specific brain structures believed to be responsible for mood-related changes following brain injury. A consensus, however, does not exist at present. Perhaps one of the first and most well-recognized accounts of behavioral changes following brain injury was the report by John Harlow regarding Phineas Gage.[11] This study described how a railroad foreman changed from being well liked, honest, and dependable to vulgar, irresponsible, and offensive after sustaining a penetrating brain injury. This example served to underscore brain behavior relationships known to most students of psychology. More contemporary studies argue similarly that physical changes to the brain result in disturbances in affect and behavior.

Bigler[12] suggested that neurobiology of emotional control can be shown by injury to the brain itself increasing emotional disorders regardless of point of neurological damage. Ross[13] implied that the right hemisphere plays an important role in emotional control similar to the left hemisphere playing an important role in control of expression and receptive language. Injury to the right frontal region has been found to increase levels of anxiety and depression,[14] but does not imply necessarily that the left hemisphere does not play an important role in emotional control as well. Similarly, Jorge et al.[15] speculated that the frontal areas of the brain, which tend to have a propensity for injury in motor vehicle and acceleration/deceleration accidents, might cause depression simply from a neurological disturbance in the frontal subcortical white matter.

Max et al.[16] found that the severity of a brain injury presents a profound risk of development of psychiatric disorders and/or organic personality types of syndromes. In their study, they found higher effect sizes were evident in self-reporting of psychiatric and behavioral dyscontrol in a sample of school age students with brain injury as compared with a contrast group with less intense symptoms.

A study by Madrazo et al.[17] using the Neurologically-related Changes in Personality Inventory (NECHAPI) found that patients showed changes in three of the five factors evaluated when comparing emotional factors before and after traumatic brain injury. Their emotional vulnerability increased and their sociability decreased, as did sensation seeking. The results indicated that patients suffer a more important deterioration in their emotional life, which becomes less stable and more vulnerable. There is a change in the way the individual perceives emotions and feelings and how these are manifested in behavior. The data indicates that before suffering TBI, patients, as a group, had displayed an important tendency to sensation seeking which was reduced by 28.57% after TBI. In addition, the capacity of patients for social contact and exchange was diminished.

Research with individuals who sustained a cerebral vascular accident without traumatic brain injury (and thus with less likelihood of diffuse injury), suggests mixed results as to the impact of a brain injury secondary to stroke and its relationship to affective disturbances. Hermann and Wallesch[18] proposed that major post-stroke depression might be caused by organic factors, particularly left frontal lesions. Gainotti et al.[19] studied 58 individuals over time periods of several months, and after making adjustments of persons to follow-up, disputed this contention and stated that major post-traumatic stroke depression is caused by psychological and not neurological factors. They reported no significant relationship between lesion location, presence of major post-stroke depression, and time elapsed since stroke. Whereas there are obvious differences between the type of injury caused by a stroke and a traumatic brain injury, stroke studies may be more specific in identifying the relevance of the left frontal lobe in depression or the absence of the importance of the left frontal lesion to affective disturbances following trauma.

In a study of frontal lobe syndromes and resulting affective disturbances in a sample population of 360 individuals treated by a trauma hospital,[20] researchers examined individuals with various types of frontal lobe injuries. Of the individuals examined, only persons who met inclusion criteria as having a single lateral or medial (including interior cingulategyrus) frontal lesions, as ascertained by all raters, were studied. Persons who had a history of other neurological disorders or life-threatening physical illnesses, or CT evidence of previous brain injury were excluded from the sample. In total, 32 persons with lateral and 14 persons with medial lesions met these criteria. After some additional losses because of medical complicating factors, all remaining subjects were compared using CT scans to determine the areas of lesion and significance of neurotrauma injury. The study found "that medial-frontal lesions did not lead to higher euphoria, disinhibition, loss of emotion, or apathy than lateral lesions". The authors concluded that medial-frontal activity might be necessary to experience emotion including depressed mood, anxiety, or apathy. Medial-frontal injury may either not lead to emotional changes or may inhibit the perception of mood changes, anxiety, or apathy. Unilateral damage to lateral pre-frontal cortex may disrupt mood regulation and drive while leaving intact the ability to experience (disturbed) emotions.

Gainotti et al.[19] summarizing the controversies argued in the literature, proposed the possibility that the "difference between the right and left hemispheres in the regulation of emotions may be qualitative rather than quantitative and that the two sides of the brain may play complementary roles in emotional behavior". They further hypothesized that the "right hemisphere might be involved mainly in more basic and automatic components of the emotional response, whereas the left hemisphere might play a more important role in control functions". Control over emotional expression, therefore, would fall in this domain.

In a study on the relatively long-term effects of brain injury on mood disturbance conducted by researchers from the University of Leeds, UK, 77 subjects were studied at both 6 and 12 month follow-ups. Bowen et al.[21] reported that the "rates of clinically significant mood disorders of the 77 TBI individuals completing both the 6 and 12 month follow-ups were 39% and 35% respectively". They did not find evidence that mood disorders increased with time since injury, nor did they decrease significantly. Three-quarters of the subjects reported the same level of emotional distress and mood disorder at both assessments. Those reporting a change were just as likely to experience positive as opposed to negative alterations in emotional state as time went on.

The findings of Bowen et al.[21] were consistent with those of Jorge et al.[22] who years earlier reported that likelihood of depression following brain injury does not increase with time since injury. Both of these studies argue that their data are not consistent with the findings of Varney et al.[23] and Harrick et al.[24] that implied emotional difficulties increased with time since injury following TBI. León-Carrión[8] suggested the possibility that the samples in more recent studies, if re-examined at a later date, may show increased depression. Presumably, increased insight and the realization that additional changes and improvements may not occur may result in further depression.

A recent study reported by Friboes et al.[25] examined sleep disturbances and EEG abnormalities several months after traumatic brain injury as a contributor to affective disturbances. Their study found that sleep disturbances and changes in hormone secretion are frequently observed following brain injury. They also reported that similarly, in depression, abnormalities of sleep and neuroendocrine regulation are common. This study reported that the changes in metabolism, hormone secretion, and resulting sleep disturbances all had stressful effects on individuals including mood disturbances and personality changes for several years after brain injury. The authors hypothesized that the "persistence of sleep-endocrine changes in patients who have recovered from depression might represent a biological scar resulting from the metabolic aberrations during acute illness". Changes in hormonal and chemical levels in the brain were speculated to be similar in recurrent depression and traumatic brain injury, and the authors suggest that disturbances in sleep patterns of individuals with brain injuries may be an important factor to examine in order to assess potential for occurrence of depression or other affective disturbances following brain injury.

Other factors contributing to mood disturbances following brain injury

A brain injury, whether it is mild or severe in regard to resulting functional limitations and cognitive changes, can cause a great deal of stress on the individual and their family.[3] There are a number of possible negative consequences that may occur as a result of the brain injury, such as physical disability and pain, financial hardships, life-style changes, as well as occupational, social, and personal changes. Changes in any areas of physical, financial, or self-sufficiency can affect a person's sense of well-being, confidence, and security.[26] Emotional reactions and adjustment problems may also interact with medications being used to treat biological and chemical changes that result from the brain injury.

Adjustment to a physical disability can produce changes in mood including anxiety or panic-like symptoms, depression, or severe stress-related symptoms.[27] Cognitive changes such as decreased efficiency in mental processing, slowing of processing speed, inefficient memory, and forgetting information vital to day-to-day functioning can also produce mood-related symptoms.[3] Certainly, individuals who had a pre-morbid history of anxiety, depression, anger-related difficulties, or any type of pre-existing personality disorder may be at risk of increased symptoms following the brain injury.[28]

A study conducted by Malec et al.[29] suggested that simple day-to-day stressors, caused by cognitive deficits and made worse by financial and family stressors, could cause short-term changes in mood and emotional adjustment. In their study of participants in the Mayo Clinic Outpatient Brain Injury Program, subjects who tended to greatly underestimate their cognitive and psychosocial problems relative to staff opinions were less frequently found to be depressed and had more difficulty on a measure of executive cognitive function than did other subjects in their sample. The authors stressed, however, that a degree of dysphoria might represent an appropriate reaction to disability, impaired executive cognitive function, and impaired self-awareness subsequent to brain injury. Those with dysphoria were regarded as having a better grasp of their true situation, and their reactions were posited to likely interfere with normal emotional adaptation. Impaired self-awareness, however, was reportedly not a predictor of employment.

Prigatano and Schacter extensively studied the role of impaired self-awareness in individuals with brain injury and eventual emotional maladjustment, which in turn creates changes in the person's social, family, and work-related relationships. They argue that "unawareness of deficits, especially those of a psychosocial nature contribute dramatically to difficulties in vocational situations, marriage and family, and can also interfere with neuropsychological treatment".[30] Lezak, a pioneer in the study of family reactions and adjustment, also suggested that stress created by behavioral and relationship changes following brain injury are likely to affect people and family relationships in a wide variety of ways. Some family members learn new roles in their relationship, while others learn to tolerate the behaviors that have become commonplace following a brain injury, and in fact tend to perpetuate the behaviors that are causing the problems.[31] Maladaptive behaviors may include explosiveness in a verbal or physical sense, which causes disruption within families, or actions that appear as "child-like". Family members may choose to ignore the behaviors or to deny that they are creating problems because the family has habituated or become accustomed to the behaviors. Therefore, they may abandon attempts to change or redirect such behaviors and in effect, add additional stress within the family.

Prigatano argues that unawareness that they have changed and that persons with brain injuries consequently are interacting differently with others is the sole reason responsible for the majority of divorces and work-related problems following brain injury.[7] Since people with brain injury often view themselves as having the same skills, abilities, and personality traits as they did prior to the brain injury, they tend to become more frustrated when they are treated differently by others, when they have changes in their job or loss of job, and when family members begin to socially alienate themselves from friends and loved ones. The loss of friends, the changes in the number of visits from family members, and feelings of isolation are among the most common family-related difficulties that tend to occur following a brain injury.[32]

Suicide precautions and intervention strategies

The possibility that an individual may consider or attempt suicide following a traumatic brain injury has been identified as a critical factor to examine in neuropsychological rehabilitation programs.[33] Several published studies suggested that changes in the serotonin (5HT) system and to the ventral pre-frontal cortex are the neurobiological abnormalities most consistently associated with suicide.[1,34,35] Other studies have shown that dysregulation of the hypothalamic–pituitary–adrenal (HPA) axis can be found in suicide victims. The HPA is the neuroendocrine system that responds to stress and whose final product, corticosteroids, targets components of the limbic system, particularly the hippocampus.[36] The use of medication that can reduce the stress response, and/or decrease HPA activation, will be useful in the pharmacological treatment of anxiety, depression, and perhaps, in suicidal behavior.

A study by Tondo et al.[37] reviewed evidence of possible anti-suicide action of lithium maintenance treatment in mood disorders and reviewed studies involving over 17,000 patients with major affective illnesses. Most yielded supportive evidence that the risk of suicides and attempts averaged 3.2 vs. 0.37/100 patients/year without versus with lithium treatment. Lithium maintenance treatment in recurring major mood disorders appears to offer anti-suicide effects not demonstrated with other mood stabilizers.

In a study of individuals who were provided with neuropsychological rehabilitation services, León-Carrión et al. studied 39 individuals after hospital discharge. All were voluntarily seeking neuropsychological assessment and recommendations, and all came because more than a year and a half after discharge from the hospital they continued presenting with adaptation, behavioral, and cognitive problems. Using the depression index from Exner's Rorschach system, all individuals were examined in regard to depressive symptoms, as well as for suicidal tendency or ideation.

In total, 33% of the clinical population of brain injury patients seeking neuropsychological care was determined to be at risk for committing suicide. León-Carrión et al. suggested that approximately half of the people surviving a severe traumatic brain injury and seeking care might suffer from depression more than one year after discharge.[33] Among the persons with a brain injury diagnosed as having depression, approximately two-thirds had suicidal ideation and tendencies. People judged to be at a higher potential suicidal risk were seen as having problems interpreting reality and finding the true meaning of their perceptions and were concrete in their reasoning processes. Poor coping skills, difficulties with stressful and conflict-type situations, and feeling trapped in the present situation were commonly reported. The importance of examining suicidal ideation was identified as an important part of any neuropsychological rehabilitation assessment program.

Depression and suicidal thinking should be assessed early in the evaluation process. One approach may involve the assessment of cognitive and vegetative symptoms of depression during a clinical interview. Another approach involves collection of collateral information from significant others and family members. One way to approach such an assessment is to ask that a family member or significant other accompany the person with a brain injury to intakes and follow-up sessions as appropriate, and to ask individuals for permission to include them in discussions and to see their family members separately if necessary.

Risk factors to examine include feelings of helplessness and hopelessness, past indications of suicidal attempts, presence of a means to follow through (such as access to potentially lethal drugs, access to weapons or other means of committing suicide), past family history of suicide attempts, history of physical or sexual abuse, and a stated deadline for committing a suicidal act. Alcohol and drug abuse or dependence may also increase the risk of suicidal thinking.[38]

When assessing these features, it is important to let family members and individuals with a brain injury speak candidly about their thoughts and feelings. It may be important to normalize the thought of depression occurring following severe physical and cognitive changes, and to report that having suicidal ideation is an indication of the severity level and desperateness that they feel. Developing a crisis plan in the event that emotional dyscontrol or feelings of isolation and desperation increase is also an important consideration.

Means of assessing for depression levels and suicidal tendencies vary widely, but an objective means for assessing such traits is important. As in an aforementioned example, the Rorschach may be one manner of approaching assessment of suicidal and depressive tendencies. The Minnesota Multiphasic Personality Inventory-2 (MMPI-2)[39] has also been cited as an important tool for examining such characteristics in the US literature. Other objective tests such as the Milan Clinical Multiphasic Inventory[40] have also been found to be a means of objectively identifying symptoms associated with thought disturbances, affective disturbances, and personality variables that are important to consider. Any personality tests used with persons with a brain injury must be interpreted cautiously, since there is a tendency to show clinical scale elevations if physical symptoms, fatigue, sleep disturbances, and cognitive processes have been affected. The clinician should be thoroughly familiar with the testing protocols being used as well as the literature in regard to using any type of personality assessment instruments with a brain injury population.

Depression inventories such as the Beck Depression Inventory,[41] the Beck Hopelessness Scale,[42] the Beck Anxiety Scale,[43] and the Hamilton 77 and 22 Item Depression Scales,[44] as well as depression inventories using care staff or significant others as informants may be of value in this regard. Although a review of the numerous standardized instruments suitable for use with this population is beyond the scope of this chapter, no one instrument is presently universally used.

Methods of treating depression and intervention strategies

Several authorities in the field of brain injury rehabilitation have argued that a holistic approach to treating the residuals of brain injury is important, including treatment not only of the physical and cognitive related deficits but also affective related changes that occur.[8,30,45–47] The majority of all researchers and clinicians, who embrace the holistic treatment model of brain injury rehabilitation, support the notion of providing neuro-psychological treatment as well as cognitive and physical restorative services, although all authors do not agree on the best means of providing such services. Miller and Keitner[48] suggested several possible positive effects of combining medications with psychotherapy, including the following:

1   Medications increase the effectiveness of psychotherapy by making the person more accessible due to a decrease in symptoms.
2   Psychotherapy enhances compliance with a medication regime (and therefore compliance).
3   The two may produce a faster overall response.
4   Psychosocial intervention, particularly family intervention, decreases the amount of stress and disruption for the patient.

Several authors have suggested that because physical changes in the structure of the brain and resulting neurochemical changes that occur may be an important aspect of affective disturbances, the treatment of affective disorders may require the use of medications.[2,15,49,50] Although it is beyond the scope of this chapter to discuss the pharmacological treatment of brain injury, a brief review of some current trends in this area will be discussed below.

Gaultieri[50] suggests that moodiness and irritability following a brain injury, even a mild brain injury, can produce changes in a person's emotional state. He hypothesized that moodiness and irritability can give way to deeper, more pervasive feelings of sadness, discouragement, and despair. Sleep disturbances commonly result, and internalization of stress may cause muscular tension as well as tiredness, irritability, and depression that are already experienced. Low doses of antidepressants such as amitryptiline or trazodone are often used to treat sleep disturbances and pain.

If depression emerges, more aggressive treatment may be recommended by the person's physician or psychologist, including the use of modern antidepressants, such as serotonin reuptake inhibitors (SSRIs).[2] At times, other medications can be added to antidepressants to augment their effect. Lithium is the only true augmenting Rx. Amantadine may help cognitive and motor deficiency, but not depression. Ritalin is not for depression but inattention, hyperactivity, and emotional lability/impulsivity. Other medications are sometimes used, depending on side-effects, physical factors, and the discretion of the physician.

The management of treatment-resistant depression in the traumatic brain-injured person is a complex process. Some persons with a brain injury who are depressed do not respond to psychotherapy and to the adequate doses of medication, or both. These individuals are a challenge to the treatment team who must consider alternative methods of treatment. Most people who are resistant to the treatment efforts run an increased risk of suicide attempts. There are several general principles to consider before starting treating depression in these patients.[1,51–53]

1 Recognize whether or not the physical illness is inducing the depression and assess what is being done to treat or minimize the features of the original disorders.
2 Explore whether or not the medications or treatments used for physical illness may be the precipitant or contributed to the depression and what substitution might be considered.
3 Determine if a treatment such as an antidepressant should be prescribed and which would be the most effective and safest choice.

Franco-Bronson[51] reported (not specifically for people with brain injury):

One of the most common misdiagnoses of treatment-resistant depression occurs in persons who are medically ill and have not been given adequate doses of medication. Physicians tend to be fearful of initiating cardiac arrhythmias, causing urinary retention, or setting off other highly unpleasant effects in persons who are already physically ill. Newer-generation antidepressants have largely avoided the quinidine-like, anticholinergic, and anti-adrenergic influence. It is also possible to avoid antihistaminic appetite increase and weight gain, a problem for persons with hypertension, cardiovascular disease, and diabetes mellitus. As both our knowledge about how to safely use the older choices has been joined by a new variety of selections, the physicians are less tempted to under treat.

Some antidepressants (non-SSRI antidepressants) used in patients resistant to other antidepressants may increase seizure risk, especially when using monoamine oxidase inhibitors (MAOIs), tricyclic antidepressant agents (TCAs), atypical heterocyclic agents (amoxapine, maprotiline and bupropion), because all are known to lower seizure threshold. To use these medications in depression-resistant patients may require higher therapeutic levels of anticonvulsants. Thus, the higher the antidepressant dosage, the higher the risk of seizure. Valproate (valproic acid) has been shown to have a positive response in persons with seizures and brain injury[54] (Valproate does not treat depression, it is a mood stabilizer). Selegaline is an MAOI lowering seizure threshold. Bomocriptine may help cognitive features but not depression.

For treatment of agitation, some authors have suggested the use of neuroleptic medication, although they are known to have a side-effect that may have long-term consequences for cognition and motor recovery.[55] Medications such as Haldol or Zyprexa may be used. For post-traumatic agitation, medications typically used for treatment of seizures may be used, such as Depakote, as well as Tegretol – however, *post-traumatic* agitation suggests a more acute event, such as re-emergence belligerence, and needs something faster acting, like propranol. Sedation and resistance to taking such medications may be a complaint and at times individuals with brain injuries have a difficult time accommodating to such medications.

Yudofsky et al.[56] have also suggested the use of beta-blockers such as Inderal as a means of treating explosive personality characteristics if they are related to a known neurological trauma. In an excellent review article, Burnett et al.[55] discussed the use of many of the above-mentioned medications, and indications for use as well as side-effects. They conclude that the "lack of consensus in defining and managing TBI-related agitation requires interdisciplinary work to classify its manifestation". They further report that an interdisciplinary team should include at a minimum physicians, psychiatrists, and other rehabilitation professionals such as neuropsychologists in order to balance the team and provide a broader approach to treatment. The authors report that continued research is necessary to identify which neuroleptic drugs would have the greatest reduction of TBI-related agitation and the best benefits for treatment of such disturbances. The serotonin/dopamine antagonists seem to be quite available and offer promise for effective treatment without compromising cognitive functioning.

Literature published in the area of treatment of depression for persons with a brain injury, using SSRI medications has stirred controversy in the field of psychology and psychiatry. A recent article discussed a previously published study that showed little difference in a non-brain injury population between those receiving antidepressant medications (such as SSRIs or tricyclic medications), when compared to cognitive behavioral therapy interventions. This article relayed the results of a subsequent study that did not support this finding,[57] but instead pointed out that some people in the previous study were resistant to certain medications and likely would have benefited from trials of a different type of antidepressant. Using a crossover design in their study, these researchers found that indeed the medications were as effective as or better than only psychotherapy, and that the previous study, as well as theirs, did not allow adequate time and dosing to show an optimal effect on the people being treated.

A more recent article discussed the use of SSRI agents for a person with a BI and concluded: "SSRIs have been effective in the treatment of several psychiatric disorders, mainly depression, and have been found to be effective in the treatment of psychiatric conditions following TBI".[58] The authors also advised that care be used when combining agents, and rapid withdrawal avoided.

Another recent study discussed the promising effects of amantadine, a tricyclic water-soluble amine salt. The authors of this study suggest that this substance "affects the synthesis, accumulation, release, and uptake of catecholamines in the central nervous system". Although a large multicenter double-blind trial of amantadine has not been completed, preliminary evidence found "a consistent trend toward a more rapid functional impairment of TBI cases if treated within the first three months after injury".[59]

Clearly, additional studies are needed to assess the effectiveness of medications versus various types of psychotherapy. Use of one of several types of possible antidepressant medications in addition to psychological treatment modalities may be most effective for treatment of depression and related affective disorders. Studies of this nature, specifically with persons with brain injury, are suggested in future research in order to draw more definitive conclusions about treatment effectiveness with brain injured persons.

Talk therapy in neurorehabilitation

Perhaps the least controversial method of treating the depression, anxiety, and related affective disturbances following brain injury is that of individual neuropsychological treatment or individual and group psychotherapy. In traditional holistic brain injury programs, treatment in groups is often a preferred modality. This is often the most available means of treating individuals because it tends to be cost effective, promotes coherence within the group, and is an effective means of providing feedback.[60] Group approaches can be used to provide feedback to individuals who, because of impaired self-awareness, may not benefit ultimately from having one therapist relate their impressions of how they are functioning, whereas they may react differently to their peers providing such feedback. The process of professional and peer feedback, tends to shape behaviors over time, with continuous reinforcement and modeling used to identify appropriate responses to various social and interpersonal situations.[7] Providing an atmosphere that is supportive, permissive, yet structured enough to focus on central activities such as appropriate assertiveness, goal-directed conversations, and "in the moment" experiences is a critical part of this process.[47]

In addition to the holistic multidisciplinary team approach, individual psychotherapy is also a common approach to treatment of depression and anxiety-related symptoms. Whereas there may be a potential ethical dilemma to consider if treating individuals both in a group and individually, the importance for providing a supportive therapeutic outlet to discuss the emotional attachment that they have to certain ideas or changes in their life is a critical part of the treatment process. Often, delicate issues may not be appropriate to discuss in group situations, or in the milieu of a holistic brain injury program. These may include issues related to sexual functioning, real or potential changes in the family structure due to cognitive physical and emotional changes of the brain injury, or to issues regarding suicidal thinking and appropriate intervention planning.

León-Carrión,[1] in a chapter on the treatment of affective disorders and suicidal tendencies after traumatic brain injuries, offers valuable suggestions on how to provide emotional support for individuals following a neuropsychological treatment approach, as can be seen in Table 7.1. Nonetheless, the importance of careful planning of all aspects of therapy should not be overlooked. León-Carrión,[1,17] considers that people at high risk for suicide will generally make an attempt when they are experiencing cognitive improvement, and the therapist may not be aware of the potential risk. Cognitive improvement brings with it an end to an unawareness of deficits, which until that time, in a way, protected the person from suicidal acts. However, as the person experiences a growing awareness of his or her situation, the risk of suicide increases. Given that a person in this process may need additional help in coping with his or her new personal situation, feelings and emotions, the authors recommend that cognitive and psychotherapy be carried out in concert with medication.

Table 7.1 Suggestions for the rehabilitation of patients with emotional sequelae after acquired brain injury

The 10 steps of emotional therapy for TBI patients

1. Offering hope, always
2. Offering affection explicitly, especially on the part of relatives and close friends
3. Promoting self-esteem
4. Seeing what is affectively relevant for patients
5. Providing, insofar as patients can, opportunities for participation in group therapy, group discussion, or group activities
6. Providing some weekly individual therapy sessions where patients can express their most intimate feelings or needs, which can and should be worked on at the individual level more than at the group level
7. Carrying out adjustment therapies to reality rather than interpretative or figurative therapies of reality. In the therapy, reality should be clear. Therapy should favor "awareness," not confusion
8. Involving the family in treatment. In case it may be necessary, it is advisable to carry out family therapy with the rebuilding of the family affective system as the main objective
9. Trying to find the patient's strong side, that which he/she has preserved best and what he/she does best, reinforcing it, and from this point, expanding to other areas. Finding points of motivation and interests
10. Developing the expression of emotions so that they are socially appropriate and not socially disabling.

Reproduced by permission from (1).

Other treatment modalities to treatment of depression and anxiety

The nature and types of other treatments that go beyond the neuro-psychological approach or group dynamics and milieu therapy have also been approached in the literature. McKenna and Haste[61] reported the clinical effectiveness of dramatherapy and the recovery from neurotrauma. They examined ten patients in a neurorehabilitation unit, and each participant received five individual one-to-one therapy sessions over a 5 week period. A semi-structured interview was carried out with each participant following the course of the dramatherapy. In the therapy, various forms of artistic and creative expression were used. The use of visual images, objects, music, arts and crafts, maps, myths, and legends, as well as poetry and relaxation exercises were used. The authors found that dramatherapy made an important contribution to the healthy adjustment of some patients both to hospital life and to acquired disability. The various approaches allowed individuals to interact comfortably with media that they felt were relevant to their own style of interaction and acquired deficits.

Biofeedback has also been a means of assisting and controlling anxiety-related symptoms and for gaining better control over medical symptoms, as well as for improving physiological awareness. In one of the few published articles in the use of biofeedback-assisted relaxation training for brain-injured individuals in the acute stages of recovery, Holland et al.[62] found this approach to be very useful. The cases profiled in their article suggested that the concrete and direct nature of biofeedback may help even severely cognitively impaired individuals gain control over anxiety reactions when other techniques for relaxation training or anxiety remain too complex or too abstract for a confused patient.

Similar means of anxiety reduction have been identified in the literature including the use of breathing techniques for managing anxiety-related symptoms.[47] Exercises, especially while still in the hospital and in the alert but pre-stages of rehabilitation, may prove valuable for teaching methods of self-control. When individuals begin to react to stress, breathing also often becomes shallow, fast, and may produce other physiologic symptoms.[63] By simply focusing on the fact that a person can have better control over their physiologic status by monitoring their breathing, regulating their breath by taking control over what otherwise may be a simple physiologic response, anxiety symptoms can often be managed very quickly. Diaphragmatic breathing is one rapid way to teach people a brief yet simple method of controlling symptoms.

Concluding remarks

The occurrence of depression, anxiety, and other affective disturbances is a complex issue that must be dealt with in any comprehensive neuropsychological treatment program. There is evidence to suggest that the neurotrauma injury in itself may produce altered states of mood, and the cascading chemical events that occur following brain injury contribute to additional physiologic and emotional changes as well. Perhaps the most important aspect of behavioral change that occurs following stabilization of the physical and medical aspects of an acquired brain injury occur as a result of realizing the losses, adjusting to the new sense of self, and finding a new direction to follow in the future.

The changes in family structure, changes in finances, and changes in the person's role not only in the family but also in the community and, most importantly, in the workforce, can cause great discomfort and changes in self-image.

A number of theories as to why depression, anxiety, and other symptoms may occur have been presented, as well as varying points of view for treatment, including pharmacological medication, neuropsychological approaches to treatment, and involvement of the family as a critical part of the treatment team.

Some additional points to consider when developing treatment plans for individuals with an acquired brain injury include issues relative to dignity and empowerment. After having things "done to them", during the medical recovery phase, it is important to begin to restore control over their environment back to the individual. This does not mean that they will have total control over all aspects of their treatment, but they should have choices and options wherever feasible which can be communicated to them in a manner that they can understand. This principle of informed consumer choice should be an essential element in any neuropsychological treatment approach.

Included in this approach is the need to treat each person with dignity and respect, which a recent study found to be the most important consideration of individuals entering community-based rehabilitation programs.[64] Beyond any physical changes, monetary changes due to improvement in work status or living situations, the desire to be treated with dignity and respect and, to be actively involved in all aspects of their treatment programs as appropriate given the level of cognitive ability, was cited as the single most important factor in the treatment and rehabilitation program.

Much is left to be discovered regarding the efficacy of various treatment approaches to persons with brain injury, especially in the area of treatment of depression, anxiety, and related disorders. With the rapid advancements in medical technology, biochemical research and high technology, dramatic changes in treatment methods for affective-related disturbances in the future are expected. This provides not only hope for treating clinicians, but should be a critical aspect that the clinician can also relate to the people they serve. Even though we may not be able to achieve our greatest successes in today's treatment environment, the hope that improved knowledge and techniques will be able to provide better answers and better solutions in the future is an important aspect to relate to all individuals seeking treatment for affective disorders.

References

1. León-Carrión, J. (1997). An approach to the treatment of affective disorders and suicide tendencies after TBI. In J. León-Carrión (Ed.), *Neuropsychological rehabilitation: Fundamentals, innovations, and directions* (pp. 415–429). Delray Beach, FL: GR/St. Lucie Press.
2. Gaultieri, C. T. (1999). The pharmacologic treatment of mild brain injury. In N. R. Varney & R. J. Roberts (Eds.), *The evaluation and treatment of mild traumatic brain injury* (pp. 411–419). Mahwah, NJ: Lawrence Erlbaum Associates.
3. Perlesz, A., Kinsella, G., & Crowe, S. (2000). Psychological distress and family satisfaction following traumatic brain injury: injured individuals and their primary, secondary, and tertiary carers. *J. Head Trauma Rehabil., 15*, 909–929.
4. Thomsen, I. V. (1992). Late psychosocial outcome in severe traumatic brain injury. *Scand. J. Rehabil. Med. Suppl., 26*, 142–152.
5. Willer, B. S., Allen, K. M., Liss, M., & Zicht, M. S. (1991). Problems and coping strategies of individuals with traumatic brain injury and their spouses. *Arch. Phys. Med. Rehabil., 72*, 460–464.
6. Schlund, M. W., & Pace, G. (1999). Relations between traumatic brain injury and the environment: feedback reduces maladaptive behavior exhibited by three persons with traumatic brain injury. *Brain Inj., 13*, 889–897.
7. Prigatano, G. P. (1997). The problem of impaired self-awareness in neuropsychological rehabilitation. In J. León-Carrión (Ed.), *Neuropsychological rehabilitation: Fundamentals, innovations, and directions* (pp. 301–312). Delray Beach, FL: GR/St. Lucie Press.
8. León-Carrión, J. (1998). Neurologically-related changes in personality inventory (NECHAPI): a clinical tool addressed to neurorehabilitation planning and monitoring effects of personality treatment. *NeuroRehabilitation, 11*, 129–139.
9. Malec, J. F., & Basford, J. S. (1996). Postacute brain injury rehabilitation. *Arch. Phys. Med. Rehabil., 77*, 198–207.
10. Malec, J. F., & Thomas, D. F. (1993) Brain injury rehabilitation in small towns and rural communities. In D. F. Thomas, F. E. Menz and D. C. McAlees (Eds.), *Community-based employment following traumatic brain injury* (pp. 83–112). Menomonie, WI; University of Wisconsin–Stout, Research and Training Center.
11. Harlow, J. M. (1868). Recovery from the passage of an iron bar through the head. *Publ. Mass. Med. Soc., 2*, 327–347.
12. Bigler, E. D. (1988). On the neuropsychology of suicide. *J. Learn. Disabil., 22*, 180–185.
13. Ross, E. D. (1985). Right-hemisphere lesions in disorders of affective language. In A. Kertesz (Ed.), *Localization in neuropsychology* (pp. 493–508). New York: Academic Press.
14. Grafman, J., Vance, S. C., Weingartner, H., Salazar, A. M., & Armin, D. (1986). The effects of lateralized frontal lesions on mood regulation. *Brain, 109*, 1127–1148.
15. Jorge, R. E., Robinson, R. G., & Arndt, S. V. (1993). Depression after traumatic brain injury: a 1 year longitudinal study. *J. Affect. Disord., 27*, 233–243.
16. Max, J. E., Koele, S. L., Smith, W. L. Jr, et al. (1998). Psychiatric disorders in children and adolescents after severe traumatic brain injury: a controlled study. *J. Am. Acad. Child Adolesc. Psychiat. 37*, 832–840.
17. Madrazo-Lazcano, M., Machuca-Murga, F., Barroso y Martín, J. M.,

Domínguez-Morales, M. R., & León-Carrión, J. (2000). Emotional changes following severe brain injury. *Revist. Española Neuropsicología, 2*(4), 75–82.

18. Hermann, M., & Wallesch, C. W. (1993). Depressive changes in stroke patients. *Disabil. Rehabil. 15*, 55–66.

19. Gainotti, G., Azzoni, A., & Marra, C. (1999). Frequency, phenomenology and anatomical–clinical correlates of major post-stroke depression. *Br. J. Psychiat., 175*, 163–167.

20. Paradiso, S., Chemerinski, E., Yazici, K. M., Tartaro, A., & Robinson, R. G. (1999). Frontal lobe syndrome reassessed: comparison of patients with lateral or medial frontal brain damage. *J. Neurol. Neurosurg. Psychiat. 67*, 664–667.

21. Bowen, A., Chamberlain, M. A., Tennant, A., Neumann, V., & Conner, M. (1999). The persistence of mood disorders following traumatic brain injury: a 1 year follow-up. *Brain Inj., 13*, 547–553.

22. Jorge, R. E., Robinson, R. G., & Arndt, S. V. (1993). Are the depressive symptoms specific for a depressed mood in traumatic brain injury? *J. Nerv. Ment. Dis., 181*, 91–99.

23. Varney, N. R., Martzke, J. S., & Roberts, R. J. (1987). Major depression in patients with closed head injury. *Neuropsychology, 1*, 7–9.

24. Harrick, L., Krefting, L., Johnston, J., Carlson, P., & Minnes, P. (1994). Stability of functional outcomes following transitional living programme participation: 3-year follow-up. *Brain Inj., 8*, 439–447.

25. Frieboes, R., Müller, U., Murck, H., von Cramon, D. V., Holsboer, F., & Steiger, A. (1999). Nocturnal hormone secretion and the sleep EEG in patients several months after traumatic brain injury. *J. Neuropsychiat. Clin. Neurosci. 11*, 354–360.

26. Kosciulek, J. F. (1994). Relationship of family coping with head injury to family adaptation. *Rehabil. Psychol., 39*, 215–230.

27. Bryant, R. A., Marosszeky, J. E., Crooks, J., Baguley, I. J., & Gurka, J. A. (1999). Interaction of postraumatic stress disorder and chronic pain following traumatic brain injury. *J. Head Trauma Rehabil., 14*, 588–594.

28. Hibbard, M. R., Uysal, S., Kepler, K., Bogdany, J., & Silver, J. (1998). Axis I psychopathology in individuals with traumatic brain injury. *J. Head Trauma Rehabil., 13*, 24–39.

29. Malec, J. F., Machulda, M. M., & Moessner, A. M. (1997). Differing problem perceptions of staff, survivors, and significant others after brain injury. *J. Head Trauma Rehabil., 12*, 1–13.

30. Prigatano, G. P., & Schacter, D. L. (1991). *Awareness of deficit after brain injury: Theoretical and clinical issues.* New York: Oxford University Press.

31. Lezak, M. D. (1983). *Neuropsychological Assessment* (2nd ed.). New York: Oxford University Press.

32. Thomas, D. F. (1990). Vocational evaluation of persons with traumatic head injury. In D. Corthell (Ed.), *Traumatic brain injury and vocational rehabilitation* (pp. 111–140). Menomonie, WI: University of Wisconsin–Stout, Research and Training Center.

33. León-Carrión, J., Serdio-Arias, M. L., Cabezas, F. M., et al. (2001). Neurobehavioral and cognitive profile of traumatic brain injury patients at risk for depression and suicide. *Brain Inj., 15*, 175–181.

34. Mann, J. J. (1987). Psychobiologic predictors of suicide. *J. Clin. Psychiat. 48*(Suppl.), 39–43.

35. Mann, J. J., Arango, V., Marzuck, P. M., Theccanat, S., & Reis, D. J. (1989).

Evidence for the 5-HT hypothesis of suicide: a review of post-mortem studies. *Br. J. Psychiat. 8*, 7–14.

36. Lopez, J., Vazquez, D. M., Chalmers, D. T., & Watson, S. J. (1997). Regulation of 5-HT receptors and the hypothalamic–pituitary–adrenal axis: implications for the neurobiology of suicide. In D. H. Stoff and J. J. Mann (Eds.), *The neurobiology of suicide: From the bench to the clinic. Ann. N. Y. Acad. Sci., 836*, 106–134.

37. Tondo, L., Jamison, K. R., & Baldessarini, R. J. (1997). Effect of Lithium maintenance on suicidal behavior in major mood disorders. In D. M. Stoff & J. J. Mann (Eds.), *The neurobiology of suicide: From the bench to the clinic. Ann. N. Y. Acad. Sci., 836*, 339–351.

38. Tate, R. L., Simpson, G., Flanagan, S., & Coffey, M. (1997). Completed suicide after traumatic brain injury. *J. Head Trauma Rehabil., 12*, 16–28.

39. Butcher, J. N., Dahlstrom, W. G., Graham, J. R., Tellegen, A. T., & Kaemmer, B. (1987). *MMPI-2 manual for administration and scoring*. Minneapolis, MN: University of Minnesota Press.

40. Millon, T. (1987). *Manual for the MCMI-II*. (2nd ed.). Minneapolis, MN: National Computer Systems.

41. Beck, A. T., Steer, R. A., & Brown, G. K. (1996). *BDI-II, Beck depression inventory: Manual* (2nd ed.). Boston, MA: Harcourt, Brace & Co.

42. Beck, A. T., & Steer, R. A. (1988). *Beck hopelessness scale manual*. San Antonio, TX: The Psychological Corporation.

43. Beck, A. T., & Steer, R. A. (1990). *Beck anxiety inventory manual*. San Antonio, TX: The Psychological Corporation.

44. Reynolds, W. M., & Kobak, K. A. (1995). *A self-report version of the Hamilton depression rating scale*. Odessa, FL: Psychological Assessment Resources, Inc.

45. Prigatano, G. P., Bruna, O., Mataro, M., Junoz, J. M., Fernandez, S., & Junque, C. (1998). Initial disturbances of consciousness and resultant impaired awareness in Spanish patients with traumatic brain injury. *J. Head Trauma Rehabil., 13*, 29–38.

46. Ben-Yishay, Y. (1979). Structured group techniques for heterogeneous groups of head trauma patients. *NYU Rehabil Monogr., 60*, 39–88.

47. Malec, J. F., & Moessner, A. M. (2000). Self-awareness, distress, and postacuate rehabilitation outcome. *Rehabil Psychol., 45*, 227–241.

48. Miller, I. W., & Keitner, G. I. (1996). Combined medication and psychotherapy in the treatment of chronic mood disorder. *Psychiat. Clin. N. Am., 19*(1), 151–171.

49. Neppe, V. M., & Goodwin, G. T. (1999). Neuropsychiatric evaluation of the closed head injury of transient type (CHIT). In N. R. Varney and R. J. Roberts (Eds.) *The evaluation and treatment of mild traumatic brain injury* (pp. 261–284). Mahwah, NJ: Lawrence Erlbaum Associates, Inc.

50. Gaultieri, C. T. (1993). Traumatic brain injury. In B. S. Fogel and A. Stoudemire (Eds.) *Psychiatric care of the medical patient* (pp. 517–535). New York: Oxford University Press.

51. Franco-Bronson, K. (1996). The management of treatment-resistant depression in the medically ill. *Psychiat. Clin. N. Am., 19*(2), 329–350.

52. Cohen-Cole, S. A., & Stoudemire, A. (1987). Major depression and physical illness: special considerations in diagnosis and biological treatment. *Psychiat. Clin. N. Am., 10*, 1–17.

53. Metzger, E. D., & Freedman, R. S. (1994). Treatment-related depression. *Psychiat. Ann., 24*, 540–544.

54. Stoll, A. L., Banov, M., Kolberner, M., et al. (1994). Neurologic factors predict a

favorable valproate response in bipolar and schizoaffective disorders. *J. Clin. Psychopharmachol., 14*, 311–313.

55. Burnett, D. M., Kennedy, R. E., Cifu, D. X., & Levenson, J. (1999). Using atypical neuroleptic drugs to treat agitation in patients with brain injury: a review. *NeuroRehabilitation, 13*, 165–172.

56. Yudofsky, S. C., Silver, J. M., Jackson, M., Endicott, J., & Williams, D. (1986). The overt aggression scale: an operationalized rating scale for verbal and physical aggression. *Am. J. Psychiat. 143*, 35–39.

57. Thase, M. E., Friedman, E. S., Fasiczka, A. L., et al. (2000) Treatment of men with major depression: a comparison of sequential cohorts treated with either cognitive-behavioral therapy or newer generation antidepressants. *J. Clin. Psychiat., 61*, 466–472.

58. Meythaler, J., Brunner, R., Johnson, A., & Novack, T. (2002). Amantadine to improve neurorecovery in traumatic brain injury-associated diffuse axonal injury: a pilot double-blind randomized trial. *J. Head Trauma Rehabil., 17*, 300–313.

59. Zafonte, R., Cullen, N., & Lexell, J. (2002). Serotonin agents in the treatment of acquired brain injury. *J. Head Trauma Rehabil., 17*, 322–334.

60. Ben-Yishay, Y., & Gold, J. (1990) Therapeutic milieu approach to neuropsychological rehabilitation. In R. L. Wood (Ed.), *Neurobehavioural sequelae of traumatic brain injury* (pp. 194–215). London: Taylor & Francis.

61. McKenna, P., & Haste E. (1999). Clinical effectiveness of dramatherapy in the recovery from neurotrauma. *Disabil Rehabil., 21*, 162–174.

62. Holland, D., Witty, T., Lawler, J., Lanzisera, D. (1999). Biofeedback-assisted relaxation training with brain injured patients in acute stages of recovery. *Brain Inj., 13*, 53–57.

63. Bonica, J. J., & Loeser, J. D. (1990). Medical evaluation of the patient with pain. In J. J. Bonica (Ed.), *The management of pain* (Vol. 1, pp. 563–579). Philadelphia, PA: Lea & Febiger.

64. Thomas, D. F., Menz, F. E., & Rosenthal, D. A. (2001). Employment outcome expectancies: consensus among consumers, providers, and funding agents of community rehabilitation programs. *J. Rehabil., 67*, 26–34.

8   Sleep disorders in patients with traumatic brain injury

Antonio Vela-Bueno, E. O. Bixler, and A. N. Vgontzas

Introduction

Sleep disorders are common clinical manifestations of brain traumas. For example, many patients who have sustained mild brain traumas complain of insomnia or excessive daytime sleepiness. Also, the most severely injured patients may have different sleep disorders as part of their clinical picture. Sleep disorders can be part of both the acute and the chronic behavioral consequences of traumatic brain injuries (TBI). In the latter case, they may be a symptom of a well-defined clinical condition, such as an anxiety disorder, a mood disorder or a psychotic disorder. In some cases, sleep and wakefulness disturbances are the primary complaint or one of the most important ones presented by a patient with a TBI.

The etiology of sleep disorders in TBI patients may be related to the brain lesion itself, the psychopathology associated with the trauma or the use of medication commonly prescribed in brain injured subjects. An example of the first catagory is that of hypersomnia related to a lesion of the structures involved in the regulation of sleep and wakefulness, such as the reticular activating system in the brainstem. Psychopathological factors are well exemplified by the post-traumatic stress disorder that is commonly found among patients after traffic accidents. The use of drugs with central nervous system (CNS) depressant or stimulant effects can contribute to the appearance of excessive daytime sleepiness or insomnia respectively.

The presence of a sleep disorder in a TBI patient may have an adverse impact on the clinical course of the traumatic sequelae. In this regard, the neuropsychological consequences of various sleep disorders are well known, particularly those of the sleep apnea syndrome.[1] Also insomnia and the use of hypnotics may cause cognitive (especially memory) impairment.[2,3]

The evaluation of a patient with a sleep disorder associated with a TBI should be accomplished following the same model recommended for the sleep-disordered patient in general, i.e., a multidimensional approach.[4] The first step is a thorough clinical history that includes a detailed sleep history, and a general medical, mental, and drug history. The diagnostic process should also include a complete physical examination and a mental status assessment. The use of brain imaging and polygraphic sleep studies, when indicated, completes the evaluation.

There is a dearth of information regarding sleep disorders in TBI patients in spite of their potential impact on the clinical presentation and course, as well as treatment and rehabilitation of the behavioral consequences of TBI. One reason for this underreporting could be that in this type of patient, especially when severe sequelae are present, sleep disorders are not considered a priority.

In this chapter we shall summarize the available literature and experience on sleep disorders in TBI patients. The chapter is organized following the two major categories of sleep disorders according to DSM-IV sleep nosology: dysomnias and parasomnias.

Dysomnias consist of disorders due to inadequate duration and/or quality of sleep or of misplacement of the major sleep period within the 24-hour period. Since they are associated with either disturbed, nocturnal sleep or impaired daytime wakefulness, their manifestations are insomnia or excessive sleep. Generally speaking, they involve the mechanisms underlying the regulation of sleep and wakefulness.

Parasomnias are episodic disorders associated with the transition between wakefulness and sleep, or vice versa, or with specific sleep stages, and involve various motor, autonomic, psychic, and behavioral functions. They do not involve the regulatory mechanisms of sleep and wakefulness per se.

Dysomnias

The dysomnias summarized here are: insomnia, the disorders of excessive sleepiness and the disorders of the circadian sleep–wakefulness rhythm. For the main ones such as insomnia, excessive sleepiness in general, sleep apnea and narcolepsy in particular, we include a relatively detailed description of the condition.

Insomnia

General issues

Insomnia literally means lack of sleep, although in clinical practice the term is used to refer to complaints of insufficient sleep duration and poor quality. Insomnia is characterized by three types of difficulties: falling asleep (the most common), staying asleep and early final awakening.

Insomnia can be of short duration (transient) or chronic. When chronic, especially if severe, the patient can consider the sleep problem a disease in itself.[2]

The prevalence of persistent chronic insomnia in adult general populations is about 10–11%.[5,6] It is more common among women, elderly individuals and those of lower socioeconomic status and poorer health.

Etiological factors contributing to the appearance of insomnia are multiple.[2] A variety of diseases can be associated with it both due to their somatic manifestations (e.g., pain, fever, general distress) and to the psychological reactions to the disease (e.g., anxiety and depression symptoms). The environment, especially that of the hospital, can be a source of insomnia. The use of CNS stimulant substances and drugs as well as continued use and withdrawal of CNS depressants can be factors in the development of insomnia. This is a frequent symptom of different psychiatric conditions such as anxiety, mood and psychotic disorders, among others. Patients with a primary complaint of chronic insomnia have high levels of psychopathology (both state and trait). Thus the vast majority of those patients present with minor or subsyndromal depressions, anxiety and personality disorders or traits.[2]

Stressful life events in vulnerable individuals who cope inadequately with stress through internalization of emotion lead to emotional arousal, and then to physiological hyperarousal, as shown by hyperactivity of the neuroendocrine system of stress and the autonomic functions controlled by the sympathetic system. This hyperarousal state is responsible for the difficulty in falling asleep at night (both at sleep onset and following nocturnal awakenings) and during the daytime. The fear of sleeplessness increases the emotional arousal closing the vicious circle that perpetuates insomnia.

The evaluation of the insomniac patient starts with a thorough clinical history. Table 8.1 summarizes some guidelines for obtaining it. The diagnosis must be completed with the somatic examination and the psychological assesment. The polygraphic study of sleep is not systematically indicated in the diagnosis of insomnia unless the coexistence of another sleep disorder, such as sleep apnea, is suspected.

The treatment of transient insomnia is based on helping the patient to cope in an adaptive manner with stressful situations and/or dealing with other etiological factors (somatic and pharmacological among others) contributing to insomnia. The treatment of chronic insomnia is a much more complicated task, and needs to be done based on a multidimensional approach that includes several therapeutic modalities: general hygiene measures, psychotherapy, cognitive-behavioral measures and pharmacological treatment.[2] Table 8.2 summarizes the hygiene measures. Psychotherapy used in the treatment of insomnia is one that combines different technical modalities. Cognitive-behavioral therapy is based on restriction of time in bed, stimulus control, and changes in the ideas and beliefs about sleep and the consequences of insomnia.

The pharmacological treatment of insomnia is mainly based on the use of agonists of the supramolecular receptor complex GABA A-benzodiazepine that belong to four groups: benzodiazepines, cyclopirrolones, imidazopyridines, and pirazolopyramidines. The administration of hypnotics should be done following the guidelines summarized in Table 8.3. However, because this class of medication is associated with a relatively rapid onset of tolerance and

Table 8.1 Clinical history of the sleep-disordered patient

General history
• Demographic information
• Chief complaint

Sleep history
• Assess sleep–wakefulness patterns
• Identify the sleep disorder
• Assess its clinical course
• Differentiate between disorders
• Determine impact of the disorder on patient's life
• Ask the bed partner
• Family history

Medical history
• Symptoms of any present illness
• Past medical history
• Family history

Psychiatric history
• Obtain biographic and developmental history
• Assess premorbid personality
• Assess previous adjustment
• Assess presence of stressful life events
• Assess coping mechanisms
• Family history

Drug history
• Ask about caffeine and nicotine consumption
• Assess alcohol use patterns
• Investigate use of illegal drugs
• Assess manifestations of drug withdrawal
• Rule out causative role of prescription drugs

---

loss of efficacy, sedative antidepressants are increasingly used by clinicians in the treatment of insomnia.

Hypnotics should be used cautiously in patients with severe TBI because of the enhanced likelihood of adverse reactions. Of particular concern are those involving cognitive functions. These are more common with the short-acting, high-potency compounds.[3] Also, antidepressants with strong anticholinergic activity may adversely affect the cognitive functions of these patients and even cause delirium.

In the presence of a definite depressive disorder, a sedative antidepressant, administered at bedtime, is the drug of choice. If insomnia is a symptom of a psychotic condition, a sedative antipsychotic is preferred. In both cases, attention has to be paid to the potential for lowering the convulsive threshold in a brain-damaged patient and to the anticholinergic side-effects.

Table 8.2 Sleep hygiene measures

Daytime
• Avoid long naps
• Exercise properly and regularly
• Minimize or avoid the use of caffeine, nicotine, and alcohol
• Eat at regular times
• Manage stress properly

Bedtime
• Avoid alcohol and other drugs
• Use sleep-inducing drugs only if prescribed by a physician
• Develop and practice bedtime rituals
• Avoid worrying; set aside worry time
• Bedtime snacks may be helpful
• Relaxation techniques, e.g., tapes, books
• Go to bed when sleepy

Sleep environment
• Be aware of "adaptation effect" in unfamiliar environments
• Minimize the disruptive effects of light and noise
• Regulate humidity, ventilation, and temperature

Sleeptime
• Do not try to force sleep
• Avoid other activities (except sex) other than sleep in the bedroom
• Avoid too much time in bed
• Avoid extremes in sleep duration
• Sleep the hours that allow you good daytime functioning
• Avoid watching the clock if you wake up at night
• Go to bed and get up at regular times 7 days a week

Table 8.3 The use of hypnotic drugs

• Rule out the presence of sleep apnea
• Rule out the presence of COPD
• Assess the presence of organic brain syndromes
• Use hypnotics as an adjunctive treatment
• Use the lowest effective dose
• Assess the development of tolerance
• Be aware of expected adverse reactions, i.e., daytime sedation
• Be aware of unexpected adverse reactions, i.e., daytime anxiety and delayed amnesia
• Be aware of withdrawal reactions, i.e., rebound insomnia

Insomnia in TBI

Most studies on sleep disorders in patients with traumatic brain injury have focused primarily or exclusively on insomnia. A common finding is that it is very frequent among patients with injuries of various levels of severity. Thus, in a group of 102 adult patients with a TBI representing a broad range of severity,[7] a total of 36% complained of insomnia 1 month after suffering the trauma compared to 18% of the controls. There were no differences among the TBI subgroups based on severity.

A large epidemiological survey on high school and university students found that more than one-third of the subjects interviewed reported having experienced a head injury, mostly mild, and close to 12% reported multiple head injuries.[8] In one of the two high school subsamples and in the university group, sleep difficulties were significantly more prevalent among those subjects who suffered a traumatic brain injury than in those who did not (32% vs. 25%, respectively). Also, multiple brain injuries were associated with more sleep difficulties in the same high school subsample and in one university subsample. In all of the subsamples mentioned above, brain injury and multiple brain injuries were independent predictors of sleep difficulties after controlling for age, gender, and depression.

Several clinical studies have confirmed that insomnia is a frequent finding in patients who had minor traumatic brain injuries. In one of them, insomnia was among the most common sequelae of concussion[9] with 15.2% of 145 patients complaining of it six weeks after the injury. A more recent study of 39 patients interviewed an average of two years after suffering a minor injury[10] found high proportions of patients complaining of various aspects of their sleep: problems with sleep initiation (52.6%), frequent nocturnal awakenings (64.9%), sleep duration complaints (53.8%), problems with early awakening (92.3%), complaints of restless sleep (55.9%) and complaints of shallow sleep (97.4%). However, only sleep initiation problems and sleep duration complaints were significantly more frequent in these patients than in the control group that consisted of orthopedic surgery patients. Another study found significant changes in the reported sleep patterns of a sample of 75 patients who were questioned 3 months after experiencing a minor head injury.[11] Compared with 3 months before the accident, they had significantly more sleep complaints, poorer quality of sleep, more sleep interruptions, and more difficulty returning to sleep. These changes were related to the scores on the Glasgow Coma Scale (GCS) with subjects with lower scores reporting more sleep complaints.

Patients with moderate to severe traumatic brain injury also complain frequently of insomnia. In one study that included 20 subjects with severe traumatic brain injury,[12] 45% of the patients had insomnia. Insomnia was more frequent in those with diffuse bilateral cortico-subcortical injury, loss of consciousness and intracerebral hemorrhage. The polygraphic recordings in this study showed abnormal temporal distribution of REM sleep and short REM latency, a finding associated with depression and other psychiatric conditions.[13] Another study showed that the frequency of insomnia declines with time.[14] Thus, 59% of a sample of 22 hospitalized patients who suffered a recent traumatic brain injury reported insomnia, whereas less than 4% of a sample of 77 patients who had suffered the trauma approximately two-and-a-half years before complained of insomnia. More than half of the hospitalized patients with insomnia attributed a causative role to the hospital environment.

Finally, a recent study of 86 patients consecutively admitted to a rehabilitation unit reported that 1 year after discharge,[15] about two-thirds of them (64%) complained of waking up too early, whereas 45% had difficulty falling asleep. Subjects with higher scores (equal to or above seven) on the GCS reported more sleep difficulties; median score for the whole sample was four. Also, those with immediate memory scores average or above had more sleep problems than those with impaired memory scores. The logistic regression analysis showed that sleep difficulties were more likely if the person was older, female or with a history of alcohol abuse. There was no relationship with the medications being used.

Sleep problems are more common among those brain-injured individuals with pain including headaches.[16,17] Both insomnia and pain (56.4% and 58.9%, respectively) were significantly more frequent among patients with TBI as compared to neurological patients with various conditions.[16] The average time post-injury was about 2 years, whereas the time elapsed after the neurologic patients'[16,17] symptoms started was almost 3 years. The most common sleep difficulty was that of maintaining sleep. Patients complaining of pain were twice as likely to report difficulties falling asleep and maintaining sleep, as well as overall insomnia, compared to those without pain, Thus, TBI subjects with pain had significantly more complaints of insomnia than those without pain. Subjects with a mild injury reported about 50% more complaints of insomnia than those with a moderate to severe injury without pain. Also, those patients with mild injury and no pain had twice as many complaints of insomnia as compared to those with moderate to severe injury. There was a decrease of both insomnia and pain complaints over time (follow-up of 5 years or more). The temporal evolution of patients with a TBI without pain differed depending on whether it was mild or moderate to severe. In the mild group, the decrease of complaints was gradual, whereas in the moderate to severe group there was an increase between the second and the fourth year and then a decrease.

The role of depression in insomnia among TBI patients has been addressed in several studies. In one study that included 91 consecutive patients admitted to an outpatient rehabilitation program, the strongest association of insomnia was with depression, as measured by the Beck Depression Inventory (BDI) and milder brain injury severity as assessed by the GCS and the lack of positive findings (lesions) in the CT scan. The presence of pain was significantly associated with insomnia. When logistic regression analysis was performed with a model including BDI, the pain item of the Pittsburgh Sleep Quality Index, GCS and litigation status, it correctly classified 87% of the cases having the presence or absence of insomnia. Only depression and severity of injury made unique contributions to the prediction of insomnia.[18]

Furthermore, it appears that the various insomnia complaints contribute to delineate, along with a cluster of symptoms, the type of depressive disorders associated with traumatic brain injury.[19] Thus, difficulty falling asleep in addition to anxiety symptoms, diurnal mood variation (morning depression), decreased appetite and weight loss appear to be significantly associated with depression 3 months after the injury. Also, early morning awakening along with loss of libido, difficulty concentrating and inefficient thinking distinguish depressed from non-depressed TBI patients 6 months to a year after the injury.

As for the treatment of TBI insomnia in patients with traumatic brain injury, there is a lack of systematic information and there are only isolated reports in the literature of severe persistent insomnia following traumatic injury.[20,21] In the first case study, the patient had a brainstem lesion and a marked reduction of total sleep time; the administration of 5-hydroxy-tryptophan substantially increased the amount of time he spent asleep.[20] The other patient was clearly depressed and showed signs of basal ganglia dysfunction.[21] Different therapeutic strategies (pharmacological and non-pharmacological) failed, whereas some improvement was noticed with the use of a combination of neuroleptic and antihistamine drugs. The latter were discontinued because of the concerns about adverse reactions.

To summarize, data from several sources have clearly shown that insomnia is a common complaint among individuals who sustained traumatic brain injuries of varying severity. As shown in the previous paragraphs, virtually all the existing evidence was obtained from subjective reports. This approach might be insufficient in research focusing on patients with cognitive impairment. For example, when memory impairment was taken into account in some studies, those with poorer memory reported fewer sleep difficulties. Therefore, adding objective sleep measures to assess sleep patterns is of utmost importance in these patients who most likely underreport their symptoms.

Disorders of excessive sleepiness

The presence of excessive sleepiness after a TBI, in addition to being a clinical problem, often constitutes a public safety and a medico-legal problem.[22] In this section we will review the general aspects of excessive sleepiness in TBI patients, as well as three specific subtypes of disorders of excessive sleepiness (DES) occurring in these patients: sleep apnea, narcolepsy, and periodic hypersomnias. Although excessive daytime sleepiness is not always associated with an increase in total sleep time throughout the 24 hours (hypersomnia), we will not differentiate between excessive sleepiness and hypersomnia.

Excessive sleepiness in TBI patients

Head injuries may be one of the factors leading to symptomatic hypersomnias.[23,24] The lesions most likely to cause hypersomnia are those of the mesencephalic tegmentum, the posterior and lateral hypothalamus, third ventricle and posterior fossa. However, excessive sleepiness can be present in cases without clear-cut lesions. Finally, psychopathology may contribute to the manifestation of excessive daytime sleepiness (EDS) in TBI patients.

The EDS may appear at varying time intervals following the TBI. When hypersomnia occurs immediately after the TBI, it needs to be differentiated from coma. The differentiation is mainly based on the severity of sleepiness, its depth and associated reactivity. When sleepiness is mild, the patient is easily awakened, although he or she may fall asleep again easily. In other cases, it will be more difficult to wake up the patient. When it is not possible to wake up the patient, the state is better defined as coma rather than hypersomnia. An oscillation from one state to the other is possible.

Subjective complaints of excessive sleepiness by patients who sustained TBI are frequent. In one study, patients with mild TBI were found to complain of excessive sleepiness (worded as "inappropriate napping") significantly more often (20%) than their controls (0%).[10] Another study found that "drowsiness" was among the most common post-concussion sequelae 48 hours after the trauma, decreasing from 13% to 9% 1 week after the trauma.[24]

Studies with patients who suffered moderate to severe TBIs have also reported more frequent excessive sleepiness. In one of them, 12 (20%) of the subjects had EDS. The frequency of complaints of excessive sleepiness appears to depend on the time elapsed after the trauma took place.[14] Thus, whereas only 3 out of 22 patients (13.6%) with a recent brain injury complained of EDS, 29 out of 77 (37.6%) subjects complained of EDS two and a half years after the injury. Finally, another subjective study[15] reported that 25% of the subjects slept more than usual after experiencing the TBI and this was not found to be related to the use of any medication.

According to some authors, the clinical characteristics of the post-traumatic hypersomnias are not different from those of the other hypersomnias.[23] In general, the sleepiness of variable intensity is part of a more general post-traumatic syndrome. It is uncommon that EDS occurs as the only or main symptom.

Other authors have pointed out that the severity of sleepiness that can be incapacitating is mainly related to the severity of the TBI, as defined by the duration of the coma and the degree of neurological deficits.[22,25] Another factor that may contribute is the use of anticonvulsant medications.

There have been attempts to objectively document excessive daytime sleepiness in patients with TBI. Thus, one study reported that patients with a post-concussional syndrome were more likely than normal subjects to show signs of drowsiness during routine EEG recordings.[26] Another study that recorded the EEG both in conditions that favored wakefulness and sleep (darkness) found that the post-concussional subjects showed more EEG signs of sleepiness.[27]

The evaluation of the sleepy patient after a TBI should include a thorough clinical assessment as well as auxiliary techniques and tests. Several polygraphic recording techniques (continuous recording, or one or more naps taken ad lib or scheduled after a full night recording) have been used to objectively document the daytime sleepiness of TBI patients.[22,25] The most commonly used, the so called Multiple Sleep Latency Test (MSLT) that consists of giving the subject several opportunities to take a nap at 2-hour intervals,[28,29] has shown limitations in this regard.

There are no controlled studies on the pharmacological treatment of EDS following TBI. However, there is a report stating that when hypersomnia following head trauma becomes chronic, especially in cases in which the patients were in coma more than 1 week, the response to stimulant medications can be unsatisfactory.[25] Thus, other pharmacological strategies should be tried, including the use of energizing antidepressants.

Sleep apnea–hypopnea syndrome (SAHS)

GENERAL ISSUES

The sleep apnea–hypopnea syndrome (SAHS) is characterized by the presence during sleep of numerous apneas and hypopneas lasting at least 10 s each.[30,31] There are three types of apneas: central, with a complete cessation of air flow and ventilatory effort; obstructive, with cessation of air flow and persistence of ventilatory effort; mixed, starting with a central component and ending as obstructive. There is no consensus on the definition of hypopnea, but it is generally accepted that it is present whenever there is a decrease of the air flow of 50% and a drop of oxygen saturation of more than 4%. The diagnosis of the syndrome is based on the presence of clinical symptoms, i.e, daytime sleepiness and an apnea/hypopnea index of more than ten.

The symptoms of SAHS are nocturnal and diurnal.[30,31] The most typical nocturnal ones are: respiratory pauses, intense snoring, snorting and gasping. Night-time sleep usually is restless, with nocturia (sometimes enuresis) excessive sweating, sleeptalking (sometimes sleepwalking) headaches, gastro-esophagical reflux and excessive salivation. After getting up, patients are usually fatigued, with headaches and dry mouth and throat, among other symptoms. During the daytime typical symptoms include: excessive sleepiness and even sleep attacks; impairment of attention, concentration and memory (sometimes with automatic behavior); anxiety and depression, irritability and even aggressivity; sexual dysfunctions are also common.

Most patients with SAHS (75%) present systemic arterial hypertension.[32] Often the most severe also show right heart failure and left ventricular hypertrophy.

Snoring often precedes by many years the onset of SAHS.[33] The temporal sequence of appearance of the symptoms as obtained by a clinical history is usually: (1) snoring; (2) excessive daytime sleepiness; (3) systemic arterial hypertension; (4) obesity; (5) nocturnal respiratory pauses; (6) daytime sleep attacks.[33]

The prevalence of SAHS in the general adult population is 4% for men and 1% for women.[34,35] There is an increase of prevalence until middle age (55 for men and 65 for women) followed by leveling off. In women there is an increase in prevalence after menopause.[35]

The etiology of SAHS is not well known.[31] There seems to be some genetic predisposition. Other contributing factors are obesity, particularly central, and in some cases anatomical abnormalities (micrognatia, retrognatia, tonsilar and/or amygdalar hypertrophy and deviated nasal septum among others). Some skeletal malformations (both cranial and thoracic) as well as some muscular diseases may increase the risk. SAHS is associated with acromegaly and hypothyroidism in a certain proportion of cases. The use of alcohol and other CNS depressants has a temporary worsening effect on SAHS.

The obstructive mechanism underlying apneas and hypopneas involves several sites in the pharyngeal area.[31] Factors such as the muscular hypotonia, the supine decubitus and pre-existing narrowings favor the obstruction.

The diagnosis of SAHS is made based on a thorough clinical history obtained with the cooperation of the patient's bed partner. The physical examination should preferably be completed with an exploration of the maxilofacial structures as well as the upper airways. The suspicion of SAHS should always be confirmed with a polygraphic study of nocturnal sleep including electroencephalogram, electrooculogram and electromyogram, as well as recordings of the nasal and oral air flow, respiratory movements and oximetry. This type of study assesses the severity of the condition based on the number of apneas and hypopneas per hour of sleep (apnea/hypopnea index), as well as the degree of oxygen desaturation associated with them.

The treatment of SAHS starts with some general measures such as weight loss and abstinence from alcohol, and CNS depressants.[36] Whenever possible, all the contributing factors, i.e., hypertrophic tonsils or adenoids, deviated septum, etc., should be corrected.[36] However, these measures are insufficient in most cases. The treatment of choice is the application of continuous positive pressure through the nares (a method known as nasal-CPAP).[37] This procedure maintains the upper airways patent and suppresses apneas, hypopneas and snoring. This procedure will also normalize the sleep organization (that is often severely disturbed in these patients) and the levels of O_2 saturation. Surgical procedures such as uvulopharyngopalatoplasty are associated with a low success rate (40–50%). The success rate tends to be lower in obese patients and 2 years after surgery. In very severe cases, tracheostomy with a permanent cannule can be indicated.[38] In mild to moderate cases, oral appliances may be helpful. They work by expanding the pharyngeal space.[39]

SHAS IN TBI PATIENTS

There are a few reports of cases of sleep apnea syndrome appearing after significant head trauma. In one of them, eight patients presented typical apnea syndromes ranging in severity from moderate to severe, as shown by an apnea/hypopnea index in all patients of more than 20 and in six of them of more than 30, the predominant type of apnea being mixed, with a marked obstructive component.[25] Oxygen desaturation was marked, and all patients presented fragmented nocturnal sleep. During the daytime, excessive sleepiness was objectively documented with polygraphic recording of naps. Slow improvement without treatment was reported in 5/8 subjects over periods of 18–24 months. Follow-up polygraphic sleep recordings showed an average apnea/hypopnea index of 6 (range 1–8). One subject who complained of marked excessive daytime sleepiness 34 months after the trauma had an index of 35. This patient was treated with stimulants and clomipramine with no improvement. Of these eight patients, four complained of whiplash, two reported loss of consciousness and others mentioned significant head/neck trauma without major loss of consciousness. None of them presented odontoid or cervical fractures or significant cervical hernias.

In another study, 50 out of a total sample of 184 patients who presented excessive sleepiness following head–neck trauma were diagnosed with SAHS, with an apnea/hypopnea index of 31.[22] The vast majority (94%) of the respiratory events were obstructive or mixed. The patients had a mean body mass index of 26.7. Another nine patients with an apnea/hypopnea index of less than five were diagnosed with an upper airway resistance syndrome (UARS). This condition is characterized by the presence in the polysomnogram of multiple brief arousals (as shown by the appearance of alpha or theta rhythm in the EEG) associated with increases in respiratory effort.[40]

Of the total 59 patients with SAHS or UARS of the above-mentioned study,[22] 49 had maxillomandibular and orofacial features that are considered "risk factors" (see the section on general aspects). An interesting finding that extends previous observations of the same group of authors (see above) is that all 16 patients with whiplash had either SAHS or UARS.

A challenging question is whether SAHS or UARS precedes the trauma, considering that patients with those conditions have an increased risk of having accidents.[41,42] In the above-mentioned study,[22] that possibility was shown to be quite unlikely since 52 of the 59 patients did not provide a previous history of those conditions. Six patients were identified to be snorers prior to the accident, but without excessive sleepiness, whereas the remaining patients' histories of sleep-disordered breathing was unobtainable.

Another report described the case of an 11-year-old boy who developed a very severe central sleep apnea syndrome after suffering a traumatic brain injury that caused extensive multilevel lesions: left occipital and parietal areas; left thalamic area; and bilateral lesions in the posterior and lower medulla.[43] The lesions at the medullary level were responsible for the central sleep apnea syndrome. Treatment with continuous positive airway pressure (CPAP) in association with a negative pressure ventilator suppressed all the apneas and normalized the O_2 saturation.

In summary, the presence of an SAHS should always be ruled out after a person suffers a traumatic brain injury. In addition to being a life-threatening condition, the well-known cognitive impairment associated with SAHS might interfere with neuropsychological rehabilitation.[1] Another issue that deserves attention is whether the SAHS might have preceded the accident.

Narcolepsy

GENERAL ISSUES

The main clinical features of narcolepsy are manifestations of excessive sleepiness and the so-called "auxiliary symptoms", i.e., cataplexy, sleep-paralysis and hypnagogic hallucinations. The four symptoms together are known as the "narcoleptic tetrad".[32,44-46]

Excessive sleepiness expresses itself as a general trend to fall asleep or as sleep attacks. These occur more easily in circumstances that involve monotony or inactivity and can last between a few seconds and half an hour.[32,44-46] Cataplexy consists of a brief and sudden loss of muscle tone without loss of consciousness. It is triggered by strong emotions and its intensity ranges from drooping of the jaw to complete bilateral loss of the muscle tone that provokes a fall.[32,44-46] Sleep paralysis consists of the inability to move any muscle (other than the respiratory ones) during the transition between wakefulness and sleep.[32,44-46] Hypnagogic hallucinations consists of vivid pseudoperceptions (mainly visual and auditory) occurring between the transition between wakefulness and sleep.[32,44-46] The nocturnal sleep of narcoleptic patients is often disturbed with multiple awakenings, and, in some patients, with difficulty falling asleep.[32,44-46]

The onset of the symptoms of narcolepsy usually occurs before 25 years of age. The first symptoms to appear are those of excessive sleepiness, followed, months or years later, by cataplexy and/or the other auxiliary symptoms. Narcolepsy is a chronic disorder without lasting remissions. The auxiliary symptoms tend to improve over the years.[32,44-46]

The prevalence of narcolepsy in the general population is about 0.05%.[47] It is somewhat more common among men than among women.[45]

The etiology of narcolepsy is unknown, although both genetic and environmental factors seem to be involved.[46] The genetic contribution seems to be well documented by several facts. These include: (1) a high proportion of first degree relatives are affected; (2) a high degree of association of the disease with HLA-DR2 and DQW1; (3) it has been shown that the susceptibility for narcolepsy is related to HLA DQB1* 0602 and DQA1*0102.[48] Environmental factors, especially those of a stressful nature through their interaction with genetic ones, seem to contribute to the development of the disease.[46]

The pathophysiology of the symptoms of narcolepsy seems to be related to abnormalities in the mechanisms maintaining wakefulness and those involved in the regulation of REM sleep.[44-46,48] Sleepiness is specifically associated with a failure to maintain wakefulness during sleep attacks and auxiliary symptoms with REM sleep abnormalities. Sleep in the narcoleptic frequently begins in REM sleep (both during the day and at night). Cataplexy and sleep paralysis involve muscle atonia, and hypnagogic hallucinations, oniric activity.

The diagnosis can be made based on the clinical history, especially when cataplexy is present along with excessive sleepiness. The polygraphic recording of sleep both at night and during the day (with multiple nap recordings or continuous 24 h recording) help to confirm the diagnosis. Two findings that are diagnostic of narcolepsy are a short sleep latency and two or more sleep onsets in REM sleep (SOREMP) periods. The inmunogenetic tests (HLA) do not have a well-established predictive value.[48]

The treatment of narcolepsy is based on both pharmacological and non-pharmacological measures. Pharmacological treatment of somnolence is based on the use of stimulant drugs, such as amphetamines, methylphenidate and, more recently, modafinil, a drug with a better benefit to risk ratio.[44,45,49] For the auxiliary symptoms the drugs of choice are antidepressants, ranging from tryciclics to the SSRI and, more recently, venlafaxine and reboxetine.

Non-pharmacological measures include: regularizing sleep habits, increasing activity and taking several regular, planned short naps. Supportive psychotherapy may be indicated in some cases, particularly those associated with secondary psychopathology.

POST-TRAUMATIC NARCOLEPSY

There have been reports suggestive of cases of narcolepsy following head trauma.[50] More recently there have been descriptions of definite narcolepsy in patients who sustained a TBI, although this is an uncommon finding even when dealing with general samples of excessive sleep disorders following TBI.[22,25] In one series of 20 patients, only one presented definite narcolepsy,[25] whereas in a much larger sample (n = 184) the same group[22] did not report any definite case, although five patients had two or more SOREMPs during the five MSLT naps and two of the five were positive for the HLA haplotypes commonly found in narcolepsy. No patient presented cataplexy.

Post-traumatic narcolepsy has also been reported in nine patients who suffered mild to moderate closed head injury.[51] Except in two cases, all of them presented at least one "auxiliary symptom", whereas all of them except one (who had only one) showed two or more SOREMs in the MSLT. In a group of six patients, HLA was considered to be DR2 positive in three patients, one DQw1 positive and two DR4 positive. In a clinical follow-up of up to 5 years, all remained symptomatic. They were treated with a combination of stimulants and/or tricyclic antidepressants and showed some response.

There are a few isolated case reports of post-traumatic definite narcolepsy. In one,[52] a 19-year-old man started to develop the symptoms of the narcoleptic tetrad 4 months after suffering a head trauma that involved a brief loss of consciousness; in the MSLT, two SOREMPs were found. Another case[53] was that of a 37-year-old man who developed the full narcoleptic tetrad 18 months after the TBI. He also showed three SOREMs in the MSLT and was HLA-DR2 positive. He was partially responsive to a combination of methylphenidate and nortryptiline.

A 27-year-old man suffered a severe TBI and developed the full tetrad several weeks after being discharged, following a coma which lasted 19 days.[54] In addition, he had several SOREMPs in the MSLT. The administration of methylphenidate improved both excessive daytime sleepiness and cataplexy. Another interesting observation was that of a 37-year-old man who had coexisting narcolepsy and delusions of jealousy.[55] The narcoleptic symptoms (sleep attacks, cataplexy and sleep paralysis) appeared several months after the trauma. Behavior (impulsivity, irritability, and accusations towards his wife) improved and cataplexy and sleep paralysis disappeared with 20 mg of fluoxetine although objective signs of sleepiness persisted in the MSLT. Finally, there has been a report of a patient who presented all the clinical features of narcolepsy-cataplexy, but not excessive sleepiness nor SOREMPs in the polygraphic studies. The HLA typing was negative for DR2.[56]

In summary, although post-brain-injury narcolepsy is a rare finding, the specialist dealing with TBI should be aware of this condition. When present in such patients, it raises interesting questions about the pathophysiology of narcolepsy, in addition to the clinical and medico-legal issues.

Periodic hypersomnias

The course of chronic symptomatic hypersomnia is usually of the short-cycle type,[23] i.e., having episodes of sleepiness every day: however, some cases follow the evolution of long cycle or periodic. A few cases of periodic hypersomnia following head injury have been documented in the literature. Some of them are associated with mood and eating disorders.[23]

The most typical periodic hypersomnia is the Kleine–Levin syndrome, a rare condition characterized by periodic hypersomnolence, hyperphagia, sexual disinhibition, irritability and aggressiveness, as well as other psychopathological manifestations.[57] The condition is mostly found in male adolescents and its etiology is unknown. Although head trauma has been considered as one of the possible etiological factors since its initial description,[58–60] in only 2.3% of 162 observations in the literature[57] was "a blow in the face" associated with the onset of the condition. There are also reports of cases in which the symptoms appeared in close temporal relationship with the brain injury. In one report, 2 patients out of a series of 14 developed periodic hypersomnia following mild head traumas.[61] The patients were a woman and a man. In both cases the symptoms did not appear immediately after the injury. The woman presented a typical Kleine–Levin syndrome, whereas in the case of the man, it was considered to be atypical. In the other report,[62] the patients were two male adolescents who developed the typical symptomatology of Kleine–Levin syndrome a few weeks and one day, respectively, after a traumatic brain injury. Both improved with the administration of lithium carbonate, a drug that has been useful in patients with idiopathic Kleine–Levin syndrome.

Circadian rhythm sleep disorders

These types of conditions have in common a mismatch between the patient's sleep timing and the one that is desired or considered socially normal.[63] Their pathophysiology is believed to be related to a dysfunction in the patient's endogenous circadian timing system or to its relative lack of capacity to adjust to unusual schedules due to social demands.[63] Current classifications of sleep disorders include at least six subtypes of circadian disorders.[63] In this section, we will focus on the three that have been reported to occur in association with traumatic brain injury: the delayed sleep-phase syndrome, the advanced sleep-phase syndrome, and the irregular sleep–wake pattern.

The three circadian rhythm disorders mentioned may occur with either the complaint of insomnia or excessive sleepiness. Thus, it is not unlikely that a substantial number of patients included in the studies described in the sections on insomnia and excessive sleepiness might have had this type of disorder. In trying to understand the pathophysiology of these diagnoses, the role of a dysfunction of the endogenous circadian system is emphasized. However, environmental, psychological, and behavioral factors should always be taken into consideration.

Delayed sleep-phase syndrome

The main symptom of this disorder is a marked difficulty in initiating sleep and in awakening at the desired times. The result is a marked delay in the timing of the major sleep episode, which is of normal duration when the patient is allowed to sleep freely. Average times of falling asleep and of waking up are between 2 am and 6 am and around noon, respectively. The daytime consequences are significant delays at school or at the workplace. If the patient tries to fulfill his or her obligations, partial sleep deprivation occurs with the ensuing daytime sleepiness. Adolescence is an age of increased vulnerability to suffering from this disorder.[63]

There have been a few case reports of delayed sleep-phase syndrome following traumatic brain injury without adequate chronobiological assessment, both in two male adolescents[64,65] and an adult man.[66] The brain injuries in the adolescents were mild, whereas in the adult they were moderate to severe. None of the two patients who were evaluated from a psychiatric standpoint showed psychopathology.[64,66] In the case of the adolescent,[64] the authors described a dysfunctional family and secondary gain on the part of the boy. In these two patients, chronotherapy was attempted without success. This method consists of delaying the bedtime and getting up time 3 hours daily with the goal of realigning the patient's sleep schedule with the desired one.[63] The active cooperation of the patient and family are crucial for this treatment to succeed. In these two patients, it failed. Factors such as the secondary gain and dysfunctional family might have accounted for the failure in the case of the adolescent,[64] whereas refusal of the request for permanent disability filed by the adult[66] could have contributed to the failure in the adult.

In the best-documented case report, a 15-year-old girl who suffered head trauma 3 days before experiencing the symptoms of delayed sleep-phase syndrome was administered melatonin, which normalized her circadian rhythms.[67] Markers studied were: endogenous melatonin and body temperature rhythms, wrist actigraphy and sleep polygraphy.

In another report (published as an abstract) more than half of 15 patients with minor traumatic brain injury suffered a delayed sleep-phase syndrome.[68] No other details (such as age, sex, and treatment) were provided.

Advanced sleep-phase syndrome

This disorder is characterized by an advance of both sleep onset and final awakening, resulting in a marked advance of the major sleep episode. The patient feels very sleepy in the evening, falling asleep, when allowed, not later than 9 pm and waking up as early as 3 am.[63]

There is only one report of a case of post-traumatic advanced sleep-phase syndrome.[65] The patient was a 53-year-old man; no information on psychiatric evaluation or treatment was provided.

Irregular sleep–wake pattern

In this disorder, the episodes of sleep and wakefulness are variable in duration and disorganized in their temporal presentation. The patient may complain of either insomnia or excessive sleepiness.[63]

There is only one report of a case of post-traumatic irregular sleep-wake pattern.[68] In a group of 15 patients with minor traumatic brain injury, less than half presented the disorder. No demographic or therapeutic information was provided.

Parasomnias

Several clinical studies have reported the frequency of parasomnias in TBI patients. In one study of patients with a minor brain injury,[10] the patients reported relatively high rates for their age of nightmares (36.8%), sleepwalking (10.2%), and sleep talking (31.5%), although not statistically significantly higher than their controls in the study. The role that psychological factors might have played in their occurrence is unclear. In a more recent study on post-traumatic hypersomnia,[22] 41.3% of patients reported nightmares, 16.8% night terrors, and 8.7% abnormal behavior during sleep that the authors equated with "REM behavior".

There are two clinical case reports in the literature of parasomnia following traumatic brain injury. One is the case of a 16-year-old girl with jactatio nocturna after a severe head injury.[69] This condition, also known as rhythmic movement disorder, is characterized by repetitive movements of large muscular groups, most commonly of the head and neck, that typically occur immediately before sleep onset and are sustained into light sleep. The disorder usually affects infants and toddlers and usually disappears by the third year of life, although it may be present even into adulthood in rare cases. In the above-mentioned case,[69] the episodes disappeared with imipramine administered at bedtime. The mechanism by which the drug exerted its effect is unknown.

There was only one post-traumatic case of REM sleep behavior disorder out of the 280 cases reported in world literature until 1995.[70] This was a parasomnia characterized by a complaint of violent or injurious behavior during REM sleep associated with dream mentation. The patient behaved as if he or she were acting out the dream content. Polygraphic studies of sleep show the loss of the muscle atonia typical of REM sleep, in addition to demonstrating the episodes (in conjunction with the video monitoring). The treatment of choice for this disorder is the use of clonazepam at bedtime. The drug seems to maintain its efficacy even in long-term treatments.

In summary, there is little information about the occurrence of parasomnia following traumatic brain injury. However, its presence should always be elicited and, when necessary, differentiated from epileptic seizure. Also, its occurrence should be ascertained to help in the identification of a post-traumatic stress syndrome.

Other sleep disorders

In a sample of subjects with minor head injuries,[10] 50% complained of "sleep kicking". This figure was not significantly higher than that of the controls. A recent study[22] reported "leg and body jerks during sleep" in 18.5% of their sample. Subjects were patients referred for hypersomnia after head–neck trauma.

There are two case reports regarding periodic leg movements as sequelae of head injury. One of them described periodic leg movements occurring during wakefulness and nocturnal arousals in two patients who suffered severe traumatic brain injury.[71] In both patients the movements disappeared at sleep onset.

The other report[72] included three patients, two adults who suffered a mild traumatic brain injury and a 6-year-old child who was in coma after the trauma. The adults complained of difficulty in initiating and maintaining sleep and daytime fatigue, whereas the child complained of daytime somnolence. In all of them, periodic leg movements during sleep were present; although the author mentioned restless legs symptoms, it is not clear if he considered those movements to be sufficient for diagnosing this syndrome. The three patients were treated with clonazepam for their symptoms. It is unclear from the report if the child had disturbed nocturnal sleep.

Once it is decided that a polygraphic nocturnal sleep recording is justified, the evaluation of a patient with sleep disorders should include electrodes on the limbs (especially the legs) to rule out periodic leg movements. However, the causative role of these movements is questioned in the occurrence of insomnia and daytime somnolence.

Sleep complaints and sleep patterns: relation to cognitive and behavioral outcome

One of the most important issues in traumatic brain injuries is prognosis of the cognitive, affective and behavioral outcome. Several studies, both clinical and polygraphic, have addressed the issue of the possible correlation between sleep complaints and sleep patterns and the cognitive, behavioral and affective outcome of the injured patients.

One study[14] reported that the presence of cognitive, affective and behavioral disorders was unrelated to that of sleep complaints in patients with a recent brain injury. However, patients with sleep complaints were dependent on others in activities of daily life and had aphasia. In contrast, 2 to 3 years after the injury, those with sleep complaints had more anxiety, depression, apathy, and aggression. Also, they had poorer occupational outcome. Communicative and cognitive disorders tended to be more common among those with sleep complaints.

A consistent relationship between REM sleep and cognitive outcome has been shown in several studies using polygraphic recordings. In one of them,[73] none of the patients who initially had their REM sleep extremely reduced recovered a normal cognitive performance at follow-up (14 months after the trauma took place). Those who initially showed a complete suppression of REM sleep still had severe cognitive deficits at follow-up and severe or mild REM sleep abnormalities. The patients who showed normal REM sleep 4 weeks after the injury completely recovered their cognitive functions. The authors pointed out that the sooner the polygraphic features of sleep are restored, the earlier the cognitive normalization.

In another study with a larger sample, the same group of authors[74] confirmed and extended their results. They concluded that patients with severe residual cognitive defects had an initial complete suppression of stages REM and 4. In addition, they showed that almost 90% of those with initial REM suppression had some degree of neuropsychological deficit 2 years later.

Another study found a positive correlation between cognitive improvement and the increase of amount of REM sleep in seven out of the nine patients they studied.[75] No correlation was found with other sleep stages. In the two patients in whom the correlation between REM and cognition was negative, the damage was thought to be in the brainstem.

Finally, another study found a negative correlation between the percent of REM sleep and ratings in hyperactivity.[76] In addition, the number of awakenings during the night showed a positive correlation with the ratings of global psychopathology.

The findings of the polygraphic studies we have summarized in this section generally agree with what is known about patients with various sleep disorders and neuropsychiatric syndromes. For example, the cognitive sequelae of various disorders of excessive sleepiness are well known[77] and the possible association of the disturbances in REM sleep with cognitive deficits has been documented.[78]

The above-mentioned polygraphic studies have some methodological limitations that might have influenced their results. One is the potential effect of pharmacological treatment. The drug status of their patients was not clear from their description both initially and at follow-up. Also, none of them included respiratory recordings ruling out the presence of sleep apnea. This syndrome is well known for causing important cognitive deficits.[1] It has been shown that some patients with traumatic brain injury developed sleep-related breathing abnormalities that spontaneously resolved with time.[22]

References

1. Kales, A., et al. (1985). Severe obstructive sleep apnea II: associated psychopathology and psychosocial consequences. *J. Chron. Dis., 38*, 427–434.
2. Kales, A., & Kales, J. (1984). *Evaluation and treatment of insomnia.* New York: Oxford University Press.
3. Kales, A., Vgontzas, A. N., & Bixler, E. O. (1995). Hypnotic drugs. In A. Kales (Ed.), *Pharmacology of sleep* (Chapter 13). Berlin: Springer.
4. Kales, A., & Madow, L. (1987). Office management of sleep disorders patients. *Psychiat. Ann., 17*, 479.
5. Ford, D. E., & Kamerow, D. B. (1989). Epidemiologic study of sleep disturbance and psychiatric disorders: an opportunity for prevention 2. *M. J. Am. Hed. Assoc., 262*, 1479–1484.
6. Vela-Bueno, A., de Iceta, M., & Fernández, C. (1999). Prevalence of sleep disturbance in the city of Madrid. *Gac. Sanit., 13*, 441–448.
7. McLean, A., et al. (1984). Psychosocial functioning at one month after head injury. *Neurosurgery, 14*, 393–399.
8. Segalowitz, S. J., & Lawson, S. (1995). Subtle symptoms associated with self-reported mild head injury. *J. Learn. Dis., 28*, 309–319.
9. Rutherford, W. H., Merrett, J. D., & McDonald, J. R. (1977). Sequelae of concussion caused by minor head injuries. *Lancet, 8001*, 1–4.
10. Perlis, M. L., Artiola, L., & Giles, D. E. (1997). Sleep complaints in chronic postconcussion syndrome. *Percept. Motor Skills, 84*, 595–599.
11. Parsons, L. C., & Ver Beek, D. (1982). Sleep–wake patterns following cerebral concussion. *Nurs. Res., 31*, 260–264.
12. Askenasy, J. J., & Rahmani, L. (1988). Neuropsychosocial rehabilitation of head injury. *Am. J. Phys. Med., 66*, 315–327.
13. Benca, R. M., Obermeyer, W. H., Thisted, R. A., & Gillin, J. C. (1992). Sleep and psychiatric disorders: a meta-analysis. *Arch. Gen. Psychiat., 49*, 657–668.
14. Cohen, M., Iksenberg, A., Snir, D., Stern, M. J., & Grosswasser, Z. (1992). Temporally related changes of sleep complaints in traumatic brain injured patients. *J. Neurol. Psychiat., 55*, 313–315.

15. Clinchot, D. M. (1998). Defining sleep disturbance after brain injury. *Am. J. Phys. Med. Rehabil., 77*, 291–295.

16. Beetar, J. T., Guilmette, T. J., & Sparadeo, F. R. (1996). Sleep and pain complaints in symptomatic traumatic brain injury and neurologic populations. *Arch. Phys. Med. Rehabil., 77*, 1298–1302.

17. McBeath, J. G., & Manda, A. (1994). Use of dihydroergotamine in patients with postconcussion syndrome. *Headache, 34*, 148–151.

18. Fichtenberg, N., Mills, S. R., Mann, N. R., Zafonte, R. D., & Millard, A. E. (2000). Factors associated with insomnia among post-acute traumatic brain injury survivors. *Brain Inj., 14*, 659–667.

19. Jorge, R. E., Robinson, R. G., & Arndt, S. (1993). Are there symptoms that are specific for depressed mood in patients with traumatic brain injury? *J. Nerv. Ment. Dis., 181*, 91–99.

20. Guilleminault, C., Cathala, J. P., & Castaigne, P. (1973). Effects of 5-hydroxytryptophan on sleep of a patient with a brainstem lesion. *Electroencephalogr. Clin. Neurophysiol., 34*, 148–151.

21. Tobe, E. H. (1999). Persisting insomnia folowing traumatic brain injury. *J Neuropsychiat. Clin. Neurosci., 11*, 504–506.

22. Guilleminault, C., Yuen, K. M., Gulevich, M. G., Karadeniz, D., Leger, D., & Philip, P. (2000). Hypersomnia after head–neck trauma: a medicolegal dilemma. *Neurology, 54*, 653–659.

23. Roth, B. (1980). *Narcolepsy and hypersomnia* (Chapter 18). Basel: S. Karger.

24. Coonley-Hoganson, R., Sachs, N., Desai, B. T., & Whitman, S. (1984). Sequelae associated with head injuries in patients who were not hospitalized: a follow-up survey. *Neurosurgery, 14*, 315–317.

25. Guilleminault, C., Faull, K. F., Miles, L., & van den Hoed, J. (1983). Post-traumatic excessive daytime sleepiness: a review of 20 patients. *Neurology, 33*, 1584–1589.

26. Lairy-Bounes, G. C., & Benbanaste, J. V. (1953). Quelques aspects EEG des syndromes subjectifs posttraumatiques. *Rev. Neurol., 89*, 440.

27. Meurice, E. (1966). Les signes d'endormissement diurne dans un groupe de malades post-commotionnels comparé à un groupe de sujets normaux. *Rev. Neurol., 115*, 524.

28. Carskadon, M. A., Dement, W. C., Mitler, M. N., Roth, T., Westbrook, P. R., & Kenan, S. (1986). Guidelines for the multiple sleep latency test (MSLT): a standard measure of sleepiness. *Sleep, 9*, 519–524.

29. Carskadon, M. A., & Dement, W. C. (1981). Cumulative effects of sleep restriction on daytime sleepiness. *Psychophysiology, 18*, 107–113.

30. Coccagna, G. (2000). *Il sonno e i suoi disturbi* (Chapter 6). Padova: Piccin.

31. Bassiri, A. G., & Guilleminault, C. (2000). Clinical features and evaluation of obstructive sleep apnea–hypopnea syndrome. In M. H. Kryger, T. Roth, and W. C. Dement (Eds.), *Principles and practice of sleep medicine* (Chapter 74). Philadelphia, PA: Saunders.

32. Kales, A., Vela-Bueno, A., & Kales, J. D. (1987). Sleep disorders: sleep apnea and narcolepsy. *Ann. Int. Med., 106*, 434–443.

33. Kales, A., et al. (1985). Severe obstrutive sleep apnea–I: onset, clinical course, and characteristics. *J. Chron. Dis., 38*, 419–425.

34. Bixler, E. O., Vgontzas, A. N., Ten Have, T., Tyson, K., & Kales, A. (1998). Effects

of age on sleep apnea in men I. Prevalence and severity. *Am. J. Resp. Crit. Care Med., 157,* 144–148.

35. Bixler, E. O., et al. (2001). Prevalence of sleep-disordered breathing in women: effects of gender. *Am. J. Resp. Crit. Care Med., 163,* 608–613.
36. Kryger, M. H. (2000). Management of obstructive sleep apnea–hypopnea syndrome: overview. In M. H. Kryger, T. Roth, and W. C. Dement (Eds.), *Principles and practice of sleep medicine* (Chapter 79). Philadelphia, PA: Saunders.
37. Grunstein, R., & Sullivan, C. (2000). Continuous positive airway pressure for sleep breathing disorders. In M. H. Kryger, T. Roth, and W. C. Dement (Eds.), *Principles and practice of sleep medicine* (Chapter 76). Philadelphia, PA: Saunders.
38. Riley, R. W., et al. (2000). Surgical therapy for obstructive sleep apnea–hypopnea syndrome. In M. H. Kryger, T. Roth, and W. C. Dement (Eds.), *Principles and practice of sleep medicine* (Chapter 77). Philadelphia, PA: Saunders.
39. Lowe, A. A. (2000). Oral appliances for sleep breathing disorders. In M. H. Kryger, T. Roth, and W. C. Dement (Eds.), *Principles and practice of sleep medicine* (Chapter 78). Philadelphia, PA: Saunders.
40. Guilleminault, C., Stoohs, R., Clerk, A., Cetel, M., and Maistros, P. (1993). A cause of excessive daytime sleepiness: the upper airway resistance syndrome. *Chest, 104,* 781–787.
41. Terán-Santos, J., Jiménez-Gómez, A. & Cordero-Guevara, J. (1999). The association between sleep apnea and the risk of traffic accidents. *N. Engl. J. Med., 340,* 847–851.
42. Masa, J. F., et al. (2000). Habitually sleepy drivers have a high frequency of automobile crashes associated with respiratory disorders during sleep, *Am. J. Resp. Crit. Care Med., 162,* 1407–1412.
43. Quera-Salva, M. A., & Guilleminault, C. (1987). Posttraumatic central sleep apnea in a child. *J. Pediat., 110,* 906–909.
44. Vgontzas, A. N., & Kales, A. (1999). Sleep and its disorders. *Ann. Rev. Med., 50,* 387–400.
45. Guilleminault, C., & Anagnos, A. (2000). Narcolepsy. In M. H. Kryger, T. Roth, and W. C. Dement (Eds.), *Principles and practice of sleep medicine* (Chapter 60). Philadelphia, PA: Saunders.
46. Billiard, M., Dauvilliers, Y., & Carlander, B. (1998). La Narcolepsie. In M. Billiard (Ed.), *Le sommeil normal et pathologique: Troubles du sommeil et de l'eveil* (p. 278). Paris: Masson.
47. Partinen, M., & Hublin, C. (2000). Epidemiology of sleep disorders. In M. H. Kryger, T. Roth, and W. C. Dement (Eds.), *Principles and practice of sleep medicine* (Chapter 47). Philadephia, PA: Saunders.
48. Mignot, E. (2000). Pathophysiology of narcolepsy. In M. H. Kryger, T. Roth, and W. C. Dement (Eds.), *Principles and practice of sleep medicine* (Chapter 59). Philadelphia, PA: Saunders.
49. Carlander, B. (1998). Traitements de la narcolepsie et autres troubles primaires de l'eveil. In M. Billiard (Ed.), *Le sommeil normal et pathologique: Troubles du sommeil et de l'eveil* (p. 313). Paris: Masson.
50. Autret, A., Lucas, B., Henry Lebras, F., & de Toffol, B. (1994). Symptomatic narcolepsies. *Sleep, 17,* 521–524.
51. Lankford, D. A., Wellman, J. J., & O'Hara, C. (1994). Posttraumatic narcolepsy in mild to moderate closed head injury. *Sleep, 17,* S25–8.

52. Macario, M., Ruggles, K. H., & Meriwether, M. W. (1987). Posttraumatic narcolepsy. *Milit. Med., 152*, 370–371.
53. Good, J. L., Barry, E., & Fishman, P. S. (1989). Posttraumatic narcolepsy: the complete syndrome with tissue typing. *J. Neurosurg., 71*, 765–767.
54. Francisco, G. E., & Ivanhoe, C. B. (1996). Successful treatment of posttraumatic narcolepsy with methylphenidate. *Am. J. Phys. Med. Rehabil., 75*, 63–65.
55. Wing, Y. K., Lee, S., Chiu, H. F., Lo, C. K., & Chen, C. N. (1994). A patient with coexisting narcolepsy and morbid jealousy showing favourable response to fluoxetine. *Postgrad. Med., 70*, 34–36.
56. Billiard, M., et al. (1993). Posttraumatic hypersomnia associated with cataplexy, hypnagogic hallucinations, sleep paralysis and disturbed nocturnal sleep but not with SOREM episodes and HLA DR2. *Sleep Res., 22*, 171.
57. Billiard, M. (1998). Les hypersomnies récurrentes. In M. Billiard (Ed.), *Le sommeil normal et pathologique. Troubles du sommeil et de l'eveil* (p. 298). Paris: Masson.
58. Levin, M. (1936). Periodic hypersommolence and morbid hunger: a new syndrome. *Brain, 59*, 494–504.
59. Critchley, M. (1962). Periodic hypersomnia and megaphagia in adolescent males. *Brain, 85*, 627–656.
60. Orlosky, M. J. (1982). Kleine–Levin syndrome. *Psychosomatics, 23*, 609–612.
61. Smolik, P., & Roth, B. (1988). Kleine–Levin syndrome. Ethiopathogenesis and treatment. *Acta Univ. Carol Med.* (Monograph 128). Prague: Charles University.
62. Will, R. G., Young, J. P. R., & Thomas, D. J. (1988). Kleine–Levin syndrome: report of two cases with onset of symptoms precipitated by head trauma. *Br. J. Psychiat., 152*, 410–412.
63. Wagner, D. R. (1996). Disorders of the circadian sleep–wake cycle. *Neurol. Clin., 14*, 651–670.
64. Patten, S. B., & Lauderdale, W. M. (1992). Delayed sleep phase disorder after traumatic brain injury. *J. Am. Acad. Child Adolesc. Psychiat., 31*, 100–102.
65. Govidan, S., & Govidan, E. (1993). Brain imaging in post-traumatic circadian rhythm sleep disorders. *Sleep Res., 24A*, 308.
66. Quinto, C., Gellido, C., Chokroverty, S., & Masdeu, J. (2000). Posttraumatic delayed sleep phase syndrome. *Neurology, 54*, 250–252.
67. Nagtegaal, J. E., Kerkhof, G. A., Smits, M. G., Swart, A. C., & van der Meer, Y. G. (1997). Traumatic brain injury-associated delayed sleep phase syndrome. *Funct. Neurol., 12*, 345–348.
68. Schreiber, S., et al. (1997). Polysomnographic and actigraphic findings of patients with minor traumatic brain injury. *J. Neuropsychiat. Clin. Neurosci., 9*, 640.
69. Drake, M. E. (1986). Jactatio nocturna after head injury. *Neurology, 36*, 867–868.
70. Schenck, C. H., & Mahowald, M. W. (1996). REM sleep parasomnias. *Neurol. Clin., 14*, 697–720.
71. Broughton, R., Willmer, J., & Skinner, G. (1987). Posttraumatic insomnia with rhythmic leg movements. *Sleep Res., 16*, 466.
72. Buda, F. B. (1996). Periodic leg movement syndrome: a newly described sequela of head trauma. *Sleep Res., 25*, 402.
73. Alexandre, A., Rubini, L., Nertermpi, P., & Farinello, C. (1979). Sleep alterations during posttraumatic coma as possible predictor of cognitive defects. *Acta Neurochir. Suppl., 28*, 188–192.

74. Alexandre, A., Colombo, F., Nertempi, P., & Benedetti, A. (1983). Cognitive outcome and early indices of severity of head injury. *J. Neurosurg., 59*, 751–761.
75. Ron, S., Algom, D., Hary, D., & Cohen, M. (1980). Time-related changes in the distribution of sleep stages in brain injured patients. *Electroencephalogr. Clin. Neurophysiol., 48*, 432–441.
76. Prigatano, G., Stahl, M. L., Orr, W. C., & Zeiner, H. K. (1982). Sleep and dreaming disturbances in close head injury patients. *J. Neurol. Neurosurg. Psychiatry., 45*, 78–80.
77. Ramos-Platón, M. J. (1996). Alteraciones neuropsicológicas en los trastornos del sueño. In M. J. Ramos-Platón (Ed.), *Sueño y procesos cognitivos* (Chapter 8). Madrid: Sintesis.
78. Bliwise, D. L. (2000). Dementia. In M. H. Kryger, T. Roth, and W. C. Dement (Eds.), *Principles and practice of sleep medicine* (Chapter 89). Philadelphia, PA: Saunders.

9 Rehabilitation of equilibrium and posture control after brain injury
The NeuroBird method

José León-Carrión, Eugene Mikhaelenov, María del Rosario Domínguez-Morales, and Olga Voronina

Introduction

Balance dysfunction and problems of postural control are commonly observed in people with acquired brain injury, causing problems in the control of body position in space and dificulties in stability and orientation. This chapter offers a conceptualization and protocolization of an effective system of functional re-education of problems of balance and stability associated with neurological injury. Different studies note the importance of treating balance at the beginning of rehabilitation due to the fact that the degree of balance dysfunction upon admission to rehabilitation would be a significant predictor of the need for assistance at discharge. Routine assessment of balance at admission to inpatient rehabilitation may enhance the ability to predict rehabilitation outcomes beyond that provided by assessment of functional status alone. Emphasis on rehabilitation techniques to treat balance dysfunction in the patient with traumatic brain injury will be considered in this chapter.

Different studies point out the importance of the rehabilitation of balance. In a study by Juneja et al.[1] it was found that balance scores in the Berg Balance Scale at admission accounted for more variation than scores on the FIM instrument. A multicenter analysis made by Greenwald et al.[2] assessed sitting and standing balance within 72 hours of admission to inpatient rehabilitation, and found that patients under 50 years of age had a significant association with normal sitting and standing balance. Measures of severity of traumatic brain injury (admission Glasgow Coma Score, length of post-traumatic amnesia, length of coma, and acute care length of stay) were each significant in relation to impaired sitting but not standing balance. The presence of intracraneal hemorrhages did not have a significant relationship with either sitting or standing balance. Intracraneal compression had a significant relationship with standing but not sitting balance. Another study involving 237 cases of patients sustaining traumatic brain injury admitted to a rehabilitation unit[3] found that the combination of age, initial admission Glagow Coma Score, rehabilitation admission strength, standing balance and sitting balance accounted for 29% of the variance in the Discharge total FIM score. Among these, sitting balance was the second most powerful predictor of both selected elements of the discharge FIM motor score and Discharge FIM-T. Sitting balance predictive capacity was exceeded in importance only by age. The authors conclude that impairments in sitting balance appear to have a significant impact in functional outcome.

Motor control and stability

The concept of stability is closely related to that of equilibrium: the resistence to both linear and angular acceleration. The ability of an individual to assume and mantain a stable position is referred to as balance. Stability is achieved when an equilibrium between destabilizing and stabilizing forces is established.[4] To obtain postural control for stability and orientation, people need to integrate sensory information for assessing the position and motion of the body in space, and have the ability to generate the strength necessary to control the body position. Postural control requires a complex interaction of muscoskeletal and neural systems. *Musculoskeletal components* are the joint range of motion, spinal flexibility, muscle properties, and biomechanics among linked body segments. *Neural components* are: motor processes, sensory processes, sensory strategies to organize the multiple inputs, internal representations for the mapping of sensation to action, and higher cognitive processes for the adaptive and anticipatory aspects of motor control.[5]

A patient has motor control when he or she has good posture and balance as well as correct movements in his or her personal and interpersonal space. Motor control is a whole process including sensitive, perceptual, cognitive, and motor abilities. In acquired brain injury patients it is very important to obtain progress in cognitive functioning in order to gain or increase motor control. Motor control is not only related to physical training, but also to cognitive and emotional rehabilitation (see Figure 9.1). Some patients could do better in movement control with concurrent cognitive rehabilitation sessions. Without cognitive rehabilitation, in those patients who need it, there will not be motor control. This is a basic principle for our method of rehabilitation of motor control disorders. Fong et al.[6] found that cognitive abilities such as judgement, comprehension, and repetition have a positive relationship to functional performance. Tappan[7] argues that we need to determine the interaction between balance and attention in patients with brain injury and effective treatment for patients with decreased balance related to attention impairments. In a study trying to investigate whether balance is associated with mental functioning after mild traumatic brain injury (mTBI), Geurts et al.[8] found a possible association of balance with cognitive performance

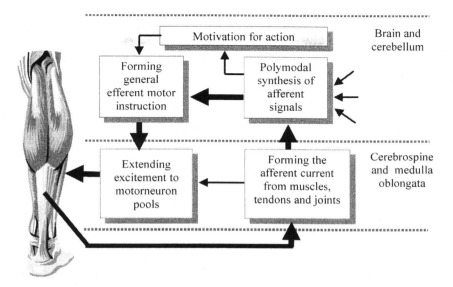

Figure 9.1 The main functional brain blocks participating in generating movements. The cause of most motor problems is a break in the interaction of brain structures responsible for motor control. As a result of the influence of pathological factors (such as trauma, blood vessel pathology, the aftermath of operations, etc.), the process of transferring efferent signals transmitted by the brain to motorneurons may be impaired. The process of afferent current from muscle sensor apparatus, tendons and joints to the supraspinal organs can be badly affected. Such a process leads to the impossibility of effective efferent instructions to muscles. Various combinations of afferent and efferent defects can occur depending on the type of the pathological process and its localization.

but not with emotional well-being: these data suggested to the authors an organic rather than a functional cause of postural instability.

There are different theories about the control of movement [for a more detailed explanation of these theories, see Shumway-Cook and Woollacott[5]].

The *classic theory of motor control* by Sherrington: in an intact nervous system, reflexes are combined into greater actions, which constitute the behavior of the individual as a whole. Reflexes work together or in sequence to achieve the common purpose of building complex behavior. This theory is very limited, especially because it is not able to explain the novel movements, and cannot explain and predict movements that occur in the absence of a sensory stimulus. Today, reflexes are not accepted as the sole determinant of motor control. Reflex theories seem to be useful only in explaining certain stereotyped patterns of movement.

The *hierarchical theory* from Hughling Jackson: specific brain impairments from disease and physical injury clearly affect the use of limbs and other parts of the body. The brain contains a motor area amidst its functional regions that governs the movements of an individual person. The nervous system has a hierarchical structure that is *top down*. The motor function has a complex vertical organization that is: first, represented in the lower level (spinal or brain stem); second, is re-represented in the medium level of the motor (or sensorial) areas of the cerebral hemisphere; third, re-re-represented in the upper level of the frontal lobes. That is to say each successively higher level exerts control over the level below it, and there is never bottom up control, so that is why a lesion does not necessarily lead to the complete loss of a function. Today the idea of a strict hierarchy in motor control is not totally accepted. It seems that each level of the nervous system can act upon other levels (higher and lower) in some way.

Motor programming theories come mainly from psychology. While reflex theory explains certain patterns of movements, motor programming theories propose the concept of motor patterns in the brain. That is, there are higher level motor programs representing actions in more abstract terms in the brain, storing the rules for generation of movements. So, when you want to perform a movement reversal as usual, you can do it more or less efficiently because you have the motor program stored in your brain. That means that patients with acquired brain injury (ABI) may have the patterns of the movements but they are not able to retrieve them. However, this may not always be true. As Shumway-Cook and Woollacott[5] suggest: "In patients whose higher levels of motor programming are affected, motor program theory suggests the importance of helping patients relearn the correct rules for action. In addition, treatment should focus on retraining movements important to functional task, not just on reeducating specific muscles in isolation."

Other theories are the *systems theories* which argue that movement control is the consequence of the work of different systems of the body in order to achieve the desired movement. To restore movement control, the therapist must know how the body works as a whole. *The task-oriented theories* propose that motor control has to be goal directed to the specific motor function to be rehabilitated.

The NeuroBird method: system and strategies

The fundamentals of the NeuroBird method rely on sophisticated electronic computerized feedback signals allowing patients to know what happens in their muscles when performing a movement in order to achieve motor control. The patient trains his or her muscles according the information he or she is continuously receiving about the functioning of the muscle or muscles affected. The clinical effect of training the patient how to do it is considerably higher when the feedback signal information is optimal. The aim of the biofeedback (BFB) technologies used for restoring motor functions is an attempt to normalize the afferent–efferent relations between the brain and the motor system. The treatment using BFB technologies is directed towards forming, as well as increasing the afferent current to the patient's CNS during his or her attempts to perform a motor action. It promotes the formation of new functional ties, serving as a basis for restoring and forming new motor skills and coordination (Figure 9.2).

The Neurocrecer biofeedback system consists of a stabilometric platform in which the patient is connected to a system of movement control and gravity center. The system is designed to show the patient the skills of arbitrary

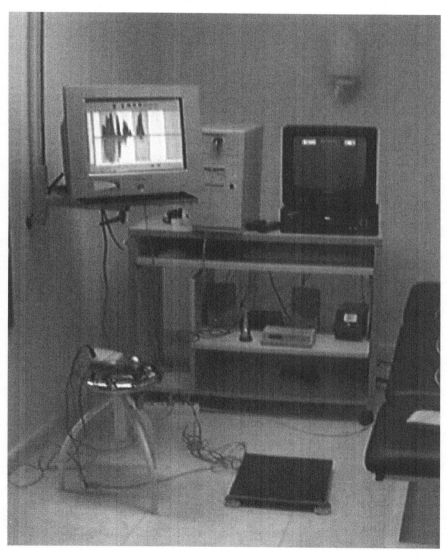

Figure 9.2 NeuroBird system for rehabilitation of equilibrium and posture control.

and non-arbitrary control over muscular contraction. First of all, an analysis is made after a certain time (normally, 1 minute) of how the patient's weight is distributed between his lower extremities. After this analysis, a graphic and numeral representation (in the X and Y axes) of weight distribution appear on the computer screen. Axis X shows anteroposterior movement and axis Y shows lateral movement of weight distribution. In horizontal training, a symmetrical distribution of weight between the lower right and left limbs is intended. In vertical training, symmetry of weight between the front and back of the foot is attempted. In training the center, a combination of the two training procedures is examined.

Apart from the visual (graphic) and the sound feedback, there is an opportunity to create a higher level of motivation by showing a movie. It achieves the aim (making the height of the columns the same, or the size of the circles the same or not crossing the circle boundaries) of making it possible to watch a film. If a mistake is made, the screen goes off. This approach not only allows making a treatment session exciting, but helps transfer the control of balance into the non-conscious system which easily permits automatization of the process of the movement. The latter guarantees a stable fixing of a newly acquired habit and makes its realization in all motor actions easier. Another technique of stimulating the patient's motivation is to offer the patient a special children's computer game in which the film character's movements on the screen are controlled by tensing or relaxing one's muscles (Figure 9.3 and Table 9.1).

Protocol for restoration of equilibrium with the NeuroBird system

Assessment

Before starting to work with the biofeedback system to recuperate equilibrium, it is necessary to assess the impairments in the patient's musculature that control gait and posture control, and also to assess carefully which specific alterations of equilibrium the patient has.

To assess the *musculature*, the NeuroBird EMGraphic biofeedback system is used, allowing an evaluation of the activity of the groups of muscles by means of different functional tasks. The results obtained allow knowing which deficits prevent the functioning of groups of muscles from carrying out efficient equilibrium actions. The design for the protocol of rehabilitation must take into consideration the deficits found in the examination.

Assessment of equilibrium begins with a detailed analysis of the patient's posture control and afterwards evaluates equilibrium. In order to evaluate *posture control*, the NeuroBird screen is used to observe the two axes of space, horizontal and vertical. The patient is asked to remain standing without trying to correct his or her normal posture. After an assessment (usually not more than 2 minutes), the system displays the data: mean and typical deviation of each of the axes and the percentages of the time of correct

Table 9.1 Cognitive involvement in motor control

Intention	Sensation	Perception	Analyzing	Executive planning	Action
Prefrontal cortex/limbic system	Peripheral nervous system	Sensory cortex	Association cortical areas (parietal, occipital and temporal)	Prefrontal cortex	Frontal motor areas/ basal ganglia/ cerebellum

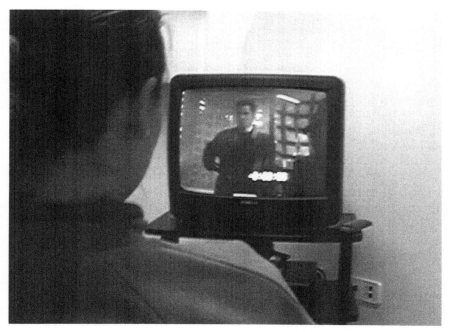

Figure 9.3 Instead of training with graphic circles, movies can be used to train a patient's correct posture. Clarity of the screen image depends on correct performance of the exercises. If the patient does the task badly, the screen darkens and the film cannot be seen. In order to be able to continue watching it, the patient has to do the exercises over again and maintain the required posture for a specific period of time.

performance. These data give the therapist a clear idea of the patient's posture control (as far as posture and imbalances exhibited during the evaluation).

Analyzing the *patient's area of equilibrium* is determined by the convergence of all points of space (marked by X and Y) towards which the patient is able to confidently project his or her center of gravity without moving their feet on the balance platform. Therefore, the patient can execute efficient equilibrium actions in this area. This evaluation thus requires the patient's active collaboration. In order to carry out a correct evaluation of the area of equilibrium, a study should be made of the total surface area and the location of the area of equilibrium in space. This analysis offers data which is essential for knowledge of the specific difficulties the patient has with gait. This type of evaluation is made in this way, as walking is a continuous adjustment of a state of imbalance in which it is necessary to have efficient equilibrium reactions in a large area, marked by different weight distribution in each phase of walking. Once assessment has been made of these three aspects, the training procedure begins.

Preparing the patient for the training

The process of restoring equilibrium starts with increased contractibility of the muscles engaged in walking. Successive involvement of muscles in the activity is an individual procedure. Working should start with muscles less affected by the pathology. It is then followed by working with the antagonist muscles to suppress spasticity and pathological synergies. Usually this phase of the work is a responsible and lengthy one. A specific step in the rehabilitation process for patients with walking pathologies consists of restoration of control over the gravity center projection. To obtain this control, the stabiloplatform connected to the NeuroBird system has to be used. The pressure sensors in its base allow visualization of the patient's gravity center projection and conduct the training. It is done in the following way. The patient is settled on the platform and an analysis is made of his or her gravity center projection (coordinates and the dispersion) (Figure 9.4). The patient is then prepared to be trained in the next three steps.

FIRST PHASE: CONTROLLING HORIZONTAL AXIS

During the first step the patient is taught to control his or her own gravity center along a horizontal axis. The height of the left and right-sided columns on the monitor screen depend on the shift of the gravity center to the right or to the left. The aim of the training is to sustain the same height of the columns for a considerably long period of time (Figure 9.5). If the difference in the height between the columns exceeds a preset level, a sound signal is heard. Depending on the gravity of the case, this phase may take anything from 2–3 days to 2 weeks.

SECOND PHASE: CONTROLLING SAGITTAL AXIS

The second phase aims at controlling one's gravity center projection along the sagittal axis. As illustrated in Figure 9.6, a shift of the gravity center to the front or back enlarges the upper or lower circle on the monitor screen. The patient's aim is to make the size of the circles the same. Like the previous one,

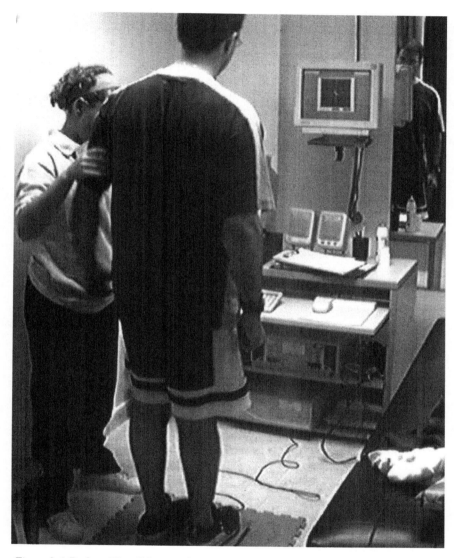

Figure 9.4 Patient JP walking on the stabiloplatform paying attention to the screen to maintain the correct center of gravity.

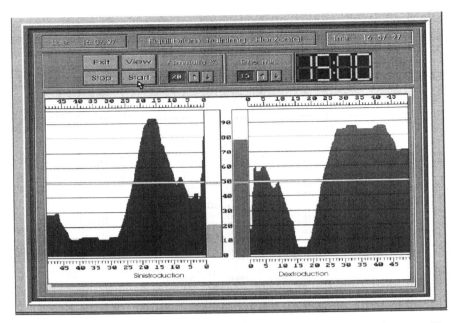

Figure 9.5 The patient has to sustain the same height of the columns for a specific period of time.

this variant of the program makes use of a sound signal as an indicator of a mistake.

THIRD PHASE: CONTROLLING BOTH AXES

When the patient has mastered the skill of sustaining his or her own gravity center along the horizontal and the sagittal axes separately, he or she is offered the third step of the training which will teach the patient to control his or her gravity center projection on the full surface of the base along both axes simultaneously. Displayed in Figure 9.7, the screen shows the gravity center projection and the circle which must not be overstepped. Overstepping the circle is considered a mistake and is accompanied by a sound signal. The size of the circle can be set automatically, based on the preliminary analysis of the coordinates of the gravity center or its dispersion, or manually.

IMPROVING WALKING FUNCTION

The walking function is now improved with the help of the "phase movements" program. Recommended steps of the process are as follows:

1   *The patient is seated on a chair.* The assignment is to support one foot on

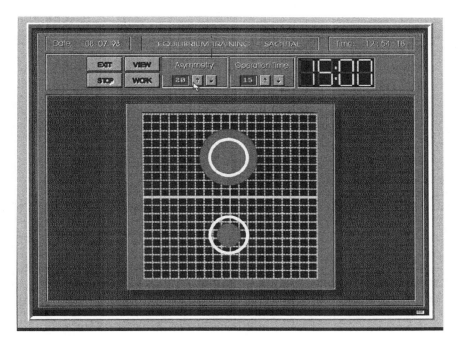

Figure 9.6 Depending on the posture of the patient, the upper or lower circle on the screen will enlarge.

its toes (thus activating m. gastrocnemius et soleus) and the other on the heel (thus activating m. tibialis ant.), illustrated in Figure 9.8. With the EMG electrodes fixed on the projection of m. tibialis ant. and m. gastrocnemius, the first foot should be the one more affected by the pathology (first 15 min of training) and then the second, if needed.

2   *The patient is seated on a chair.* The task is to successively extend one's thighs from the coxofemoral joints. The EMG electrodes are fixed to the proximal parts of m. rectus femoris dext. et sin.

3   *The patient is standing using back-of-chair support.* His or her task is to perform successive extension of the left and right foot. The EMG is registered from the left and right m. tibialis ant.

4   *The patient is standing supported by the back of the chair.* The task is the same as in (2).

5   *The patient is standing with the back of the chair as support.* He or she is performing successive flexions of his or her knee joints. The EMG electrodes are fixed on m. biceps femoris (caput lonum) dext. et sin.

6   *The patient is standing using the back of the chair as support.* The electrodes are fixed on the putter surface quadrants of m. gluteus maximus dext. et sin. The patient's task is to extend his or her thighs in turn.

7   *The patient is standing on the moving track of the simulator (the running*

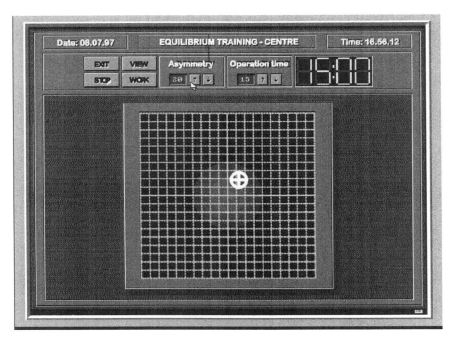

Figure 9.7 The small circle should not overlap the big circle to maintain correct posture.

track). Both passive (set into motion by muscular effort) and active (using an electro-engine capable of working at low speed of about 0.5 km/h) simulators can be used. One can perform three types of exercises on this simulator (Figure 9.9).

(a) The EMG electrodes are fixed on the right and left m. tibialis ant.
(b) The EMG electrodes are fixed on the projection of m. tibialis ant. et gastrocnemius. The electrodes are fixed first on the foot affected worse by pathology (first 15 min of training), and then, if needed, on the other.
(c) The EMG electrodes are fixed on the proximal parts of m. rectus femoris dext. et sin.

When working with the phase movements program, one should be careful in setting temporal parameters of movements as well as individual thresholds. The tempo of movements should be realistic for a particular patient (Figure 9.10). If possible, the patient should be offered the possibility of performing the exercise without the support of their hands after several training sessions.

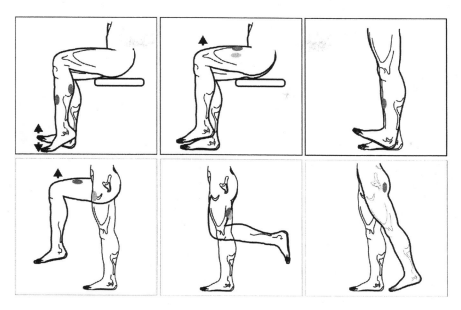

Figure 9.8 Exercises with the NeuroBird system for improving the walking function (see text for explanation).

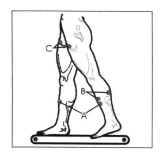

Figure 9.9 Exercises on the simulator.

Presentation of a case of rehabilitation of balance with the NeuroBird method

We present JB, 22 years old, who after an automobile accident had the following injuries: traumatic brain injury with thalamic damage and diffuse axonal injury, fracture of the right scapula, fractured right iliac wing, fractured left pubic rami, fractured right rib and ruptured right kidney. He was admitted to the intensive care unit in a state of deep coma with several lung and kidney complications that evolved favorably. Two months later, he was in hospital in a vegetative state with general hypertonia, more accute in the right MS. Eight months after the accident, he recovered consciousness with correct

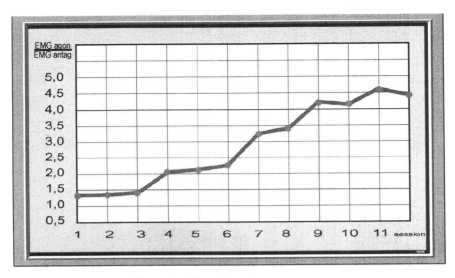

Figure 9.10 Progress of the patient in each session.

time–space orientation and limited comprehension of oral and written language. He had accute dysarthria, diplopia which forced alternate eye occlusion, and a more severe tetraparesis in the right side of the body. Nineteen months after the accident, the patient was referred to a specialized center for brain injury rehabilitation.

Somatosensory assessment

The Rivermead Assessment of Somatosensory Performance[9] was used and results from all subtests indicated a normal state of sensitivity. The correct score was 54 for the sharp/dull discrimination subtest; 58 the correct score for the surface pressure touch subtest; 57 for the surface localization subtest; 10 for the sensory extinction subtest; the total score was pass in both hands for the two-point discrimination subtest; for the temperature discrimination subtest the total score was 56; and for the proprioception movement and direction discrimination subtest the total movement detected correctly was 60.

Static balance

According to the Berg Balance Scale[10] the score before intervention was 8 (maximum 56). The results showed that the risk of falling was significantly high.

Turning over, as well as posture changes in general, show a deficiency in support from the right side of the body. When seated, there is good control of the trunk with the appearance, however, of an extensor reflex which elevates the MMII (with or without extending the knee). In the prone position, support on the right elbow after elevating the left MS makes the patient retract, and the hand is shaped in a claw.

During the assessment of quadruped balance, the lack of support of the right MSD and MID was noted in the elevation of the left side of body (which makes patients lose their balance), like in an arm or leg alternatively, which forces the hand into a claw position. The patient is able to remain kneeling, even with alternate pressures, although there is evidence of wavering of the stabilizers on the right side of the pelvis (especially the medius and maximus glutei).

Dynamic balance

It was not posible to quantitatively or qualitatively evaluate independent ambulation before intervention. Autonomous ambulation was not possible. A walker was used and supervision or personal assistance was needed, especially when turning. In the support phase, recurvatum in the knee of the lower limb supporting the weight was observed.

The patient could ascend and descend stairs with assistance, but had serious difficulties doing so. He could not use his right MS to help him, standing on the right MI of one foot was deficient, the trunk was leaning to the left and, in general, balance was deficient.

In conclusion, the patient presented light tetraparesis, with mainly the right side of the body affected and was unable to walk unassisted.

Specific aim: re-establishment of balance

The patient underwent physical therapy with the aim of being able to achieve more independence in ambulation (movement). Leftover motor sequelae and spasticity were treated, trying to increase active as well as passive limb movements in the right MS and, in general, retraining and maximizing normal balance and muscle tone. Sessions of static balance training were centered around the NeuroBird system of biofeedback with the aim of achieving a symmetrical, balanced distribution of weight ("sway balance") that reduces the risk of falling.

Results

Table 9.2 shows data obtained by the patient at admission and discharge. The results show a reduction of amplitude of weight shifting and a reduction of the results of symmetry in the distribution of weight.

Table 9.2 Results JP obtained at admission and at discharge after 90 sessions of 30 min each were carried out

Date	Analysis	Horizontal training	Vertical training	Central training
Admission	H: 16 ± 13.0	H: 16 ± 13.0	H: −4 ± 6.5	H: 2 ± 4.2
	V: 28 ± 6.4	V: 28 ± 6.4	V: 32 ± 6.0	V: 12 ± 5.2
Discharge	H: 0 ± 2.3	H: 0 ± 1.2	H: −4 ± 5.2	H: 0 ± 2.2
	V: 0± 4.0	V: 0 ± 5.3	V: 0 ± 4.8	V: 0 ± 2.4

H, horizontal axis; V, vertical axis.

Conclusion

An improvement is also observed in another variable: dynamic equilibrium. According to the Berg Balance Scale, the score after the intervention is 40 (maximum 56) while the score in the Berg Balance Scale before training with the NeuroBird method was 8 (maximum 56). The patient shows five times more equilibrium than he showed at the beginning of the treatment. While falling was common when JP tried to walk now, the risk of falling decreased and was more unlikely (see Figure 9.11).

Concluding remarks

The majority of patients with traumatic brain injury and severe cerebro-vascular disorders have balance and posture dysfunctions which seriously limit their possibilities of recovering an independent and autonomous life style. As different studies of balance retraining have demonstrated, this is fundamental for being able to recuperate independent functioning in every-day activities. Stability and orientation are two necessary conditions for a person to be able to control his or her body in space. In the process of recovering from balance disorders, different techniques have traditionally been used.[11,12] In this chapter we have presented a sophisticated computer-ized instrument for retraining balance based on the techniques of bio-feedback which is, at present, one of the most efficient, precise and controlled systems in restoring balance and postural control in neurological patients, as can be observed in the case we have described and in our clinical experience. The type of training consists in recuperating the ability to control the projec-tion of the center of gravity in the vertical position of the body, making control mechanisms automatic via feedback in the static form of posture as well as the dynamic form of locomotion.

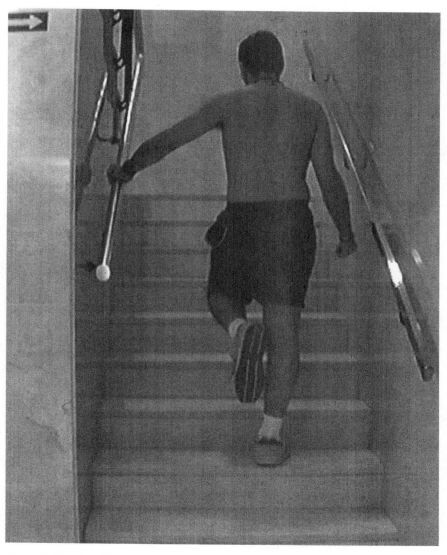

Figure 9.11 After 90 sessions of 30 min each, the patient goes from a score of 8 at the beginning to 40 (maximum 56) in the Berg Balance Scale, allowing him/her to climb stairs independently and correctly.

Acknowledgements

We thank Maria Isabel Garcia Bernal and Montserrat Altemir Lara, physiotherapists at the Center for Brain Injury Rehabilitation (CRECER) in Seville,

Spain, for helping collect data of the case presented in the chapter, and Jill Snow for helping with the English translation.

References

1. Juneja, G., Czyrny, J. J., & Linn, R. T. (1998). Admission balance and outcomes of patients admitted for acute inpatient rehabilitation. *Am. J. Phys. Med. Rehabil.*, 77, 388–393.
2. Greenwald, B. D., Cifu, D. X., Marwitz, J. H., et al. (2001). Factors associated with balance deficits on admission to rehabilitation after traumatic brain injury: a multicenter analysis. *J. Head Trauma Rehabil.*, 16, 238–252.
3. Black, K., Zafonte, R., Millis, S., et al. (2000). Sitting balance following brain injury: does it predict outcome? *Brain Inj.*, 14, 141–152.
4. Hamil, J., & Knutzen, K. M. (1995). *Biomechanical basis of human movement.* Media, PA: Lippincott, Williams & Wilkins.
5. Shumway-Cook, A., & Woollacott, M. H. (1995). *Motor control: Theory and practical applications.* Baltimore, MD: Williams & Wilkins.
6. Fong, K. N., Chan, C. C., & Au, D. K. (2001). Relationship of motor and cognitive abilities to functional performance in stroke rehabilitation. *Brain Inj.*, 15, 443–453.
7. Tappan, R. S. (2002). Rehabilitation for balance and ambulation in a patient with attention impairment due to intracranial hemorrhage. *Phys Ther.* 82, 473–484.
8. Geurts, A. C., Knoop, J. A., & van Limbeek, J. (1999). Is postural control associated with mental functioning in the persistent postconcussion syndrome? *Arch. Phys. Med. Rehabil., 80,* 144–149.
9. Winward, E., Halliigan, W., & Wade, T. (2000). *Rivermead assessment of somatosensory performance.* Hove, UK: Psychology Press.
10. Berg, K., Wood-Dauphinee, S., & Williams, J. I. (1995). The balance scale: reliability assessment for residents and patients with an acute stroke. *Scand. J. Rehab. Med., 27,* 27–36.
11. Barroso y Martín, J. M., García-Bernal, M. I., Domínguez-Morales, R., Mikhailenok, E., & Voronina, O. (1999). Total functional recovery in hemiparetic left post-brain injury patient through a neuromuscular bio-feedback computerized program, Remicord-2. *Rev. Esp. Neuropsicol., 1*(2–3), 69–88.
12. Domínguez-Morales, R., & León-Carrión, J. (2001). Impact of intensive, integral and multidisciplinary treatment in the economical compensation of traumatic brain injury patients. Monografias de la *Revist. Española Neuropsicol.*; Neuropsicologia legal y forense del daño cerebral. *Rev. Esp. Neuropsicol., 3*(1–2), 77–84.

10 Neuropharmacologic management of impairment after traumatic brain injury

Nathan D. Zasler, Michael F. Martelli and Treven C. Pickett

Introduction

The use of neuropharmacologic interventions to modulate impairment in persons with acquired brain injury (ABI) has become a mainstay of good neurorehabilitation care. Unfortunately, there has been a historical dearth of consolidated information on the pharmacologic approaches and their rationale relative to their application in this subset of neurological patients. In fact, there is likely to be better consensus among physicians in the field of neurorehabilitation regarding the psychopharmacologic management of ABI-related neurobehavioral impairments than there is for neuropharmacologic management, with the exceptions of pharmacologic approaches to epilepsy and spasticity management.

The basic tenet of positively affecting neurologic outcome and functional status after brain injury through the use of pharmacologic agents is not a product of the "Decade of the Brain" but rather a practice which has its roots in the early part of the last century.[1,2] Nonetheless, most rehabilitation professionals have historically relied almost exclusively on non-pharmacologic modalities to address neurophysical and related neuromedical impairments following ABI.

Until recently, there was little to any evidence that medications could make a difference in either the rate or plateau of neurological and functional recovery following brain injury. There is now good evidence that many acute, subacute and chronic neurologic and functional sequelae resulting from brain injury can be lessened and potentially even abated through the thoughtful and appropriate use of pharmacologic agents.[3–6] More specifically, drugs that are proadrenergic seemingly facilitate recovery while agents that deplete central norepinephrine through either receptor blockade, decreased production or increase in turnover may impede neural recovery.[7,8] The mechanisms by which proadrenergic agents affect recovery in a positive fashion remains theoretical. Concepts such as diaschisis and facilitation of plasticity seem to remain at the forefront of the potential explanations. Although, historically, best demonstrated with proadrenergic agents, other drugs used to modulate impairment following ABI typically result in rapid modulation of the previously fixed neurologic deficit (when the drug is effective), may have long-lasting effects (even after discontinuation, implying underlying neurochemical and plastic changes having occurred) and seemingly are "therapeutically augmented" often by concurrent behaviorally relevant training.[9,10]

Clearly, physicians must be aware of drugs to avoid or minimize given the available information germane to potential inhibition of behavioral recovery after brain injury as demonstrated in numerous animal studies, as well as a few human studies. Potentially detrimental agents include neuroleptics and other central dopamine receptor antagonists, benzodiazepines, and certain anticonvulsants.[8]

Although more and more practitioners, in part based on patient as well as family request, are prescribing naturopathic and homeopathic agents for ABI-related impairments, these agents are not without side-effects and/or drug:drug interactions. This fact must be appreciated by prescribing physicians, particularly given the propensity for persons with ABI to be on polypharmaceutical regimens. Interestingly, there has been little formal investigation of these latter agents relative to their application in ABI aside from one study in persons with mild traumatic brain injury that suggested positive functional gains with this interventional strategy relative to placebo.[11]

This chapter will provide an overview of neuropharmacologic management of select impairments after ABI with primary emphasis on the post-acute period or chronic phase of care. An overview of basic neurochemical systems and commonly utilized classes of neuropharmacologic agents precedes the discussion of current treatment options.

Neurotransmitter receptors

Three broad categories will be discussed in order to provide a foundation for the clinical application of neuropharmacologic principles to treatment of persons with ABI-related impairments: receptor types, neurotransmitter gated receptors and voltage gated ion channels. Ligand gated receptors are categorized into two broad types: ionotropic and metabotropic. Binding agonists to these receptors produce conformational changes of channel components that alter ionic conductance and modify intracellular processes requiring specific ions. The binding of ligands to metabotropic receptors activates GTP-binding proteins (so-called G proteins) that subsequently modulate various intracellular second messenger systems. Neurotransmitter gated receptors include gamma-aminobutyric acid, glutamate, AMPA and NMDA receptors, acetylcholine (muscarinic versus nicotinic), dopamine, norepinephrine and epinephrine and serotonin. Voltage gated ion channels include sodium, calcium, potassium, and chloride.

Although there are presently theorized to be a cornucopia of putative neurotransmitters in the mammalian CNS, most that have been identified can be grouped into four main categories: acetylcholine, monoamines, peptides, and amino acids. The number of putative neurotransmitters now exceeds 40, most of which are thought to be small peptides. Neurotransmitters are chemicals that are released from the nerve terminal (pre-synaptic neuron) as the result of changes in membrane potential generated by the arrival of an action potential. The process of "normal" neuronal function relies greatly on appropriate synthesis and release from the pre-synaptic neuron, successful crossing of the synaptic cleft, binding to the post-synaptic receptors, and termination of receptor stimulation by either removal or degradation.[12]

Cholinergic neurons (nerves that release acetylcholine) are distributed throughout a variety of areas in the central nervous system including the ventral forebrain, upper brainstem, and striatal interneurons.[13–15] There are two major subclasses of cholinergic receptors: nicotinic and muscarinic. Functionally, cholinergic systems have been theorized to play a role in learning/memory processes, motor control, stress, affective disorders, and arousal.[16]

Monoaminergic systems tend to have long branched ascending and descending axons and are mainly associated with the more diffuse neural pathways in the CNS. Their cell bodies are typically in small groups of neurons, primarily located in the brainstem. While noradrenaline, adrenaline, and dopamine are chemically classified as catecholamines, serotonin is an indoleamine.

Dopaminergic projections are typically divided into three categories based on length: long, short and ultra-short. The long tracts emanate from the substantia nigra (nigrostriatal tract) and the ventral tegmentum (mesolimbic/mesocortical tracts). The intermediate length systems include the tuberoinfundibular system, the incerto-hypothalamic neurons, and the medullary periventricular group. Ultra-short systems are found in the retina and olfactory bulb[13,15,16] It is presently theorized that there are several subtypes of dopaminergic receptors.[14,15,17] It should be noted that the exact interrelationship between D1 and D2 receptors remains unclear; however it is theorized that activation of both receptors is necessary for full expression of dopaminergically mediated motor behaviors.[18,19] Functionally, dopaminergic systems have been theorized to be involved with behavior, motor control, hypothalamic function, and arousal.[16]

Noradrenergic cell bodies in the CNS are found in the locus ceruleus and lateral tegmental nuclei, all in the pons and medulla. Noradrenergic axons innervate multiple structures, both caudally and rostrally, including the forebrain, medulla, spinal cord, and cerebellum. Adrenergic cell bodies are found in the dorsal and lateral tegmentum in the lower brainstem and innervate limbic as well as spinal structures.[13,15,16] Noradrenergic and adrenergic systems act at both alpha (alpha 1 and alpha 2), as well as beta receptors (beta 1 and beta 2). Functionally, central noradrenergic pathways have been postulated to be involved with sleep/wake cycle regulation, learning and memory, anxiety-nociception, behavioral vigilance, and affective disturbance. There is still a lack of knowledge about the functional role of adrenergic systems within the CNS.[16]

Serotonergic cell bodies are also confined to the brainstem, mostly within the raphe nuclei. These axons project into the forebrain, cerebellum, and spinal cord.[13,15,16,20] Multiple subtypes of CNS serotonergic receptors have been identified.[17] Functionally, serotonergic systems have been theorized to be involved with arousal, sleep/wake cycle regulation, mood and emotion including aggression, feeding, thermoregulation, ataxia, and sexual behavior.[16]

Peptidergic neurons have recently been the focus of intense research with regard to their potential role as putative neurotransmitters. Neuropeptides are widely distributed in the CNS and are also expressed in various types of glial cells. A characteristic of neuropeptides is the plasticity in their expression and their typical coexistence with one or more classic transmitters suggesting involvement in modulatory processes and other functions such as trophic effects.[21] In recent years, the opioid peptides and their precursors have probably received the most attention of all the neuropeptides secondary to their role in stress and pain mediation within the central nervous system. These neurochemical systems, including beta-endorphins, enkephalins, and dynorphins, have their cell bodies in deeper, more primitive regions of the brain such as the limbic system, reticular formation, medulla and hypothalamus.[13,15,16] There are several subtypes of opiate receptors that have been proposed including mu, delta, and kappa receptors.[14,17] Other CNS peptides which have been postulated to have a neurotransmitter or neuromodulator role include: galanin, melanocortins, orexin, substance P, vasopressin, oxytocin, somatostatin, and thyrotropin-releasing hormone to name just a few. The exact roles for all of the peptidergic substances has not been fully clarified.[13–15] However, recent reviews have concluded that they serve a particular role in responding to CNS stress, challenge or disease.[21]

Amino acids are thought to be the most common of all putative neurotransmitters. Some of the more common amino acid neurotransmitters are γ-aminobutyric acid (GABA) and glycine (both inhibitory), as well as glutamate and aspartate (both excitatory).[22,23] Glutamate may in fact be involved with post-ABI chronic neurodegeneration which further belies the need for development of receptor antagonists. GABA which serves as the major inhibitory neurotransmitter is concentrated in Purkinje cells within the cerebellar cortex and in the striatum. GABA-A receptors are heterogeneous multimeric ligand-gated Cl channels and postsynaptic, whereas GABA-B receptors which are coupled to G-proteins occur on presynaptic autonomic and central nerve terminals.[14,15,24] Functionally, gabaminergic systems have been theorized to be involved with the control of spinal reflexes, movement, nociception, anxiety states, and epilepsy.[16,24]

It was long assumed, in accordance with Dale's principle, that one neuron secreted one neurotransmitter at all its terminals. However, we now know that there are several examples of neurons that contain and secrete more than one biologically active substance. In the central nervous system this most often takes the form of mixed monoamine and peptide neurons.[25] The exact biological significance of this phenomenon is as yet unclear but is presently an active area of research given the obvious clinical treatment implications. In fact, this factor of neuronal "hardwiring" may often explain atypical responses to medications that are frequently assumed by practitioners to be fairly specific for a particular neurotransmitter system.

Principles of therapeutics

Inherent in applying neuropharmacologic principles to treatment of impairment in the context of neurorehabilitation, practitioners must be familiar with the medication preparation alternatives, bioavailability, titration, distribution, biotransformation, and pharmacogenetics of the agent in question. Additionally, drug interactional issues must always be appreciated including the role of physiologic variation and drug elimination (biotransformation and elimination).

Inherent in achieving optimal response to neuropharmacologic interventions, the treating physician must make a correct diagnosis of the impairment in the first place. Knowledge of the therapeutic index and mechanism of action simplify selection of the most appropriate drug for the condition in question. Generally, a drug should be chosen that has the least number of actions required to effectively treat the specific ABI-related impairment. Practitioners should also keep in mind the cost efficacy of the particular proposed prescription, the drug delivery format for the particular agent, the ease of titration for the particular drug, the side-effect profile (particularly with regard to potential cognitive suppressant effects) and last but not least the dosing frequency, the latter as related to implications for prescription compliance.

Optimal drug response in part requires knowledge on the part of the practitioner regarding a particular drug's bioavailability that may be limited by its uptake mechanism. Additionally, it is just as important to be aware of what other drugs may impact on uptake, both in a positive and a negative fashion, as well as how the presence of food may facilitate or impede bioavailability. Understanding titration issues is also an important component of achieving optimal drug response in the context of neuropharmacologic management. Specifically, one must understand the rate at which a dose of a particular medication can be increased, as well as the amount by which the dose can be increased with any specific upward titration. The titration rate is generally considered to be an inverse function of the half-life or elimination rate. A steady state should be reached before the clinical efficacy of the particular drug trial is determined. Steady state levels are achieved after five half-lives from the dosage increase or initiation. There are clearly implications with regard to dosing schedules with drugs that have relatively short half-lives; specifically, the drug will have to be dosed more frequently the shorter the known half-life. Lastly, drug:drug interactions must be understood by the prescribing clinician so as to minimize the potential for iatrogenic polypharmaceutical complications. Clearly, an exhaustive discussion detailing the principles of neuropharmacologic therapeutics is beyond the scope of this chapter. However, there are numerous resources for this information in the neuroscience and pharmacologic literature. The reader is referred to the *Physician's Desk Reference* or an equivalent source, among other reference texts, for this information.

Overview of pharmacologic agents by class

Many pharmacologic agents exist which may have potential utility in altering function following brain injury. Much of what is known regarding pharmacologic rehabilitation of this patient population is based on theories derived from work done at the basic science level with animal models, individual clinical experience, and/or studies in persons with other neurologic disease entities. The peer-reviewed scientific literature as it presently stands does not provide one with much useful information regarding well-controlled, methodologically sound, prospective research data regarding neuropharmacologic intervention following acquired brain injury. Nonetheless, clinicians should be aware of the major pharmacological agents in each neurotransmitter class in order better to grasp what effect if any they may have, positive or otherwise, on neurological recovery and/or impairment.

Catecholaminergic agonists

The major drugs in this class include L-dopa, amantadine, bromocriptine, pergolide, lisuride, cabergoline, and pramipexole, as well as some of the more "classic" stimulant drugs such as dextroamphetamine, methylphenidate, and pemoline,[26,27] as well as some of the newer atypical stimulants such as modafinil.[28]

The "classic" dopamine agonist has historically been levodopa (L-dopa). A combination formulation of L-dopa and carbidopa is also available. The use of the combination drug minimizes peripheral (non-CNS) side-effects of the drug and increases the amount available for central nervous system incorporation. L-dopa has its action pre-synaptically and is agonistic at both the D1 and D2 receptor sites.[29] Side-effects are numerous but the more frequent ones include dyskinesias, various bradykinetic episodes (i.e. "on–off" phenomena), psychiatric disturbances, gastrointestinal disturbances (nausea, vomiting, anorexia, and slowing of gastric motility), as well as orthostatic hypotension.[30] Carbidopa–levodopa is available in ratios of 1:10 (100 mg levodopa: 10 mg carbidopa) and 1:4 (100 mg levodopa: 25 mg carbidopa). Most patients with clear clinical evidence of dopaminergic deficiency will respond to a 1:10 ratio provided the daily dosage of carbidopa is 70 mg or more. When the 1:4 ratio is used, the usual starting dose is one tablet three times a day, increasing by one tablet every 2 days up to a maximum dosage of six tablets daily. If the 1:10 ratio is used, the usual starting dose is one tablet three to four times/day, increasing by one tablet every 2 days, to a maximum of eight tablets daily.[31] In addition to carbidopa, other enzyme inhibitors such as benserazide and L-deprenyl (a monoamine oxidase Type B inhibitor) have been used in conjunction with L-dopa in an attempt to increase therapeutic efficacy.[29]

Amantadine hydrochloride has been utilized clinically as an antiviral agent, as well as an anti-Parkinsonian agent. Its exact mechanism of action is still not fully elucidated. However, it has been theorized to have a pre-synaptic action, as well as a possible post-synaptic action with at least partial non-competitive NMDA receptor antagonism.[29,32] Some authors have speculated that amantadine may also increase central cholinergic and gabaminergic activity. Therapy can be initiated at 50–100 mg/day and increased to a maximum of 400 mg/day. Recent research has confirmed a possible role of amantadine in facilitating neurorecovery following diffuse TBI.[33] Since the drug is not metabolized and is excreted unchanged in the urine, dosage adjustments must be made when there is concurrent decreased renal function such as in the elderly or in patients with renal disease. Peripheral side-effects include but are not limited to peripheral edema, lightheadedness, orthostatic hypotension, hot and dry skin, rash, lowering of seizure threshold, and livedo reticularis. Livedo reticularis is a discoloration of the skin that occurs in a reddish-blue to purple blotchy pattern. The reaction tends to occur after at least one month of treatment and it may occur more commonly at higher doses. Livedo reticularis is totally benign and the medication does not need to be discontinued unless the cosmetic aspects outweigh the therapeutic benefit.[29,31] Central side-effects that may be seen in the geriatric population include confusion and hallucinations. Seizures have also reportedly been induced by amantadine in patients with lowered seizure threshold.

Due to levodopa's "indirect" mechanism of action, researchers have pursued and developed several direct dopamine-receptor stimulating agents, all of which happened to be of the ergot-alkaloid class. These direct agents include bromocriptine, lisuride, pergolide, quinpirole, carmoxirole, ropinirole, and pramipexole.[34] Both bromocriptine and lisuride are antagonistic at the D1 receptor and agonistic at the D2 receptor. Pergolide, on the other hand, is agonistic at both the D1 and D2 receptor sites. Bromocriptine mesylate tends to produce fewer problems with dyskinesias, but more problems with mental side-effects, orthostasis, and nausea than L-dopa.[29] Clinical results have demonstrated a triphasic response to bromocriptine with dopamine agonism occurring only in the midrange doses.[31] Dosing should start with a test dose of 1.25 mg and if tolerated then the patient can begin at a dose of 2.5 mg daily, increasing to a three to four times/day dose fairly quickly. Once at 10 mg/day, the dose can be increased every 4 days by 2.5 mg. Typically, clinical experience has dictated that doses higher than 60 mg/day are unnecessary in patients with acquired brain injury. As a point of interest, the manufacturer has not established safety limits for dosages greater than 100 mg/day.

Pergolide and lisuride are relatively new agents in the USA and there is little literature on their utility in the pharmacologic rehabilitation of the individual with brain injury. It should be noted that pergolide is an extremely potent dopamine agonist and only very small doses are required. Pergolide can be sedating, so it should be titrated slowly and appropriate dosing should be followed. Lisuride is also extremely potent and therapeutic effects are typically seen with daily doses of 4–10 mg/day.[29] Most of the ergot alkaloids also have concommitant central serotonergic receptor agonism which might explain the high incidence of mental status changes with this class of dopamine agonists. Pramipexole and ropinirole are dopamine agonists that do not possess the ergot structure. Pramipexole is a full dopamine agonist with high selectivity for the D2 dopamine receptor.[35] Ropinirole may offer some advantages over levodopa and the adverse effects are generally the same as the dopmine agonist class on the whole.

The classic "psychostimulant" drugs include dextroamphetamine, methylphenidate, pemoline, adderall, and to a lesser extent activating tricyclic antidepressants. These agents have typically been theorized to possess mixed dopaminergic and noradrenergic agonist activity.[27,36] Dextroamphetamine has been theorized to produce noradrenergic agonism via blocking of the re-uptake mechanism for norepinephrine. In higher doses, it is also dopaminergic via a similar mechanism of dopamine re-uptake blockade.[15] Dosing of dextroamphetamine should be initiated at 5 mg once to twice daily. The maximum recommended dose of dextroamphetamine is 60 mg/day.[30] There is little to any data addressing dosing limits in individuals following brain injury. To avoid problems with insomnia the last dose of medication should be given at least 6 h before going to sleep. There is some evidence that "pulsed" dosing of noradrenergic agonists via standard formulations rather than extended release dosing may be preferential with regard to the resultant psychostimulant effects. Generally, adults are fairly sensitive to psychostimulant therapy, particularly so after brain injury. Relative or absolute "toxicity" may be manifested by anxiety, dysphoria, increased irritability, cardiovascular symptoms, headache, palilalia, sterotypical thoughts, cognitive impairment, hallucinations, insomnia, and motor disorders including dyskinesias, tics, and worsening of spasticity.[30,37]

Methylphenidate hydrochloride is a mixed dopaminergic, noradrenergic agonist whose pharmacologic action is similar to amphetamines. The main sites of action appear to be the cerebral cortex and subcortical structures such as the thalamus. Dosing typically should be initiated at 5 mg twice a day and titrated up to a maximum dose of 60 mg/day. An extended release formulation is also available. The adverse effects of this drug are analogous to those of dextroamphetamine.

Pemoline is a oxazolidinone derivative stimulant with pharmacologic actions qualitatively similar to dextroamphetamine and methylphenidate. Evidence suggests that pemoline may have its stimulatory effect via dopaminergic mechanisms. The drug is typically dosed initially at 37.5 mg daily as a morning dose with increases of 18.75 mg made weekly as appropriate. The effective dose is typically in the range 56.25–75 mg/day. The most frequently encountered adverse effects include insomnia and anorexia, both being dose related.

Serotonergic agonists

The major drugs in this class include trazodone hydrochloride, fluoxetine, as a parent compound in its class, and other selective serotonin reuptake inhibitors, buspirone and L-tryptophan. Trazodone hydrochloride is a triazolopyridine derivative that selectively inhibits serotonin uptake. Initial dosing should begin at low doses (50–150 mg), typically at bedtime with light food. The dose should be on the lower end of the dosing range in geriatric patients secondary to more common side-effects such as sedation and orthostatic hypotension. The dose may be increased by 50 mg/day every 3–4 days to a maximum of approximately 400 mg/day. If closely monitored, as in an inpatient setting, the maximum dose may be as high as 5 mg/kg/day.

Fluoxetine is also a selective serotonin reuptake inhibitor (SSRI) but it tends to be more activating than other serotonergic drugs such as trazodone. Initial dosing should be 20 mg/day given as a morning dose. Doses above 20 mg/day should ideally be given on a twice a day schedule with a maximum daily dose of no more than 80 mg. The major reported side-effects include headache, nausea, nervousness, sexual dysfunction, and insomnia.[30,38] There are now multiple SSRI agents available including but not limited to sertraline, paroxetine, fluvoxamine, citalopram, and escitalopram.[39] Medications should be chosen based on specific impairment(s) being treated and side-effect profile and tolerance in the particular patient in question.

Buspirone is a novel benzodiazepine anxiolytic which is theorized to work through its serotonergic agonist activity at the 5-HT$_1$ receptor.[30] It should also be noted that this medication is pre-synaptically antagonistic at the D2 dopaminergic receptor.[40] The medication should be initiated at a dose of 10–15 mg twice a day and increased over 4–6 weeks to a maximum of 60 mg/day based on patient response and tolerance.[41] The main side-effects with buspirone are dizziness, headache, nervousness, and light-headedness.[42]

L-tryptophan is a serotonergic precursor which has received quite a bit of attention as of late secondary to the incidence of eosinophilic myalgia syndrome. This syndrome was purportedly traced to a bad batch of this pharmacologic agent produced in Japan.[43] This agent may be effective secondary to its modulation of CNS serotonin in regulation of sleep, depression, anxiety, aggression, appetite, temperature modulation, sexual behavior, and pain.[44]

Opioid antagonists

The two most commonly used opioid antagonists are naloxone and naltrexone, the latter being preferred secondary to its oral route of administration and prolonged mode of action.[45] Dosing typically starts low with a 12.5–25 mg daily dose with titration up to 150 mg/day with an average daily dose of 50 mg.[30] Exact dosing schedules and upper limits have not been well established in TBI. The major side-effects relate to gastrointestinal complaints and hepatocellular injury.

Gabaminergic agonists

A variety of pharmacologic agents that are commonly used in the general rehabilitation setting fall into this category. It should be noted, however, that only a few of them can be recommended for use in the patient with concommitant brain injury. Classic antispasticity agents such as valium and baclofen are gabaminergic agents, GABA-A and GABA-B, respectively. Many of the presently available anticonvulsant agents are also gabaminergic; specifically, valproate, gabapentin, barbiturates, and benzodiazepines. Other commonly utilized anticonvulsants such as phenytoin and carbamazepine are felt to mediate their anticonvulsant effect through other neurochemical systems.[46] From a clinical standpoint, many gabaminergic agents tend to be overly sedating in persons with acquired brain injury and may be associated with concommitant suppression of cognitive function. The use of these agents in the subacute and chronic phases following brain injury should be examined carefully given their potential side-effects.[4]

The prototypical agent for this class, valproic acid, is typically dosed at 15 mg/kg/day. Dosages may be increased by 5–10 mg/kg/day at weekly intervals until clinical efficacy is achieved or adverse side-effects prevent further increases. Due to potential adverse gastrointestinal side-effects it is recommended to administer the drug in two or more divided dosages. The maximum daily recommended dose is 60 mg/kg.[30] Side-effects are generally dose dependent.

Review of treatment options for specific clinical deficits

Appetite dysregulation

Alterations in appetite are not uncommon in patients with brain injury. The hyperphagic patient or "bulimic-type" must be contrasted with the hypophagic or "anorectic-type". Presumptive central neurochemical and neurophysiologic mechanisms responsible for alterations in appetite regulation form the basis of drug treatment for these functional sequelae.[47,48] The present consensus based on animal as well as human studies suggests that serotonergic agonists (trazodone, fluoxetine, and fenfluramine), opioid antagonists (naltrexone) and possibly corticotropin releasing factor (CRF) may all inhibit feeding behavior.[49,50] A recent case suggests that risperidone may be effective in insatiable appetite following hypothalamic injury.[51] Central serotonergic antagonists such as cyproheptadine can be utilized when there are problems with anorexia/hypophagia.[49]

Ataxia

Various forms of brain injury can result in cerebellar ataxia including trauma, stroke, tumor, degenerative conditions, and inherited ataxias such as Freidrich's ataxia. Several authors have reported that the serotonergic precursor L-tryptophan can significantly improve cerebellar ataxia due to a variety of primary etiologies.[52,53] Hydroxytryptophan (5-HTP) has several advantages over L-tryptophan including the fact that it bypasses the conversion of L-trytophan into 5-HTP by the enzyme tryptophan hydroxylase, which is the rate-limiting step in the synthesis of serotonin.[44] Other agents that have been utilized with some success include amantadine, buspirone, propranolol, clonazepam, gamma-vinyl GABA, acetazolamide, and phthalazinol.[54] Oral thyrotropin-releasing hormone also appeared to be a promising agent in the recent past.[55] Rohr et al. found that citalopram, an SSRI, improved symptoms of ataxia.[56] Some practitioners use low doses of clonazepam starting at 0.25 mg at bedtime, increasing the dosage to 1.5–5 mg/day in divided doses over several weeks.[54]

Autonomic dysregulation

One of the most challenging clinical conditions to treat following severe central nervous system injury is that of autonomic dysregulation with associated symptoms of hyperthermia,[57] diaphoresis, tachycardia, and tachypnea. There have been numerous neurochemical systems theorized to be involved with central control of temperature regulation. Hypothalamic dopaminergic systems seem to play a very significant role in thermoregulation.[58,59] Hyperpyrexia following brain injury has been successfully treated at a central level with dopaminergic agonists.[60,61] Dantrolene sodium has also been utilized to help decrease peripheral systemic effects such as rigidity commonly associated with this condition. Lastly, intrathecal baclofen has also been shown to be effective in alleviating autonomic dysfunction in severe brain injury.[62]

Hemi-inattention/neglect

Ascending dopaminergic pathways have been experimentally implicated in mediation of attentional processes including hemi-spatial neglect. Two small studies have demonstrated a potential utility of dopamine agonists: specifically, bromocriptine in the treatment of neglect secondary to cerebrovascular accident[63] and traumatic brain injury.[60] Both studies utilized an ABA paradigm and demonstrated significant differences in testing performance as well as functional capabilities while patients were receiving dopamine agonist pharmacotherapy. Further prospective studies are obviously warranted based on the encouraging results of these two studies.

Motor impairments

The major motor impairment encountered in the care of persons with ABI is spasticity. Spasticity is a velocity dependent increase in stretch reflex activity that is commonly seen after both focal and certain types of diffuse brain injury. Often it is severe enough to produce significant impairment and functional disability. Generally speaking, interventions may be directed at spasticity modulation for functional (e.g., better use of a limb in functional activities) versus non-functional (e.g., positioning, hygiene, comfort) purposes. Spasticity management has evolved to a great extent in the last decade with the introduction of newer management strategies and honing of older techniques. The following brief review will examine some of the current pharmacologic techniques utilized in spasticity management in persons with ABI.

Neurorehabilitationists have generally espoused focal treatment in cases where there is localized as opposed to diffuse spasticity. Treatments that have been found successful for such localized spasticity include neuromuscular blockade and perineural blockade. Local anesthetics may be used to block both afferent and efferent pathways and serve as a means of assessing the potential functional benefit of longer lasting interventions such as botulinum toxin and/or alcohol-based preparations (e.g., phenol and ethanol). Short acting local anesthetic blockade may also be useful in assessing the differential contributions of spasticity relative to contracture in the impaired extremity. Alcohol-based preparations, although highly effective in skilled hands, can produce an array of complications when used for perineural injection, including but not limited to dysesthesia (both chronic and transient), compartment syndromes, intravascular toxicity, and local infection, pain and/or bleeding. Neurolytic agents such as pheno are, for the present, cheaper, easier to titrate relative to antispasticity effect at the time of injection, as well as longer lasting. Botulinum toxin has its advantages relative to being easier to use for small muscles, e.g., distal muscles such as hand and foot intrinsics and/or extraocular musculature. Injection in certain areas such as the anterior neck must be done cautiously with botulinum toxin due to diffusional properties of the agent and the potential complication of dysphagia.[64] A recent review demonstrated that botulinum toxin may ameliorate spasticity and improve multiple aspects of ADLs and mobility in addition to decreasing medical morbidity associated with a variety of spasticity related disorders without significant adverse side-effects.[65]

When spasticity is more diffuse in nature as in spastic quadriparetic conditions following ABI, then systemic or enteral pharmacotherapy may be indicated, often in conjunction with focal treatment. Generally, the most commonly used enteral agents are baclofen, dantrolene sodium, diazepam, and tizanidine. However, multiple other drugs have been used to act synergistically with the aforementioned agents to enhance antispasticity effects. A recent review provided algorithmic approaches to enteral as well as chemodenervation techniques in spasticity modulation.[66] Some have argued that predominantly peripherally acting agents such as dantrolene sodium should be the drug of choice for spasticity management in cerebrally mediated spasticity whereas centrally acting drugs would be preferable for spinal mediated spasticity.

Intrathecal administration of antispasticity agents such as baclofen has been most effective in persons with intractable, severe and/or diffuse spasticity and/or non-ambulatory patients with predominantly lower extremity tonal abnormalities. Clearly, this is an expensive albeit often very effective treatment intervention which carries with it risks associated with long-term implantation and monitoring of a foreign device and risk for mechanical failure.[67]

Movement disorders

A variety of movement disorders have been treated with some success following brain injury. These include dystonia, tremors, parkinsonism, tics, akathisia, myoclonus, and dyskinesias such as chorea, ballismus, and athetosis.[68]

Dystonia, whether focal, segmental or generalized, has been treated with a variety of agents but generally with mixed results. Early onset dystonia following trauma tends to have a better prognosis than late onset dystonia which tends to be more persistent.[69] Dopaminergic agonists and antagonists, anticholinergics, baclofen, benzodiazepines, and carbamazepine have all been utilized in the treatment of this class movement disorders.[70,71]

Tremors are typically of the postural and/or kinetic type following traumatic brain injury whereas resting tremors are typically seen with nontraumatic degenerative cerebral disorders resulting in dopaminergic deficiency. Pharmacologic treatment tends to work better for non-traumatically induced tremor than for tremor resulting from trauma. A variety of drugs have been utilized including β-adrenergic blocking agents, benzodiazepines, dopaminergic agents, valproic acid, and anticholinergics.[72-74] Isoniazid has been used for treating cerebellar tremor related to multiple sclerosis.[75] Clonazepam has also been shown to be effective for post-traumatic rubral tremor.[76] One must always consider drug-induced tremor as a result of iatrogenic prescription and/or patient use of nicotine.[77]

Parkinsonism, when a result of trauma, can generally be treated fairly well with pharmacologic intervention. Numerous authors have reported Parkinson-like symptoms following diffuse brain injury such as bradykinesia, dysarthria, decreased facial expression, and rigidity.[78-81] Drugs that have been shown to be affective for "post-traumatic parkinsonism" include dopaminergic agonists such as L-dopa/carbidopa, bromocriptine and cabergoline, and to a lesser extent anticholinergics.[79] Rigidity associated with diffuse axonal injury has also been reported responsive to L-dopa leading to amelioration of functional motor disturbances associated with TBI.[82]

Tics are rare consequence of acquired brain injury.[70,71] The drugs used to treat tics include gabaminergic agonists, dopamine antagonists, and to a lesser extent noradrenergic drugs such as clonidine.[71] More recent work has shown potential promise with some of the newer atypical neuroleptics, as well as with other agents such as clonidine, guanfacine, tetrabenazine, pergolide, and botulinum toxin injections.[83]

Akathisia has been reported following brain injury and is thought to be associated in animal models with a relative dopaminergic deficiency in the prefrontal area.[84] Successful treatment of akathisia after brain injury with bromocriptine has been reported.[85] Other drugs that have been utilized but with fairly limited success include benzodiazepines and β-adrenergic blockers.[86]

Myoclonus is a common sequelae of severe hypoxic ischemic brain injury but can also be seen after non-hypoxic brain injury. Cortical myoclonus must be differentiated from epilepsy partialis continua.[87] A variety of drugs including benzodiazepines (clonazepam), serotonergic agonists such as trazodone and L-tryptophan, valproic acid, primidone, levetiracetam, and piracetam have all been reported effective.[88–90] Only a small percentage of patients respond to 5-HTP therapy. Of note is the fact that benzodiazepines tend to produce tolerance.[91]

Dyskinesias can occur in a variety of conditions and be manifested as ballismus, chorea, or athetosis. These types of movement disorders can result from thalamic and/or striatal injury as a result of trauma. Advances in drug treatment will likely evolve from recent developments in GABA and glutamate receptor pharmacology.[92] Typically, the drugs that have shown some utility for dyskinesias associated with traumatic brain injury include dopaminergic antagonists, as well as a variety of anticonvulsants including carbamazepine, phenobarbital, valproic acid, and phenytoin.[70,93–95] A few pharmacotherapies address the underlying pathophysiology of the dyskinesia itself, these agents include immunomodulators, antioxidants, cofactors, metabolic inhibitors and chelators.[92] It should be noted that certain dyskinesias may actually be atypical presentations of post-traumatic epilepsy.

Akinesia can be seen as a result of frontal brain involvement from trauma or anterior communicating artery aneurysmal hemorrhage. Due to the close association of dopamine systems with the neural pathways for kinesis (nigral projections to the basal ganglia, mesocortical projections to the anterior cingulate gyrus and the medial forebrain bundle projection to cortical and limbic sites), dopamine agonist drugs have been noted to be potentially beneficial in treatment of akinetic disorders.[96]

Neurogenic heterotopic ossification

Although the exact mechanism underlying neurogenic heterotopic ossification is unclear, recent reports suggest that insulin-like growth factor type 1 and growth hormone may play a etiologic role.[97] The only pharmacologic therapies presently available to minimize the extent of morbidity associated with neurogenic heterotopic ossification following brain injury involve the use of etidronate disodium and non-steroidal anti-inflammatory agents (NSAIDs).[98] Didronel presumptively works by interfering with biological calcification; specifically, impairing the calcification of osteoid. When there is still an acute phase to the condition, NSAIDs have been advocated to decrease the suspected inflammatory component of this pathologic process.

Didronel therapy is typically initiated at 20 mg/kg and the dose is subsequently lowered after several weeks to months to 10 mg/kg. There are no well-controlled, prospectively sound trials examining the use of this agent in "homogeneous" brain injury populations. Therefore, many if not all of the recommendations are based on the spinal cord injury literature. The main side-effect of the medication involves gastrointestinal complaints in the form of diarrhea and nausea.

Seizure disorders

Most neurosurgeons continue to use either phenytoin or phenobarbital for early management of seizures and/or seizure prophylaxis due to the fact that these medications can be administered parenterally (by intravenous route in the acute care setting). Prophylactic anti-epileptic drugs (AED) are considered to be effective in reducing early seizures, but there is no evidence that treatment with prophylactic anti-epileptic drugs reduces the occurrence of late seizures. Additionally, there is no data to support a role for prophylaxis in modulating the extent of impairment or death rate.[99,100]

There is now a trend within the field of brain injury rehabilitation to advocate for the utilization in the post-acute setting of specific anticonvulsants following brain injury (traumatic or non-traumatic); specifically, carbamazepine and valproic acid.[101–103] In general, carbamazepine should be a first line agent for treatment of partial seizures, whether simple or complex. On the other hand, valproic acid should be the agent of choice for multi-focal epilepsy and generalized tonic–clonic seizures. It should be noted, that valproic acid has been reported to be associated with encephalopathy and alterations in consciousness most likely secondary to hyperammonemia.[104–106]

Obviously, side-effects of the various anticonvulsant medications must be taken into consideration, particularly with patients with altered levels of consciousness and/or significant cognitive impairment. Various studies have demonstrated significant negative effects on cognitive function secondary to phenytoin and phenobarbital.[107–109] There is a recent study questioning this general consensus opinion bringing to light the need for further research in this area.[110] Recently, practice parameters on the use of anti-epileptic drugs for post-traumatic seizures have been published which recommend that use of prophylactic AED treatment not extend beyond the first week post-injury in patients with no history of seizures following non-penetrating TBI.[111] Other studies have demonstrated that other agents such as valproate show no benefit over short-term phenytoin therapy for prevention of early seizures and that neither treatment prophylaxes against the development of late post-traumatic seizures.[112] Although valproate is a potentially reasonable choice for controlling established seizures or stabilizing mood due to its relatively "clean" neuropsychological side-effect profile, it may have a propensity to produce more deaths compared to other agents such as phenytoin. A variety of newer agents such as oxcarbazepine, neurontin, lamotrigine, topiramate, zonisamide, tiagabine, and levetiracetam are presently being studied in an attempt to develop more effective drugs with fewer cognitive and systemic side-effects.[113,114]

Sleep disorders

A variety of sleep problems have been reported following brain injury. Many of these disorders are treatable with appropriate pharmacologic interventions. A good history is critical in eliciting appropriate information to determine the indicated diagnostic testing, as necessary, and subsequent best treatment including as apropos pharmacologic prescription. Various disorders have been described in the literature, particularly after traumatic brain injury, including but not limited to hypersomnia due to sleep disordered breathing, e.g. sleep apnea,[115] narcolepsy and/or CNS hypersomnia including excessive daytime sleepiness (EDS), wake–sleep cycle abnormalities, agrypnia (e.g. organic insomnia), parasomnias and dream state abnormalities.[116]

Post-traumatic narcolepsy has been successfully treated with methylphenidate.[117] Delayed sleep-phase syndrome, probably underdiagnosed in ABI, has been recognized and can be treated with both medication such as melatonin and behavioral therapies such as light therapy.[118,119] Depending on the clinical scenario, physicians must consider use of medications that may be atypical, such as risperidone.[120] The use of behavioral interventions, including "sleep hygiene" education, diet and environmental modifications, cannot be excluded from holistic management of this class of post-traumatic disorders.[121]

Speech–language and related disorders

A number of different medications have been used successfully for a variety of speech–language disorders in patients with brain dysfunction. Bromocriptine has been reported to improve speech dysfunction in patients with diffuse brain injury following trauma with dosages ranging from 20 to 40 mg/day.[122] Another series of studies demonstrated the efficacy of bromocriptine in the treatment of dysphasia; specifically the transcortical motor variant.[123,124] A more recent study showed efficacy of bromocriptine for crossed non-fluent aphasia following a right frontal stroke, and more interestingly continued positive effects on modulation of verbal initiation impairment even after discontinuation.[125,126] Amphetamine has also been reported to be efficacious in facilitation of aphasia recovery when paired with speech–language pathology in the subacute period following stroke.[127] Piracetam has also been reported to augment the response to speech therapy and improve activated blood flow as measured by cerebral PET in a prospective double-blind, placebo-controlled study done in patients post-stroke.[128] These former results were later questioned in a Cochrane review which found that drug treatment with piracetam may be effective in the treatment of aphasia after stroke.[129]

Animal studies have yielded some support for the role of dopaminergic pathways in both spontaneous and reflex swallowing[130,131] leading to human studies supporting the potential efficacy of DA agonist therapy for dysphagia following brain injury utilizing L-dopa/carbidopa.[132] Parkinsonian hypokinetic dysarthria has been treated with low-dose clonazepam (0.25–0.5 mg/day). The presumptive mechanism for its efficacy being striatal gabaminergic agonism.[133] Benzodiazepines have been reported to be effective in ameliorating traumatic mutism after severe brain injury.[134] A recent review of mutism etiologies concluded that the drug that seemed to be most effective for mutism was fluoxetine.[135]

Neurogenic stuttering, albeit rare, has been described following ABI. A case of post-traumatic adult onset stuttering responsive to anticonvulsant treatment has been reported suggesting that ictal speech disorders should always be considered in this patient population.[136] A more recent report by Schreiber and Pick noted beneficial effects for secondary stuttering presumed to be on the basis of a serotonergic–dopaminergic interaction.[137]

Sexual dysfunction

It is not uncommon for persons to have problems in the area of sexuality following brain injury. One of the most common complaints is alteration in libido.[138] Hyposexuality can be treated pharmacologically with a number of different agents including activating antidepressants, yohimbine (a noradrenergic agonist), dopamine agonists, and hormonal supplementation.[139–142] Hypersexuality, on the other hand, is a relatively rare clinical condition which is more difficult to broach from a pharmacotherapeutic standpoint. Hormonal agents, specifically medroxyprogesterone acetate, have been utilized to "chemically castrate" individuals with severe hypersexuality problems.[143–147] For patients who have bitemporal involvement and associated hypersexuality as seen in Kluver–Bucy syndrome, carbamazepine is generally considered to be the treatment of choice.[148] Other agents that may hold potential utility for treatment of the hypersexual patient following brain injury include serotonergic agonists, gabaminergic agonists, and opioid agonists. There are obviously significant ethical and medicolegal ramifications to the utilization of agents affecting sexual drive in this population.[149]

Conclusions

It is obviously of great importance for neurorehabilitation professionals treating individuals with brain injury to appreciate the potential benefits of neuropharmacotherapeutic interventions. This appreciation is necessary to truly maximize neurological and functional outcome in our patients with ABI-related impairments. It is critical, therefore, to have a good understanding of CNS neurochemical systems, both anatomically and physiologically, as well as basic pharmacologic issues prior to instituting any type of pharmacologic therapies in this patient population. Judiciously utilized medication prescription can significantly enhance treatment option armamentarium and discretionarily used can facilitate modulation of both impairment and functional disability.

References

1. Chavany, J. A. (1928). Role des causes occasionelles dan le déterminisime du ramolissenment cerebral (reflections therapeutiques à le propos). *Pratique Méd. Franç., 7.*
2. Sciclounoff, F. (1934). L'acetylcholine dans le traitement de l'ictus hemiplegique. *Presse Med., 42*, 1140.
3. Sutton, R. L., Weaver, M. S., & Feeney, D. M. (1987). Drug-induced modifications of behavioral recovery following cortical trauma. *J. Head Trauma Rehabil., 2*, 50.
4. Feeney, D. M., & Sutton, R. L. (1987). Pharmacotherapy for recovery of function after brain injury. *CRC Crit. Rev. Neurobiol., 3*, 135.
5. Goldstein, L. B. (1999). Pharmacological approach to functional reorganization: the role of norepinephrine. *Rev. Neurol., 155*(9), 731.
6. Gladstone, D. J., & Black, S. E. (2000). Enhancing recovery after stroke with noradrenergic pharmacotherapy: a new frontier? *Can. J. Neurol. Sci., 27*, 97.
7. Hornstein, A., et al. (1996). Amphetamine in recovery from brain injury. *Brain Inj., 10*(2), 145.
8. Goldstein, L. B. (1995). Prescribing of potentially harmful drugs to patients admitted to hospital after head injury. *J. Neurol. Neurosurg. Psychiat., 58*(6), 753.
9. Feeney, D. M. (1997). From laboratory to clinic: noradrenergic enhancement of physical therapy for stroke or trauma patients. *Adv. Neurol., 73*, 383.
10. Shiller, A. D., et al. (1999). Treatment with amantadine potentiated motor learning in a patient with traumatic brain injury of 15 years duration. *Brain Inj., 13*(9), 715.
11. Chapman, E. H., et al. (1999). Homeopathic treatment of mild traumatic brain injury: a randomized, double-blind, placebo-controlled clinical trial. *J. Head Trauma Rehabil., 14*(6), 521.
12. Frazer, A., & Hensler, J. G. (1994). In G. J. Siegel, et al. (Eds.), *Basic neurochemistry* (5th ed.). New York: Raven.
13. Gilman, S., & Newman, S. W. (1987). *Manter and Gatz's essentials of clinical neuroanatomy and neurophysiology*. Philadelphia, PA: F. A. Davis.
14. Seigel, G. J. (1989). *Basic neurochemistry: Molecular, cellular, and medical aspects*. New York: Raven.

15. Cooper, J. R., Bloom, F. E., & Roth, R. H. (1986). *The biochemical basis of neuropharmacology*. Oxford, NY: Oxford University Press.
16. Bradley, P. B. (1989). *Introduction to neuropharmacology*. Boston, MA: Wright.
17. Hyman, S. E. (1988). Recent developments in neurobiology: Part II. Neurotransmitter receptors and psychopharmacology. *Psychosomatics, 29*, 254.
18. Gershanik, O., Heikkila, R. E., & Duvoisin, R. C. (1983). Behavioral correlations of dopamine receptor activation. *Neurology, 33*, 1489.
19. Koller, W. C., Herbster, G. (1988). D_1 and D_2 Dopamine receptor mechanisms in dopaminergic behaviors. *Clin. Neuropharmacol., 11*, 221.
20. Julius, D. (1991). Molecular biology of serotonin receptors. *Ann. Rev. Neurosci., 14*, 335.
21. Hokfelt, T., et al. (2000). Neuropeptides – an overview. *Neuropharmacology, 39*(8), 1337.
22. Barnes, J. M., & Henley, J. M. (1992). Molecular characteristics of excitatory amino acid receptors. *Prog. Neurobiol., 39*, 13.
23. Lipton, S. A., & Rosenberg, P. A. (1994). Excitatory amino acids as a final common pathway for neurologic disorders. *N. Engl. J. Med., 3*, 613.
24. Fakuda, H., & Ito, Y. (1998). Pharmacology of the GABA receptor functions in the central nervous systems. *Yakugaku Zasshi, 118*(9), 339.
25. Siegel, G. J., et al. (Eds.) (1994). *Basic neurochemistry* (5th ed.). New York: Raven.
26. Montastruc, J. L., Rascol, O., & Senard, J. M. (1999). Treatment of Parkinson's disease should begin with a dopamine agonist. *Mov. Disord., 14*(5), 725.
27. Solanto, M. V. (2000). Clinical pharmacology of AD/HD: implications for animal models. *Neurosci. Biobehav. Rev., 24*(1), 27.
28. Elovic, E. (2000). Use of provigil for underarousal following TBI. *J. Head Trauma Rehabil., 15*(4), 1068.
29. Cedarbaum, J. M. (1987). Clinical pharmacokinetics of anti-Parkinsonian drugs. *Clin. Pharmacokinet., 13*, 141.
30. *Physician's desk reference*. (2001). Montvale, NJ: Medical Economics/Thomson Healthcare.
31. Berg, M. J., et al. (1987). Parkinsonism – drug treatment: Part I. *Drug Intell. Clin. Pharm., 21*, 10.
32. Gualtieri, T., et al. (1989). Amantadine: a new clinical profile for traumatic brain injury. *Clin. Neuropharmacol., 12*, 258.
33. Meythaler, J. M., Brunner, R. C., Johnson, A., & Novack, T. A. (2002). Amantadine to improve neurorecovery in traumatic brain injury-associated diffuse axonal injury: a pilot double-blind randomized trial. *J. Head Trauma Rehabil., 17*(4), 300–313.
34. Velasco, M., & Luchsinger, A. (1998). Dopamine: pharmacologic and therapeutic aspects. *Am. J. Ther., 5*(1), 37.
35. Hubble, J. P. (2000). Pre-clinical studies of pramipexole: clinical relevance. *Eur. J. Neurol., 7*(1), 15.
36. Kraus, M. F. (1995). Neuropsychiatric sequelae of stroke and traumatic brain injury: the role of psychostimulants. *Int. J. Psychiat. Med., 25*(1), 39.
37. Gualtieri, C. T. (1988) Pharmacotherapy and the neurobehavioural sequelae of traumatic brain injury. *Brain Inj., 2*, 101.
38. Sommi, R. W., Crismon, M. L., & Bowden, C. L. (1987). Fluoxetine: a serotonin-specific, second-generation antidepressant. *Pharmacotherapy, 7*, 1.

39. Bezchlibnyk-Butler, K., Aleksie, I., & Kennedy, S. H. (2000). Citalopram – a review of pharmacological and clinical effects. *J. Psychiat. Neurosci., 25*(3), 241.
40. Kastenholz, K. V., & Crismon, M. L. (1984). Buspirone, a novel nonbenzodiazepine anxiolytic. *Clin. Pharm., 3,* 600.
41. Eison, A. S., & Temple, D. L. (1986). Buspirone: review of its pharmacology and current perspectives on its mechanism of action. *Am. J. Med., 80,* 1.
42. Newton, R. E., et al. (1986). Review of side-effect profile of buspirone. *Am. J. Med., 80,* 17.
43. Slutsker, L., et al. (1990). Eosinophilia–myalgia syndrome associated with exposure to tryptophan from a single manufacturer. *J. Am. Med. Assoc., 264,* 213.
44. Birdsall, T. C. (1998). 5-Hydroxytryptophan: a clinically effective serotonin precursor. *Altern. Med. Rev., 3*(4), 271.
45. Calvanio, R., Burke, D. T., Kim, H. J., et al. (2000). Naltrexone: effects on motor function, speech, and activities of daily living in a patient with traumatic brain injury. *Brain Inj., 14*(10), 933–942.
46. Bleck, T. P., & Klawans, H. L. (1990). Convulsive disorders: mechanisms of epilepsy and anticonvulsant action. *Clin. Neuropharmacol., 13,* 121.
47. Rolls, E. T. (1985). Psychopharmacology and food. In M. Sandler and T. Silverstone (Eds.), *The neurophysiology of feeding* (p. 1). British Association for Psychopharmacology Monograph No. 7. New York: British Association for Psychopharmacology.
48. Halford, J. C., & Blundell, J. E. (2000). Pharmacology of appetite suppression. *Prog. Drug. Res., 54,* 25.
49. Morley, J. E. (1989). An approach to the development of drugs for appetite disorders. *Neuropsychobiology, 21,* 22.
50. Childs, A. (1987). Naltrexone in organic bulimia: a preliminary report. *Brain Inj., 1,* 49.
51. Bates, J. B. (1997). Effectiveness of risperidone in insatiable appetite following hypothalamic injury. *J. Neuropsychiat. Clin. Neurosci., 9*(4), 626.
52. Sandyk, R., & Iacona, R. P. (1989). Post-traumatic cerebellar syndrome: response to L-tryptophan. *Intern. J. Neurosci., 47,* 301.
53. Trouillas, P., Brudon, F., & Adeleine, P. (1988). Improvement of cerebellar ataxia with levoratory form of 5-hydroxytryptophan. A double-blind study with quantified data processing. *Arch. Neurol., 45,* 1217.
54. Perlman, S. L. (2000). Cerebellar ataxia. *Curr. Opin. Neurol., 2*(3), 215–224.
55. Bonuccelli, U., et al. (1988). Oral thyrotropin-releasing hormone treatment in inherited ataxias. *Clin. Neuropharmacol., 11,* 520.
56. Rohr, A., Eichler, K., & Hafezi-Moghadam, N. (1999). Citalopram, a selective serotonin reuptake inhibitor, improves symptoms of Friedreich's ataxia. *Pharmacopsychiatry, 32*(3), 113.
57. Rudy, T. A. (1980). Pathogenesis of fever associated with cerebral trauma and intracranial hemmorrhage. Thermoregulatory mechanisms and their therapeutic implications. In *4th International symposium on the pharmacology of thermoregulation, Oxford, 1979* (pp. 75–81). Basel: Karger.
58. Lipton, J. M., & Clark, W. G. (1986). Neurotransmitters in temperature control. *Ann. Rev. Physiol., 48,* 613.
59. Yamawaki, S., Lai, H., & Horita, A. (1983). Dopaminergic and serotonergic mechanisms of thermoregulation: mediation of thermal effects of apomorphine and dopamine. *J. Pharmacol. Exp. Therap., 227,* 383.

60. Zasler, N. D., & McNeny, R. (1989). Neuropharmocologic rehabilitation following traumatic brain injury via dopamine agonists. *Arch. Phys. Med. Rehabil., 70,* A12.

61. Russo, R. N., & O'Flaherty, S. (2000). Bromocriptine for the management of autonomic dysfunction after severe brain injury. *J. Paediatr. Child Health, 36*(3), 283.

62. Cuny, E., Richer, E., & Castel, J. P. (2001). Dysautonomia syndrome in the acute recovery phase after traumatic brain injury: relief with intrathecal baclofen therapy. *Brain Inj., 15*(10), 917–925.

63. Fleet, W. S., et al. (1987). Dopamine agonist therapy for neglect in humans. *Neurology, 37,* 1765.

64. Gracies, J. M., et al. (1997). Traditional pharmacological treatments for spasticity. Part I. Local treatments. *Muscle Nerve Suppl., 6,* S61.

65. Simpson, D. M. (1997). Clinical trials of botulinium toxin in the treatment of spasticity. *Muscle Nerve Suppl., 6,* S169.

66. Elovic, E. (2001). Principles of pharmaceutical management of spastic hypertonia. *Phys. Med. Rehabil. Clin. N. Am., 12*(4), 793–816.

67. Rawicki, B. (1999). Treatment of cerebral origin spasticity with continuous intrathecal baclofen delivered via an implantable pump: long-term follow-up review of 18 patients. *J. Neurosurg., 91*(5), 733.

68. Krauss, J. K., Trankle, R., & Kopp, K. H. (1996). Post-traumatic movement disorders in survivors of severe head injury. *Neurology, 47*(6), 1488.

69. Silver, J. K., & Lux, W. E. (1994). Early onset dystonia following traumatic brain injury. *Arch. Phys. Med. Rehabil., 75*(8), 885.

70. Koller, W. C., Wong, G. F., & Lang, A. (1989). Post-traumatic movement disorders: a review. *Mov. Disord., 4,* 20.

71. Katz, D. I. (1990). Movement disorders following traumatic head injury. *J. Head Trauma Rehabil., 5*(1), 86.

72. Biary, N., et al. (1989). Post-traumatic tremor. *Neurology, 1,* 103.

73. Ellison, P. H. (1978). Propranolol for severe post-head injury action tremor. *Neurology, 28,* 197.

74. Samie, M. R., Selhorst, J. B., & Koller, W. C. (1990). Post-traumatic midbrain tremor. *Neurology, 40,* 62.

75. Hallett, M., et al. (1985). Controlled trial of isoniazid therapy for severe postural cerebellar tremor in multiple sclerosis. *Neurology, 35,* 1374.

76. Jacob, P. C., & Pratap-Chand, R. (1998). Posttraumatic rubral tremor responsive to clonazepam. *Mov. Disord., 13*(6), 977.

77. Zdonczyk, D., Royse, V., & Koller, W. C. (1988). Nicotine and tremor. *Clin. Neuropharmacol., 11,* 282.

78. Sohn, D. G., Hoerning, E., & Kaplan, P. E. (1987). Carbidopa–levodopa therapy for movement disorders. *Arch. Phys. Med. Rehabil., 68,* 745.

79. Santosh, L., Merbtiz, C. P., & Grip, J. C. (1988). Modification of function in head-injured patients with Sinemet. *Brain Inj., 2,* 225–233.

80. Eames, P. (1989). The use of Sinemet and bromocriptine. *Brain Inj., 3,* 319.

81. Della, S. S., & Mazzini L. (1990). Post-traumatic extrapyramidal syndrome: Case report. Servizio di Neuropsicologia Clinica, Centro Medico De Veruno, Fondazione Clinica del. Lavoro. *Ital. J. Neurol. Sci., 1,* 65.

82. Koeda, T., & Takeshita, K. (1998). A case report of remarkable improvement of motor disturbances with L-dopa in a patient with post-diffuse axonal injury. *Brain Dev., 20*(2), 124.

83. Seahill, L., et al. (2000). Pharmacological treatment of tic disorders. *Child Adolesc. Psychiat. Clin. N. Am., 9*(1), 99.

84. Carter, C. J., & Pycock, C. J. (1980). Behavioral and biochemical effects of dopamine and noradrenaline depletion within the medial prefrontal cortex of the rat. *Brain Res.*, 192.

85. Stewart, J. T. (1989). Akathisia following traumatic brain injury: treatment with bromocriptine. *J. Neurol. Neurosurg. Psychiat., 52*, 1200.

86. Adler, L. A., et al. (1988). Neuroleptic-induced akathisia: propranolol versus benztropine. *Biol. Psychiat., 23*, 211.

87. Watanabe, K., Kuroiwa, Y., & Toyokura, Y. (1984). Epilepsia partialis continua: epileptogenic focus in motor cortex and its participation in transcortical reflexes. *Arch. Neurol., 41*, 1040.

88. Obeso, J. A., et al. (1989). The treatment of severe action myoclonus. *Brain, 112*, 765.

89. Marsden, C. D., & Fahn, S. (Eds.) (1987). *Movement disorders* (Vol. 2). London: Butterworth.

90. Jankovic, J., & Pardo, R. (1986). Segmental myoclonus, clinical and pharmacologic study. *Arch Neurol., 43*, 1025.

91. Snodgrass, S. R. (1990). Myoclonus: analysis of monoamine, GABA, and other systems. *FASEB J., 4*(10), 2775.

92. Pranzatelli, M. R. (1996). Antidyskinetic drug therapy for pediatric movement disorders. *J. Child Neurol., 11*(5), 353.

93. Roig, M., Monserrat, L., & Gallart, A. (1988). Carbamazepine: an alternative drug for the treatment of non-hereditary chorea. *Pediatrics, 82*, 492.

94. Robin, J. J. (1977). Paroxysmal choreoathetosis following head injury. *Ann. Neurol., 2*, 447.

95. Richardson, J. C., et al. (1987). Kinesigenic choreoathetosis due to brain injury. *Can. J. Neurol. Sci., 14*, 626.

96. Alexander, M. P. (2001). Chronic akinetic mutism after mesencephalic–diencephalic infarction: remediated with dopaminergic medications. *Neurorehabil. Neur. Repair., 15*(2), 151–156.

97. Wildburger, R., Zarkovic, N., Leb, G., et al. (2001). Post-traumatic changes in insulin-like growth factor type 1 and growth hormone in patients with bone fractures and traumatic brain injury. *Wien. Klin. Wochenschr., 113*(3–4).

98. Shehab, D., Elgazzar, A. H., & Collier, B. D. (2002). Heterotopic ossification. *J. Nucl. Med., 43*(3), 346–353.

99. Temkin, N. R., et al. (1990). A randomized, double-blind study of phenytoin for the prevention of post-traumatic seizures. *N. Engl. J. Med., 323*, 497.

100. Schierhout, G., & Roberts, I. (2001). Anti-epileptic drugs for preventing seizures following acute traumatic brain injury. *Cochrane Database Syst. Rev., 4*, CD000173.

101. Glenn, M. B., & Wroblewski, B. (1986). Anticonvulsants for prophylaxis of post-traumatic seizures. *J. Head Trauma Rehabil., 1*, 73.

102. O'Shanick, G. J., & Zasler, N. D. (1989). In J. Kreutzer and P. Wehman (Eds.), *Neuropsychopharmcological approaches to traumatic brain injury in community integration following traumatic brain injury.* Baltimore, MD: Paul H. Brookes.

103. Pellock, J. M. (Ed.). (1989). Who should receive prophylactic antiepiliptic drug following head injury? *Brain Inj., 107*.

104. Gaskins, D., Holt, R. J., & Postelnick, O. (1984). Non-dosage-dependent valproic acid-induced hyperammonemia and coma. *Clin. Pharm., 3,* 313.
105. Jones, G. L., et al. (1990). Valproic acid-associated encephalopathy. *West. J. Med., 153,* 199.
106. Marescaux, C., et al. (1982). Stuporous episodes druing treatment with sodium valproate: report of seven cases. *Epilepsia, 23,* 297.
107. Collaborative Group for Epidemiology of Epilepsy (1986). Adverse reactions to anti-epileptic drugs: a multicenter survey of clinical practice. *Epilepsia, 27,* 323.
108. Thompson, P. J., & Trimble, M. R. (1982). Comparative effects of anticonvulsant drugs on cognitive functioning. *Br. J. Clin. Pract., 18,* 154.
109. Trimble, M. R. (1987). Anticonvulsant drugs and cognitive function: a review of the literature. *Epilepsia, 28,* S37.
110. Hernandez, T. D. (1997). Preventing post-traumatic epilepsy after brain injury: weighing the costs and benefits of anticonvulsant prophylaxis. *Trends Pharmacol. Sci., 19*(7), 59.
111. Brain Injury Special Interest Group (1998). Practice parameter: antiepileptic drug treatment of posttraumatic seizures. Brain Injury Special Interest Group of the American Academy of Physical Medicine and Rehabilitation. *Arch. Phys. Med. Rehabil., 79*(5), 594.
112. Temkin, N. R, et al. (1999). Valproate therapy for prevention of posttraumatic seizures: a randomized trial. *J. Neurosurg., 91*(4), 593.
113. Loring, D. W., & Meador, K. J. (2001). Cognitive and behavioral effects of epilepsy treatment. *Epilepsia, 42*(Suppl. 8), 24–32.
114. Asconape, J. J. (2002). Some common issues in the use of antiepileptic drugs. *Semin. Neurol., 22*(1), 27–39.
115. Webster, J. B., Bell, K. R., Hussey, J. D., et al. (2001). Sleep apnea in adults with traumatic brain injury: a preliminary investigation. *Arch. Phys. Med. Rehabil., 82*(3), 316–321.
116. Mahowald, M. W. (2000). Sleep in traumatic brain injury and other acquired CNS conditions. In A. Culebras, (Ed.), *Sleep disorders and neurological disease* (p. 365). New York: Marcel Decker.
117. Francisco, G. E., & Ivanhoe, C. B. (1996). Successful treatment of post-traumatic narcolepsy with methylphenidate: a case report. *Am. J. Phys. Med. Rehabil., 75*(1), 63.
118. Nagtegaal, J. E., et al. (1997). Traumatic brain injury-associated delayed sleep phase syndrome. *Funct. Neurol., 12*(6), 345.
119. Quinto, C., Gellido, C., Chokroverty, S., & Masdeu, J. (2000). Post-traumatic delayed sleep phase syndrome. *Neurology, 54*(1), 250–252.
120. Schreiber, S., et al. (1998). Beneficial effect of risperidone on sleep disturbance and psychosis following traumatic brain injury. *Int. Clin. Psychopharmacol., 13*(6), 273.
121. Rao, V., & Rollings, P. (2002). Sleep disturbances following traumatic brain injury. *Curr. Treatm. Options Neurol., 4*(1), 77–87.
122. Crismon, M. L., et al. (1988). The effect of bromocriptine on speech dysfunction in patients with diffuse brain injury (akinetic mutism). *Clin. Neuropharmacol., 11,* 462.
123. Bachman, D. L., & Morgan, A. (1988). The role of pharmacotherapy in the treatment of aphasia: preliminary result. *Aphasiology, 2,* 225.

124. Albert, M. L., et al. (1988). Pharmacotherapy for aphasia. *Neurology, 38,* 877.
125. Raymer, A. M., et al. (2001). Effects of bromocriptine in a patient with crossed nonfluent aphasia: a case report. *Arch. Phys. Med. Rehabil., 82,* 139.
126. Gold, M., VanDam, D., & Silliman, E. R. (2000). An open-label trial of bromocriptine in non-fluent aphasia: a qualitative analysis of word storage and retreival. *Brain Lang., 74*(2), 141–156.
127. Walker-Batson, D., Curtis, S., Natarajan, R., et al. (2001). A double-blind, placebo-controlled study of the use of amphetamine in the treatment of aphasia. *Stroke, 32*(9), 2093–2098.
128. Kessler, J., Thiel, A., Karbe, H., & Heiss, W. D. (2000). Piracetam improves activated blood flow and facilitates rehabilitation of post-stroke aphasic patients. *Stroke, 31*(9), 2112–2116.
129. Greener, J., Enderby, P., & Whurr, R. (2001). Pharmacological treatment for aphasia following stroke. *Cochrane Database Syst. Rev., 4,* CD000424.
130. Bieger, D., Giles, S. A., & Hockman, C. H. (1977). Dopamingeric infuences on swallowing. *Neuropharmacology, 6,* 245.
131. Bieger, D., Weerasuriya, A., & Hockman, C. H. (1978). The emetic action of L-dopa and its effect on the swallowing reflex in the cat. *J. Neur. Transm., 42,* 87.
132. Rucker, K. S., et al. (1988). Resolution of swallowing disorder with L-dopa and evaluation of CSF neurotransmitters in brain injury. *Arch. Phys. Med. Rehabil., 69,* 734.
133. Biary, N., Pimental, P. A., & Langenberg, P. W. (1988). A double-blind trial of clonazepam in the treatment of parkinsonian dysarthria. *Neurology, 38,* 255.
134. Caradoc-Davies, T. H. (1996). Traumatic mutism in severe head injury relieved by oral diazepam. *Disabil. Rehabil., 18*(9), 482.
135. Gordon, N. (2001). Mutism: elective or selective and acquired. *Brain Dev., 23*(2), 83–87.
136. Baratz, R., & Mesulam, M. (1981). Adult-onset stuttering treated with anticonvulsants. *Arch. Neurol., 38*(2), 132.
137. Schreiber, S., & Pick, C. G. (1997). Paroxetine for secondary stuttering: further interaction of serotonin and dopamine. *J. Nerv. Ment. Dis., 185*(7), 465.
138. Kreutzer, J., & Zasler, N. D. (1989). Psychosexual consequences of traumatic brain injury: methodology and preliminary findings. *Brain Inj., 3,* 177.
139. Zasler, N. D., & Horn, L. J. (1990). Rehabilitative management of sexual dysfunction. *J. Head Trauma Rehabil., 5,* 14.
140. Segraves, R. T. (1988). Drugs and desire. In S. R. Leiblum and R. C. Rosen (Eds.), *Sexual desire disorders.* New York: Guilford.
141. Morales, A., et al. (1982). Nonhormonal pharmacological treatment of organic impotence. *J. Urol., 128,* 45.
142. Kockott, G. (1983). Sexual disorders. In H. Hipius and G. Winokur (Eds.), *Clinical psychopharmacology, Part 2* (p. 345). Lawrenceville, NJ: Excerpta Medica-Princeton.
143. Zasler, N. D. (1990). In P. Wehman and J. S. Kreutzer (Eds.), *The role of the physiatrist in vocational rehabilitation for persons with traumatic brain injury.* Rockville, MD: Aspen.
144. McConaghy, N., Blaszczynski, A., & Kidson, W. (1988). Treatment of sex offenders with imaginal desensitization and/or medroxyprogesterone. *Acta Psychiatr. Scand., 77,* 199.

145. Lehne, G. K. (1986). Brain damage and paraphilia: treated with medroxyprogesterone acetate. *Sexual. disabil., 7*, 145.
146. Berlin, F. S., & Meinecke, C. F. (1981). Treatment of sex offenders with antiandrogenic medication: conceptualization, review of treatment modalities, and preliminary findings. *Am. J. Psychiat., 137*, 782.
147. Britton, K. R. (1998). Medroxyprogesterone in the treatment of aggressive hypersexual behavior in traumatic brain injury. *Brain Inj., 12*(8), 703.
148. Stewart, J. T. (1985). Carbamazepine treatment of a patient with Kluver–Bucy syndrome. *J. Clin. Psychiat., 46*, 496.
149. Zasler, N. D., & Martelli, M. F. (in press). Sexuality issues in TBI. In J. M. Silver, S. C. Yudofsky, and T. W. McAllister (Eds.), *Neuropsychiatry of traumatic brain Injury*. (2nd ed.).

11 Spasticity of cerebral origin

John S. Hong and
Christopher G. Zitnay

Background

Introduction and epidemiology

Spasticity is a very important medical as well as social issue because it can greatly affect a person's health, function, comfort, care delivery, and self-image. Medical issues that can arise secondarily to spasticity include contractures, skin ulcers, pain, and even subluxation. Although the exact prevalence and incidence of spasticity in acquired brain injury (ABI) is not known, the prevalence of spasticity has been estimated to be approximately 500,000 to over 2 million in USA and 12 million in world.[1,2] Traumatic brain injury (TBI) in itself is very common in the USA with approximately 2 million episodes per year.[3]

Definition of spasticity

Because spasticity has been hard to characterize, there are several definitions seen in the literature.[4] Spasticity has been defined as follows:

> A condition in which stretch reflexes that are normally latent become obvious. The tendon reflexes have a lowered threshold to tap, the response of the tapped muscle is increased, and usually muscles besides the tapped one respond; tonic stretch reflexes are affected in the same way.[5]

> A motor disorder characterized by a velocity-dependent increase in tonic stretch reflexes (muscle tone) with exaggerated tendon jerks, resulting from hyperexcitability of the stretch reflex, as one component of the upper motoneuron syndrome.[5]

> A disorder of spinal proprioceptive reflexes, manifested clinically as tendon jerk hyperreflexia and an increase in muscle tone that becomes more apparent the more rapid the stretching movement.[6]

As we can see from these definitions, spasticity involves muscles that are extraordinarily prone to contracting, especially when the muscle is trying to be stretched.

Spasticity is a hallmark component of a syndrome called upper moto-neuron (UMN) syndrome. In UMN syndrome, there are two main "positive" symptoms: (a) enhanced stretch reflexes (spasticity); (b) released flexor reflexes in the lower limbs; and two "negative" symptoms: (a) loss of dexterity; (b) weakness.[7]

Pathophysiology

In the segmental reflex arc there are muscle receptors: the afferent nerve to the spinal cord, and the motoneuron back to the muscle. Primary afferent Ia fibers surround intrafusal fibers of the muscle spindle. When the muscle stretches, the muscle spindles are excited. This stimulus travels up the Ia nerve to the spinal cord. There are two different synaptic connections made there: (a) α-motoneuron back to the muscle of origin as well as synergistic muscles (i.e., quadriceps); (b) inhibitory interneuron which inhibits the α-motoneuron to the antagonistic muscle (i.e. hamstrings).[4,8] Hence, the stretched muscle begins to oppose the stretch by contracting itself.

In ABI, the basis of spasticity lies in abnormal proprioceptive reflexes. Some theories state that the increased stretch reflex is due to hyperexcitability of the α-motoneuron pool at the segmental level. This condition may result from an imbalance between inhibitory (reduced) and excitatory (increased) inputs and/or the motoneurons fire below their normal threshold. In ABI, the normal inhibition at the primary afferent nerve terminals may be reduced, especially the reticulospinal pathway. On the other hand, the motoneurons may be more excited due to increased depolarization from a supraspinal pathway, such as the lateral vestibulospinal pathway.[4,9,10]

Spastic muscles are flaccid during rest phase (though this is of some debate due to definition problems of spasticity). The reflex of spasticity occurs from a fast stretch of the muscle involved because the spasticity is dependent upon the velocity of stretch. In fact, the spastic reflex response is proportional to the speed of the stretch. Therefore, the examiner needs to deliver a brisk passive stretch to the muscles in question. If the examiner stretches the muscle too slowly, spasticity may not be elicited.[9,11] "Clasp-knife phenom-enon" is one characteristic sign of spasticity, as seen in the biceps and quadri-ceps muscles. To the examiner, a "catch-and-give" sensation occurs. The "catch" is due to muscle contraction from the reflex. The "give" occurs as the examiner succeeds in stretching out the spastic muscle.[12] So as the examiner tries to passively stretch out a muscle, the muscle will gather resistance as the reflex develops due to the stretch, in particular due to the *velocity* of the stretch occurring. When the muscle stops stretching due to the spastic con-traction, the reflex diminishes and the examiner is able to further stretch out the muscle. Virtually it is analogous to opening a clasp-knife (Swiss Army knife) in which it is initially difficult to open the blade but then it snaps out easily. As the muscle is increasingly stretched out, an inhibitory effect to the reflex begins to develop. In the quadriceps, there is a threshold in which when the knee is flexed past the "clasp-knife" position, the reflex cannot be elicited. In this case, the spasticity reflex is a balance between velocity-dependent excitation and position-dependent suppression of the reflex.[9] Interestingly however, unlike the quadriceps which has less reflex response as it is stretched more, the hamstring muscles develop more reflex activity to stretch.

Clinical

History and physical examination

The history and physical examination are crucial to diagnose the patient and to decide which treatment modalities will best benefit the patient. In addition to spasticity, UMN syndrome includes hyper-reflexia, clonus, rigidity, incoordination, and weakness. Therefore, the clinician needs to see how all these factors play in the role of the patient's condition. Also, because other neurological and medical conditions can easily complicate the picture, the clinician needs to be detailed with the history and physical examination to learn the exact etiology of the patient's condition. For example, noxious stimuli can cause or exacerbate spasticity; e.g., an ingrown toenail can lead to lower extremity spasticity. A past medical history of polio or rheumatoid arthritis can increase the difficulty in diagnosing spasticity. Furthermore, the clinician needs to distinguish between a contracture versus spasticity because in the brain injury population (especially stroke patients) contractures are commonly seen. Lastly, the patient's current and past medicine regimen needs to be reviewed, as well as drug allergies.

EMG, Electrical Stimulation, and Motion Analysis are valuable instruments to help the clinician diagnose spasticity and decide upon treatment modalities. However, in this section we will focus on the physical examination itself. Below are the most common spasticity syndromes seen.[13,14]

The Modified Ashworth Scale

The Modified Ashworth Scale (MAS)[15] is the current clinical assessment tool used to measure the level of spasticity in a patient:

- 0 = no tone.
- 1 = slight increase in muscle tone, manifested by a catch and release or by minimal resistance at end of range of motion when affected parts moved in flexion or extension.
- 1+ = slight increase in muscle tone, manifested by a catch, followed by minimal resistance throughout the remainder (< 50%) of range of motion.
- 2 = more marked increase in muscle tone through most of range of motion, but affected part is easily moved.

- 3 = considerable increase in muscle tone, passive movement difficult.
- 4 = affected part is rigid in flexion or extension.

Syndromes of spasticity

ADDUCTED/INTERNALLY ROTATED SHOULDER

In this syndrome, the four common muscles involved are: pectoralis major (clavicular and sternal heads), latissimus dorsi, teres major, and/or subscapularis. The humerus is pulled against the chest wall and internally rotated so that combined with the typically flexed elbow, the forearm lies across the middle of the anterior chest. The glenohumeral joint does allow the hand to move spherically. The adducted/internally rotated shoulder can create difficulties in axillary hygiene, getting dressed, and shoulder/arm movement restrictions.

During passive ROM testing, the clinician may see prominence in the tendinous insertions of the pectoralis major, latissimus dorsi, and/or teres major. Observe the resting position of the shoulder and elbow in sitting, standing, and walking positions because spasticity may occur during one or more of these situations. The examiner should test for potential functional use by having the patient touch the mouth, back of the neck, pants pocket, tip of contralateral shoe, and four quadrants of a tabletop. Latissimus dorsi and teres major should be suspected of spasticity if there is hyperextension posturing of the shoulder, especially during walking.

Dynamic EMG and diagnostic nerve blocks are useful when the examination does not help distinguish between volitional, spastic and contractural etiologies. To liberate muscles that are restricted by spasticity, the clinician must see if any muscles are capable of voluntary movement. For this shoulder problem, adductor muscles that will work need to be found. Temporary nerve blocks (e.g., lidocaine) of the medial and lateral pectoral nerves or thoracodorsal nerve may show improvement if all the shoulder adductors have poor EMG activity during voluntary movement. Spastic latissimus dorsi or teres major muscles can be diagnosed with a block of the thoracodorsal nerve or lower subscapular nerve. Although the pectoralis major tendon insertion is prominent when spastic, an EMG reading is useful to see which head/heads need to be diagnostically injected (though one could inject lidocaine to both the medial and lateral pectoral nerves for diagnosis).

FLEXED ELBOW

The three muscles involved in this syndrome are brachioradialis, biceps, and/or brachialis. The flexed elbow syndrome is considered to be the most common motor dysfunction. Patients usually complain that while standing up from sitting position or while walking their elbow starts to ride up, even to the point of hitting their throats. Also, the elbow forms a "hook" and will catch on objects such as doorframes, people, or furniture. Obviously, it is difficult for them to get dressed or even put on a jacket. Skin breakdown in the antecubital fossa can occur.

As with the shoulder examination, the elbow is observed during sitting, standing, and walking. The elbow should be examined during passive and active range of motion. If the patient is able to voluntarily move his or her elbow, chances are that they will be able to flex their elbow much faster than they can extend it (due to weak triceps, to spastic flexors, or a combination of the two). The brachioradialis is spastic more often than biceps and brachialis. EMG can help to determine where the dyssynergy is occurring among the elbow muscles. The brachioradialis, biceps, brachialis, and three heads of the triceps can then be injected accordingly for diagnosis and treatment.

PRONATED FOREARM

The two muscles involved in this syndrome are pronator quadratus and/or pronator teres. The pronated forearm is more common that a supinated forearm because voluntary supination is one of the last movements to recover after a CVA.[16] Patients with this syndrome can encounter difficulty using feeding and grooming utensils, fastening clothing, and reaching for a place that requires supination.

During the resting stage, the forearm is usually pronated. The examiner will be able to palpate the pronator teres but not the pronator quadratus. Pronator dyssynergy is suspected when passive range of motion exceeds active range of motion during supination. Dynamic EMG studies of the pronator quadratus, pronator teres, and even the biceps are helpful. (Spastic biceps often accompany the pronated forearm.) Once again, a diagnostic motor point block with Lidocaine to each muscle can be performed.

FLEXED WRIST

The muscles involved in this syndrome are flexor carpi radialis, flexor carpi ulnaris, flexor digitorum superficialis, and/or flexor digitorum profundus. Patients complain that grasping an object can be very difficult since they cannot extend their fingers and wrist. Inserting their hands through sleeves can also be hard. Other complications include carpal tunnel syndrome, radial deviation, ulnar deviation, clenched fist, and wrist subluxation.

During rest, radial deviation is indicative of flexor carpi radialis spasticity, ulnar deviation is indicative of flexor carpi ulnaris spasticity, clenched fist is indicative of extrinsic finger flexors spasticity, fingernails digging into the palm are indicative of flexor digitorum profundus spasticity, and markedly flexed PIP joints without DIP flexion are indicative of flexor digitorum superficialis spasticity. On physical examination, passive range of motion is usually painful and very difficult to perform due to strong resistant muscles. Dynamic EMG studies may be helpful, but they are not easily predictable from the physical examination. Also, EMG activity does not correlate with force production; hence, diagnostic nerve blocks are usually required. Furthermore, the extensor muscles need to be evaluated as well because flexors are much stronger than extensors. So after blocking the spastic flexor muscles, you may end up with wrist hyperextension if the extensor muscles are spastic too. With a hyperextended wrist, the flexor muscles of the fingers tighten up leading to a clenched fist deformity.

CLENCHED FIST

The muscles involved in this syndrome include various muscle slips of flexor digitorum profundus and/or various muscle slips of flexor digitorum superficialis. One or more fingers can be involved. With this condition, the patient is unable to grasp objects easily or release grasped objects. From the fingers being clasped in the palm, palm skin breakdown may occur as well as nailbed infections and fingernail lacerations.

If accompanied by a flexed wrist in this syndrome flexor digitorum superficialis and flexor digitorum profundus are the main spastic muscles involved. As mentioned above, if PIP is flexed but DIP is not flexed, then flexor digitorum superficialis is spastic rather than flexor digitorum profundus. On examination, the examiner should flex the wrist as much as possible to try to get the fingers to be less curled. If this technique fails, joint contracture must be considered. The examiner must individually test each joint with the wrist in flexion and in extension.

To test for intrinsic muscle spasticity, the wrist is flexed to relax the extrinsic muscles. To stretch the intrinsic muscles, the examiner must flex the PIP joint while extending the MCP joint. If the intrinsic muscles are spastic, resistance will be felt. If this intrinsic muscle stretch is done with enough velocity, clonus may even be produced. Diagnosis of spastic intrinsic muscles is important to prevent an Intrinsic Plus Hand deformity (flexion of MCPs with extension of DIPs/PIPs) after treatment of spastic extrinsic muscles but not spastic intrinsic muscles. Dynamic EMG studies and diagnostic nerve blocks are recommended on flexor digitorum profundus, flexor digitorum superficialis, extensor digitorum communis, lumbricals, and samples of the interossei.

THUMB-IN-PALM DEFORMITY

The muscles involved in this syndrome are adductor pollicis, flexor pollicis longus, and/or the thenar group (especially the flexor pollicis brevis). In this condition, patients usually have difficulty in grasping objects, or picking things up with their thumb in opposition. The thumb cannot function during key grasp (opposition with index finger) or three-jaw chuck (opposition with third finger).

In appearance, the DIP joint is usually flexed, and the MCP and CMC joints may or may not be flexed. Often, though, the patient will have a clenched fist.

However, if the patient can extend their thumb when their wrist is flexed, the spastic muscle may be the flexor pollicis longus. Therefore, passive range of motion needs to be tested during wrist extension and flexion to measure the tightness of the flexor pollicis longus. To test the intrinsic muscles, the wrist should be flexed. A spastic thenar muscle will feel tight while the MCP is actively flexed. Contractures may be present in the thumb IP joint and the skin web space. Dynamic EMG studies and nerve blocks once again are useful to determine the potential effectiveness of treatment.

EQUINOVARUS FOOT

In this syndrome, curled toes or claw toes are due to muscle spasticity seen in medial gastrocnemius, lateral gastrocnemius, soleus, tibialis posterior, tibialis anterior, extensor hallucis longus, long toe flexors, and/or peroneus longus. This condition is the number one pathologic posture of the lower limbs due to TBI. While standing, the foot and ankle are plantarflexed and inverted so that the distal lateral foot is pressed against the floor, which can lead to pain (and even skin breakdown) over the fifth metatarsal head. Toe curling is another phenomenon commonly seen in this condition.

Initial contact with the floor occurs on the forefoot with the weight primarily on the lateral aspect of the foot. During early push-off, the patient will hyperextend the knee due to the lack of dorsiflexion of the foot. The forward swing phase of the leg can be difficult with the inverted and dorsiflexed foot. Dynamic EMG and Lidocaine injections are useful for diagnosis.

VALGUS FOOT

In this syndrome, the muscles involved are peroneus longus and brevis, gastrocnemius, soleus, tibialis anterior, and/or long toe flexors. The patient usually has pain over the medial aspect of the foot since the foot and ankle are everted. The toes may be flexed. The patient could even develop genu valgum in the future from the forces upon the knees.

Opposite to equinovarus, the valgus foot makes initial contact with the floor on the forefoot and the weight is mostly over the medial aspect of the foot. If the patient cannot dorsiflex the foot, hyperextension of the knee will occur as described in equinovarus, as well as difficulty in swinging the leg forward. Dynamic EMG and nerve blocks to differentiate the muscles, such as peroneus longus and peroneus brevis, are useful.

STRIATAL TOE (HITCHHIKER'S GREAT TOE)

The extensor hallucis longus is responsible for holding the great toe up due to spasticity, although flexor hallucis longus can be involved. Because the extensor hallucis longus can also invert the foot, ankle equinus and varus can occur. Because the great toe is extended, it rubs against the shoe and causes pain at the tip of the toe and under the first metatarsal head while standing. Also, balance and push-off are affected during walking. EMG is useful to locate this thin muscle in diagnosis and treatment.

STIFF KNEE (EXTENDED)

The muscles involved in this syndrome are gluteus maximus, rectus femoris, vastus lateralis, vastus medialis, vastus intermedius, hamstrings, gastrocnemius, and/or iliopsoas. Walking is difficult since the knee stays extended throughout the gait cycle, and the patient may complain of tripping from dragging the toes.

Dynamic EMG is necessary to locate the spastic muscles involved. The EMG can determine if all the quadriceps muscles are spastic, or if the vastus intermedius and rectus femoris are involved with or without opposing hamstrings. Dynamic EMG is also useful to rule out a spastic hamstring, for the extensor muscles could be guarding against flexing the knee. The differential diagnosis includes a weak iliopsoas or spastic hip extensors that prevent good hip flexion during gait. Calf muscle spasticity can also produce an extended knee during the stance phase.

FLEXED KNEE

In this syndrome, the muscles involved are medial hamstrings, lateral hamstrings, quadriceps, and/or gastrocnemius. Because full knee extension cannot occur, the patient must stand and walk in a crouched position to compensate (bilateral hip flexion and contralateral knee flexion).

The medial hamstrings are usually the cause of this condition. The quadriceps may be simultaneously tight and this makes flexion even worse. If the knee has a contracture, the quadriceps may be weak and therefore need strengthening after therapy. If the patient has the flexed knee only during stance, this is suggestive of a gastrocnemius-soleus weakness. Dynamic EMGs are important in diagnosis, including ruling out spasticity in hip flexion since the patient is in a crouched position.

ADDUCTED THIGHS (SCISSORING THIGHS)

The muscles involved in this spastic syndrome are adductor longus, adductor magnus, gracilis, iliopsoas, and/or pectineus. Patients may have problems with groin hygiene, dressing, sexual function, transfers, gait, and balance. The thighs have a scissors-like motion with sitting or walking.

Dynamic EMG are needed again to assist in diagnosis. A diagnostic obturator nerve block is used to see if there is a contracture and to see if the patient will be able to walk if the adductors are treated for spasticity (in case the other leg muscles do not function well enough to walk).

FLEXED HIP

In this syndrome, the muscles involved are rectus femoris, iliopsoas, pectineus, adductor longus, adductor brevis, and/or gluteus maximus. Patients may have difficulties with positioning, sexual function, perineal care, and gait. During gait, the contralateral step is shortened. This syndrome can lead to a knee flexion deformity.

Dynamic EMG and nerve blocks are needed to aid in diagnosis. The hamstrings need to be studied as well with EMG. Heterotopic bone formation must be ruled out.

Treatment decisions

For the clinician, making a decision on the modality of treatment will depend on a variety of factors. In the past, the treatment paradigm followed a step-ladder approach as follows: positioning, modalities, casting/braces, oral medicines, injections, intrathecal baclofen or rhizotomy, surgery. Today, clinicians will choose a composition of these treatments to best suit the patient. Usually, a patient will require at least two kinds of therapy. For example, injecting Botulinum toxin A alone will often be ineffective without physical therapy and casting. Therefore, a multidisciplinary team approach offers the best care to the patient. This team includes physiatrists, neuro-surgeons, orthopedic surgeons, physical therapists, occupational therapists, speech pathologists, and psychologists.

While taking the history, the clinician needs to learn who this patient is and what areas are being affected by spasticity: pain, functionality, hygiene, cosmesis, etc. For example, in the case with intrathecal baclofen therapy (IBT), if the patient lives in a rural area and has difficulty in traveling to a medical facility, he or she may not be a good candidate for an intrathecal baclofen pump because of the care that is required for maintenance. The clinician also needs to know what the functional goals are in treatment. For example, in the case with Botulinum toxin A injections, if the patient has difficulty walking but is more concerned about his or her adducted shoulder with flexed elbow, the clinician needs to discuss with the patient about which body parts to treat first. The clinician may want to treat the gait disturbance first, but if the patient has more pain and suffering due to the arm problem, treatment should be directed at the upper extremity first. (In fact, treating the upper extremity spasticity could actually improve gait problem!)

There is always the question of what consequences will occur after treatment. With oral medications (especially baclofen), sedation, weakness, and cognitive impairment can occur within the brain-injured population. The clinician always needs to rule out contractures and also must differentiate between spasticity and dystonia. Without correct diagnosis, treatment can fail or even be detrimental to the patient's functionality. This is why in most cases, an EMG with or without electrical stimulation is needed to ensure that the correct muscle(s) is selected.

In the case with neurolysis, once the spastic muscle is treated the clinician needs to consider how the patient will compensate for that. If the antagonist muscles of the treated spastic muscle are spastic as well, there is a risk that the patient's antagonist muscles could overcompensate. Or if the non-spastic muscles around the spastic muscles are weak, after therapy the patient may lose all function of that joint (e.g., a sprained ankle could occur because the spastic muscle no longer supports the ankle). Therefore, bracing and strengthening are important in rehabilitation.

IBT can be very effective, but is dependent upon accessibility (enough abdominal adipose tissue to place the pump in), reliability of patient, drug use, and other mechanical devices already in. The three Cs in deciding on IBT are: common goal, compliance, and commitment (by the patient, caregiver, and healthcare provider). In children, the question of IBT is often difficult for the parents of the patient and for the child, but more children are successfully using IBT today. In large muscle groups, especially the lower extremities, IBT is more efficient than numerous injections of neurolysis. However, IBT is not as effective in upper extremity spasticity, which may be due to catheter placement in the lower part of the spinal column.

The treatment of spasticity has been under study for decades, but most of the treatment has focused on the treatment of spasticity due to spinal cord disorders. However, because the manifestation and treatment of spasticity are the same regardless of the origin, most of the modalities discussed here will be in the context of brain injury, but may work just as well with spinal injuries.

The treatment of spasticity needs to take into account the location of the spastic muscles, the impact that the spastic muscle has on day-to-day functioning, the degree of pain due to the spasticity, and the degree of dependence on the spasticity the person has on his or her movements. This is important for treating spasticity of the lower limbs because many individuals use the "locked" spastic muscles to support their weight when transferring or when ambulating, and the decrease of the spasticity may result in more difficult movement for the person.

The amount of pain the spasticity induces should not be underestimated. This pain often induces further spasticity, and with the appropriate treatment the pain will subside, and secondary spasticity will be eliminated.

Treatment of spasticity involves a multidisciplinary group composed of the physician, the physical and occupational therapists, the patient, and the family. Without the proper cooperation and planning, the treatment will fail.[17]

Medical treatment of spasticity

There are a number of medications that have been used to treat spasticity of cerebral origin, but most of these medications have limited value because of side-effects of the doses required to achieve a therapeutic effect on the spasticity. The most commonly used medications are baclofen, diazepam, clorazepate clonidine, dantrolene, ketazolam, and tizanidine (see Table 11.1 for side-effect comparisons). In the USA the Food and Drug Administration has approved four agents for the treatment of spasticity of cerebral origin baclofen, diazepam, dantrolene, and tizanidine.

GABA ANALOGUES

γ-amino butyric acid (GABA) and glycine are the main inhibitory neuro-transmitters in the CNS. GABA acting via pre-synaptic inhibition of the Ia afferent neuronal terminal will reduce the motor neuron output without direct motor neuron inhibition. Thus agents that increase GABA release or bind to the GABA receptor will reduce the neuronal overdrive, which is present in spasticity of cerebral origin. Since GABA does not cross the blood-brain barrier, analogs have been developed to achieve this affect.

Baclofen (Lioresal®*) is a structural analogue of GABA (*registered trademark of Novartis). It binds to the $GABA_B$ receptor as opposed to the classic $GABA_A$ receptor. Since the $GABA_B$ receptor is found both pre- and post-synaptically, there is an increased effect of baclofen to reduce the pre-synaptic inhibition. In addition, by inhibiting the gamma motor neuron activity baclofen may reduce the sensitivity of the muscle spindle, and thus reduce both monosynaptic and polysynaptic spinal reflexes.

When taken orally baclofen has a number of unpleasant and possibly detrimental side-effects. Baclofen can increase somnolence, and reduce the attention span and memory in brain-injured individuals. Baclofen can reduce muscle strength, which can be a problem as the brain-injured individual becomes more functional. It can also cause hypotonia, ataxia, and parasthesias. It can potentiate the effects of antihypertensive medications. Finally, because of its side-effects, baclofen is a medication that may be stopped by the patient abruptly. This can be devastating to an individual with a brain

Table 11.1 Side-effects of oral medications

	Decreased ambulation speed	*Muscle weakness*	*Sedation*	*Toxicities/ precautions*
Baclofen	+	+	+	Seizure difficulty, hypotension
Diazepam	+	±	++	Cognitive dysfunction
Clorazepate		±		
Ketazolam		+		
Clonazepam		++		
Piracetam				Nausea
Dantrolene	+	+		Hepatotoxicity
Tizanidine		±	+	Hepatotoxicity

injury because of the increased risk of seizures, confusion, hallucinations, and severe muscle hypertonicity, including diaphragm spasm. This should also be taken into account when treating individuals with deceased stomach motility. Oral baclofen has been shown to work best for treatment of spasticity of spinal pathology, but a few studies have shown benefit in spasticity of cerebral origin.[18]

Baclofen can be initiated with 5 mg three times a day and titrated gradually by 5 mg increments every 4–7 days, until a therapeutic level has been reached. The maximum dose is 80 mg/day; however, doses as high as 150 mg have been used successfully.[18]

BENZODIAZEPINES

Diazepam (Valium®*) and clorazepate (Tranxene®**) (*registered trademark of Roche Laboratories, **registered trademark of Abbott) are benzodiazepines and act via the coupled benzodiazepine-$GABA_A$ receptor chloride ionophore complex. Benzodiazepines exert their actions via postsynaptic increase in $GABA_A$ activity and thus, when GABA transmission is intact; benzodiazepines reduce both mono- and polysynaptic reflexes.

Diazepam is one of the first anti-spasticity medications and is still in widespread clinical use. It is effective in treating spasticity due to cerebral palsy and in spasticity of spinal cord origin. In other forms of spasticity, diazepam is less effective, mostly due to side-effects. The side-effects of diazepam include somnolence, decreased muscle strength, impaired motor coordination, impaired intellect, and decreased behavioral arousal. Also, with chronic use true physiologic addiction may occur. Thus, if diazepam is tapered too rapidly, withdrawal symptoms can appear 2–4 days after diazepam is stopped.

Clorazepate dipotassium (Tranxene®) is a benzodiazepine analogue that is transformed into desmethyldiazepam in the gastric juices of the stomach. The half-life of desmethyldiazepam is up to 106 h. It is felt that the antispasticity effect is greater than that of diazepam. In one study on clorazepate's use in multiple sclerosis there is decease in the phasic stretch reflexes and there is less drowsiness compared to diazepam.[19,20] When first started clorazepate needs to be given as a loading dose because of its long delay until steady state.[18]

Ketazolam is an excellent muscle relaxant for use in patients with stroke. It is better tolerated with fewer side-effects than diazepam in both CVA and MS patients. It however has more sedation in MS than in CVA.[18] It is not available in the USA but is available in Canada. It can be given as a once a day dose once therapeutic steady-state levels have been reached.

Clonazepam (Klonopin®*) is widely used in the USA for suppression of myoclonic, akinetic, or petite mal seizure activity and for control of dystonia (*registered trademark of Roche Laboratories). In the treatment of spasticity it is most commonly use for the treatment of night-time spasms rather than daytime functional treatments. It is too severely sedating and causes too much confusion and other cognitive impairments to be used effectively in individuals with brain injury.

PIRACETAM

Piracetam is chemically related to GABA and crosses the blood–brain barrier effectively. It is available in Europe but not the USA. It has been studied mainly in children with cerebral palsy and it has been shown to improve movement and reduce spasticity. It has few side-effects. It has not been extensively studied since it was first released.

DANTRIUM

Dantrolene sodium (Dantrium®*) reduces spasticity by acting on the peripheral muscle fiber (*registered trademark of Procter & Gamble Pharmaceuticals). In the muscle fiber it uncouples the motor nerve excitation of the muscle by reducing the action potential release of calcium from the sarcoplasmic reticulum. This reduces the force produced by the excitation–contraction coupling. Dantrolene reduces the phasic stretch reflexes more than the tonic reflexes in a dose dependent manner. Dantrolene works best on fast twitch fibers, at slow neuronal stimulation frequencies. It is thought that at high stimulation frequencies and in slow twitch fibers there is calcium build-up which partly neutralizes the effectiveness of dantrolene. To the benefit of dantrolene, the decreased force of contraction produced can be overcome by voluntary contraction. Because dantrolene affects both extrafusal and intrafusal fibers, it may also reduce spasticity by altering the spindle sensitivity.

Despite the fact that dantrolene is good at reducing muscle tone, tendon reflexes, and clonus, while also increasing the passive range of motion, it is not very good at improving ADL functioning. However, in a direct comparison of dantrolene with diazepam at controlling spasticity in several different populations, dantrolene appeared to better improve spasticity, and had fewer side-effects.[18]

TIZANIDINE

Tizanidine (Zanaflex®*) is an agonist at the α2-agonist receptor (*registered trademark of Athena Neurosciences). It reduces spasticity by increasing pre-synaptic inhibition of motor neurons. It has no direct effect on skeletal muscle fibers or the neuromuscular junction. It also has minimal effect on monosynaptic spinal reflexes but has great effect on polysynaptic pathways and thus reduces facilitation of spinal motor neurons.[21]

The maximal effect of tizanidine is seen in 1 h and wears off by 6 h. The dosage of tizanidine is started at 4 mg/day and titrated up as necessary with the maximal dose not to exceed 36 mg/24 h given at 6–8 h intervals.

The side-effects of tizanidine include sedation, mental status changes including hallucinations, and hepatocellular injury (resolves with discontinuation of the drug). Monitoring of the aminotransferase levels for the first 6 months is recommended. Tizanidine should be used with caution in patients with renal impairment (creatinine clearance less than 25 ml/min) as the clearance is reduced up to 50%. Women using oral contraceptives should use tizanidine with caution as the clearance of tizanidine is reduced by about 50%.

There are a number of agents that are used parenterally to treat spasticity. Many of these agents are short-lived and are useful mainly as evaluation tools. Some of the earliest agents to be injected included anesthetic agents such as lidocaine or bupivocaine. These agents work to block neuronal functioning by depolarizing the neurons, and thus reduce the stimulus for muscle contraction. Ethanol and phenol are locally active agents that work to destroy the motor endplate and thus stop neuronal input to the muscle and reduce spasm.

Injections

LOCAL ANESTHETICS

There are three local anesthetics that are commonly used for the treatment of spasticity: lidocaine, bupivocaine, and etidocaine. All three are depolarizing agents that block the conduction of nerve transmission as well as muscular contraction. The main difference between the three anesthetic agents listed is the duration of action with lidocaine being the shortest lived, and bupivocaine and etidocaine being the longest. Because of the short duration of action, these agents are used as assessment agents rather than long-term treatment agents. Etidocaine is preferred by clinicians because of its propensity for blocking motor fibers more than sensory fibers and because its longer duration of action can allow a better assessment of function. Lidocaine is dosed at 7 mg/kg while etidocaine is dosed at 6 mg/kg. Table 11.2 shows doses of these medicines as well as risks, indications, and methods. The duration of action can be prolonged by the addition of epinephrine to the injection, provided the injection is not into an organ with end arteries such as the fingers or toes.[18]

Side-effects of these agents include CNS stimulation with restlessness and tremor progressing to convulsions. This can be treated with a benzodiazepine. Cardiovascular side-effects include arteriolar dilation with subsequent decrease in blood pressure. Finally, since these agents are metabolized through the liver, extensive use should be avoided in patients with hepatic insufficiency.

Local anesthetic agents block both the afferent and efferent messages in a muscle. The use of these agents requires that resuscitation equipment is available. These agents are useful to assess mechanisms of functional impairment and help predict the effect of long-term blockade.

Table 11.2 Parenteral therapy

	Maximum dose	Risks	Indications	Method
Anesthetics	Lidocaine (0.5–2%) < 4.5 mg/kg Bupivocaine (0.25–0.75%): < 3 mg/kg	CNS and cardiac toxicity Hypersensitivity	Testing of spasticity cessation and relaxation for casting	Stimulation motor point? Resuscitation equipment available
Ethyl alcohol	10–50%	Pain at injection (intramuscular*) Chronic dysesthesia and pain (perineural*) Vascular complications Permanent peripheral nerve palsy	Proximal and large muscles Sensory integrity not a primary concern Hygiene and comfort purposes? Combination with Botulinum toxin	Stimulation motor Point? Intramuscular "wash"?
Phenol	< 1 g (10 ml 5% phenol)	Pain at injection (intramuscular*) Chronic dysesthesia and pain (perineural*) Vascular complications Permanent peripheral nerve palsy	Proximal and large muscles Sensory integrity not a primary concern Hygiene and comfort purposes? Combination with Botulinum toxin	Stimulation motor point?
Botox	≤ 400 U within 3 months (for Botox)	No major risk	Muscles accessible for i.m. injection Sensory integrity indispensable Purposes of active function Combination with neurolytic agents	Stimulation endplate targeting? Dilution 100, 50, or 20 U/ml?
Intrathecal baclofen	10 mg/20 ml 10 mg/5 ml 0.05 mg/ml 1000 µg/day**	Drowsiness Increased weakness Seizures Coma	Lower limb spasticity and mild effect on upper limbs	Intrathecal infusion

* Indicates a serious risk.
** Over 1000 µg/day becomes too expensive.

ALCOHOL AND PHENOL

Alcohol and phenol have been used as chemical neurolytics for years. Ethyl alcohol has been used more for treatment of pain or sympathectomy than for the treatment of spasticity. It can be injected into the nerve or the muscle itself. In neuronal injections there is neuronal degeneration and fibrosis with some regeneration. The effect of injecting into the nerve lasts weeks to months depending on the concentration used. Intramuscular injection causes a dose-dependent coagulation necrosis followed by granulation and fibrosis.

For the treatment of spasticity 45% alcohol is used, and most authors agree that there is a reduction of spasticity without a reduction in strength. The effects last 6–12 months. Most reports on the use of ethyl alcohol in the treatment of spasticity are in patients with cerebral palsy.

Side-effects include pain at the injection site, phlebitis or other vascular complications, permanent nerve palsy, skin irritation, painful muscle necrosis, and intoxication.

Phenol (benzyl alcohol) was first used intrathecally as a treatment for spasticity. This has serious and undesired side effects on bowel and bladder function. Phenol is now almost exclusively used in percutaneous or open muscle or nerve blocks. Like ethyl alcohol, phenol causes local destruction and tissue necrosis. It is used in a concentration of 3–6%. For percutaneous injections between 0.1–5.0 ml 3% solution has been used with the usual being 2.0 ml. For motor point blocks, a volume of 1.0–5.0 ml is used. The maximum dose of phenol has not been established. The effects of phenol last from 4–6 months and are almost immediately seen. The effects of phenol can be augmented by the use of electrical stimulation.[22,23] Phenol is a very potent agent and it can be associated with permanent nerve damage. Like ethyl alcohol it can cause local phlebitis, pain and irritation, and painful muscle necrosis.[24]

BOTOX®* (*REGISTERED TRADEMARK OF ALLERGAN)

Botulinum toxin type-A (BTX-A) is one of a series of different neurotoxins (A, B, C1, D, E, F, and G) produced by different strains of *Clostridium botulinum*. Its mechanism of action is due to reducing muscle spindle activity by inhibition of the γ-motor neuron cholinergic junction on the intrafusal fibers.[25] The overall effect is to reduce the muscle stretch receptor activity and reduce spasticity.

At the current time there are two commercially available sources of BTX, BOTOX and a BTX-B preparation. The most commonly used form is BTX-A, which is actually called new BOTOX® because a new strain of bulk toxin source has been developed. The new BOTOX® is said to have a higher specific potency than the original BOTOX®. There is an additional form of BTX-A called Dysport®, which is less potent and more immunogenic than new BOTOX®.

New BOTOX® is a safe medication with excellent safety margins, having better safety margins than Dysport®. Possible side-effects of BOTOX® include weakness, fever, constipation, dysphasia, and weight loss. There are some individuals who initially respond to BOTOX® but who over time become less responsive, despite increasing doses of medication. This secondary non-responsiveness is very low, approximately 5%.[26,27] It is thought that secondary non-responsiveness may be due to neutralizing antibodies. The incidence of antibodies to BTX-A has been measured in several studies and found to be 0% in naive volunteers, 15–25% in responders, and 60–74% in secondary non-responders.

BTX-A is used for the treatment of spasticity in cerebral palsy, traumatic brain injury, cerebral vascular accidents, torticollis, and in spinal cord injury.[28] BTX-A is injected directly into the affected muscle. The dosage of BTX-A is dependent on the body weight, the size of the muscle injected, and the level of spasticity in the injected muscle. In larger muscles multiple injections are usually required because the largest single injection is 50 units (5 U/kg in gastrocnemius, 4.3 U/kg hamstring, 2.7 U/kg for adductors, 1 U/kg for forearm and wrist flexors).[29] The injections are done using 27-gauge Teflon®* coated needles and is usually guided by the use of electromyographic readings or electrical stimulation of the muscle injected (*registered trademark of E.I. du Pont de Nemours & Co. Inc., Wilmington, DE).

Once injected the BOTOX® will begin to show effects in two to three weeks with the treatment effects lasting 3–6 months. BOTOX® is most effective when used in a multidisciplinary approach, in combination with at least twice weekly physical therapy, splinting/casting, and other orthotics. Without the proper communication and interaction between the members of the treatment team, the patient will not get maximal benefit from the injections. Side-effects of BOTOX® include infections at the injections site, bleeding, flu-like syndrome for several days post injection, or excessive weakness.

Intrathecal Baclofen®(ITB)

Baclofen®, an analogue of GABA has numerous side-effects when taken orally that limit its usefulness in long-term treatment of spasticity. This is primarily true because of the poor levels of drug that are achieved by the oral route. When delivered by continuous intrathecal infusion, Baclofen® becomes a wonderful agent for the treatment of spasticity of cerebral origin. The system consists of a subcutaneously placed pump and reservoir attached to an intarsia catheter. The pump can be programmed to deliver various rates of medication via the catheter in the subarachnoid space in the lumbar/thoracic region of the spine. By placing the catheter in the thoracic region (T6) there appears to be some improvement in the spasticity of the upper extremities as well as the usual improvements seen in the lower extremities with the usual lumbar catheters. In nearly all studies of intrathecal Baclofen®, there are reductions in the Ashford ratings of at least two points, and marked improvement in the quality of life and ability to perform ADLs.[30,31]

Patients must be properly screened prior to the implantation of the ITB pump. Patients with Ashworth scores of ≥ 3 and who are intolerant or refractory to oral medications are appropriate candidates for screening. Patients must be weaned from oral baclofen prior to screening trial. Screening trials consist of the infusion of a bolus of 50 µg of Baclofen® in the L3–L4 or L2–L3 spinal segment. In children the dose is reduced to 1 µg/kg.[32]

After infusion serial Ashworth scores are taken over a 6 h period. The peak effect is at 4 h after injection. A good response is considered a reduction of 1–2 points in the most involved muscle groups of one limb and the reduction is maintained for two consecutive assessments. If no response is seen at 50 µg, then a repeat dose of 75 µg is performed. If there is still no response, there is a final bolus of 100 µg. Each of these boluses is separated by at least 24 h.[32]

Once screened, patients and their families need to be counseled about what to expect with the chronic infusion of Baclofen and the need for dosage adjustments over time as well as drug holidays. Most patients do require increased dosages over time, but usually the ITB is still effective after one year if not longer.[33]

Side-effects are usually due to mechanical or technical difficulties with placement, programming, or equipment failure. However, side-effects can include seizures from abrupt withdrawal, possible infections of the implanted pump or catheter, respiratory depression, lethargy, dizziness, or headache. Most of the latter side-effects are for a limited time or can be treated with a dose reduction. In some patients, particularly with spinal disorders, urogenital side-effects can be seen such as decreased reflexive penile erection and ejaculation, and possible bladder dysfunction.[34,35]

While medications such as ITB, BOTOX®, and tizanidine can help with the treatment of spasticity, none of these medications is successful without the proper use of physical therapy, occupational therapy, and appropriate orthoses. Depending upon the medication chosen, the therapy should begin 1–3 days after the initiation of therapy and should be continued indefinitely. Occasionally surgical interventions are needed such as tendon lengthening, despite the use of appropriate medications and splinting. It is the cooperative effort of the entire treatment team consisting of the patient, the family, therapists, orthotists, and physicians that will create an environment for the patient to improve and be able to function more independently.

References

1. Brin, M., & Group, T. S. S. (1997). Spasticity: etiology, evaluation, management, and the role of botulinum toxin A. *Muscle Nerve*, Suppl 6.
2. Francisco, G. (2000). *An integrated approach to the management of spasticity of cerebral origin*. Charlottesville, VA: 17–18 March.
3. Kant, R., Duffy, J., & Pivovarnik, A. (1998). Prevalence of apathy following head injury. *Brain Inj.*, *12*(1), 87–92.

4. Katz, R., & Rymer, W. (1989). Spastic hypertonia: mechanisms and measurement. *Arch. Phys. Med. Rehabil., 70*, 144–155.
5. Nathan, P. (1973). Some comments on spasticity and rigidity. In J. E. Desmedt (Ed.), *New developments in electromyography and clinical neurophysiology.* Basel: Karger.
6. Lance, J. (1980). Symposium synopsis. In R. G. Feldman, R. R. Young and W. P. Werner (Eds.), *Spasticity: Disordered motor control.* Chicago, IL: Year Book Medical Publishers.
7. Lance, J. (1984). Pyramidal and extrapyramidal disorders. In D. Shahani (Ed.), *Electromyography in CNS disorders: Central EMG.* Boston, MA: Butterworth.
8. Delwaide, P. (1984). Contribution of human reflex studies to the understanding and management of the pyramidal syndrome. In B. Shahani (Ed.), *Electromyography in CNS disorders: Central EMG.* Boston, MA: Butterworth.
9. Burke, D. (1988). Spasticity as an adaptation to pyramidal tract injury. *Adv. Neurol., 47*, 401–423.
10. Deseilligny, E., & Mazieres, L. (1985). Spinal mechanisms underlying spasticity. In P. J. Delwaide and R. R. Young (Eds.), *Clinical neurophysiology in spasticity.* Amsterdam: Elsevier.
11. Gormley, M. J., O'Brien, C., & Yablon, S. (1997). A clinical overview of treatment decisions in the management of spasticity. *Muscle Nerve,* Suppl. 6, 14–20.
12. Herman, R. (1970). The myotatic reflex: clinico-physiological aspects of spasticity and contracture. *Brain, 93*, 273–312.
13. Mayer, N., Esquenazi, A., & Wannstedt, G. (1996). Surgical planing for upper motoneuro dysfunction: the role of motor control evaluation. *J. Head Trauma Rehabil., 11*(4), 37–56.
14. Mayer, N., Esquenazi, A., & Childers, M. (1997). Common patterns of clinical motor dysfunction. *Muscle Nerve, 20*(Suppl. 6), S21–S35.
15. Bohannon, R., & Smith, M. (1986). Interrater reliability of a modified Ashworth scale of muscle spasticity. *Phys. Ther., 67*, 206–207.
16. Twitchell, T. (1951). The restoration of motor function following hemiplegia in man. *Brain, 74*, 443–480.
17. Moore, D. (1998). Helping your patients with spasticity reach maximal function. *Postgrad. Med., 104*(2), 123–136.
18. Gracies, J.-M., Elovic, E., McGuire, J., & Simpson, D. (1997). Traditional pharmacological treatments for spasticity, part II: General and regional treatments. *Muscle Nerve, 20*(Suppl. 6), S92–S120.
19. Lossius, R., Dietrichson, P., & Lunde, P. (1980). Effect of diazepam and desmethyldiazepam in spasticity and rigidity. A quantative study of reflexes and plasma concentrations. *Acta Neurol. Scand., 61*(6), 378–383.
20. Lossius, R., Dietrichson, P., & Lunde, P. (1985). Effect of clorazepate in spasticity and rigidity: a quantative study of reflexes and plasma concentrations. *Acta Neurol. Scand. 3*, 190–194.
21. RxList.com.: Tizanidine. Internet. Mosby, Inc 1998; http://www.rxlist.com/cgi/generic/tizanidine.htm (accessed 21 March 2000).
22. Apkarian, J., & Naumann, S. (1991). Stretch reflex inhibition using electrical stimulation in normal subjects and subjects with spasticity. *J. Biomed. Eng., 13*, 67–74.
23. Vodovnik, L., Bowman, B., & Winchester, P. (1984). Effects of electrical stimulation on spasticity in hemiparetic patients. *Int. Rehab. Med., 6*(64), 153–156.

24. Botte, M., Abrams, R., & Bodine-Fowler, S. (1995). Treatment of acquired muscle spasticity using phenol peripheral nerve blocks. *Orthopedics, 18*(2), 151–159.

25. Aoki, K. (1999). Preclinical update on BOTOX (*Botulinum* toxin type A)-purified neurotoxin complex relative to other *Botulinum* neurotoxin preparations. *Eur. J. Neurol., 6*(Suppl. 4), S3–S10.

26. Greene, P., Fahn, S., & Diamond, B. (1994). Development of resistance to *Botulinum* toxin type-A in patients with torticollis. *Mov. Disord., 9*, 213–217.

27. Jankovic, J., & Schwartz, K. (1991). Clinical correlates of response to *Botulinum* toxin injections. *Arch. Neurol., 48*, 1253–1256.

28. Delgado, M. (1999). The use of *Botulinum* toxin type A in children with cerebral palsy: a retrospective study. *Eur. J. Neurol., 6*(Suppl. 4), 11–18.

29. Molenaers, G., Desloovere, K., Decat, J., Jonkers, I., & De Cock, P. (1999). *Botulinum* toxin type A treatment of cerebral palsy: an integrated approach. *Eur. J. Neurol., 6*(Suppl. 4), 51–57.

30. Becker, R., Alberti, O., & Bauer, B. (1997). Continuous intrathecal baclofen infusion in severe spasticity after traumatic or hypoxic brain injury. *J. Neurol., 244*, 160–166.

31. Meythaler, J., Guin-Renfroe, S., Grabb, P., & Hadley, M. (1999). Long-term continuously infused intrathecal baclofen for spastic–dystonic hypertonia in traumatic brain injury: 1-year experience. *Arch. Phys. Med. Rehabil., 80*, 13–19.

32. Albright, L., Meythaler, J., & Ivanhoe, C. (1997). *Intrathecal baclofen therapy for spasticity of cerebral origin: Patient selection guidelines*. Minneapolis MN: Medtronic Inc.

33. Meythaler, J., Guin-Renfro, S., & Hadley, M. (1998). Continuously infused intrathecal baclofen (ITB) for spastic hypertonia in adult cerebral palsy [abstr.]. *Am. J. Phys. Med. Rehabil., 77*, 173.

34. Steers, W., Meythaler, J., Haworth, C., & Park, T. (1992). Effects of acute bolus and chronic continuous intrathecal baclofen on genitourinary dysfunction due to spinal cord pathology. *J. Urol., 148*, 1849–1855.

35. Denys, P., Mane, M., Azouvi, P., Chartier-Kastler, E., Thiebault, J., & Bussel, B. (1998). Side effects of chronic intrathecal baclofen on erection and ejaculation in patients with spinal cord lesions. *Arch. Phys. Med. Rehabil., 79*, 494–496.

12 Rehabilitation in water

A practical guide

*Gianpietro Salvi, Annamaria
Quarenghi, and Paola Quarenghi*

Introduction

Rehabilitation in water lets one carry out therapeutic exercises in water.

The idea of treating patients affected by injuries caused by cranial trauma in a swimming pool first came to mind as a result of the observation that patients relaxed during routine baths, leading to reduction in the spastic condition, which lasted for some time after the bath.

The practice was then introduced to give patients a full hydromassage before each physiotherapy session, resulting in greater relaxation and easier rehabilitation for the physiotherapist. On the strength of these positive and encouraging results, patients began to be treated during the actual hydromassage with passive mobilizing exercises, with even better and longer-lasting results. Unfortunately, conventional hydromassage pools offered little chance for movement owing to the confined space.

Thus, traumatized patients began to be immersed in a butterfly-shaped pool, with encouraging results given that the physiotherapist could actually enter the pool and move the patient in a larger space. Once more autonomous, the patient could then continue these exercises in a normal swimming pool.

After the exercises in water had been worked out, these were entered in a rehabilitation plan as an autonomous program or integrated in the gym rehabilitation plan.

Effects of immersion on the human body

When a body is immersed in water, it becomes subject to the following laws:

- *Hydrostatic pressure:* where a body immersed in water receives pressure from part of the water equal to the weight of the column of water above it. This pressure is directly proportional to the depth of immersion and the density of the water.
- *The Archimedean principle:* where a body immersed in water receives a thrust upwards equal to the weight of the fluid it displaces. Thus the apparent loss in weight when the full body is immersed is roughly 97%,

dropping to 93% with the head out of the water, 66% if the water only comes up to the chest and just 20% with only the lower limbs in water.

- *Water viscosity:* given that water is 800 times denser than air, moving an object in water at the same speed becomes 800 times more difficult. This viscosity drops as the temperature rises and, in salty water, it also rises as the water becomes saltier.[1,2]

The effect of water on the human body

As a result of the above laws, the immersion of a patient in water[3-5] has the following effects:

1 There is an apparent loss in the weight of the body, with movement in complete or partial weightlessness.
2 Facilitates movement of muscles with reduced motor units.
3 Water is an unbalancing factor, increasing the difficulty of the exercise.
4 The hydrostatic pressure associated with the viscosity of the water provokes exteroceptive and, during movement, proprioceptive stimuli responsible for greater perception of the position of the limbs in space and a better awareness of the body at rest and during movement in water.
5 Hydrostatic pressure and the thermal effect are responsible for stimulation of the pressure and thermal receptors that, according to some, offer an explanation for the antalgic effect of water, especially in terms of articulation, based on the gate control theory, whereby intense proprioceptive stimuli inhibit the formation of nocioceptive impulses in the spinal cord, with the production of endorphin.
6 Hydrostatic pressure acts on the abdomen by offering resistance to the movement of the diaphragm, and on the chest by offering resistance to the rib muscles, thus affecting the respiratory processes.
7 Hydrostatic pressure acts directly on the blood circulation via the veins and lymph vessels.
8 The thermal effect of water above 34–35 °C provokes peripheral vascular dilation, a reduction in muscle tone, and an analgesic effect according to the same gate control theory.
9 Movement of the body in water creates turbulence that, together with hydrostatic pressure, creates an enervating and relaxing hydromassage effect on muscle, capsule, and tendon tissues.
10 Water offers resistance to movement of the immersed body, which increases as the speed and the advancing body surface increase.
11 On a psychological level, all these benefits create a sense of well-being in the patient, plus awareness of less disability and thus a desire for greater movement.

Therapeutic effects of water on the human body

The following benefits are possible for organs within the human body when it is immersed in water at 34–35 °C.[6–8]

1   *Cardiovascular system:* an increase in cardiac input, cardiac output with a drop in heart rate, peripheral vasodilation, arterial hypotension, reduced edema in the veins and lymph system.
2   *Urinary system:* an increase in diuresis with elimination of toxins.
3   *Respiratory system:* an increase in the respiratory capacity and reduced expiratory reserve volume.
4   *Bone system:* reduced weight, stress on joints and pain, an increase in articulation range.
5   *Muscle system:* an increase in muscle vascularization with elimination of toxins from muscles, an increase in muscle, tendon and capsule elasticity, a reduction in muscle tone.
6   *Nervous system:* an increase in exteroceptive, thermal, proprioceptive and pressure point stimuli, with an analgesic effect, improvement in the body scheme and balance, a relaxing and sedative effect.

Structures and means

For correct water rehabilitation treatment, well-ventilated, heated rooms with pools of suitable size fitted with the necessary equipment to immerse even severely ill patients (in a coma, paraplegics or tetraplegics) are needed. Equipment must include a full range of accessories for the various exercises, for balance and walking, plus simple but effective safety systems such as alarm bells and lights.[9]

An efficient water purification and hygiene system is also indispensable. The pools, showers, relaxation beds for before and after the water therapy session and the space for maneuver must be separated from the rest of the rehabilitation structure.

Role of the physiotherapist

A physiotherapist uses rehabilitation in water with the aim of improving the specific pathology and the patient's motor capacities of balance.

Following the doctor's instructions, he must select the patients, assess their level of aquatic ability (i.e., their ability to move in water without fear), assess their clinical, neuromotor and neuropsychological situation, prepare a personalized therapy plan, prepare the individual or group treatment plan, establish the length and frequency of the sessions, follow the treatment plan and progress made in the sessions and assess the results.

Indications for rehabilitation in water

Rehabilitation in water is of great importance in any rehabilitation program for patients affected with the results of cranial trauma and completes neuro-motor and neuropsychological rehabilitation treatment.[10,11] There are various indications and exercises to suit the stage of evolution of the cranial trauma:

- *Vegetative state:* the patient's eyes are open, with spontaneous eye movement, sleep/awake pattern, uncontrolled limb movements, no contact with the surrounding environment.
- *Minimum response:* the patient's eyes are open, follows objects with his eyes, sleep/awake pattern, limb movements may be controlled, contact with the surrounding environment, but only occasionally and not constant.
- *Results:* the patient can experience full contact with the surrounding environment, may collaborate with the physiotherapist. Motor and cognitive deficits require additional rehabilitation.

Contraindications for rehabilitation in water

Special attention needs to be paid in the case of patients with one or more of the following pathologies or complications:[12,13]

- Septic or febrile states.
- Urinary or fecal incontinence.
- Severe respiratory failure.
- Severe cardiac failure.
- Unstable coronary disease.
- Uncontrolled hypertension or hypertension.
- Uncontrolled epilepsy.
- Hydrophobia.
- Burns.
- Infectious and parasitic dermatitis.
- Perforated eardrum.
- Catheters in veins.

Objectives of treatment in water of patients with traumatic brain injury (TBI)

The aims of physiotherapists using treatment in water are as follows:[14,15]

- Restore and improve the overall postural reactions of the patient when seated, on his knees or standing.
- Restore and improve the body scheme, motor coordination, balance, upright position, walking.

- Restore and improve the articulation of the spine, the shoulders, the elbows, the hands, the hips, the knees, and the feet.
- Restore and improve the elasticity of muscles, tendons and capsules, plus skin trophism.
- Restore and improve the proprioceptive and exteroceptive sensitivity.
- Reduce pain symptoms.
- Restore and improve levels of consciousness.
- Improve respiratory function.

Treatment in water must differ to suit the stage of evolution of the post-trauma coma (vegetative state, minimum response, and post-TBI patients).[16–18]

Patients in vegetative state

Hydrotherapeutical treatment of patients in the *vegetative state* has the following objectives:

- To improve the level of consciousness.
- To regain joint flexibility.
- To reduce spasticity.
- To improve skin trophism.
- To reduce edema.
- To improve respiratory activity.
- To improve sensitivity.
- To increase exteroceptive and proprioceptive reception.

Treatment should last for 1 h a day, unless there are contraindications, and should continue throughout the patient's stay in hospital.[19] The patient is accompanied to the hydrotherapy section, undressed and placed on a steel seat (Figure 12.1a), then given an initial shower to accustom him to the water before being slung and transferred to the butterfly pool using an electrically powered hoist. The physiotherapist must check whether the patient has any neurovegetative reactions (sweating, hair erection, tachycardia, urination, and even muscle contractions), as the patient cannot communicate and so it is up to the physiotherapist to keep an eye on his general condition. Facial expressions may indicate discomfort due either to the new situation or possible joint pains during the exercises, but equally a state of well-being and relaxation during treatment. There are no contraindications to treatment in water if the patient has a nasogastric tube (closed), bed sores, provided these are protected by an impermeable medication (duoderm), or suffers from incontinence, provided a urine collection device is used (uridon). It is important that the immediate environment is quiet to avoid disturbing the patient and that the therapist's voice is not shrill, but low and reassuring, thus encouraging the patient's trust in the therapist. The treatment is enforced by verbalizing the movement that therapist intends to make. Simple orders are

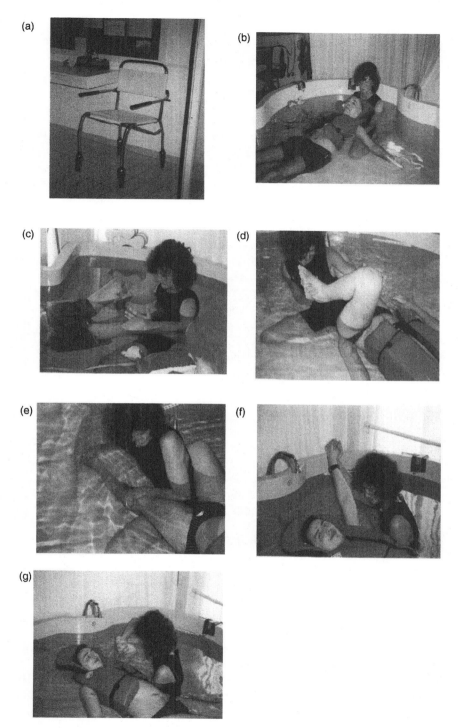

Figure 12.1 Exercises in hydrotherapy.

preferable in order to get even minimum motor responses. Moreover, only one order should be given at a time followed by a sufficient delay, awaiting the expected response.

Before entering the water, the patient is made to wear a lifejacket (as on boats) so that he can relax and not be afraid of the water, plus some floats on his legs (generally hypertonic). The temperature of the water is also important, as this must never exceed 34–35 °C to avoid the risk of drops in blood pressure, nor fall below 32 °C, as cold leads to a rise in spasticity. Opinions vary as to temperature: ranging from 28–35 °C, most between 30–34 °C. In our experience, we have found that the ideal temperature for these patients is 34–35 °C. It is worth noting that this procedure is the same for all types of patients entering the water.

The treatment starts with backwards movement holding the patient around the chest (Figure 12.1b) to relax the muscles around the lumbar vertebrae and the lower limbs. By backwards movement we mean movement of the patient with side-to-side movement of the trunk.

The next step is passive mobilizing of the lower limbs. It should be stressed that unlike treatment on a bed, where the body rests and is immobile at all times, one of the hardest problems to solve in water is the difficulty in keeping the patient's body still, which tends to move in the absence of support and so makes segmented mobilizing of the joints particularly difficult.

The treatment starts by stretching the adductors, especially if these are very contracted (Figure 12.1c): the therapist moves to the patient's feet, grips his ankles and tries to move his legs apart. On obtaining good bilateral abduction, with the therapist between the legs, the next step is to mobilize the hip, knee, tibia and tarsus joints via triple flexion (Figure 12.1d). To mobilize the patient's right leg, the therapist bends his left knee (left foot on the bottom of the pool) and places this under the patient's back to get a fixture point.

The therapist now stretches the iliopsoas. The therapist returns to the previous position and places his right hand on the patient's right knee to extend his hip and so stretch his right iliopsoas, holding the position for a few seconds (Figure 12.1e). The ischiocrural muscles are then stretched by placing the heel on the bottom of the pool and holding the position for a few seconds. If patient is not in too much pain, the therapist can shift his knee towards the patient's right gluteus and place his hand on the patient's sole and so stretch also the triceps surae (Figure 12.1f).

The palm grip is effective in mobilizing the upper limbs: the therapist lies alongside the patient and intertwines his fingers with the patient's, while his other hand is placed on the trapezius on that side and his elbow rests at lumbar height. The arm can thus be mobilized by abducting and adducting, flexing and extending the shoulder (Figure 12.1g).

The forearm can also be mobilized using the same grip by flexing and extending this, turning it to face upwards and downwards, to get deviation of the radius and ulna. The wrist can also be flexed and extended using the same grip. To mobilize the hand, the therapist moves to the side of the patient and mobilizes the metacarpals, flexing and extending all the fingers together, before mobilizing each finger in turn (flexion and extension) and finally the thumb.

It is important to mobilize the shoulderblades. The therapist moves behind the patient's head and tries to grasp the median of the shoulderblades and abduct these. Initially, there will be a lot of resistance and the patient will be in some pain, but the attrition and rigidity will lessen with time.

It is also possible to mobilize the head in water, taking care that the patient does not swallow any water as this would make him stiffen up.

Patients with minimum responses

In treating patients with minimum responses (Figure 12.2a), all the exercises described above are needed, followed by others with a higher degree of difficulty, requiring the active participation of the patient, where possible. The treatment should last for 1 h a day throughout the patient's stay in hospital, unless problems arise. Suitable exercises here include:

- With the patient seated, the therapist helps from behind to support his trunk (Figure 12.2b).
- Still seated, the patient is asked to abduct his arms and then adduct them until they touch the bottom (Figure 12.2c).

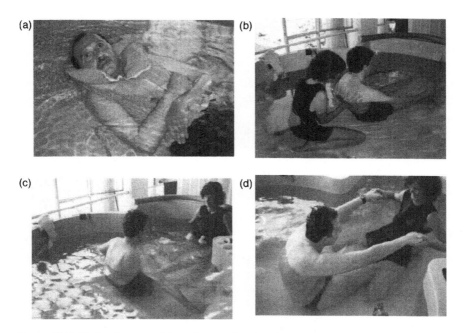

Figure 12.2 Hydrotherapy with patients in low level status.

- Still seated, the therapist moves in front of the patient holding his hands and asks him to push his chest forwards (Figure 12.2d)
- Finally, the patient is asked to grab certain plastic objects (fish and balls).

Treatment of post-TBI patients

As the patient's level of consciousness increases, exercises requiring more participation are made possible. Here the treatment varies to suit the evolution of the pathology:

- Spasticity.
- Symptoms of cerebellar dysfunction and balance.
- Proprioceptive difficulty.
- Stiff joints.
- Stenosis due to injury to the central or peripheral nervous systems.

The treatment should last for 1 h three times a week throughout the patient's stay in hospital.

To reduce the *spasticity*, the treatment starts with rear chest movement, as described above (Figure 12.1b), to allow the patient to become used to the water and relax. To reduce the spasticity in the upper limbs in terms of adduction and flexion of the elbow and wrist, the therapist moves to the side of the patient and, using the palm grip, starts to mobilize the shoulder by flexing this. If this is very stiff to begin with, there will be some resistance, but this will gradually diminish. Next, the therapist reduces the spasticity of the biceps by extending the elbow, before stretching the wrist and the fingers.[20,21]

In addition to the classic stretching of the iliopsoas adductors, ischiocrural muscles and triceps surae described for the vegetative state, the following exercises can be useful in reducing *spasticity in the legs*:

- With patient seated and limbs apart: the more the patient keeps his legs apart, the greater the stretching of the adductor muscles and those at the rear of his thighs and leg (Figure 12.3a).
- As above, but the therapist forces the position by moving to behind the patient's shoulders and placing his hands behind his back, gently pushing the patient's trunk down.
- Patient seated, he brings his legs up against his chest, then joins the soles of his feet, opening his knees outwards and towards the bottom of the pool, trying to keep the position and, if possible, pressing his knees down (Figure 12.3b).
- On all fours: to stretch the muscles around the lumbar vertebrae, the patient brings one knee under his chest and holds the position for a few seconds, then switches leg (Figure 12.3c).
- To stretch the ischiocrural muscles and adductors, the hurdle-jumper

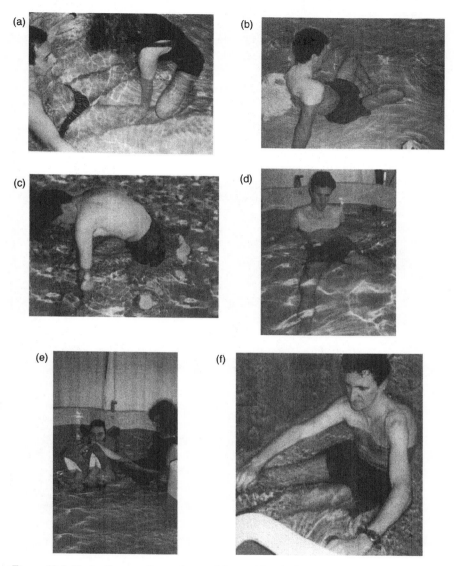

Figure 12.3 Hydrotherapy for patients with good level of consciousness.

position: seated with upright trunk and legs stretched out in front, the patient bends one knee and turns his leg so that the knee rests on the bottom, then abducts this to get an angle of 90° between his thighs, holding the position for a few seconds and then switches leg (Figure 12.3d).

Exercises to reduce *trunk spasticity* are:

- Patient floating on his back: the therapist helps him bring his knees up to his chest and hold for a few seconds (Figure 12.3e).
- Patient seated with legs extended: the therapist immobilizes the legs at the ankles and asks the patient to turn his trunk to the right and then to the left (Figure 12.3f).

Symptoms of cerebellar dysfunction problems and balance

Exercises can be done in a semi-floating position to correct cerebral problems and improve balance. Starting position: feet placed on the bottom of the pool, knees bent, pelvis extended, upper limbs abducted, head supported by a float (Figure 12.4a).

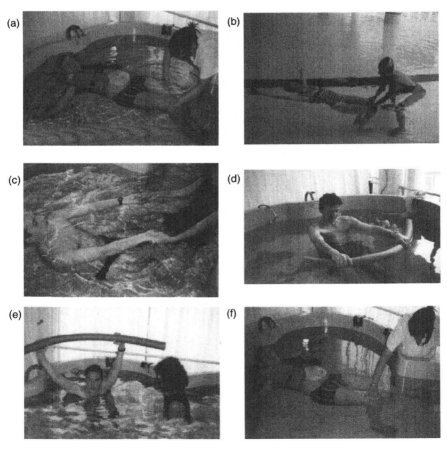

Figure 12.4 Provoking intensive stimulation in the proprioceptive circuits.

The entire kinetic chain works in this position, as the patient needs to make continuous adjustments in his posture to stay in the right position, thus provoking intense stimulation in the proprioceptive circuits. If the patient finds it difficult to keep his feet on the bottom, the therapist should block his feet or even his knees, if necessary.[22–25] Possible exercises in this position for the *upper limbs* are:

- In the semi-floating position, with upper limbs abducted, the patient lifts an arm close to his ear and keeps the position for as long as he can, then switches arm (Figure 12.4b)
- Position recognition: starting with arms abducted, the patient assumes different positions (from 0 to 5) with one arm at a time and elbow extended, as indicated by the therapist.

Exercises to *strengthen the abdominals* are as follows:

- Patient seated, legs extended, arms at 90° with elbows extended, trunk slightly forwards. The therapist, sitting on the ankles to immobilize the legs, takes hold of the patient's hands and helps the patient to flex his trunk (Figure 12.4c).
- Patient seated, legs extended, trunk slightly forwards. The patient grasps hold of a float (rod shape) and moves this forwards by flexing his trunk (Figure 12.4d).
- As above, but patient turns his trunk to the right and left after flexing forwards, keeping his arms flexed at the shoulder and with his elbows extended (Figure 12.4e).
- Bicycle exercise.
- Flex and extend the legs, keeping the hands resting on the bottom of the pool with elbows extended.

To *strengthen the glutei*:

- In the semi-floating position, ask the patient to contract his glutei.

For the *lower limbs* the following exercises are possible:

- To control the recruitment of the knees, with the feet immobilized on the bottom of the pool, the therapist asks the patient to move his knees to different positions (from 0 to 5) by moving his body along the sagittal axis.
- The same exercise, but using only one leg: the leg not resting on the bottom is extended and lifted to the height of the bent knee (Figure 12.4f). Not only is the success of the actual exercise important in this position, but also the control of the starting position, avoiding any rotation in the shoulders, trunk or pelvis.

Once the patient can control the position well when semi-floating, he can pass to the exercises while *seated*. The exercise can be made easier or more difficult to suit the motor capacity of the patient. A sequence of increasingly difficult exercises could be:

- The trunk is gently held from behind to limit retropulsion.
- The patient can hold his arms outwards and keep the position (Figure 12.5a)
- The patient can flex an arm at a time with the elbow extended and then switch arms.
- The patient can flex both arms with the elbows extended (Figure 12.5b).
- The patient can abduct his arms and hold the position (Figure 12.5c).
- The therapist can complicate the position by provoking turbulence in all directions to recruit both the extending trunk muscles and the abdominal muscles.

Exercises are also possible *on all fours*. From the starting position:

- Flex one arm with the elbow extended, hold the position for a few seconds and then switch arms (Figure 12.5d).
- Abduct an arm, trying to move the head and trunk in the required sense of rotation (Figure 12.5e).
- Bring one knee up to the chest, hold the position for a few seconds and then switch legs (Figure 12.5f).
- Extend the right arm and the left leg at the same time, trying to hold the position for a few seconds and then switch (Figure 12.5g).
- Abduct a leg, bending this at the knee, and hold for a few seconds before switching legs (Figure 12.5h).

Exercises are also possible *kneeling on both knees*, close to the edge of the pool if the patient needs something to hold on to. Below is a sequence of typical exercises of increasing difficulty:

- Take one hand away from the edge.
- Take both hands away from the edge.
- Flex one arm with the elbow extended (Figure 12.5i).
- Flex both arms with the elbows extended (Figure 12.5j); repeat the last three exercises in turbulent water.

Exercises are also possible *kneeling on one knee*. Starting by kneeling on both knees, the patient shifts his weight to just one knee, bending the other leg at the hip to rest the sole of his foot on the ground. The patient can then:

- Remove both hands from the edge of the pool and try to hold the position.
- Withstand turbulence created by the therapist.

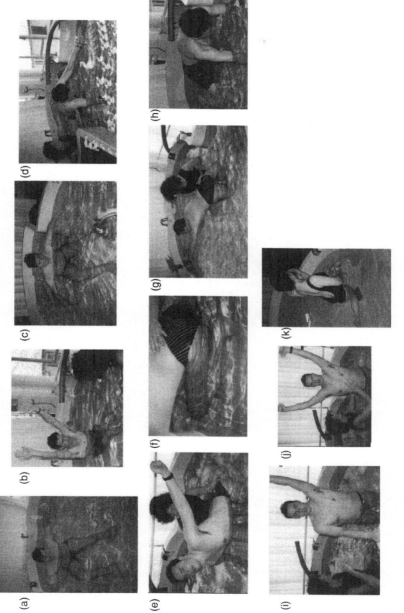

Figure 12.5 Exercises for cerebellar and balance dysfunction.

- Flex an arm with the elbow extended (Figure 12.5k).
- Flex both arms with the elbows extended.
- Repeat the last exercise, trying to withstand turbulence created by the therapist.

Once the patient has gained sufficient confidence in shallow water and meets the above objectives, he can pass to the exercises in the upright position and when walking *in deep water* (c. 120 cm). To improve his aquatic ability, the patient may be asked to walk close to the edge of the pool. Next, the patient may try the following:

- Facing the edge of the pool, with his hands on this: bend his hips in turn, staying still (Figure 12.6a).

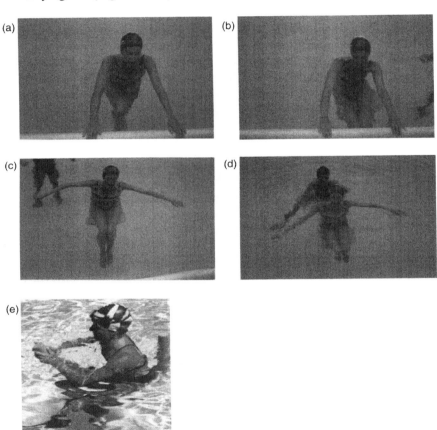

Figure 12.6 Walking in deep water.

- As above, but moving through the water.
- Edge of pool: abduct and adduct one leg at a time.
- Edge of pool: extend his hip, with the knee extended, one leg at a time.
- Hands on edge of pool, seated with glutei on a square float: ask the patient to use his pelvis to keep the square float horizontal (Figure 12.6b).
- Again seated on a square float, but without his hands on the edge of the pool (Figure 12.6c).
- As above, but the therapist creates turbulence to off-balance the patient (Figure 12.6d).
- Lateral ambulation: abduct and adduct the legs sideways.
- Crossed ambulation.
- Ambulation with one leg in front of the other.
- Ambulation on tiptoes.
- Backwards ambulation.
- Jumping with feet together.
- Hopping.
- Abduct and adduct the legs while jumping.
- Patient in deep water with a float (sausage-shaped) between his legs, pedalling as though on a bicycle (Figure 12.6e).
- Try to run, with good coordination of the arms.

Proprioceptive difficulty

Exercises aimed at position recognition are possible, with the patient floating on his back, seated or on all fours.[26,27]

Floating on back: arms

- Starting position: arms abducted and relaxed, legs relaxed, resting on a float. The patient is asked to move the affected arm to his side and then the therapist indicates the positions he should adopt (e.g., from 0 to 8 depending on the ease of articulation of his shoulder) with the elbow extended and eyes open. The patient is made to feel the positions and then is told to adopt the relevant position.
- The same exercise is possible with the eyes closed: on removing his vision, the patient's recognition becomes more difficult.
- To improve kinematic sensitivity of the fingers, the therapist flexes and extends one finger at a time in a random sequence. The therapist then asks the patient to say which finger is moving and how it is moving (flexed, stretched or rotated).

Floating on back: legs

- Starting position: arms abducted and legs adducted with floats at the feet. The patient is asked to abduct the extended leg to reach certain positions indicated by the therapist (e.g., from 0 to 5). First with his eyes open, then with eyes closed. The therapist asks the patient to recognize the position.

- To improve kinematic sensitivity of the toes, the therapist flexes and extends one toe at a time in a random sequence. To improve the patient's proprioceptive sensitivity, the therapist then asks the patient to say which toe is being touched.

Seated: arms

- Starting position: patient seated against the edge of the pool, with arms adducted along the sides of the body: the patient is asked to abduct an arm with the elbow extended to reach certain, previously felt positions. With eyes open and then eyes closed.
- As above, but the patient is asked to flex his shoulder, with elbow extended, to reach set positions with his eyes open and then closed.

On all fours: arms

- From the starting position, the patient is asked to flex an arm with the elbow extended. The patient is asked to adopt certain previously felt positions (e.g., from 0 to 8). With eyes open and then closed.
- From the starting position, the patient is asked to draw numbers 1 to 10.
- From the starting position, the therapist asks him to write the letters of the alphabet.
- From the starting position, the patient must control a square float placed under his hand and reach positions 0 to 8 (Figure 12.7a).

On all fours: legs

- From the starting position, the patient is asked to adopt certain positions (e.g., from 0 to 5) until the knee is fully extended (Figure 12.7b).

(a)   (b)   (c)

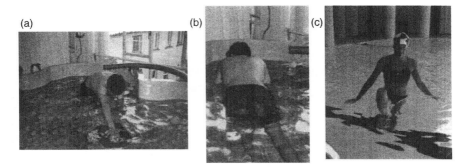

Figure 12.7 Exercises for proprioceptive difficulties.

Upright position

- Standing in the upright position, the patient places a square float under his feet and is asked to adopt certain previously indicated positions (e.g., from 0 knee extended to 5 knee bent). In addition to recognition of the position, the problem here is to keep the square float under control, as this tends to fly out from under the patient's feet (Figure 12.7c).

Stiff joints

To reduce stiffness in the joints, the following are possible for all those joints requiring such treatment:

- Forced passive mobilization.
- Active mobilization.
- Forced active mobilization.
- Alternating rhythmical stabilization.

Forced passive mobilization

Shoulders: with the patient floating on his back, the therapist holds his hand, intertwining the fingers, and tries to flex the shoulder, holding the position.

Active mobilization

Rotations are suitable for releasing the *shoulder* and *pelvic girdles*. These rotations can start from either the craniocaudal area or the legs.

Craniocaudal rotation

- Starting position: floating on back, arms abducted, legs relaxed (Figure 12.8a).
- Rotation starts with sideways rotation of the head: if the head turns to the right, the left arm moves to the opposite shoulder with the elbow bent, while the right arm moves to the opposite gluteus, the left arm is then moved towards the right edge of the pool; at the same time, the left knee is bent slightly in the same direction, to cross the other.
- The rotation of the head and the movement of the arm guide the rotation of the entire body.
- The right arm is used to release the position and move to the prone position with arms abducted. The final position is reached when the patient is floating, face down (180°).

(a)

(b)

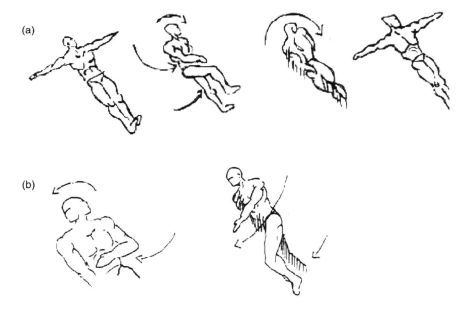

Figure 12.8 Rotating the body.

Rotation starting from legs

- Starting position: floating on back, arms abducted, legs relaxed (Figure 12.8b).
- Rotation starts with the legs: the hip is bent and turned, one knee bent to cross the other; the arm on the same side as the bent knee is bent at shoulder height, with the hand resting on the opposite shoulder; the other arm is bent at the elbow and turned behind the back, to touch the opposite gluteus; the arms help release the pelvis from the trunk, extending the elbow on the side of rotation; the head is the last to move in the sense of rotation; the final position is reached when the patient is floating, face down (180°).

Forced active mobilization

Shoulders

- Shallow water: the patient kneels, rests his wrists on the edge of the pool and bends his trunk forwards (Figure 12.9a)
- Patient on all fours: arm bent at the shoulder, elbow extended, hand holding a foam or rubber ball (depending on the patient's strength). The patient is asked to take the ball to the bottom of the pool and then control it as it returns to the surface: the thrust of the ball favors flexion in the shoulder (Figure 12.9b)

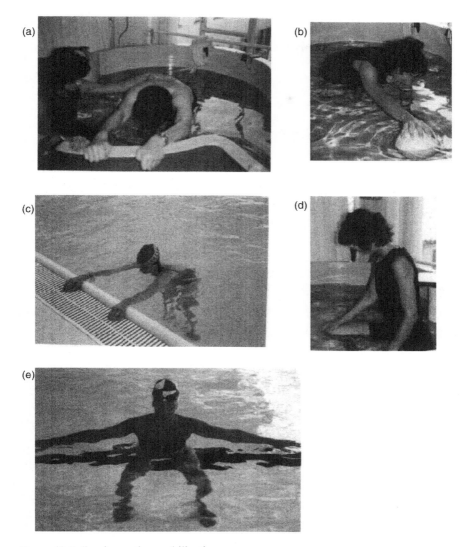

Figure 12.9 Forcing active mobilization.

- Deep water: the patient bends his trunk and rests his wrists on the edge of the pool, legs extended. The patient is asked to bend his trunk further (Figure 12.9c).

Knees

- Kneeling on one knee: force the flexion of the knee by pushing the pelvis forwards (Figure 12.9d).

- Upright position: try to bend the knees and hold the position for a few seconds (Figure 12.9e).
- Upright position: with a square float under his feet, the patient is asked to adopt certain positions, from 0 knee extended to 6 knee bent. As the stiffness gradually diminishes, the positions can be increased (Figure 12.7c).

Alternating rhythmical stabilization

Elbow joints

- Patient seated, shoulder bent at 90°, elbow bent at 90°, held by therapist: the patient is asked to extend his elbow while the therapist applies resistance at the wrist. He is then asked to bend his elbow, with the therapist applying resistance at the distal end of the radius.

Stenosis due to injury to the central or peripheral nervous systems

The exercises that can be used to favor recruitment of the muscles in the *arms* with the patient seated at side of pool[28–30] are:

- The patient wears floats on his wrists and is asked to abduct his arms and make small circles with these (Figure 12.10a).
- The patient wears floats on his wrists and tries to do breaststroke with his arms.
- The patient holds a pool buoy with both hands and is asked to push it underwater, flexing and extending his elbows as though he were drawing a circle (Figure 12.10b)
- The patient holds a rod fitted with floats and "paddles" with this (Figure 12.10c)
- With arms abducted, the patient holds a couple of pool buoys and adducts them to touch the bottom of the pool.
- The patient holds a long, narrow float and flexes and extends his shoulder until the float touches his knees.

Legs: patient floating on his back:

- The therapist places an elastic band (soft, to start with) around the patient's ankles and asks the patient to abduct his legs (Figure 12.10d).
- As above, but the patient must bend one hip with the knee extended and extend the other hip with the knee bent (Figure 12.10e).
- Lying on his side, the patient is asked to make "scissors" movements with his legs.
- Lying on his side, the patient is asked to abduct one leg with the elbow extended.

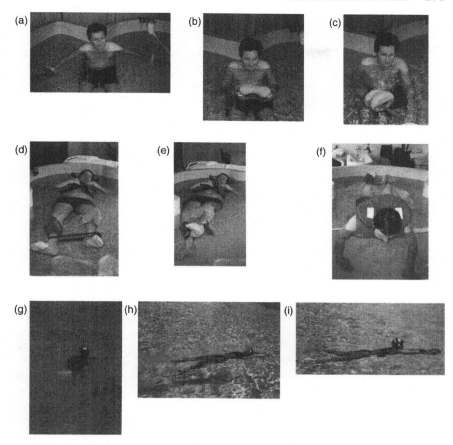

Figure 2.10 Exercises for stenosis.

- Floating face down, the patient is asked to abduct one of his legs with the knee extended (Figure 12.10f).
- As above, but the patient is asked to extend his hip with the knee extended.

Once the patient has gained a good level of aquatic ability and motor independence, the following swimming pool exercises may be done, thus starting the preliminaries for swimming.

Floating on his back:

- The patient wears palmar devices and is asked to do backstroke using just his arms.
- The same, but using both arms at the same time.
- Proper backstroke.
- Backstroke, but using only his legs, keeping his arms at his sides (Figure 12.10g).

- Arms bent at the shoulders, elbows extended, fingers intertwined, "beating" his legs (Figure 12.10h).
- Arms bent at the shoulders, elbows extended, fingers intertwined: "beating" his legs with flippers on his feet.

Floating face down:

- Holding a square float in his hands, elbows extended, head resting out of the water: "beating" his feet (Figure 12.10i).
- As above, but with breathing exercises, breaststroke.
- As above, but with palmar devices.

Stretching exercises for legs:

- Starting position: legs abducted, knees extended, soles touching the bottom, arms straight, hands resting on edge of pool: hold position (Figure 12.11a).
- Starting position: legs adducted, knees extended, soles touching the

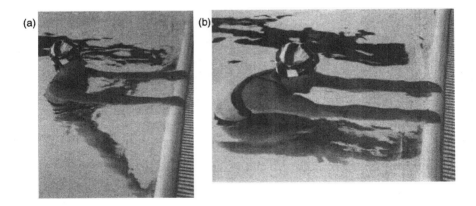

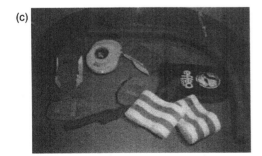

Figure 21.11 Exercises for legs and material for hydrotherapy.

bottom, arms straight, hands resting on edge of pool: hold position (Figure 12.11b).

The aim of these exercises is to improve the patient's overall motor ability, coordination and respiration. Moreover, the patients can be treated in groups to favor socializing and to have the opportunity to compare their progress.

Conclusion

Considering our 20 years of experience in the rehabilitation in water of patients affected by cranial trauma, we can assert that with this therapy we have managed to obtain the following results:

- A quicker improvement in the relaxation of the muscles and of the articular range when compared to the traditional treatment.
- Facilitation of the execution of the requested movements.
- An improvement in the coordination of the balance and of the perception of the body scheme.
- An important reduction of articular and neurogenic pain.
- A psychological, relaxing effect, well appreciated by patients.
- A positive, supporting psychological effect, related to a better consciousness of one's own motor potentials.

The benefits we have just described reward our effort and support our determination to continue our research towards new satisfactory programs and new successful therapeutical exercises.

References

1. Campion-Reid, M. (1990). *Adult hydrotherapy: A practical approach*. Oxford: Heinemann.
2. Davis, B. C., & Harrison, R. A. (1988). *Hydrotherapy in practice*. London: Churchill Livingstone.
3. Debergue, J. C. (1992). *Gimnastique aquatique*. Paris: Amphora.
4. Duffield, M. H. (1983). *Exercise in water*. London: Baillière Tindall.
5. Esnault, M. (1991). *Rééducation dans l'eau, étirements et renforcement musculaire du tronc et des membres*. Paris: Masson.
6. Becker, B. (1994). The biologic aspects of hydrotherapy. *J. Back Musculoskel. Rehabil., 4*, 255–264.
7. Cassady, S. L., & Nielsen, D. H. (1992). Cardiorespiratory responses of healthly subjects to calisthenics performed on land versus in water. *Phys. Ther., 72*, 532–538.
8. Eyestone, E. D., Fellingham, G., George, J., & Fisher, A. G. (1993). Effect of water running and cycling on maximum oxygen consumption and 2-mile run performance. *Am. J. Sports Med., 21*, 41–43.
9. Aspinall, S. T., & Graham, R. (1989). Two sources of contamination of a hydrotherapy pool by environmental organisms. *J. Hosp. Infect., 14*, 285–292.

10. Franchimont, F., Juchmes, J., & Lecomte, J. (1983). Hydrotherapy, mechanisms and indications. *Pharmacol. Ther., 20*, 79–84.
11. Hall, J., Bisson, D., & O'Hare, P. (1990). The physiology of immersion. *Physiotherapy, 76*, 517–521.
12. Moschetti, M., & Cole, A. (1994). Aquatics: risks management strategies for the therapy pool. *J. Back Musculoskel. Rehabil., 4*, 265–272.
13. Revel, M., Maydoux-Benhamou, M. A., & Medicis, P. (1987). Les contreindications de l'hydrokinésithérapie. In C. Hérisson and L. Simon (Eds.), *Hydrothérapie et kinébalnéothérapie* (pp. 12–16). Paris: Masson.
14. Minaire, P. (1986). Pathologie de l'immobilité. *Ann. Réadapt. Med. Physic., 28*, 409–424.
15. Johnston, M. V., & Hall, K. M. (1994). Outcomes evaluation in TBI rehabilitation. Part 1: Overview and system principles. *Arch. Phys. Med. Rehab., 75*, SC 2–9.
16. Boldrini, P., & Basaglia, N. (1994). *La riabilitazione del grave traumatizzato cranio-encefalico.* Milan: Masson
17. Rappaport, M., Allison, M. D., & Kelting, D. L., (1992). Evaluation of coma and vegetative states. *Arch. Phys. Med. Rehab., 73* 628–634.
18. Katz, D. I., Alexander, M. P. (1994). Traumatic brain injury – predicting the course of recovery and outcome for patients admitted to rehabilitation. *Arch. Neurol., 51*, 661–670.
19. Skinner, A. T., & Thomson, A. M. (1985). *La rieducazione in acqua: Tecnica Duffield.* Rome: Marrapese.
20. Booth, B. J., Doyle, M., & Montgomery, J. (1983). Serial casting for the management of spasticity in the head-injured adult. *Phys. Ther., 63*, 1960–1966.
21. Glenn, M. (1994). Nerve blocks. In R. T. Katz (Ed.), *Spasticity. State of the art.* Philadelphia, PA: Hanley & Belfus. Reviews in *Phys. Med. Rehabil.* (Vol. 8).
22. Massion, J. (1992). Movement, posture and equilibrium: interaction and coordination. *Progr. Neurobiol., 38*, 35–56.
23. Massion, J., Fabre, J. C., Mouchnino, L., & Obadia, A. (1995). Body orientation and regulation of the center of gravity during movement under water. *J. Vestib. Res., 5*, 211–221.
24. Dietz, V., Horstmann, G. A., Trippel, M., & Gollhofer, A. (1989). Human postural reflexes and gravity – an under water simulation. *Neurosci. Lett., 106*, 330–335.
25. Nelson, J. G. (1968). Effect of water immersion and body position upon perception of gravitational vertical. *Aerospace Med., 39*, 806–811.
26. Wood, R. L., Winkowski, T. B., Miller, J. L., Tierney, L., & Goldman, L. (1992). Evaluating sensory regulation as a method to improve awareness in patients with altered states of consciousness: a pilot study. *Brain Inj., 6*, 411–418.
27. Wood, R. L., Winkowski, T. B., & Miller, J. L. (1993). Sensory regulation as a method to promote recovery in patients with altered states of consciousness. *Neuropsychol. Rehab., 3*, 177–190.
28. Hérossp, C., & Simo, L. (1987). *Hydrothérapie et kynéobalnéothérapie.* Milan: Masson.
29. Oda, S., Matsumoto, T., Nakagawa, K., & Moriya, K. (1999). Relaxation effects in humans of underwater exercise of moderate intensity. *Eur. J. Appl. Physiol., 80*(4), 253–259.
30. Morelli, A., & Calligaris, A. (1999). L'esercizio terapeutico in acqua. *Le scienze dell'allenamento.* Rome: Società Stampa.

13 Neuropsychological assessment of persons with acquired brain injury

José Léon-Carrión, Paul J. Taaffe, and Juan Manuel Barroso y Martín

Introduction

This chapter reviews the most relevant aspects of neuropsychological assessment of persons with acquired brain injury. Changes in cognition, emotions and behavior occur as a result of acquired brain injury (traumatic brain injury, stroke, brain tumors, etc.), and these changes have to be detected as objectively as possible. Neuropsychological techniques, methods and instruments allow the expert neuropsychologist to detect which main impairments a patient has as a result of an injury to the brain. Neuropsychological assessment is a changing discipline and probably has to change even more dramatically in the next decade as a result of a changing world and new developments in administering health programs. This chapter offers a review of this state-of-the-art discipline, trying to combine classic neuropsychological assessment with new tendencies.

Quantitative and qualitative assessment

"Assessment" refers to the purposeful gathering of information about an individual to include clinical interview material, psychometric data, formal observations, and past medical records. Generally speaking, the purpose of an assessment is to generate a diagnosis, to provide direction for treatment planning, to assist in patient care, and to advance research efforts. "Neuropsychological assessment", then, implies that these methods of study are utilized to evaluate and intervene with regard to brain–behavior relationships. Traditionally, there have been two main models of neuropsychological assessment, namely the quantitative method and qualitative method.

For the neuropsychologist who comes from the quantitative perspective, a fixed battery is used. The product of the evaluation – or the data, per se – is more important than the process the patient goes through to provide the data. The quantitative neuropsychologist is primarily interested in the numbers directly derived from answers to questions and comparisons to reference groups. Scores are viewed as having some intrinsic meaning upon which assumptions are made as to the existence of a lesion, its location, and associated deficits. There is a focus on problem areas, and a causal relationship is drawn between the suspected lesion site and measured weaknesses. The treatment plan emanating from the test results calls for a return to the premorbid level of functioning. Progress toward that end must be measurable. In contrast, for the neuropsychologist who operates from a qualitative vantage point, there is a theoretical foundation that underlies the approach through which flexibility in the choice of instruments administered is extremely important. The evaluation is process oriented rather than being data driven. Latitude exists for the inclusion of indirect observations, and obtained scores are thought to be meaningful only in a broad context. The patient's relative strengths as well as weaknesses are considered with respect to treatment efforts. Furthermore, the goal of rehabilitation is to assist the patient in achieving an optimal level of coherence, not necessarily a return to normalcy.

Whereas the quantitative neuropsychologist is mainly concerned with the mathematics and statistics of the functional impairment, the qualitative neuropsychologist endeavors to know the procedural breakdowns implicit in the loss of functional integrity. Quantitative neuropsychological assessment developed out of the work of Ward Halstead, an American who was trained in physiological psychology and worked side by side with neurosurgeons. He sought to bring empirical order to the evaluation. The Halstead–Reitan Neuropsychological Test Battery (HRB)[1] that bears his name is likely the most thoroughly researched and widely used instrument primarily geared toward quantitative assessment. Qualitative neuropsychological assessment, on the other hand, recognizes Alexander Luria, a Russian psychologist and neurologist, as its founder. He was much more interested in the three principal functional units of the brain and the dynamic processes involved in the organization of mental activity.[2] Luria[2] also provided descriptions of lobe specific functions and syndromes. Christensen[3] was successful at documenting Luria's investigational methods. Golden et al.[4] formalized such procedures into psychometric form, i.e., the Luria–Nebraska Neuropsychological Battery (LNNB), although it lost its qualitative format and interpretation. The Luria/Christensen Diagnostic Examination is, at the moment, the only test battery whose items are based on a human model of functioning brain.

Over the years, neuropsychologists have seemed most comfortable with tests that might be categorized as being quantitative in nature.[5] The Wechsler intelligence measures and memory scales, along with the HRB and the Bender-Gestalt Test, have been cited in surveys of popular test use.[6] With proper motivation and a touch of creativity on the part of the neuropsychologists who develop and utilize testing instruments, science and art could combine to make for a fuller and richer assessment experience. Most of these tests have strong psychometric properties, as is the custom of North American neuropsychologists. Nonetheless, there is some merging of quantitative and qualitative methods, perhaps in an effort to be more universally appealing and comprehensive.

The clinical interview

Just as a well-thought-out rehabilitation program evolves, in part, from the results of a carefully chosen test battery, the selection of testing instruments emanates from a thorough clinical interview. However, before the clinical interview is undertaken, the neuropsychologist is encouraged to keep in mind the purpose of the evaluation which, typically, occurs for diagnostic, planning, descriptive, legal, and/or research reasons.[7] It may be necessary to clarify the purpose with the referral source and, in this age of managed healthcare, to gather some preliminary information from the referral source so that insurance company pre-authorization for the assessment can be secured. In many cases, an initial interview may be permitted in order to generate hypotheses about the patient and to decide on diagnostic procedures. Again, pre-approval from the managed care company may be required prior to testing proper.

In keeping with prior discussion of quantitative and qualitative approaches to neuropsychological assessment, the clinical interview phase of the assessment will produce objective data as well as subjective material. Furthermore, the neuropsychologist may want to consider having "private" interviews with the patient, and the significant other, respectively. Each person may be reluctant to talk openly with the other listening in. The patient who has suffered a brain injury may not understand the questions being asked, may not be able to respond verbally, may not make sense if a verbal response is given, and/or may not remember the material of inquiry. Difficulties with aphasia and memory are quite common in the brain-injured population and, usually, can be spotted shortly into the interview. Another reason for interviewing a significant other is that the patient may not be inclined to answer due to decreased initiation. It is conceivable that a patient may be less than forthcoming because of secondary gain and/or forensic entanglements.

As a first step before starting a test battery, it is necessary to obtain information about the patient and his or her premorbid functioning. A baseline can then be established with respect to his or her cognitive functioning, and personality, emotional, social and behavioral characteristics that were present before the accident and assist in determining which changes were due to the neurological damage. This can be done by screening various yet specific areas. To begin, information is needed about the accident itself and the severity of the trauma. Results of the Glasgow Coma Scale, the length of post-traumatic amnesia, the duration of the coma, neuroimages, as well as details about the lesion, are essential components of the screening. It is also helpful to know how the patient's condition has changed from the time of the injury to the present moment.

The data collection proceeds and takes into account the psychological aspects of the patient regarding his or her behavioral functioning and premorbid cognition. There must be an assessment of whether the patient's neurocognitive and behavioral deficits are due to the present traumatic neurological condition or, on the contrary, they already existed before the trauma or recent accident. For this, the clinical interview with the patient and his family members usually provides pertinent information. Then, all relevant medical and psychological reports are considered in light of what is already known about the patient. It is often useful to compile as many medical reports as possible concerning the neurological condition as they can provide detailed references to the neurological disorders that affect the patient's central nervous system and are going to be the basis of neurocognitive functioning. If the reports are old, or if there are suspected changes in the neurological level affecting the patient, it is advisable to carry out a new neurological examination with neuroimaging tests that provide as much detail as possible of the patient's neurological condition. Once information has been obtained to establish the patient's premorbid baseline, an itemized neurocognitive, behavioral and social study should commence.

Data referring to the patient's educational level, socio-economic status, personal and family mental health history, substance abuse history, if any, should be included in order to give a thorough understanding of the patient's background.

As mentioned above, the patient's intellectual capacity before impairment should be a point of reference to help determine the extent and magnitude of the current disorder. This intellectual assessment is carried out by formulas which allow a reliable estimate of the patient's intellectual functioning prior to the disorder. It derives from an equation that takes into account data about the patient's education, race, occupation, etc. as valuable and predictive factors of his or her premorbid intellectual level.[8]

Lastly, information should be compiled about the most relevant aspects of the patient's social, family and work history to establish a premorbid baseline. On the one hand, the social aspect can shed relevant light on the patient's life style; on the other hand, the family history can indicate an increase of risk in developing certain neurodegenerative disorders such as Alzheimer's disease.[9] The patient's work history can indicate prolonged and/ or daily exposure to certain toxic substances (mercury, toluene, gasoline, etc.) that can produce serious neurocognitive disorders.

As suggested above, not all brain injury patients are ready to be interviewed. Physicians, lawyers, caregivers, insurance company personnel, and others may want a patient assessed, but until he or she is able, an inclusive evaluation will have to wait or be modified. Depending on the severity of the injury, neuropsychological assessment could begin near the moment the patient begins to communicate and interact with the neuropsychologist. In other words, the purpose of the assessment may dictate that testing proceed even if the patient's injury is relatively new and he or she cannot be interviewed in depth. When the neuropsychologist is satisfied that the assessment should move forward, the concept of confidentiality should be broached and discussed in terms of protections for the patient and legal limitations. Prior to the interview, the neuropsychologist is encouraged to apprise the patient of plans for dissemination of the assessment findings with respect to who will have access and when the results will be available. The patient may be comforted by a basic explanation of the types of tests to be given and the test administration protocol. Finally, the neuropsychologist can elicit the patient's cooperation by allowing questions and providing reassurances.

If one's preferred form of clinical interview is thought of as a favorite recipe, it is crucial to have just the right mix of ingredients. Sbordone[10] has produced an exhaustive list of clinical and background markers that constitute the neuropsychological history. The clinical markers include:

- complaints of patient and significant others
- history of injury or illness
- onset and duration of symptoms
- neurological findings
- hospitalization history
- treatment–rehabilitation history
- current residual problems
- change in patient's condition during the past year
- effect of injury on patient and significant others
- expectations of the patient and significant others
- history of medication use
- psychiatric or emotional problems since injury.

It seems likely that the clinical interview utilized by most professionals in the field could be found within the parameters set forth in Sbordone's[10] neuropsychological history. With an eye toward the upcoming months and years, and being cognizant of ultimate rehabilitation needs, the neuropsychologist will probably want to know about the patient's strengths, abilities, interests, and goals. This is particularly true if there is any possibility of the patient receiving treatment at an ecologically valid community rehabilitation program where cognitive, social, and coping skills training is woven into activities of everyday life.

Cognitive assessment

Assessment of orientation capacity

Attentional deficits are among the most frequent deriving from brain injury as this is a fundamental capacity in order to have an adequate notion of reality, of oneself and the surrounding environment. Among these, disorders in spatial and temporal orientation are frequent and appear when there are also disorders in the underlying mechanisms of attention and memory. This capacity of orientation permits the patient to know where he or she is, allowing him or her to answer questions relative to orientation in space, time and in respect to oneself, and knowing what is taking place around him or her. It is generally assessed as a part of the mental status exam. The assessment consists of asking the patient questions relative to the current date (day, month and year), time of day, location (hospital, office, city, country, etc.), what has happened to him or her, who he or she is, if married, if he or she has children, etc.

When a more detailed and complete assessment of this capacity is necessary, the *Galveston Orientation and Amnesia Test* (*GOAT*) can be used.[11] It is short, easy to use, involves some of the previously mentioned items regarding orientation of time, place and person, as well as amnesia following the neurological affectation of the brain. Scoring consists of assigning a number of points added up for each item answered correctly or within a permitted margin of error. The closer the score is to 100 points, the better the function is preserved. This test can be administered several times a day, even on successive days, which permits using graphics to show the evolution of this capacity within a certain time limit until total orientation is achieved. Some authors also use it to predict "awakening", or coming out of the coma. The authors of the test believe that it is convenient for a patient to begin neurocognitive assessment when a score of 75 points or more is attained on this test, indicating that the patient is no longer confused and disoriented.

The use of the GOAT assumes that there is some confusion in scoring as some questions may be subjective and difficult to answer for patients with more serious neurocognitive sequelae.

To avoid this confusion, the *Orientation Log* test *(O-Log)*,[12] as well as the above-mentioned test, is designed for daily use but is different from GOAT in that it does not require questions referring to the patient's personal details (name, date of birth, etc.). It can also be used for objectively estimating the patient's recovery time. The O-Log scale consists of ten items, centering on orientation of place (questions about the name of city or hospital), of time (day of the week, month, year, time of day, etc.) and personal circumstances (referring to awareness of events taking place). Verbal answers – those which need assistance and also those that are non-verbal – are scored from 0 to 30 points. A score of 24 or more correlates to the 75 points or more on the GOAT scale and can be used as the cut-off point for marking the end of the post-traumatic amnesia phase.

Dowler et al.[13] found a significant high correlation between scores obtained on the O-Log scale upon admission and those 12 months later in such factors as memory, executive functioning, and estimated IQ. These authors conclude that assessment via the O-Log scale in the acute phase reflects the severity of the injury and can serve as a predictor of cognitive evolution.

For Artiola et al.[14] losses related to the sense of orientation refer to post-traumatic amnesia and are evaluated via questions about orientation of time and space, remembering figures and the examiner's name. The duration of post-traumatic amnesia varies according to the brain injury but is usually resolved within 24 h after the lesion, within the average range from 1 h to 7 days after injury. The order of recovery observed during post-traumatic amnesia can be predicted: personal recovery is first and is more consistent than time orientation, which follows next. The last to be recovered is orientation of place.[15] The longer a patient has post-traumatic amnesia, the greater the possibility of suffering other neurocognitive deficits. When the patient is capable of giving correct answers to questions 3 days consecutively, the authors conclude that post-traumatic amnesia has disappeared and, therefore, the problems with orientation.

Improvement in orientation capacity contributes important information to brain injury recovery and can predict achievements in future rehabilitation. Frequent administration of a formal measure of orientation does not bring about recovery of this capacity: on the contrary, it progresses steadily during well-designed rehabilitation.[16]

Attention

Posner and Petersen[17] discussed attention from a physiological perspective and described alertness (i.e., CNS readiness) as being at the root of attention. Luria[2] also recognized alertness to be intimately linked to attention and postulated that both subcortical (e.g., brainstem) and cortical (e.g., prefrontal area) structures are involved in the process. It appears to be the case that activation of the left hemisphere via the internal capsule, the hypothalamus, the left basal forebrain, and the midbrain belies consciousness.[18] Often, simply observing and/or interviewing the patient provides a check of attention.

Once the neuropsychologist is satisfied that the patient is alert, the evaluation of attention may proceed to include the elements of focus–execute, sustain, encode, and shift.[19] Mirsky et al.[19] found that the Digit Symbol subtest of the Wechsler intelligence scales is a reliable measure of the focus–execute aspect of attention. It has been shown to be the Wechsler measure most sensitive to brain damage though laterality cannot be deduced.[7] Letter Cancellation techniques (see chapter 14), the Trail Making Test (1985), and the Stroop Color Word Test (1978) (see chapter 14) are recommended as well. Cancellation tests, in general, tend to demonstrate that left hemisphere patients are slow to complete the particular tasks while right hemisphere patients are more inclined to be inattentive to or neglect stimuli.[7] The Trail Making Test (1985) is good at documenting changes in cognition in dementia patients,[20] and scores have been correlated with electrophysiological measures of frontal functioning.[21] As for the Stroop (1935), the test has satisfactory reliability as reported by Spreen and Strauss.[22] However, there is a practice effect that seems to facilitate performance on a second administration.[23] As noted earlier in regard to the cancellation tests, individuals with left hemisphere lesions required more time for completion; the interference effect was evident with left-sided and right-sided patients alike.[24]

In Mirsky et al.[19] "sustain" is the next component of the attentional system. The Continuous Performance Test (CPT) as modified by Connors[25] is based on previous versions that were determined to have adequate reliability.[26] High omission rates on the Connors CPT may reflect an errant approach to testing or very slow responses. When individuals have high omission rates, inattentiveness is suspected, and when high commission rates are found, impulsivity is likely. The neuropsychologist must consider whether or not patients learn to adjust response rate over trials in an effort to self-modulate or sustain attention.

The Paced Auditory Serial Addition Test (PASAT)[27] has been employed similarly to assess sustained and divided attention. The instrument has patients listen to single-digit numbers given at different rates. The task is to add together the digit presented with the number immediately preceding it, and to state the new number before the next one is presented. Ponsford[28] has reported very good reliability percentages for the PASAT though practice effects may militate against repeated testings with the same individual.

Ponsford[28] encouraged the use of the Test of Everyday Attention (TEA)[29] to evaluate sustained attention or vigilance. This instrument attempts to be more ecologically valid than others but, as noted by Ponsford,[28] it is administered in a clinical setting rather than in the natural setting. Relevant subtests within this TEA include Elevator Counting, Telephone Search While Counting, and Lottery Task.

With respect to "encode", Mirsky et al.[19] utilized the Arithmetic and Digit Span subtests of the Wechsler intelligence tests. These researchers recognized that these tasks are more effortful, requiring mental manipulations of numbers. They are auditory tasks with visual elements. Mirsky et al.[19] suggested that this might be said of parts of the Mental Control section of the Wechsler Memory Scale as well.

The fourth part of the attentional system as posited by Mirsky et al.[19] refers to "shift". The Wisconsin Cord Sorting Test (WCST)[30] has proved helpful in measuring patients' abilities to problem solve and maintain set. The WCST is thought to be sensitive, but not necessarily specific, to frontal damage.[22] An additional means of assessing "shift" is by way of the Reciprocal Motor Programs Test.[31] Patients are asked to tap twice after the neuropsychologist taps once, and vice versa, over several trials. This task is included in the Luria battery, for example. Mirsky et al.[19] mention that this test correlates highly with the WCST and that it differentiates individuals with frontal lesions.

Executive functions

When the neuropsychologist takes it upon himself or herself to conduct an assessment of a patient's executive functions, there is the assumption that the individual under study can attend, at some level, to the evaluation procedures. In going forward with testing, the neuropsychologist would be hoping to gain insight into the patient's abilities "to control and to regulate organized behavior."[32] Over the years, executive functioning and the frontal lobes have become synonymous, although there are frontal–subcortical connections as well as temporal, parietal, and occipital association areas.[10]

As discussed in a previous section, a carefully conducted clinical interview can result in the neuropsychologist having a wealth of critical information at hand, some of which will be relevant to an understanding of the patient's executive functioning. Lezak[7] has divided the executive functions into four parts, including: (1) volition; (2) planning; (3) purposive action; and (4) effective performance. Each of these components should be covered in the neuropsychological assessment (see chapter 14).

Volition may be thought of as "the capacity for intentional behavior".[7] Again, self-reports and those of significant others, along with behavioral observations, will give the neuropsychologist clues to a patient's awareness and motivation. Sohlberg and Geyer[33] constructed the Executive Function Behavioral Rating Scale (EFBRS) that, in the first section, addresses the generation and initiation of goals. A functional approach to the assessment of volition may be in order and, with the EFBRS, the patient is asked to take part in an "Initiation of Conversation" activity. The hope is that the EFBRS has ecological validity. A new test, the Delis–Kaplan Executive Function System (D-KEFS),[34] deals with idea formulation and creativity. This instrument has encouraging correlational statistics with the California Verbal Learning Test-II, for example. Another means of assessing volition to be mentioned is the Frontal Lobe Personality Scale (FLOPS).[35] The FLOPS contains an Apathy scale that screens for abulia, or impaired initiation. An additional instrument that can be used to look at volition is the Tinkertoy Test (TTT).[7] The patient is presented with 50 pieces of a Tinkertoy set and is asked to make something. He or she is told there is a 5 min minimum for working. Clearly, other executive functions come into play as well.

The planning aspect of executive functions involves the development of "mental road maps" designed in an effort to meet certain goals. Patients also must be able to reflect on the likelihood of success given respective plans. Further, whether or not individuals can choose a plan among many to put into effect is a third component of the process. As is the case with many formal, structured tests, numbers matter. However, when evaluating a patient's planning abilities, it is incumbent upon the neuropsychologist to be attuned to the finer points of the patient's test-taking behavior. Qualitative information as to how the patient arrived at a plan, for example, can be much more meaningful than the amount of time taken to complete a task.

The planning portion of executive functions has been a focal point of assessment over the years. Although there are few if any pure planning tests, the Porteus Maze Test (PMT)[36] is used clinically to evaluate planning (and visuo-motor speed, if desired). Meier et al.[37] found that this instrument could be employed to differentiate levels of brain injury. Further, Levin et al.[38] discovered that patients with frontal damage were slower than individuals with posterior damage. Lezak[7] proposed that the WISC-III[39] mazes could be incorporated into an adult test battery. There are several "Tower Tests" in which patients must move beads, rings, or blocks, at times of varying colors from an initial position to a goal position. As with the mazes, it appears that those with anterior lesions do not perform as well as persons with posterior injuries.[7]

"Purposive action"[7] is the next step in the executive functions sequence whereby volition and planning produce goal-oriented behaviors. The neuropsychologist ought to be cognizant of the fact that his or her approach to testing can actually inhibit purposive actions.[10] This may be true, for example, when the neuropsychologist arranges the physical environment of the testing room to be relatively distraction free, and when there is an abundance of verbal reinforcers or cues put forth to enhance effort and maximize results. The specific purpose of the testing at any particular stage in the process will dictate the neuropsychologist's interaction with the patient and influence the data that is retrieved.

There are many tests that have been and can be effective at assessing purposive action. The TTT was alluded to above and gives the patient a chance to put the pieces together in a methodical or haphazard manner. The Ruff Figural Fluency Test (RFFT)[40] has patients come up with patterns in response to displays, and the strategy involved is of prime importance. Both production and perseveration are checked. According to the authors, controls did better than individuals with mild brain injuries, who did better than those with severe brain injuries. There are other techniques intended to gauge purposive actions such as those developed and refined by Luria and Christensen. The repeating pattern items of Luria's Neuropsychological Investigation[41] were designed for this reason. The Block Design, Picture Arrangement, and Picture Completion subtests of the Wechsler intelligence tests can shed light on purposive action as well.

Depending on the perspective of the neuropsychologist, effective performance may be judged by a score on a test or the way in which the patient attained the score. Ideally, there would be a merging of the two vantage points in this regard. Several questions arise when considering effective performance: (1) Did the patient achieve his or her goals? (2) Was progress made in the direction of the stated goals? (3) How able was the patient to keep track of his or her performance, to stay on track when warranted, and to alter actions if necessary? (4) What was learned for future reference?

Formal assessment of effective performance has been attempted through the use of various instruments. The EFBRS and D-KEFS are two that were introduced earlier in this section. Perhaps more familiar and more commonly utilized tests of this nature include the Wisconsin Card Sorting Test (WCST),[30] the Category Test (CT)[42] and the Trail Making Tests. A few of the other measures are thought to be ecologically valid, the Behavioral Dyscontrol Scale (BDS)[43] being one of them. In large part, the BDS follows Luria's work on frontal lobe difficulties and seeks to examine a patient's executive functioning in activities of daily living. Suchy et al.[44] reported predictive validity with respect to adjustment to living situations (i.e., independent as opposed to assisted living). Also, these researchers found that the BDS was helpful in predicting functional independence 3 months after completion of a rehabilitation program. The Behavioral Assessment of the Dysexecutive Syndrome (BADS)[45] is another test of this variety and focuses on real-world activities involving practical problem solving, following routes and directions, and adherence to rules. Questionnaires to be completed by the patient and significant others are included as well. Finally, the Behavioral Assessment of Vocational Skills (BAVS)[46] does as the name suggests and skillfully weaves components of executive functioning into vocational tasks. According to Sbordone,[10] the BAVS surpasses the WAIS-R, WISC, Trail Making Test, and sections of the WMS-R with regard to predicting effective on-the-job behaviors.

Receptive functions

With regard to receptive functions, ideally a stimulus leads to a sensation that is then perceived and, theoretically, "understood". For the individual who has had a brain injury, a breakdown in either sensation or perception can have catastrophic implications. The inability to sense a stimulus short-circuits the chain of events early on. If the patient can sense a stimulus but cannot recognize it, some form of agnosia occurs. The Tactical Performance Test, Seashore Rhythm Test, and Speech-Sounds Perception Test may be employed to check on receptive functions. Without going into great detail, the receptive functions domain of cognition has three main facets of primary importance in neuropsychological assessment (i.e., visual, auditory, and tactile perception). Visual perception encompasses a variety of skills, one of which is visual inattention. The term visual inattention is used to describe a lack of awareness of visual stimuli in the field of vision, usually on the left side.[11] A right-sided lesion, perhaps in the parietal lobe, may be the cause.[47] Over the years, many tests of visual inattention have been developed, including the Test of Visual Neglect.[48] The patient is presented with a sheet of paper containing 40 angled lines, and the task is to X out, or cross out, these lines. Research on the test has been favorable with respect to revealing right and left inattention as well as omissions in quadrants.[49] Mesulam's[50] Verbal and Nonverbal Cancellation Tasks, and Poizner et al.'s[51] Letter and Symbol Cancellations Tasks have also been utilized, and have proved to be reliable measures of inattention. More recently, as a part of the BNS, León-Carrión[52] has been successful at computerizing tests of inattention. He has been studying patients' responses to an attention task for both eyes and each one singly.

For the individual who has trouble attending to the entire visual field there is a cascade of related perceptual scanning, organization, and recognition difficulties. Scanning requires that a patient view the whole visual field with intact vision or the use of an effective compensation strategy (e.g., physically moving the head so that the eye(s) can appreciate the total array of stimuli at hand). Certainly scanning deficits can be demonstrated on some tests of inattention, while the Visual Search[53] was developed specifically for this reason. The patient looks at a large square that is made up of smaller grids, and then attempts to locate at the periphery of the square the two smaller grids that match those at the center of the square.[7] Persons with brain damage have been found to be significantly slower than either normal or psychiatric control subjects.[54] The Trail Making Test[55] is frequently employed to evaluate inattention and scanning, and is an integral part of the HRB.

Facial recognition can be very upsetting to patients with brain injury and their families, friends, and acquaintances. At times, it may be a challenge to distinguish whether the facial recognition problem is "pure" or an effect of compromised memory. Benton and Van Allen[56] purposely designed the Test of Facial Recognition without the confounding memory variable. The task has the patient match identical photographs under three conditions: (1) front view; (2) front view with side views; (3) front views with different lighting.[7] This test seems to have enjoyed clinical utility, though it does not necessarily differentiate impaired from non-impaired individuals who are older and better educated.[57]

The ability to create a gestalt from seemingly disconnected or ambiguous parts defines the organizational aspect of perception. Attending to all of the visual field for contextual purposes while systematically scanning stimuli allows for the organization of bits of information into coherent wholes. There are at least three types of visual organization tests that seek to have patients mentally complete a picture, for example, rearrange material in a more conventional form, or make sense out of inherently meaningless stimuli.[7] The Street Completion Test[58] has patients examine pictures of objects with portions missing, and bring closure to the objects by indicating what they are. This and other gestalt completion tests appear to differentiate right from left hemisphere injuries with individuals having right-sided damage faring worse.[59] As for the repositioning of visual stimuli, the Object Assembly subtest of the WAIS-III requires that disparate pieces be put together to make a butterfly, and a house, to name a couple. The Hooper Visual Organization Test (*Hooper Visual Organizational Test Manual*, 1983) contains drawings of common objects that have been cut into parts and placed on the cards. The patient tries to name each object. The Hooper has been researched and found not to discriminate lateralization of brain damage.[60] Rathburn and Smith[61] reported impairment was associated with right posterior lesions. Lewis et al.[62] found that the Hooper performance is especially vulnerable to acute lesions in the right anterior quadrant of the brain. The Rorschach Ink Blot Test (1921) is a classic projective personality test that has been used as a means of visual organization. Generally speaking, the patient is told at the start that there are no right or wrong answers and he or she is asked to tell what the ambiguous designs look like to him or her. How the patient's responses compare to the forms of the respective inkblots is one way of checking on visual organization.[63] Baker[64] determined that persons with brain damage often display perceptual disturbances on the Rorschach.

Auditory perception is a second aspect of receptive functions to be mentioned in this chapter and, as with visual perception, there are several component parts. First of all, auditory acuity can be diminished in individuals with ABI. Typically, the ear opposite to the side of the lesion is adversely affected. Lezak[7] asserts that the neuropsychologist can screen for an auditory acuity problem by purposely lowering the volume of speech and monitoring comprehension. Audiologists and ENT doctors can perform formal workups. If sufficient auditory acuity exists, auditory inattention must be evaluated. Again, the neuropsychologist can do this by rubbing together the first two fingers and the thumb to make a swishing type noise.[7] Each ear should be tested alone and both at the same time, while alternating trials. Patients who have had injuries to the temporal lobe – or to certain nerves – may very well ignore sounds produced on the side opposite to that of the lesion. Dichotic listening devices have been employed, mostly in research settings, to assist individuals for auditory inattention.[7] For the patient who has adequate hearing and attention, yet the processing of auditory information appears to be difficult, the question of comprehension arises. Perhaps he or she has Wernicke's aphasia, a condition characterized by auditory comprehension deficits[65] caused by damage to the posterior aspect of the superior left temporal gyrus. The neuropsychologist must rule out this type of aphasia, especially when assessing those with right-sided sensory impairments, or when patients seem to have trouble understanding what is being said to them. The Reitan–Indiana Aphasia Screening Test of the HRB has been a standard tool to screen for symptoms of receptive and expressive aphasia.[65] The Speech Sounds Perception Test is used widely to check on perception of verbal material and the Seashore Rhythm Test addresses nonverbal auditory perception.[66] Unfortunately, there are mixed research findings in terms of what these tests really measure, as it has been reported[67] that errors in sound recognition are consistent with right temporal lobe lesions, whereas Varney and Demasio[68] attributed such deficits to left hemisphere and subcortical lesions. The Seashore Rhythm Test does not lateralize according to Reitan and Wolfson[66] and Lezak.[7] Instead, it is quite good at demonstrating difficulties with attention and concentration. The LNNB also attempts to take note of patients' auditory perception and, as above, deficits have been associated with left temporal or bilateral temporal damage.[5]

Tactile perception represents a third major receptive function that is commonly disrupted following ABI. As with visual and auditory perception, the neuropsychologist will want to examine the patient for sensation. This may be accomplished by touching the patient's hands with a pad of gauze, a pin, or a stimulator while he or she is blindfolded.[69] The HRB includes the Sensory-Perceptual Examination, a portion of which is tactile in nature and designed to check on sensation and inattention. The neuropsychologist touches the back of the patient's hands to establish sensation, with parietal damage and vascular lesions accounting for poor scores.[1] Errors in one-sided stimulation may reflect lateralization of lesion.[70] Tactile recognition tests of stereognosis are important to include in the assessment of tactile perception. Common objects are placed into the patients' hands while blindfolded and they are asked to tell what they feel. The Tactile Form Recognition Test of the HRB is utilized for this purpose and errors involving identification of the circle are most certainly indicative of brain damage.[71] Luria went to great lengths to avoid contamination errors, and had ways of partialing out true stereognosis from motor problems and/or memory deficits.[7] Regarding tactile inattention, the patient's sensation is preserved, but on examination with simultaneous stimulation of a body part on both sides, he or she will acknowledge touch on the right, typically, to the exclusion of the left. The Sensory-Perceptual Examination of the HRB test for inattention that seems to be due to a lesion in the right parietal area.[71] The Face–Hand Test[72] has been helpful in determining tactile inattention and actually calls for the neuropsychologist to touch the left cheek and right hand at the same time, for example. Also, patients can be evaluated with eyes open if there are errors with eyes closed. This instrument has differentiated patients with inattention, particularly those who have dementia.[73]

Expressive functions

Neuropsychological assessment of the receptive functions of cognition has been described in relation to the visual, auditory, and tactile domains. The complementary expressive functions will be discussed now in similar fashion.

When individuals observe stimuli and go through the processes of attending, scanning/searching, organizing, and recognizing/perceiving, often some form of motor response is warranted. The neuropsychological assessment generally includes two types of visuoconstructive tasks in which patients draw while copying a model, and by following instructions to draw a figure, object, or person.[74] The other form of visuoconstructive task has patients put together or build with various materials. Lezak[7] has noted that a patient's ability to copy relatively simple designs may be present though freehand drawing of like material might be limited. The degree of detail frequently suffers. In order to copy, at a minimum a patient must first see or feel the stimulus, take note of it if only briefly, and execute the appropriate actions. Impairment in copying per se has become associated with damage to the right parietal lobe,[75] although Lacks[74] acknowledges that the Bender actually requires several abilities and, as a result, performance reflects the status of other brain areas as well. The Bender Gestalt Test[76] has been a standard in diagnostics for many years and has the patient copy, one at a time, nine different designs that include geometric shapes, dots, and wavy lines. Heaton et al.,[77] in a meta-analysis of relevant research covering the period 1960–1975, found that the Bender correctly identified three out of four individuals with neuropsychological versus psychiatric disorders.

The Rey–Osterrieth Complex Figure Test[78] is another popular instrument for assessing visuomotor skills. The patient sets out to copy a design by using different-colored pens or pencils for component parts. In this way, the neuropsychologist can more easily follow the process the patient employed in copying the figure. After a time delay, the patient is asked to reproduce the design. This particular test, then, encourages qualitative analysis and includes a measure of visual (possibly verbally mediated) memory. Lezak[7] and Spreen and Strauss[69] provide extensive comment on the neuropsychological worth of the instrument, but suffice it to say that it succeeds largely in differentiating those with and without brain damage, and in delineating more specific functional breakdowns.

Drawing via freehand, in contrast to copying, challenges the patient to use his or her mind's eye. A mental picture of the target figure, object, or person develops, and the patient then transfers this representation onto paper. Clearly, various skills are involved in the succession of brain-driven events that have complicated the diagnostic picture. Generally speaking, right-sided lesions produce left-sided visual inattention, overworking, and a greater number of details.[79] Left hemisphere lesions tend to yield drawings lacking in details making them look incomplete.[79]

The Draw-A-Person and House–Tree–Person tests have been used extensively over the years to screen for brain damage as well as emotional disturbances. Draw-A-Clock, or the Clock Drawing Test, has been utilized in much the same way while assessing language skills, memory, perceptual-motor abilities, and executive functions.[74]

The expressive aspect of visual functions can be seen also with hands-on tasks such as the Block Design and Object Assembly subtests of the Wechsler[80] intelligence tests. There is a very definite spatial element involved in the completion of these tasks; a point that separates this type of test from the copying variety. Furthermore, patients must demonstrate an understanding of concepts, logical thinking, abstraction, constructional abilities, visuomotor speed, concentration, and frustration tolerance.[74] Block Design requires that the patient replicate model designs assembled by the neuropsychologist initially followed by designs presented on cards. Poor performance on this subtest is known to be related to lesions in the right posterior parietal area.[81] It seems that there is less reliance on abstract thinking with Object Assembly, which has the patient fit together pieces of familiar objects. Inasmuch as Object Assembly and Block Design correlate highly with one another, the fact that individuals with damage to the posterior portion of the right parietal lobe[74] have much difficulty comes as no surprise. Both the HRB and the LNNB attempt to evaluate spatial functions.

Expressive language skills are, perhaps, best evaluated by speech and language pathologists. However, in the course of conducting an assessment, the neuropsychologist should gain an appreciation for a patient's use of semantics, syntax, pragmatics, discourse, and written language.[82] The Boston Naming Test[83] is used on a regular basis and, as implied, asks patients to name items shown in pictorial form. If an individual does not name an item in 30 seconds, a cue (i.e., a description) is given. A second cue (i.e., phonemic) is provided if the patient continues to have trouble naming the object. This test has been noted to show perseveration in left posterior patients,[84] fragmentation in right frontal patients,[83] and circumlocution in older patients.[85] Semantics is concerned with the proper use of words as well as word meanings.

Tests of vocabulary, such as the Vocabulary subtest of the WAIS-III,[86] require that patients come up with definitions of stimulus words. A person's score on the Vocabulary section of the WAIS-III is a good indicator of over-all intelligence. For those who have problems with word meanings, left hemisphere damage is a distinct possibility. Syntax has to do with the grammatical aspects of sentences. Agrammatism refers to the omission of various parts of spoken or written language. Paragrammatism is the use of incorrect sequences of words, as when the noun and verb of a sentence do not agree, and an inappropriate preposition may be included as well. The Luria's tasks and the Mini-Mental Status Examination[87] are two examples of neuro-psychological instruments that include items apportioned to syntax. As for pragmatics, simply put, it is the use of language in conversation. Measures of expressive speech such as that of the Luria may address this element also. A patient's goal-directed speech certainly can be assessed informally as during the clinical interview. The patient's ability to engage in discourse can be evaluated similarly or, more clinically, by having him or her tell a story based on visual stimuli, for example. The Boston Diagnostic Aphasia Examination (BDAE):[88] allows the clinician the opportunity to gauge the patient's knowledge of the underlying rules of conversation along with pace and context. Again, discourse can be elicited by asking patients questions that call for more than a yes or no response. Because pragmatics and discourse draw on visual memory at times, localization of lesions can be more difficult to detect. Deficits in expressive language may be seen in writing numbers, phonemes, words, phrases, sentences, and so on. The HRB and Luria/Christensen Battery make provision for writing as do the BDAE and the Peabody Individual Achievement Test-Revised (PIAT-R).[89] As the complexity of the writing task increases, so does the interplay of multiple brain areas in the cerebral circuitry. The neuropsychologist surveys the cerebral circuitry in hopes of finding a "short" much the same as an electrician goes about his or her work. Rehabilitation efforts can then be more focused and effective.

The tactile modality of expressive functions has to do with motor movements of body parts secondary to sensory stimulation. Disturbances in a patient's ability to carry out such actions are known as apraxias. Constructional apraxia was alluded to during discussion of defects of visual expression. Generally, patients are required to imitate what has been shown to them, or to respond to a command.[90] Lezak[7] mentions many activities for assessing apraxia. The New England Pantomime Tests[91] include a measure of pantomime expression in which the patient must demonstrate how to use certain objects. The authors have noted that aphasic individuals performed worse than controls or patients with right hemisphere injuries. Not surprisingly, then, the BDAE examination actually contains a screening test for apraxia.

Receptive and expressive functions can be thought of as being opposite sides of the same coin. Sensory information enters the brain and a motor response follows. The process, of course, is much more complicated as learning and memory come into play.

Assessment of memory processes and learning

Of all the cognitive consequences of ABI, learning and memory difficulties certainly rate among the most common. They also happen to be cited frequently by patients as being particularly problematic in recovery and rehabilitation. After all, memory is the means by which an individual carries with him or her what has been learned in the past, and the basis on which he or she defines the person he or she is currently and aspires to be in the future. Without learning and memory, it would be as if time had an amorphous quality only to leave the person feeling lost and out of touch. The evaluation of one's abilities to absorb new material and remember it is an integral part of the neuropsychologist's assessment.

As suggested earlier in this chapter, learning presupposes that the receptive/sensory functions are, at some level, operational. Attentional factors are involved as well. Provided these are at least partially intact, possibilities exist for taking in information that can then be acted upon by other systems. Sparing discussion of the mechanics by which people learn, it should be mentioned that tests of learning often allow the patient several trials to grasp whatever is being presented, whether word pairs as in the WAIS-III, or the parallel non-language Paired Associate Learning Test.[92] The main focus of this section will be on visual, auditory, and tactile memories, and appropriate assessment techniques (see also section of memory assessment in chapter 14).

In keeping with the order of presentation up to this point in the chapter, visual memory will be addressed with the caveat that visual memory tests also measure other functions (e.g., verbal, spatial, etc.) albeit to a lesser extent. Thus, it is incumbent upon the neuropsychologist when testing to carefully observe patients in an effort to appreciate the relative contribution of visual versus verbal or spatial memory, for example. To highlight, when a patient looks at the designs of the Wechsler Memory Scale-III and simultaneously can be heard describing the features of the stimuli, the neuropsychologist must note the verbal mediation of the visual task. The Wechsler Memory Scale has been a popular test over the years for the reproduction of designs and is thought to be sensitive to right hemisphere impairment.[7] The Rey–Osterrieth Complex Figure Test is another of the reproduction tests that can be used for multiple purposes. The qualitative aspects of the drawings are extremely important in determining probable lesion location and whether or not a real memory problem is present. Certainly these reproduction tasks can be employed to look at immediate as well as delayed recall. The Luria and other batteries such as the Benton Visual Retention Test[93] also include such items. Visual memory may entail recognition of faces, for example, which also has a verbal component as when the patient views a photograph and says, "A young woman with shoulder length brown hair." Again, the Wechsler Memory Scale-III has a Faces subtest with immediate and delayed memory components. The Recognition Memory Test[94] has a measure of immediate recall for unfamiliar faces that potentially could be used for delayed memory purposes. In actuality – and with some creativity – there are many ways to assess visual memory (e.g., as with the Digit Symbol subtest of the WAIS-R or WAIS-III) but not in a pure fashion. The fact that visual memory tests have a strong verbal element demonstrates the interplay of complementary areas of the brain.

Verbal memory tests abound though only a select few seem to be used routinely by neuropsychologists. These instruments are typically chosen to examine certain content or specific areas of verbal memory. To highlight, a check on old, overlearned material may require that the patient recite the letters of the alphabet, as on the Wechsler Memory Scale. Lezak[7] believes that even one error is noteworthy and, attentional issues aside, may portend brain damage. Also, this could be the case with the individual who begins the alphabet, stops, and cannot continue the chain. The Information subtest of the Wechsler intelligence scales has been employed in a similar vein to assess semantic memory. Traditionally, this measure has been thought of as a "hold" item, being one of the most resistant to decay. Another popular way of screening for verbal memory defects is to have the person repeat digits forward and backward as on the WAIS and WAIS-III. Clearly, attention and concentration are involved along with working memory. In order to cut down on the possibility of rehearsing what has been heard, the Brown-Peterson technique has the patient listen to consonant trigrams, and to count backwards from a predetermined number just after presentation of the trigrams, and to then identify the trigrams. This is a measure of new learning. Milner[95] found that patients with left temporal lobe dysfunction and hippocampal damage recalled significantly fewer trigrams. Those with frontal lobe lesions also did poorly.

The Rey Auditory Verbal Learning Test[96] has the patient attempt to remember a list of 15 words over the course of several trials. Generally speaking, patients with frontal and left temporal damage have lower scores in the end.[97,98] Like the Rey, the California Verbal Learning Test (CVLT)[99] has the patient try to learn a "shopping list" of words. Thus, recall of verbal material is assessed as well as conceptual ability. Again, the CVLT seems to be quite sensitive to left temporal lobe difficulties with regard to fewer words learned and less categorization.[100] The Hopkins Verbal Learning Test[101] is another variation of the word-learning test as in the Selective Reminding Procedure[102] and the Verbal Paired Associate subtest of the WAIS-III.[86] In contrast, the

HRB is devoid of verbal memory tests. The Wechsler Memory Scale-III asks the patient to listen carefully to a short story and to remember as many parts as they can. Lezak[7] details a number of studies that show individuals who have sustained left temporal injuries tend to do worse on this type of task.

One final form of memory to be discussed is tactile memory. The Tactual Performance Test (TPT) of the HRB has been the instrument of choice in evaluating this function. Basically, the patient is blindfolded and must fit blocks of various sizes and shapes into holes on a board. Following the initial trials, the patient is asked to draw the board with special attention given to the shapes and their locations. Slowed or incorrect responses on the TPT have been associated with brain damage, though the exact nature of the observed deficits is unclear.[7] TPT memory and localization scores are not reliable measures of lateralization according to Reitan and Wolfson.[103] Lezak[7] considers the TPT to be too taxing for the patient and too time-consuming for the clinician.

Conceptualization and reasoning

Once an individual has sensed and perceived stimuli, has stored away information about the unique and common characteristics of the stimuli, and has the need or desire to react in some way to the stimuli, it is essential that he or she be able to perform cognitive contortions so as to respond in an effective manner. The Category Test of the HRB is employed quite often to evaluate visual concept formation. In taking the test, the patient views sets of items that are organized by an undisclosed overriding principle. On the basis of feedback telling the patient whether he or she is correct or incorrect in attempts to match, the patient hopefully figures out the various categories. Although the Category Test is thought to be extremely sensitive to the existence of brain damage,[71] it does not provide the specificity of localization (i.e., frontal lobe dysfunction) originally proposed by Halstead.[42]

The Tower of Hanoi/Seville test (see the Seville Neuropsychological Test Battery above) has been used in the simple, original Tower of Hanoi version as well as in the Seville version to evaluate the complex abilities of problem solving and capacity for conceptualizing. Shallice[36] was the first author who used this test to evaluate planning in patients who had brain damage. Shallice believed that, due to its newness, this test needed a planning strategy for arriving at the correct answer to be formulated by the patients. This plan had to include a final goal that is, in turn, broken down into various sub-solutions which should be correctly sequenced over time in order to reach the final goal. Shallice found specific deficits in the total time needed to complete the test by the patients with lesions in the left frontal lobe. León-Carrión and Barroso y Martín[104] found that patients with frontal lesions obtain worse results in all parts of the test than subjects with lesions in other parts of the brain.

Another test of some renown that has been used to assess visual patterning and reasoning is the Raven's Progressive Matrices.[105] Here the patient is presented with patterns that have a missing piece. He or she must choose one from among six to eight possible pieces to complete the pattern correctly. There are actually a number of sets of the matrices and, depending on the focus (e.g., visuospatial) of a particular set, research has reported different results in terms of lesion location.[69]

The Wisconsin Card Sorting Test (WCST)[30] is a third measure incorporating conceptualization into a visual format. With this test, the patient is told at the outset that he or she is to try to match cards from the deck to four stimulus cards on display. The only feedback to the patient is "correct" or "incorrect" as he or she strives to find the underlying ideas. Lezak[7] reviewed many studies on the WCST and seems to suggest that it documents frontal deficits, but does not localize. Picture Completion and Picture Arrangement are two additional Wechsler "visual" subtests that reflect on patients' reasoning. Parietal involvement is suspected with those who perform poorly.[106]

Assessment of sensory and motor capacity

To evaluate the sensory and tactile capacities, techniques using recognition/ discrimination are usually employed. With one's eyes closed, the patient is asked where he or she feels pressure, if it is in one or two places, if they are felt simultaneously, etc. With this type of assessment, stereognostic techniques are used in which the patient must recognize common objects by touching them, first with one hand and then with the other, while keeping the eyes closed. Results obtained from this test should not show any errors, as one sole error could indicate that this function is impaired.

In order to enhance this assessment, Luria presented a procedure of four consecutive steps to assure that the function is intact. First, put an object in the palm of the patient's hand. If it is not identified, go on to the second step that consists of moving the object to different places in the palm of the hand. The third step, if it is still unidentified, is to choose among a group of objects by touching something similar to the unidentified object. Lastly, if the patient continues to make errors, he or she tries to identify the same object with the other hand. A complementary way to obtain information about this function has been the technique of writing numbers or letters on the palm of the hand or fingertips. In any case, there are test batteries that permit detailed assessment of these functions and group these tests in a standardized way. The following are some of the tests in, first, Halstead–Reitan's test battery and then those of Luria.

In the *Halstead–Reitan Test Battery*, some tests can evaluate sensory as well as motor abilities. Thus, the *Tactual Performance Test* is one in which the subject is blindfolded and presented with ten geometric blocks which fit into corresponding holes on a board (Goddard–Segin's board). This task should be carried out with the dominant hand first, with the non-dominant hand afterwards, and with both at the end. Then the patient is asked to point out the figures he or she remembers by indicating their position on the board. The scores obtained assess the time employed in the three attempts, and the correct figures remembered and placed in position. Motor speed, tactile discrimination of forms, coordination of movements, manual skill, spatial configuration, psychomotor coordination, ability to remember objects perceived by touch and their localization are evaluated in this test, among other things.

The *Seashore Rhythm Test* is another test in this battery and contains 30 elements of sound in two rhythmic patterns for each. The patient listens and tries to ascertain if the elements are the same or different. Auditory/non-verbal perception and capacity to discriminate auditory sequences are evaluated with this test.

The Speech Sounds Perception Test is also part of this battery. This test is divided into six different parts, with ten elements per part. For each item, the patient listens to a nonsense word which must match one of four choices of letters representing the sound. Among other abilities, the capacity for audio-verbal perception is evaluated in this test.

The Finger Tapping Test evaluates motor abilities, motor speed, and differential psychomotor coordination in both hands. In the test, the index finger taps a telegraph key as rapidly as possible in five 10-second trials, alternating the dominant with the non-dominant hand.

The *Sensory-Perception Test* uses four tests, the fundamental bases of which have been described previously. These evaluate digital agnosia, recognition of writing on the skin, sensory extinction to touch, visual and auditory sensory models, and recognition of figures by touch.

Another test included in the battery is the *Test of Lateral Dominance* in which hand, eye, and foot dominance is examined, as well as the patient's capacity with the dominant and non-dominant hand.

To evaluate manual preference and measure skills of the upper extremities, the *Grooved Pegboard* is used. In this task, the patient is asked to place 25 small pegs in their corresponding slots on a 5 × 5 pegboard panel. Scores are obtained from the time it takes to complete the task using the preferred hand and then the other one.

The battery proposed by Luria/Christensen is more qualitive in nature and allows for a personalized examination. This battery is composed of a group of tasks which lead to a detailed qualitative analysis of distinct psychological functions. Normative data is not presented, permitting great flexibility in analyzing the results. The test consists of 10 parts.[107] We will only discuss the first three, since the rest are dedicated to the exploration of other superior functions not included in this section. The first part is for the study of motor functions, starting with simple praxis as a step prior to analyzing the most basic components of the motor function. The examination continues and ends with the assessment of more complex forms of praxis involving motor functions of the hands, and oral praxis and verbal regulation of motor function. Each of these is divided into different parts in order to carry out a detailed analysis of each of the group components.

The second part has to do with acoustic/motor organization, involving two series of tasks. On the one hand, perception and reproduction of tonal relations and, on the other, perception and reproduction of rhythmic structure. This is done by asking the patient to discern if pairs of tones presented are identical or different in the first group of tasks. In the second, an analysis is made of whether the patient is capable of appraising groups of signs that are presented and motor execution of different rhythmic groups. The third part evaluates the superior cutaneous and kinesthetic functions. This section is divided into three parts: cutaneous sensations, muscular and articulatory sensations, and stereognosis. All of these tests are done with the patient's eyes covered and using some of the activities that have been previously described (identifying numbers written on the palm of the hand, identifying objects in the hand, identifying where he or she has been touched, etc.).

Assessment of praxis (praxia) and gnosis

Praxia is the capacity to carry out a certain movement based on cognitive organization. Apraxic disorders are defined as "impairments in gestures, movements intended for specific ends, manipulation of a real object or by pantomime (of the capacity for intended execution of movement) which are not explained by a type of motor, sensory, perceptive or comprehensive lesion nor by intellectual impairment, detected after lesions in certain areas of the brain". Assessment of apraxia is divided into the following subtypes:

1   *Constructive apraxia.* This disorder is one in which the capacity to construct or join elements in two or three spatial planes is affected. This praxic capacity requires the ordering and control of sequential visuoperceptive and visuo-spatial elements that are carried out via motor capacity. It can be evaluated by using Benton's TRV plates.

2   *Ideomotor apraxia.* This disorder incapacitates the patient from making simple gestures without using real objects. This type of apraxia is expressed by the inability to carry out pantomimed gestures, by making unadaptable movements, by perseverating with the same gesture repeatedly, or by making tentative attempts at self-correction. For its assessment, the patient is asked to imagine different situations: how to ask the public to be quiet in an auditorium; how to express through gestures that a person is approaching; how to put out a match in gestures; or how to use different tools by gesturing (e.g., screwdriver, spade, spoon, etc.). Mistakes in these exercises determine the presence of this type of apraxia.

3   *Ideational apraxia.* This disorder is characterized by a loss of the conceptual process underlying movement. The patient cannot form a plan of movement and does not know the correct use of an object due to not knowing its purpose yet motor functioning is intact. It is generally used to assess the capacity for manipulations that involve sequences of

gestures – writing a letter, folding a piece of paper, putting it into an envelope and sticking a stamp on it.

4   *Dressing apraxia*. This disorder is an impairment observed in the absence of ideational or ideomotor apraxia. It is a special apraxia exclusive to one's own body and witnessed in the activity of getting dressed. It is easily evaluated by watching as the patient turns clothes over and over again to the right and the left. He or she looks at them, and through trial and error, ends up putting both legs into a sleeve as if putting on trousers or, after wrongly putting on a shirt with the sleeve hanging behind the back, gives up the effort and deems the task to be impossible. In the end, the patient is dressed in an odd manner as if it were a joke rather than his or her best attempt.

The Boston Naming Test for the diagnosis of aphasia presents a similar praxis assessment procedure to that described previously. Verbal praxis necessary for language is evaluated in different tests used to assess this capacity.

The term "agnosia" refers to a disorder implying an absence of the capacity to perceive and recognize. This affectation also implies an impairment in recognizing previously learned stimuli, or an incapacity to recognize stimuli routinely learned after an adequate display. This disorder should occur in absence of an impairment in perception, language, or cognitive capacity, as a consequence of an acquired brain injury lesion. It affects recognition of the types of stimuli related to the sensory canal, but not to others.

It is important to mention the mnesia component within the aspects of recognition – gnosis. In order to recognize a specific stimulus, even though it is presented in a unique sensory modality, it is necessary to evoke numerous memories. For example, tactile recognition of an orange – without seeing it – is the consequence of the union of such distant factors as form, texture, weight, and other factors such as smell, taste, color, and even emotional experiences related to it, including the agreeability/disagreeability of its acid taste or how it tastes when included in a succulent breakfast. These memories may belong to the same sensory modality or another, they may or may not be verbal, etc. This is due to the representation of each stimulus in multiple areas of the brain, therefore evoking all of them when only one part is stimulated.

There are different types of agnosia, *one for each sensory modality* – auditory, visual, tactile, and agnosia for smell and taste – or they can be grouped *according to unrecognized material* – faces, color, music, etc. Of all of them, visual agnosia has been best studied, and in greater detail.

Visual agnosias

Within these agnosias, we will center on visuo-perceptive impairments, high-lighting *cortical blindness* – other authors call it central – which is produced when the primary bilateral visual pathways are impaired. Patients affected by these calcarine lesions are capable of saying they perceive something, but do not know what it is. Perception deficits or anosognosia can be added to this impairment since patients say that they see things when they do not actually do so, not noticing that they have this perception impairment (i.e., visual agnosia, an impairment of visual recognition of objects maintaining visual sharpness and intact cognitive integrity). In this impairment, objects are detected also, but not identified (unlike the former, this impairment does not affect bilaterally the area of the occipital cortex). In this group, complete hemianopia can be identified when affecting a hemi-field or quadrantanopia if it affects only one quadrant. Prosopagnosia, or a deficit in recognizing faces, is demonstrated when patients are not able to recognize them exclusively by sight, without hearing them speak, and even oneself via a mirror or photograph. These patients can read and are capable of differentiating women's from men's faces, the approximate age one is by observing the face, and even what kind of emotions prevail. However, there is impairment in recognizing colors and textures due to the proximity of the cortical areas specializing in these capacities. Topographical agnosia refers to the incapacity to recognize specific places even though they know they are looking at a specific zone or building. This impairment is an incapacity to remember the relationship between bearings which can be identified individually although the neurocognitive capacity is preserved. Acromatopsia, or impairment in the perception of colors, is a consequence of lesions in the fusiform convolution area in both hemispheres. Perception of color is impaired while the patient maintains vision in grey tones.

For the assessment of visual agnosia, some of the tests described in the Assessment of Sensory and Motor Capacities section as well as some of those described in the Assessment of Visuoconstructive and Visuomotor aspects (in the section about visual blindness and visual agnosia) can be used. For the assessment of prosopagnosia, the test of Facial Recognition Test can be useful.[108] This test consists of 22 stimulus photographs to be used in 54 attempts. The patient must find a photograph that is the same as the stimulus among a sample of six similar photographs. This is done in three different ways. The first way shows six photographs of faces with frontal views. The second way shows the frontal-view photographs but taken from a different angle. The third has photographs with different degrees of shading on the faces. This test is carried out in 15 min. There is a shorter version using half of the stimulus material.[109]

Auditory agnosias

The same occurs in this sensory modality as in visual agnosias – from those related to the cortical perception of messages, i.e., *cortical deafness* (loss of auditory capacity due to lesion in the primary auditory areas), to those that are characterized by impairment of the capacity to recognize sounds while conserving the capacity to hear correctly, (i.e., auditory agnosia). For assessment of this section, the tests described in Assessment of Sensory/ Motor Capacity can be used.

Tactile agnosia

There is an area of the cortex, the somesthetic cortex, which specializes in recognizing objects held in the hand. It assures the reception and interpretation of proprioceptive as well as exteroceptive messages necessary for recognition of objects by touch. The incapacity to recognize objects via manual touch – feeling – is called *astereognosia* as long as no other sensory modality intervenes in perception, especially not recognizing an object by means of vision. Astereognosia is called *pure* when the patient is unable to recognize any object by touch in the absence of a sensory impairment. There is sensation but no knowledge of what it is.

Assessment of arithmetic and calculation capacities

It is important to include an assessment of these capacities in the neuropsychological examination as they are very sensitive to brain injury. There are two large groups of disorders, one of which is called acalculia,[110] referring to the loss of the ability to carry out calculus tasks as a result of some type of cerebral pathology (other authors call it acquired dyscalculia). The other group is referred to as dyscalculia, or developmental dyscalculia, and can be detected when there are defects in learning numerical skills.

At the same time, acalculias can be divided into *primary acalculia*, when there is a loss of numerical concepts and the ability to understand and/or execute basic arithmetical operations, and *secondary acalculia*, referring to the calculus deficit observed due to disorders in other cognitive capacities such as problems with memory, attention, language, etc. At present, other more complex and complete classifications can be established (see Table 13.1). To assess this function, the following aspects should be examined: if the patient has a numerical concepts (>; <; =), if he or she recognizes basic arithmetic symbols (+; –; ×; /; =), if he or she is capable of operating with them on a basic level and whether he or she can use elementary automatisms correctly (multiplication tables, putting them in correct place and order when working with paper and pencil, etc.). For this type of test it is more important to analyze the type and number of errors committed than the number of correct answers.

A test that fulfills these requirements related to arithmetic skills is *Luria's Diagnostic Neuropsychology*.[107] This subtest consists of two sections. The first section is dedicated to *comprehension of the numerical structure* and is in two parts: the first investigates comprehension, writing, and recognition of numbers in 15 different tasks; the second explores *numerical differences* with two specific tasks. The second section is *arithmetical operations*, divided into five different parts: the first has to do with *simple automatic calculations* in

Table 13.1 Classification of acalculias according to their etiology

Primary acalculia
  Anarithmetic
Secondary acalculia
  Aphasic acalculia
  Alexic acalculia
  Agraphic acalculia
  Frontal acalculia
  Spatial acalculia
Development dyscalculia
  Anarithmetic
  Alexia and agraphia
  Attentional problems
  Spatial problems
  Mixed

Reproduced by permission from Rosselli and Ardila.[111]

three tasks; the second deals with *complex arithmetic operations* and has four tasks; the third is called *arithmetic signs* and has three tasks; the fourth is *arithmetic operations series* with three tasks; and the last is called *consecutive arithmetic operations series*, with two tasks.

This section of the chapter has dealt with the major components of cognition including attention, executive functions, receptive functions, expressive functions, learning and memory, and conceptualization and reasoning.[7] Emphasis was placed on the neuropsychological assessment of each part. The intent was to be reasonably thorough, not exhaustive. Discussion will now turn to the evaluation of emotions and personality subsequent to ABI.

The assessment of emotions and personality

When a person has suffered a brain injury, naturally the main and initial concern is for his or her physical health. After all, brain injuries are often matters of life and death. For those who survive insults to the brain, attention then tends to shift toward residual deficits in bodily functioning and cognition. These can be tremendously limiting in terms of resuming one's former lifestyle. Not to be overlooked are changes in emotional well-being. According to Thomsen,[112] in the long term it is the patient's debilitated affective condition that compromises recovery from brain injury. Anxiety and depression, as well as personality disorders, are not uncommon following ABI.[113] Thus, assessment of an individual's emotional state is thought to be an integral part of a comprehensive neuropsychological evaluation.

The assessment of a patient's emotional status and personality characteristics is typically accomplished by way of examining previous records, interviewing the individual and significant others, observing verbal and non-verbal behaviors in testing sessions, and making sense of test data. Although cognitive instruments, for example, can and should be used to gather information that bears on emotions and personality, there are materials specifically designed for that purpose. Often objective personality tests are included in a neuropsychological battery, with perhaps the MMPI-2[114] being very well researched and the most frequently utilized instrument of this type. There is the legitimate argument that the MMPI-2 was not normed on individuals with documented brain damage. Also, neuropsychologically impaired patients may be at a particular disadvantage with regard to attending, comprehending, expressing, and otherwise completing the inventory in a meaningful way. Since the MMPI-2 comes equipped with validity scales, this feature certainly makes the test more appealing than alternative objective measures. At least some effort is made to understand the patient's approach to the evaluation. For example, depending on the configuration of scales L, F, and K, certain hypotheses may be generated with respect to the under-reporting or over-reporting of symptoms. Is a patient psychologically defensive or, perhaps, neurologically unaware, leading to high L and/or K? Is a patient making a "cry for help" or disinhibited given a high F and low L and K? Gass,[115] in an attempt to make the MMPI-2 more relevant to the brain-injured population, recommends that neuropsychologists employ the MMPI-2 Correction Factor for Closed Head Injury to properly interpret elevations on the clinical scales. There appear to be 14 MMPI-2 items that, when endorsed by patient with neurological disorders, confound the results of the test and, hence, the interpretation. The hope is that by being sensitive to the medical history of the patients when scoring the MMPI-2, the instrument will actually be more valid and efficacious in regard to assessing the emotional state and personality characteristics of persons with brain damage. As a rule, individuals who have had brain trauma produce elevated profiles[116] and tend to show high points on the so-called "neurotic triad" (i.e., hypochondriasis, depression, and hysteria) as well as on the schizophrenia scale.[7] Dikmen et al.[117] found the MMPI-2 useful in differentiating epilepsy patients with and without premorbid psychiatric histories. Lezak[7] has intimated that the MMPI-2 is not of assistance in localizing lesions.

The Beck Depression Inventory[118] is another objective test frequently included in a neuropsychological evaluation. Clearly, patients with brain damage are susceptible to sadness, disappointment, self-deprecation, and a whole host of symptoms that are subsumed under "depression". Suicidal thinking may also be a factor. The Beck attempts to assess many aspects of depression, but upon analysis, likely measures three main factors having to do with ideational depression, physiological depression, and behavioral depression.[119] In a similar vein, Byrne et al.[120] noted that the Beck addresses negativism, somatization, and performance difficulties. A study by Garske and Thomas[121] found that 55% of patients with severe ABI showed signs of depression on the Beck 50 months after injury. The Beck has not been advantageous in differentiating depression from dementia, however.[69] Further, the Beck has not consistently discriminated between patients with right vs.

left-sided cerebrovascular accidents.[122,123] From a test construction point of view, the Beck is considered to be face valid. Hence, malingering/dissimulation becomes a distinct possibility. The neuropsychologist must give careful consideration to the inclusion of this test in the battery.

The Symptom Check List 90-R (SCL-90-R)[124] seeks to assess patients' complaints secondary to medical and/or psychiatric illnesses. Lezak[7] has found the instrument to be helpful in highlighting individuals who have problems with attention and memory, and related obsessive-compulsive traits. Neuropsychologists are cautioned against over-interpretation of SCL-90-R data involving persons with brain injuries who have no premorbid psychiatric history.[7] As might be expected, individuals with brain damage, simply as a consequence of their current situation and not necessarily because of long-standing psychopathology, endorse certain health-related items.

There are additional objective measures of emotional state and personality as referenced by Judd.[32] The Behavior Change Inventory[125] provides an objective checklist to which patients and significant others respond with respect to personality prior to and following brain injury. Apparently few studies exist as to the neuropsychological efficacy of this test. In contrast, the Neurobehavioral Rating Scale[126] has produced favorable reliability and validity data, and attends to some functional aspects of recovery from brain injury. As the name suggests, the Coolidge Axis II Inventory[127] attempts to hone in on personality disorders in the context of neuropsychological dysfunction. The authors claim to be able to separate out mild TBI patients from normals. The Millon Clinical Multiaxial Inventory-III[128] and earlier versions, developed for use with psychiatric patients, have been employed inappropriately to check for personality disorders in the brain injury population.[69] The Neuropsychiatric Inventory[129] and The Frontal Lobe Personality Scale[35] are a couple of other objective tests neuropsychologists may want to add to their assessment armamentarium (see the Neurologically related Changes of Emotions and Personality Inventory in chapter 14).

As for projective measures of emotional state and personality, the advantage over objective tests is that patients typically have little if any idea of what they are communicating about themselves to the neuropsychologist. The underlying premise, of course, is that patients project inaccessible information from their unconscious minds. The Rorschach Ink Blot Test[130] came into existence out of Hermann Rorschach's desire to evaluate the perceptual efficiency of psychiatric patients.[69,78] The task is to examine the ambiguous stimuli and say what is seen. Certainly perception can be adversely affected by brain injury. Lezak[7] details Piotrowski's[131] system for diagnosing organic disturbances. Another standard projective personality test is the Thematic Apperception Test (TAT).[132] Patients examine a series of pictures and are asked to make up dramatic stories to explain what is currently happening, what has occurred to bring about the present situations, and what are the likely outcomes. Spreen and Strauss[69] acknowledge that the TAT is lacking in validity and reliability data though it has been included with some utility in the neuropsychological assessment. Further, patients have been known to engage in a type of catharsis by talking about themselves and their trauma as they conjecture about the characters and their lives as depicted on the TAT cards. The Incomplete Sentences Blank[133] is a third test generally considered to be a projective instrument that is more structured than both the Rorschach and the TAT. Patients are given sentence stems and finish the sentences as they wish. There are a total of 40 items with various themes, a few of which include sense of self, interpersonal relations, wishes, and regrets, and health. As with the TAT, although the test is not geared to individuals with brain damage per se, the information obtained can be quite enlightening for cognitive retraining and psychotherapeutic purposes.

Social consequences of ABI and assessment

The social consequences of moderate to severe ABI can be quite formidable. Whereas many persons with brain damage can learn to compensate reasonably well for their physical limitations and cognitive deficits, they frequently flounder when it comes to social adjustment. Changes in interpersonal relations, living arrangements, accessibility to community resources, driving, and work are generally responsible for impeding the recovery process. Adults who have experienced brain trauma to any great extent may show signs of social regression in the sense that they demonstrate self-absorption as seen in young children. Due to a neurologically based lack of awareness, they have trouble considering the needs of others and, hence, are lacking in their ability to interact in a manner that is mutually satisfying. This lack of awareness and self-absorption, unfortunately, can lead to enmity between persons with brain damage on the one hand, and family members and friends on the other. The degree to which family members feel burdened impacts upon living arrangements. Potentially, a rift may develop to the point that home healthcare, respite care, transitional living, or nursing home placements become distinct possibilities. Persons with brain damage may lose friends because the relationships become so one-sided and unrewarding.

As for assessing social aspects of ABI, Lezak and O'Brien[134] conducted a longitudinal study of 42 patients who suffered TBI. The Portland Adaptability Inventory (PAI)[135] was administered to participants. The findings indicated that difficulties in the social realm (versus the emotional or the physical) were voiced most frequently by patients as preventing improvement in their condition. The PAI seeks to measure individuals' range of social activities while containing items specific to significant relationships, residence, social contacts, self-care, leisure, and so on. Also, there are scales involving temperament and emotionality, and physical capabilities. This test may be one that the neuropsychologist would want to have in a battery as it has predictive validity.[7] Malec et al.[136] found the PAI to be more useful than strict neuropsychological test scores, for example, in estimating rehabilitation outcome.

The Katz Adjustment Scale (KAS)[137] has several forms, including those that are sensitive to behavioral symptoms and social behavior. Relatives complete the KAS, and the obtained data may be used in therapy to help alleviate the stresses and strains of life with brain injury. Further, the KAS has some utility for predicting vocational adjustment.

The Head Injury Family Interview (HIFI)[138] is a rather thorough evaluation of the individual at hand by parents, spouses, siblings, and children. Detailed information is ascertained with respect to behaviors, emotions, interpersonal skills, everyday functioning, and effects on the family. Judd[32] has reported that the HIFI has adequate reliability and encouraging validity data, making it worthy of inclusion in a neuropsychological assessment battery.

The Family Adaptability and Cohesion Scale (FACES)[139] addresses the patient's sense of integration within the family unit. As the name implies, the patient rates the family as to capacity for accommodation and degree of supportiveness. FACES has enjoyed success as both a research tool and a practical, therapeutic device.

The European Brain Injury Questionnaire (EBIQ)[140] was developed in an effort to document the emotional, personality, and social elements of patients' lives along with the consequences of cognitive dysfunction. Typically, the EBIQ is completed by the patient and a close relative for subjective accounts of the person with brain damage. The instrument also may provide a glimpse into the patient's premorbid condition versus his or her current status. At times, clinicians have been asked to fill out the EBIQ for another view of the patient. Again, this test can be very useful in individual and family psychotherapy as a stimulus for discussion around perceptions, expectations, and interpersonal issues in general. Relevant information as to the validity of the EBIQ has been reported by Teasdale et al.[141]

All of the aforementioned assessment instruments are worthy of consideration for neuropsychological evaluation purposes. They have direct application to treatment as well. Fitness for driving, with its ramifications for social consequences of moderate to severe ABI, cannot be readily assessed via neuropsychological tests. However, it would seem prudent to check the patient's performance on tasks measuring information processing speed, perceptual motor abilities, judgment, impulsivity, and frustration tolerance/anger level. Those who appear to be at risk should not only have to pass a written driving test, but ought to be checked out behind the wheel. Perhaps a "virtual" driving assessment and lessons can be offered prior to taking to the road.

Return to work is another issue with clear social ties that deserves the attention of the neuropsychologist. First of all, rather than trying to answer a global question about a patient's ability to return to work, the neuropsychologist is encouraged to assess for a specific job with appropriate vocational instruments. Referral to a vocational rehabilitation specialist may be necessary for this part of the larger evaluation. When test data is examined, the neuropsychologist must address strengths and weaknesses in the write-up with attention to social skills. The patient's interests have to be put into the mix as the neurologically impaired individual is probably less inclined to remain in a position that is boring to him or her. As with driving, a virtual work environment might be created in which the patient carries out job duties while under the supervision of trusted clinicians. Successive approximations of the actual job responsibilities can be added in as appropriate in hopes of shaping target behaviors. Scenarios that would likely tax the patient's coping skills can be simulated and worked through. Videotaping may prove to be an indispensable aid in this regard. Wehman[142] believes that experience at the job site in the form of supported employment is preferable to practice out of context. Alternatively, work trials of short duration with minimal assigned tasks may serve as a prelude to full employment. The neuropsychologist can be an invaluable resource involved in the transition process as the patient moves from unemployment, to pre-employment assessment, to work trials, to gainful employment. He or she may consult thereafter in troubleshooting and assisting the patient in efforts to remain on the job.

Concluding remarks

This chapter has integrated research findings with the classical tradition of neuropsychological assessment, trying to point out that both quantitative and qualitative methods of assessment are important for planning a rehabilitation program for acquired brain injury patients. Different tests, tasks and methods of exploring the patients are available, but the capacity to make sense out of the data resides in an expert neuropsychologist specializing in brain injury. The neuropsychologist must not forget that when using a concrete test, he or she is carrying out a practical demonstration of the theory underlying the instrument and that conceptual approach will determine the method of treating the patient. The reverse is also true: the method of rehabilitation also conditions the instruments which the neuropsychologist chooses for neuropsychological assessment. In any case, a neuropsychological assessment has to be made in order to seriously design a rehabilitation plan for a specific patient.

References

1. Broshek D., & Barth J. (2000). The Halstead–Reitan neuropsychological test battery. In G. Groth-Marnat (Ed.), *Neuropsychological assessment in clinical practice* (p. 223). New York: Wiley.
2. Luria, A. R. (1993). *The working brain: An introduction to neuropsychology*. New York: Basic Books.
3. Christensen, A. L. (1975). *Luria's neuropsychological investigation*. Copenhagen: Munskgaard.

4. Golden, C., Purisch, A. D., & Hammeke, T. A. (1985). *Luria–Nebraska neuropsychological battery: Forms I and II*. Los Angeles, CA: Western Psychological Services.

5. Sullivan, K., & Bowden, S. C. (1997). Which tests do neuropsychologists use? *J. Clin. Psychol., 53*, 657–661.

6. Piotrowski, Z., & Lubin, B. (1990). Assessment practices of health psychologists: survey of APA Division 38 clinicians. *Prof. Psychol. Res. Pract., 2*, 99.

7. Lezak, M. D. (1995). *Neuropsychological assessment* (3rd ed.). New York: Oxford University Press.

8. Barona, A., Reynolds, C., & Chastain, R. (1994). A demographic based index of premorbid intelligence for the WAIS-R+D. *J. Consult. Clin. Psychol., 52*, 885–890.

9. Mayeux, R., Sano, M., Chen, J., Tatemichi, T., & Stern, Y. (1991). Risk of dementia in first-degree relatives of patients with Alzheimer's disease and related disorders. *Arch. Neurol., 48*, 269–273.

10. Sbordone, R. J. (2000). The assessment interview in clinical neuropsychology. In G. Groth-Marnat (Ed.), *Neuropsychological assessment in clinical practice* (p. 94). New York; Wiley.

11. Levin, H. S., O'Donnell, V. M., & Grossman, R. G. (1980). The Galveston orientation and amnesia test: a practical scale to assess cognition after head injury. *J. Nerv. Ment. Dis., 167*, 675–684.

12. Jackson, W., Novak, T., & Dowler, R. (1998). Effectiveness serial measurement of cognitive orientation in rehabilitation: the Orientation Log. *Arch. Phys. Med. Rehabil., 79*(6), 718–720.

13. Dowler, R., Bush, B., Novack, T., & Jackson, W. (2000). Cognitive orientation in rehabilitation and neuropsychological outcome after traumatic brain injury. *Brain Inj., 14*(2), 117–123.

14. Artiola, L., Fortuny, L., Briggs, M., Newcombe, F., Ratcliff, G., & Tomas, C. (1980). Measuring the duration of post-traumatic amnesia. *J. Neurol. Neurosurg. Psychiat., 43*, 377–379.

15. McFarland, K., Jackson, L., & Geffe, G. (2001). Post-traumatic amnesia: consistency of recovery and duration of recovery following traumatic brain impairment. *Clin. Neuropsychol., 15*(1), 59–68.

16. Alderoso, A., & Novack, T. A. (2000). Measuring recovery of orientation during acute rehabilitation for traumatic brain injury: value and expectations of recovery. *J. Head Trauma Rehabil., 17*(3), 210–219.

17. Posner, M. I., & Petersen, S. E. (1990). The attention system of the human brain. *Ann. Rev. Neurosci., 13*, 25.

18. Salazar, A. M., Grafman, J. H., Vance, S. C., Weingartner, H., Dillon, J. D., & Ludlow, C. (1986). Consciousness and amnesia after penetrating head injury: neurology and anatomy. *Neurology, 36*, 178–187.

19. Mirsky, A. F., Anthony, B. J., Duncan, C. C., Ahearn, M. B., & Kellam, S. G. (1991). Analysis of the elements of attention: a neuropsychological approach. *Neuropsychol. Rev., 2*(2), 109–145.

20. Greenlief, C. L., Margolis, R. B., & Erker, G. J. (1985). Application of the trail making test in differentiating neuropsychological impairment of elderly persons. *Percept. Motor Skills, 61*, 1283.

21. Segalowitz, S. J., Unsal, A., & Dywan, J. (1992). CNV evidence for the distinctiveness of frontal and posterior neural processes in a traumatic brain-injured population. *J. Clin. Exp. Neuropsychol., 14*, 545.

22. Spreen, O., & Strauss, E. (1991). *A compendium of neuropsychological tests*. New York: Oxford University Press.

23. Sacks, T. L., et al. (1991). Comparability and stability of performance on six alternate forms of the Dodrill–Stroop color-word test. *Clin. Neuropsychol., 5*, 220.

24. Nehemkis, A. M., & Lewinsohn, P. M. (1972). Effects of left and right cerebral lesions on the memory process. *Percept Motor Skills, 35*, 787.

25. Connors, C. K. (1995). *Multi-health systems staff. Conners' continuous performance test*. Toronto: MHS.

26. Gordon, W. P. (1983). Memory disorders in aphasia – I. Auditory immediate recall. *Neuropsychologia, 21*, 325.

27. Gronwall, D. M. A. (1977). Paced auditory serial addition task: a measure of recovery from concussion. *Percept Motor Skills, 44*, 367.

28. Ponsford, J. L. (2000). In G. Groth-Marnat (Ed.), *Attention in neuropsychological assessment in clinical practice* (p. 355). New York: Wiley.

29. Robertson, I. H., et al. (1994). *The test of everyday attention*. Bury St. Edmunds: Thames Valley Test Company.

30. Grant, D. A., & Berg, E. A. (1948). A behavioral analysis of the degree of reinforcement and ease of shifting to new responses in a Weigl-type card sorting problem. *J. Exp. Psychol., 38*, 404.

31. Stuss, D. T., Benson, D. F., Kaplan, E. F., Della Malva, C. L., & Weir, W. S. (1984). The effects of prefrontal leucotomy on visuoperceptive and visuoconstructive tests. *Bull. Clin. Neurosci., 49*, 43–51.

32. Judd, T. (1999) *Neuropsychotherapy and community integration: Brain illness, emotions, and behavior*. New York: Kluwer Academic/Plenum.

33. Sohlberg, M. M., & Geyer, S. (1986). Executive functioning behavioral rating scale. Paper presented at Whittier College Conference Series, Whittier, CA.

34. Delis, D. C., et al. (2001). *Delis–Kaplan executive function system*. San Antonio, TX: The Psychological Corporation.

35. Grace, J., Malloy, P. F., & Stout, J. C. (1996). Assessing frontal behavioral syndromes: reliability and validity of the frontal lobe personality scale. Paper presented at the National Academy of Neuropsychology, New Orleans, LA.

36. Shallice, T. (1982). Specific impairments of planning. *Phil. Trans. R. Soc. Lond., 298*, 199.

37. Meier, M. J., Ettinger, M. G., & Arthur, L. (1982). Recovery of neuropsychological functioning after cerebrovascular infarction. In R. N. Malatesha (Ed.), *Neuropsychology and cognition*. The Hague, The Netherlands: Martinus Nijhoff.

38. Levin, H. S., Goldstein, O., Williams, O., & Eisenberg, O. (1991). The contribution of frontal lobe lesions to the neurobehavioral outcome of closed head injury. In H. S. Levin, H. M. Eisenberg, and A. L. Benton (Eds.), *Frontal lobe function and dysfunction*. New York: Oxford University Press.

39. Wechsler, D. (1991). *Wechsler intelligence scale for children* (3rd ed.). San Antonio, TX: The Psychological Corporation.

40. Ruff, R. M., Light, R. H., & Evans, R. W. (1987). The Ruff figural fluency test: a normative study with adults. *Dev. Neuropsychol., 3*, 37.

41. Christensen, A.-L. (1979). *Luria's neuropsychological investigation* (2nd ed.). Copenhagen: Munksgaard.

42. Halstead, W. C. (1947). *Brain and intelligence*. Chicago, IL: University of Chicago Press.

43. Grigsby, J., Kaye, K., & Robbins, L. J. (1990). Frontal lobe disorder, behavioral disturbance and independent functioning among the demented elderly. *Clin. Res.*, *38*, 81A.

44. Suchy, Y., Blint, A., & Osmon, D. C. (1997). Behavioral dyscontrol scale: criterion and predictive validity in an inpatient rehabilitation unit population. *Clin. Neuropsychol., 11*, 258.

45. Wilson, B. A., et al. (1996). *Behavioral assessment of the dysexecutive system.* Bury St. Edmunds: Thames Valley Test Company.

46. Butler, R. W., Anderson, L., Furst, C. J., & Namerow, N. S. (1989). Behavioral assessment in neuropsychological rehabilitation: a method for measuring vocational-related skills. *Clin. Neuropsychol., 3*, 235.

47. Golden, C. J. (1978). *Diagnosis and rehabilitation in clinical neuropsychology.* Springfield, IL: C. C. Thomas.

48. Albert, M. L. (1973). A simple test of visual neglect. *Neurology, 23*, 658.

49. Halligon, P. W., & Marshall, J. C. (1989). Is neglect (only) unilateral? A quadrant analysis of letter cancellation. *J. Clin. Exp. Neuropsychol., 11*, 793.

50. Mesulam, M.-M. (1985). *Principles of behavioral neurology.* Philadelphia, PA: F. A. Davis.

51. Poizner, H., Kaplan, E. F., Bellugi, U., & Padden, C. A. (1984). Visual–spatial processing in deaf brain-damaged signers. *Brain Cogn., 3*, 281–306.

52. León-Carrión, J. (1997). *Neuropsychological rehabilitation: Fundamentals, directions and innovations.* Del Ray Beach, FL: St. Lucie Press.

53. Lewis, R. F., & Rennick, P. M. (1979). *Manual for the repeatable cognitive–perceptual–motor battery.* Clinton Township, MI: Ronald F. Lewis.

54. Goldstein, G., et al. (1973). The validity of a visual searching task as an indication of brain damage. *J. Consult. Clin. Psychol., 41*, 434.

55. Reitan, R. M., & Davison, L. A. (1974). *Clinical neuropsychology: Current status and application.* New York: Winston/Wiley.

56. Benton, A. L., & Van Allen, M. W. (1968). Impairment in facial recognition in patients with cerebral disease. *Cortex, 4*, 344.

57. Benton, A. L., Eslinger, P. J., & Damasio, A. R. (1981). Normative observations on neuropsychological test performance in old age. *J. Clin. Neuropsychol., 3*, 33.

58. Street, R. F. (1931). *A Gestalt completion test.* New York: Bureau of Publications, Teachers' College, Columbia University.

59. McCarthy, R. A., & Warrington, E.K. (1990). *Cognitive neuropsychology: A clinical introduction.* San Diego, CA: Academic Press.

60. Wetzell, L., & Murphy, S. G. (1991). Validity of the use of a discontinue rule and evaluation of the Hooper visual organization test. *Neuropsychology, 5*, 119.

61. Rathburn, J., & Smith, A. (1982). Comment on the validity of Boyd's validation study of the Hooper visual organization test. *J. Consult. Clin. Psychol., 50*(2), 281–283.

62. Lewis, G., Campbell, A., & Takushi-Chinen, R., et al. (1997). Visual organization test performance in an African-American population with acute unilateral cerebral lesions. *Int. J. Neurosci.*, 295–302.

63. Exner, J. (1986). *Rorschach comprehensive system.* Madrid: Visor.

64. Baker, G. (1956). Diagnosis of organic brain damage in the adult. In B. Klopfer (Ed.), *Developments in the Rorschach technique.* New York: World Book.

65. Johnstone, B., Holland, D., & Larimore, C. (2000). In G. Groth-Marnat (Ed.),

Language and academic abilities in neuropsychological assessment in clinical practice. New York: Wiley.

66. Reitan, R. M., & Wolfson, D. (1989). The seashore rhythm test and brain functions. *Clin. Neuropsychol., 3*, 70.

67. Boone, K. B., & Rausch, R. (1989). Seashore rhythm test performance in patients with unilateral temporal lobe damage. *J. Clin. Psychol., 45*, 614–618.

68. Varney, N. R., & Damasio, H. (1987). Locus of lesion in impaired pantomime recognition. *Cortex, 23*, 699.

69. Spreen, O., & Strauss, E. (1998). *A Compendium of psychological tests: Administration, norms, and commentary* (2nd ed.). New York: Oxford University Press.

70. Reitan, R. M., & Wolfson, D. (1993). *The Halstead–Reitan neuropsychological test battery: Theory and clinical interpretation*. Tucson, AZ: Neuropsychology Press.

71. Jarvis, P. E., & Barth, J. T. (1994). *The Halstead–Reitan neuropsychological battery*. Odessa, FL: Psychological Assessment Resources.

72. Bender, M. B., Fink, M., & Green, M. (1951). Patterns in perception on simultaneous tests of face and hand. *A.M.A. Arch. Neurol. Psychiat., 66*, 355.

73. Storandt, M., Botwinick, J., & Danziger, W. L. (1986). Longitudinal changes: patients with mild SDAT and matched healthy controls. In L. W. Poon (Ed.), *Handbook for clinical memory assessment of older adults*. Washington, DC: American Psychological Association.

74. Lacks, P. (2000). Visuoconstructive abilities. In G. Groth-Marnat (Ed.), *Neuropsychological assessment in clinical practice* (p. 401). New York: Wiley.

75. Beaumont, J. G., & Davidoff, J. B. (1992). Assessment of visuo-perceptual dysfunction. In J. R. Crawford, D. M. Parker, and W. W. McKinlay (Eds.), *A handbook of neuropsychological assessment*. Hove, UK: Lawrence Erlbaum Associates Ltd.

76. Bender, L. (1938). A visual motor Gestalt test and its clinical use (p. 3). New York: American Orthopsychiatric Association. Research Monographs.

77. Heaton, R. K., Baade, L. E., & Johnson, K. L. (1978). Neuropsychological test results associated with psychiatric disorders in adults. *Psychol. Bull., 85*, 141.

78. Osterrieth, P. A. (1944). Le test de copie d'une figure complexe. *Arch. Psychol., 30*, 206.

79. McFie, J., & Zangwill, O. C. (1960). Visual construction disabilities associated with lesions of the left cerebral hemisphere. *Brain, 73*, 167.

80. Wechsler, D. (1981). *Wechsler adult intelligence scale*. San Antonio, TX: Psychological Corporation.

81. Black, F. W., & Bernard, B. A. (1984). Constructional apraxia as a function of lesion locus and size in patients with focal brain damage. *Cortex, 20*(1), 111–120.

82. Holland, D., Hogg, J., & Farmer, J. (1997). Fostering effective team cooperation and communication: developing community standards within interdisciplinary cognitive rehabilitation settings. *Neurorehabilitation, 1*, 21.

83. Kaplan, E. F., Goodglass. H., & Weintraub, S. (1983). *The Boston naming test* (2nd ed.). Philadelphia, PA: Lea & Febiger.

84. Sandson, J., & Albert, M. L. (1987). Perseveration in behavioral neurology. *Neurology, 37*, 1736.

85. Obler, L. K., & Albert, M. L. (1985). Language skills across adulthood. In J. Birren and K. W. Schaie (Eds.), *The psychology of aging*. New York: Van Nostrand Reinhold.

86. Wechsler, D. (1997). *WAIS-III manual*. San Antonio, TX: The Psychological Corporation.
87. Folstein, M. F., Folstein, S. E., & McHugh, P. R. (1975). Mini-mental state. *J. Psychiat. Res., 12*, 189.
88. Goodglass, H., & Kaplan, E. F. (1983). *Boston diagnostic aphasia examination (BDAE)*, Philadelphia, PA: Lea & Febiger.
89. Markwardt, F. C., Jr. (1989). *The Peabody individual achievement test*. Circle Pines, MN: American Guidance Service.
90. DeRenzi, E., Faglioni, P., & Sorgato, P. (1982). Modality-specific and supramodal mechanisms of apraxia. *Brain, 105*, 301.
91. Duffy, R. J., & Duffy, J.R. (1981). Three studies of deficits in pantomimic expression and pantomimic recognition in aphasia. *J. Speech Hearing Res., 24*, 70–84.
92. Fowler, R. S. (1969). A simple non-language test of new learning. *Percept. Motor Skills, 29*, 895.
93. Benton, A. (1974). *Revised visual retention test* (4th ed.). San Antonio, TX: The Psychological Corporation.
94. Warrington, E. K. (1984). *Recognition memory test*. Windsor, UK: NFER-Nelson.
95. Milner, B. (1972). Disorders of learning and memory after temporal lobe lesions in man. *Clin. Neurosurg., 19*, 421.
96. Rey, A. (1964). *L'examen clinique en psychologie*. Paris: Presses Universitaires de France.
97. Janowsky, J. S., Shimamura, A. P., & Squire, L. R. (1989). Source memory impairment in patients with frontal lobe lesions. *Neuropsychologia, 27*, 1043.
98. Ivnik, R. J., Sharbrough, F. W., & Laws, E. R., Jr. (1988). Anterior temporal lobectomy for the control of partial complex seizures: information for counseling patients. *Mayo Clin. Proc., 63*, 783–793.
99. Delis, D. C., et al. (1987). *California verbal learning test*. San Antonio, TX: The Psychological Corporation.
100. Hermann, B. P., Wyler, A. R., Richey, E. T., & Rea, J. M. (1987). Memory function and verbal learning ability in patients with complex partial seizures of temporal lobe origin. *Epilepsia, 28*, 547.
101. Brandt, J. (1991). The Hopkins verbal learning test: development of a new verbal memory test with six equivalent forms. *Clin. Neuropsychol., 5*, 125.
102. Buschke, H., & Fuld, P. A. (1974). Evaluation of storage, retention, and retrieval in disordered memory and learning. *Neurology, 11*, 1019.
103. Reitan, R. M., & Wolfson, D. (1993). *The Halstead–Reitan neuropsychological test battery: Theory and clinical interpretation*. Tucson, AZ: Neuropsychology Press.
104. León-Carrión, J., & Barroso y Martín, J. M. (1997). *Neuropsychology of thinking. Executive control and frontal lobe*. Sevilla: Kronos.
105. Raven, J. C. (1960). *Guide to the standard progressive matrices*. London: H. K. Lewis.
106. Chase, T. N., Fedio, P., Foster, N. L., Brooks, R., Di Chiro, G., & Mansi, L. (1984). Wechsler adult intelligence scale performance. Cortical localization by fluorodeoxyglucose F 18-positron emission tomography. *Arch. Neurol., 41*, 1244–1247.
107. Christensen, A. (1974). *Luria's neuropsychological investigation* (2nd ed.). Copenhagen: Munksgaard.

108. Benton, A., & Van Allen, M. (1968). Impairment in facial recognition in patients with cerebral disease. *Cortex, 4*, 344–358.
109. Levin, H., Hamsler, K., & Benton, A. (1975). A short form of the test of facial recognition for clinical use. *J. Psychol., 91*, 223–228.
110. Henschen, S. (1925). Clinical and anatomical contributions on brain pathology. *Arch. Neurol. Psychiat., 12*, 226–249.
111. Rosselli, M., & Ardila, A. (1997). Rehabilitation of calculation disorders. In J. León-Carrión (Ed.), *Neuropsychological rehabilitation: Fundamentals, innovations and directions.* Del Ray Beach, FL: St. Lucie Press.
112. Thomsen, I. V. (1984). Late outcome of very severe blunt head trauma: a 10–15 year second follow-up. *J. Neurol. Neurosurg. Psychiat., 47*, 260.
113. León-Carrión, J. (1997). *Neuropsychological rehabilitation: Fundamentals, directions and innovations.* Del Ray Beach, FL: St. Lucie Press.
114. Butcher, J. N., et al. (1989). *MMPI-2. Minnesota multiphasic personality inventory-2. Manual for administration and scoring.* Minneapolis, MN: University of Minnesota Press.
115. Gass, C. S. (2000). Assessment of emotional functioning with the MMPI-2. In G. Groth-Marnat (Ed.), *Neuropsychological assessment in clinical practice* (p. 457). New York: Wiley.
116. Filskov, S. B., & Leli, D. A. (1981). Assessment of the individual in neuropsychological practice. In S. B. Fiskov and T. J. Boll (Eds.), *Handbook of clinical neuropsychology.* New York: Wiley-InterScience.
117. Dikmen, S., Hermann, B. P., Wilensky, A. J., & Rainwater, G. (1983). Validity of the Minnesota Multiphasic Personality Inventory (MMPI) to psychopathology in patients with epilepsy. *J. Nerv. Mental Dis., 171*, 114.
118. Beck, A. T. (1987). *Beck depression inventory.* San Antonio, TX: The Psychological Corporation.
119. Bolon, K., & Barling, J. (1980). The measurement of self-rated depression: a multidimensional approach. *J. Genet. Psychol., 137*, 309–310.
120. Byrne, B. M., Baron, P., & Campbell, T. L. (1993). Measuring adolescent depression: factorial validity and invariance of the Beck Depression Inventory across gender. *J. Res. Adolesc., 3*, 127.
121. Garske, G. G., & Thomas, K. R. (1992). Self-reported self-esteem and depression: indexes of psychosocial adjustment following severe traumatic brain injury. *Rehabil. Counsel. Bull., 36*, 44.
122. Gordon, H. W. (1990). The neurobiological basis of hemisphericity. In Trevarthen, C. (Ed.), *Brain circuits and functions of the mind: Essays in honor of Roger W. Sperry.* Cambridge: Cambridge University Press.
123. Schramke, C., et al. (1996). Depression and anxiety following stroke: Separating distress from affective and anxiety disorders. Paper presented at the meeting of the International Neuropsychological Society, Chicago.
124. Derogatis, L. R. (1994). *SCL-90-R: Administration, scoring, and procedures manual.* Minneapolis, MN: National Computer Systems.
125. Hartlage, L. (1991). Assessment of behavioral sequelae of traumatic and chemical CNS insult. *Arch. Clin. Neuropsychol., 6*, 279.
126. Levin, H. S., et al. (1987). The neurobehavioral rating scale assessment of the behavioural sequelae of head injury by the clinician. *J. Neurol. Neurosurg. Psychiat., 50*, 183–193.
127. Coolidge, F. L., & Merwin, M. M. (1992). Reliability and validity of the

Coolidge axis II inventory: a new inventory for the assessment of personality disorders. *J. Pers. Assessm., 59,* 223–238.

128. Millon, T. (1994). *Millon clinical multiaxial inventory-III. Manual.* Minneapolis, MN: National Computer Systems.

129. Cummings, J. L. (1997). The neuropsychiatric inventory: assessing psychopathology in dementia patients. *Neurology, 48*(5) (Suppl. 6), 910.

130. Rorschach, H. (1951). *Psychodiagnostics.* New York: Grune & Stratton.

131. Piotrowski, Z. (1937). The Rorschach inkblot method in organic disturbances of the central nervous system. *J. Nerv. Ment. Dis., 86,* 525.

132. Bellack, L., & Bellack, S. (1974). *Children's apperception test.* Los Angeles, CA: Western Psychological Services.

133. Rotter, J. B., Lah, M. I., & Rafferty, J. E. (1992). *Rotter incomplete sentences blank* (2nd ed.). San Antonio, TX: The Psychological Corporation.

134. Lezak, M. D., & O'Brien, K. P. (1990). Chronic emotional, social, and physical changes after traumatic brain injury. In E. D. Bigler (Ed.), *Traumatic brain injury.* Austin, TX: Pro-ed.

135. Lezak, M. D., & O'Brien, K. P. (1988). Longitudinal study of emotional, social, and physical changes after brain injury. *J. Learning Disabil., 21,* 456–463.

136. Malec, J. F., Smigielski, J. S., DePompolo, R. W., & Thompson, J. M. (1993). Outcome evaluation and prediction in a comprehensive-integrated post-acute outpatient brain injury rehabilitation programme. *Brain Inj., 7,* 15–29.

137. Katz, M. M., & Lyerly, S. B. (1963). Methods for measuring adjustment and social behavior in the community: I. Rationale, description, discriminative validity and scale development. *Psychol. Rep., 13,* 503.

138. Kay, T., Caballo, M., Ezrachi, O., & Vavagiakis, P. (1995). The head injury family interview: a clinical and research tool. *J. Head Trauma Rehabil., 10*(2), 12–31.

139. Olsen, D. H. (1992). *Family inventories manual.* Minneapolis, MN: Life Innovations.

140. Deloche, G., Dellatolis, G., & Christensen. A.-L. (2000). The European brain injury questionnaire. In A.-L. Christensen and B. P. Uzzell (Eds.), *International handbook of neuropsychological rehabilitation.* New York: Kluwer Academic/ Plenum.

141. Teasdale, T. W., Christensen, O., & Willmes, O., et al. (1997). Subjective experience in brain-injured patients and their close relatives: a European brain injury questionnaire study. *Brain Injury, 11,* 543–563.

142. Wehman, P. H. (1991). Cognitive rehabilitation in the workplace. In J. S. Kreutzer and P. H. Wehman (Eds.), *Cognitive rehabilitation for persons with traumatic brain injury.* Bisbee, AZ: Imaginart International.

14 Sevilla Neuropsychological Test Battery (BNS) (version 2.0) for the assessment of executive functioning

José León-Carrión

Sevilla computerized Neuropsychological Test Battery (BNS) (version 2.0)

The Sevilla Neuropsychological Test Battery (BNS)[1,2] is a quantitatively and qualitatively easy-to-use tool for evaluating executive functioning of patients with neurological disorders: traumatic brain injury, cerebrovascular disorders, tumors, and adult dementia. For neurologically intact children, it is an ideal battery for assessing frontal factors which influence learning at school, as well as evaluating learning disabilities in children with neurological injury, and is very useful for designing neurological programs and for the evaluation of the rehabilitation. This battery adapts some of the classic tasks of evaluation to the computer. Some of these tasks (cancellation, Stroop and Tower of Hanoi) were adapted to the computer in other test batteries after computers appeared. The BNS version has been specifically adapted for neuropsychological assessment by means of computer. The 2.0 version is now available, having improved the 1.0 version in handling, ease, applicability, and adaption to any computer with the Windows operating system. BNS was designed to collect heterogeneous information about patients and to perform a data analysis, presenting output data in a most useful way for clinicians and investigators, thus making the possibility of constructing conclusions on clinical and experimental data essentially easier. The BNS system (Figure 14.1) allows comparison of heterogeneous data, personal medical data, testing data and parameters of brain activity. Personal medical data that are possible to store in the BNS database are:

1   Personal data about patient (name, age, profession, education), with the possibility of seeing a history of changes of basic social characteristics such as education and profession. Also, it is possible to see changes in a patient's appearance (in photographs), etc.
2   Information about drugs prescribed and taken at the moment of neuropsychological assessment.
3   Clinical record of past brain lesions.
4   Antecedents, etc.

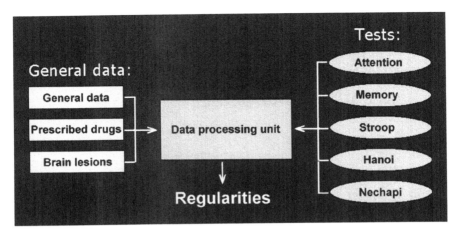

Figure 14.1 The BNS network.

The program can scan the large database with the purpose of finding a relationship between the results obtained by patients and brain lesions. This will allow finding new, undiscovered relationships and quickly obtain statistical norms for them. The data-processing unit will have a special program interface, allowing the addition of new processing tasks without recompiling the entire program. Some changes are made in version 2.0 to minimize interference of human factors in the assessment of a patient. Thus, all introductions and standard voice messages of the tests are recorded in advance and played during the test using a computer sound system: e.g., in Luria's test, the set of words is recorded and pronounced by a person with good diction. This will put all patients under the same conditions, so they will not depend on the voice, diction, and speech speed of the investigator.

The ease of handling the BNS, the possibility of obtaining a database for patients, the existence of abundant normative data, and its reliability and predictive validity, make the battery a practical instrument for neurological assessment of brain injury. In order to know the predictive validity of the battery, Pérez-Gil and Machuca[3] studied 175 subjects with and without brain injury. Results showed a high sensibility in the majority of the battery's subtests which classify subjects according to the severity of injury. The predictive value in some tasks was around 90% and never less than 65%. In the same way, these authors proved that the Tower of Hanoi/Sevilla test is the most efficient for classifying patients with brain injury according to Glasgow Coma Scale (GCS).

The use of computers for neurological evaluation should never substitute the neuropsychologist, but is fundamental as it is precise in the collection of data, with greater inter-rater reliability. The expert neuropsychologist should observe the data and the performance of the patients before giving a diagnosis or clinical judgment. The BNS facilitates the task of the neuropsychologist, providing a coherent system of evaluation to assess cognitive and emotional aspects related to the structure of the executive functioning.

The concept of executive functioning underlying the BNS

The Sevilla Neuropsychological Test Battery (BNS) stems from the evidence that the concept of executive functioning is multidimensional. That is to say, executive functions are a functional neural network that measure coherence, accuracy and meaning of the responses required of a person in life. Each subject has his or her particular way of responding to the the demands and challenges of the environment. Executive functions are described by their structure and dynamic. The structure is determined genetically (individual genes) and genomically (genes of the species), while the dynamic is their content, and depends on learning, social context and stimulation. The BNS is designed especially for the evaluation of the executive structure and not its dynamic.

The *structure* of executive functions basically depends on the prefrontal zones of the brain which are genetically configured especially in humans who, instead of having reflex reactions like animals, have varied reactions with different degrees of sophistication, creativity, and/or originality. The group of tasks or subtests comprising executive functioning are: timing, activation/inhibition, working memory, and decision making. The executive *dynamic* depends on the configuration of the subjects' limbic systems and the relationship of the limbic system with the frontal lobe.

Assessment of executive functioning (Figure 14.2) is carried out by different tasks performed by the subject (see Table 14.1). The first group of subtests assesses the attentional mechanisms, which are the basis of executive functioning. The second group assesses and appraises memory of the task and the processes of learning via a revision of Luria's original test, Luria's Memory Words (LMW). The third assesses control evaluation and cognitive interferences. The fourth evaluates the functions associated with decision making (problem solving, planning, prospectives, etc.).

Evaluation of attentional mechanisms: letter cancellation subtests

The evaluation of attention is fundamental and one of the processes that is first altered in patients with neurological injury. It plays an important role in all cognitive processes since all psychological functions consume attention. Attentional deficits can secondarily impair memory, reasoning, language, and executive functioning, among others, so it is essential to have data on the functioning of the attentional mechanism in patients who are being evaluated neuropsychologically.

Attention is one of the components of executive functions.[4,5] In concept, the BNS attentional tests evaluate the *posterior attentional system* proposed

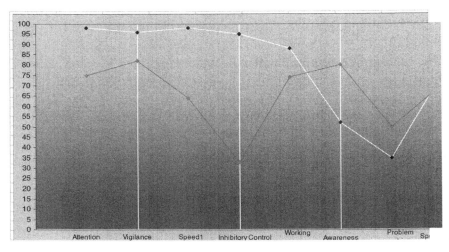

Figure 14.2 Graphic representation of the score obtained by two different patients. The two curves represent two different disorders of structural executive functioning. While the white curve reflects a person who has impairment in awareness of deficits and in the problem-solving capacity, the black curve shows a person's serious problem with inhibitory control, also affecting the problem-solving ability.

Table 14.1 Subtests for the assessment of structural executive functioning in BNS

1. Evaluation of attentional mechanisms
   1.1 Evaluation of simple attention or tonic alertness
   1.2 Evaluation of vigilance or phasic alertness
   1.3 Evaluation of centered tachitoscope attention
   1.4 Evaluation of tachitoscope attention left eye
   1.5 Evaluation of tachitoscope attention right eye
2. Evaluation of memory processes and of learning
3. Evaluation of neurocognitive interferences (Stroop effect)
4. Assessment of decision making capacity: tower of Hanoi–Sevilla
5. Assessment of neurologically related emotional/personality changes

by Posner and Petersen in 1990, which is integrated, among others, into zones of the parietal cortex, thalamic areas associated with the pulvinar and reticular nuclei and superior colliculus and/or surrounding areas. For Riccio et al.:[6] "Assessment of attention and executive control must be multifaceted, paralleling the complexity of the functional systems involved. The best any single measure can provide, including the continuous performance test, is data on specific aspects of attention and executive control that, in conjuction with other measures, can be considered in diagnostic hypothesis generation and in the monitoring of the treatment of rehabilitation process." According to Cohen and colleagues,[7] continuous performance tests (CPT) are a measure of selective attention, inhibition or filtering of attention as well as response selection and control. These authors also consider that reaction time can be viewed as cognitive efficiency and processing capability.

Attentional tests should be simple. Attentional mechanisms are evaluated in a series of tasks which measure alertness and vigilance through efficacy of perceptual and motor velocity and reaction time. The tasks are a computerized version of the classic task of cancelling letters, divided into:

1   Simple subtest of attention (tonic alertness).
2   Conditioned subtest of attention (phasic alertness).

In both subtests, the task performed consists of the patient pressing the space bar on the keyboard every time the letter O appears in the center of the screen. In the first subtest, the patient only has to be aware of the appearance of the letter O for a fixed time.

This subtest measures the patient's basic attention capacity or tonic alertness, selective visual capacity, perceptive and motor speed, and the ability to activate simple attentional mechanisms. In a study by León-Carrión and colleagues,[8] focus and execution are observed through the errors committed while doing the task and represent perceptual and motor speed. The ability to sustain one's attention is observed through the omissions made by the patient representing vigilance and alertness. Other authors[9] also found that correct hits and omission errors are indicative of alertness as well as the patient's capacity to focus on the target. This task determines the minimum attention level required for other cognitive processes.

The second subtest is basically the same as the previous one with a small modification: the patient should press the space bar when the letter O appears only when immediately preceded by the letter X. This is a sustained test of vigilance in monotonous and unappealing tasks. Errors made in this task are also related to perceptual and motor speed. Vigilance capacity requires frontal use of activation/inhibition mechanisms.

Studies of individuals with identifiable brain damage suggest a direct relationship between impairment on the CPT and the extent to which the damage/dysfunction is diffuse as opposed to focal, regardless of the etiology of the damage. Studies also consistently demonstrate sensibility to CNS dysfunction in those individuals where the brain damage is presumed rather than identifiable.[6]

Evaluation of hemianopia and hemiattention: tachitoscopic subtests of attention

In a strict sense, the phenomenon of visual inattention or negligence is the omission of visual stimuli in the left visual field which directly depends on the lesions produced in the right hemisphere, usually coinciding with lesions located in posterior zones (Figure 14.3). There are other types of disorders in

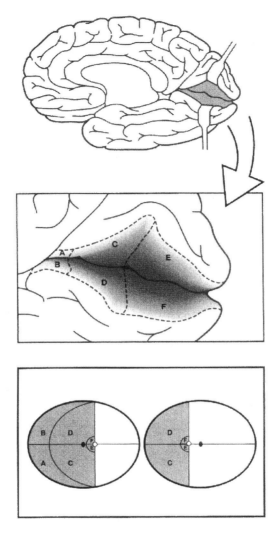

Figure 14.3 Mapping the visual field onto primary visual cortex. The posterior 50% of primary cortex (EF) encodes the central 10% of the visual field. The middle 40% (CD) encodes the peripheral field except the impaired temporal crescent of the visual field, which is encoded by the anterior 10% of visual cortex (AB) Reproduced by permission from Trobe (2001)[11].

the anterior zone, those of hemiattention, which are defects in some of the visual hemispheres not classified as negligence. Another different phenomenon is hemianopia, referring to the loss of vision in one half of the visual field. All of these disorders appear when the subject is made to focus his or her attention on a certain fixed point that appears in the center of the screen while being presented with stimuli in each of the existing visual quadrants/hemispheres (Figure 14.4).[10]

For evaluating problems of inattention and hemianopia, a letter cancellation test via a computer-adapted *tachitoscope* method is used. The patient must keep looking at a fixed point in the center of the screen while different letters appear in the center of each of the four quadrants the computer screen is divided into. The patient stares at the central point and, without deviating from it, must press the space bar only once when the letter O appears. The *hemianopic defects* are caused by lesions of the optic chiasm and retrochiasmal pathways. All lesions of the chiasm selectively damage the median bar of the chiasm where nerve fibers cross (Figure 14.5). The vulnerability of this region derives from its relatively weak arterial supply, resulting, when damaged, in a temporal visual field defect whose border occurs at the vertical meridian: a temporal hemianopia.[11] The retrochiasmal lesions produce deficits denominated homonymous (in the same side of visual space), producing homonymous hemianopia. When the defect affects only one of the quadrants of the visual fields, we find a quadrantanopia (Figure 14.6).

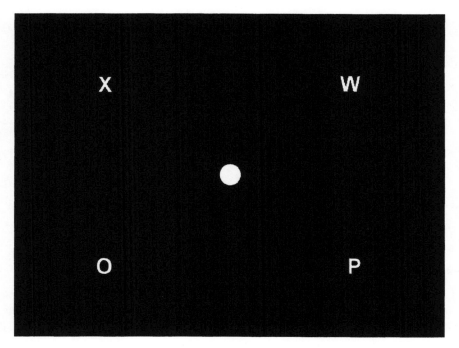

Figure 14.4 Screen showing the four quadrants where a letter appears while the patient looks at the fixed point in the center.

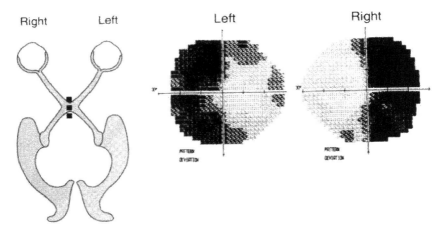

Figure 14.5 Chiasmal lesion (left), causing bitemporal hemianopia (right). Reproduced by permission from Trobe (2001)[11].

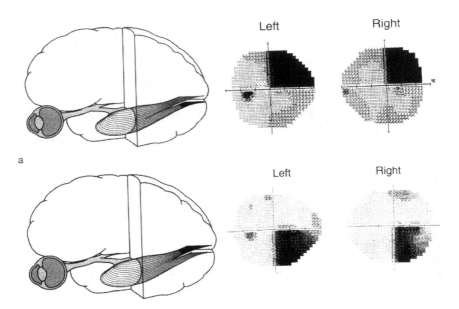

Figure 14.6 Visual field deficits associated with primary visual cortex lesions. (a) Right superior homonymous quadrantanopia (right) caused by damage to left inferior cortex (left). (b) Right inferior homonymous quadrantanopia (right) caused by damage to left superior visual cortex (left). Reproduced by permission from Trobe (2001)[11].

Evaluation of memory processes and learning

The most classic tests used for neuropsychological evaluation of verbal memory and processes of learning have consisted in giving the patient a more or less extensive list of words and in one or several tries he or she should store them and then repeat them. Based on this idea, Luria developed his "Memory Curve"[12] as a test to evaluate working memory that would later be adopted by Christensen[13] to evaluate the learning process. Different memory indexes are provided which are related to the capacity and quality of memory processes and difficulties in learning and memorizing. The Sevilla Neuropsychological Battery revises this test by adding new indexes for the learning process and different indexes of memory. The computer is used for its administration and correction, allowing qualitative and quantitative interpretation.

The subtests for the assessment of memory evaluate more than working memory (see Table 14.1). Conceptually, BNS working memory (or, in the terminology of Baddeley and Hitch,[14] the articulatory or phonological loop) refers to volume of memory, a system for the temporary holding of information necessary to perform a range of task such as comprehension, learning and reasoning. It is "on-line memory". Working memory has a limited capacity and is defined as the amount of information that can be held simultaneously and the length of time that information can be kept on-line. When we listen to other people, we are using working memory to hold the segments of sentences "on-line" millisecond by millisecond. The adjective "working" is a critical part of the definition, emphasizing as it does the *processing* of information and not its particular content. Working memory is characterized by its limited storage capacity and rapid turnover and is differentiated from the larger capacity and archival memory system traditionally defined as long-term memory. When we perform a mental arithmetic problem, recall a phone number, plan a hand of bridge or a chess move, or follow verbal instructions, we use working memory. In fact, it is difficult to think of a cognitive function that does not engage the working-memory systems of the brain. A number of different models have been proposed regarding the functional architecture of human cognition.[15] Individuals differ in the total amount of activation available to their systems. The idea that verbal working memory includes both storage and repetitive components is a cornerstone of behavioral research on working memory.[16]

In the BNS, the patient has to remember a list of ten words to be recited to the examiner or by the computer at a rhythm of one word per second. Previously, the patient has appraised the words he or she thinks they will be able to remember in each of the attempts, so that the patient's level of knowledge about his or her mnesic ability can be evaluated at the end of the test. This task is repeated ten times, independently of whether the patient is able or not to remember all the words. Thirty minutes after the last try the patient is asked to say all the words he or she can remember without the examiner reading them previously so that information can be obtained about the degree of consolidation of the patient's memory. Indices of primacy and recency effects, mnesic contamination, memory volume and mnesic gain, among others, are also obtained (Table 14.2).

The assessment of learning processes is the other objective of LMW (revised; LMW–R) included in the BNS. A study was conducted in order to find the underlying neuroanatomical site of learning processes.[17] Subjects in the study included seven severe traumatic brain injury patients with severe memory disorders after discharge from hospital. All underwent a regional cerebral blood flow measurement by Xe inhalation technique using 32 scintillation detectors placed in a helmet-type holder. All patients belong to a severe memory problem rehabilitation group and were assessed through LMW–R (Figures 14.7 and 14.8). Regional cerebral blood flow data of all patients showed a hypoperfusion in the left temporal infero-posterior lobe, more acute on the left side and slight hypoperfusion in right infero-parietal. Other zones of the brain show a normal level of CBF. All patients have poor scores in memory measures, showing a global capacity of memory of 61%. These results show evidence for criterion validity of LMW–R for the assessment of

Table 14.2 Memory processes assessed through Luria's Memory Words (revised in BNS)

Working memory	Memory volume [real memory]
Total recall	Memory volume including fabulated and or repeated material
Contamination	Quantity of remembered material but not real
Fabulation	Number of invented words
Repetition	Number of repeated words
Index of adherence	Number of words repeated in two or more consecutive trials
Index of aspiration	The volume of memory the subject believes that he/she has.
Index of self-knowledge	Difference between the index of aspiration and real memory
Index of primacy	Primacy effect
Index of recency	Recency effect
Index of learning 1	Difference of learning between the final and central part of the tests
Index of learning 2	Difference of learning between the central and initial part of the tests
Index of learning 3	Difference of learning between the final and initial part of the tests
Index of consolidation	Percentage of equal words remembered in the last three trials
Index of memory gain	Difference between what one remembers in the last three trials and the first trial

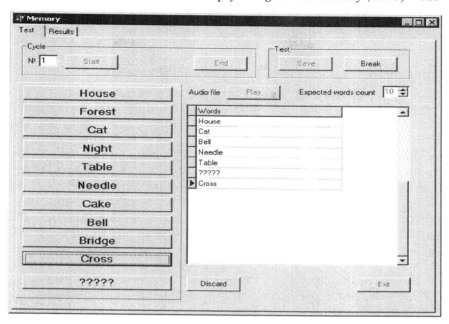

Figure 14.7 Screen of Luria's Memory Words–Revised (LMW–R). The psychologist has to click the words on the left every time the patient says one. Every word clicked appears on the right.

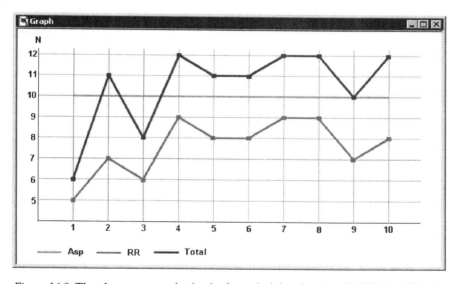

Figure 14.8 The three curves obtained after administering the LMW–R. ASP, the awareness curve; RR, the real memory curve; Total, total recall curve. These three curves do not coincide in reflecting the patient's problem.

patients with severe memory deficits associated to a functional disorder in the temporal lobes.

Evaluation of neurocognitive interferences: Stroop effect

Each of the functional systems of the brain possesses a neural network highly specialized in a balance system which is controlled between mechanisms of activation and inhibition that allow some systems to be activated at the same time, while others remain either deactivated or inhibited to maintain a level of optimum efficacy and precision in different cognitive proceses for adequate functioning.[18] The mechanisms implicated in this double process of activation/inhibition are varied. Those that stand out in importance are: the frontal lobe, which plays a central role in inhibiting irrelevant information; the prefrontal dorsolateral zone, which is important in continuously maintaining the information that requires deferred response; the basal ganglia, which are implicated in the inhibition of some automatic processes. Selectively attending to one source of information to the exclusion of others is either a separate executive process or a critical feature of many executive processes.[19] The allocation of attention is critical when there are multiple sources of information competing for processing.

The Sevilla Neuropsychological Battery (BNS) includes a computerized adaptation of Stroop's classic *Words and Colors* test (1935), originally designed for studying perceptive interference (Figure 14.9). The specialists who have presented the most relevant research on this test agree that it includes studying mechanisms of divided attention, the functioning of the activation/inhibition mechanisms and also that of the neurocognitive interference mechanism. Four subtests are used to observe these mechanisms:

1   Identification of monochromatic words.
2   Identification of blocks of color.
3   Identification of color disregarding content (both eyes).
4   Identification of content disregarding color (both eyes).

The first and second subtests introduce the patient to the mechanics of this test and appraise his or her minimum visual and reading capacities necessary for the rest of the subtests. The third and fourth subtests appraise the actual Stroop effect with the patient responding only to one of the characteristics of the stimulus (color of writing or written word) and inhibiting the other.

Positron Emission Tomography (PET) with H215O was used to further validate Stroop's test to measure frontal lobe functions by Ravnkilde et al.[20] Stroop interference was found to activate the left anterior cingulate cortex, the supplementary motor cortex, thalamus, and the cerebellum. Although the prominent anterior cingulate activation is in the frontal lobe, it is not prefrontal. The author concluded that these results bring this test closer to being a specific test of prefrontal functions. In a study by

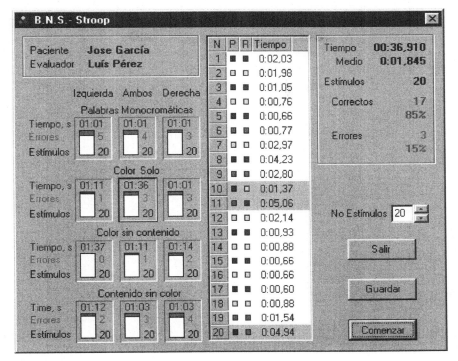

Figure 14.9 Screen showing the Stroop results of a patient in the Spanish version of the test.

MacDonald et al.[21] using event-related fMRI and the Stroop paradigm, it was found that incongruent stimuli (RED in blue ink) produce more conflict than congruent stimuli (RED in red ink); conflicting monitoring regions should activate incongruent color-naming trials. Anterior cingulate cortex (ACC) showed this pattern, and greater activation correlated with greater Stroop effects ($r = 0.41$). This suggests that Dorsolateral prefrontal cortex (DLPFC) contributes to strategic, and ACC contributes to evaluative processes in cognitive control.

Assessment of decision making capacity: the Tower of Hanoi–Sevilla

The revision of the literature specializing in problem solving, planning, prospectives, control and execution associates these functions to the frontal lobe when there is brain injury in these areas, especially in the prefrontal zones.[10,22] The classic tests used to evaluate these functions have been classifying tasks such as the *Wisconsin Card Sorting Test*,[23] tests of categories such as the *Category Test*[24] or labyrinth tests like the *Porteus Maze Test*.[25]

At present, clinical neuropsychological specialists agree that highly structured tests are not sensitive to the deficits observed when evaluating goal-oriented behavior. They defend the use of less structured tests in which the subject actively tries to discover the rules and bases that regulate them as they are the ones that can evaluate this capacity better.[26]

Following the principle of using less structured tests, together with the facility for correction and interpretation, a computerized version of the Tower of Hanoi test[27] has been used within the Sevilla Neuropsychological Battery which, due to the modifications carried out for this version, is called the Tower of Hanoi–Sevilla.[28,29] The task consists of a transformation problem in which a goal has to be achieved after execution of a series of non-routine movements where it is necessary to use orderly planning and complex abilities of problem solving. Subjects must come up with a plan to execute and reach the correct solution. This plan should include a global solution that likewise is divided into various sub-solutions sequenced in time to achieve the global objective. All of these abilities of planning for solving complex problems are seriously affected by lesions affecting the frontal lobe after TBI and can be seen when performing the Tower of Hanoi–Sevilla.[30]

The test consists of 3 parallel bars numbered 1–3, from left to right (Figure 14.10). There are discs of different sizes and colors (from 3 to 5, chosen by the person tested) on bar number 1 forming a pyramid with the largest at the base and the smallest at the top. The goal is to move the different discs by introducing the number on the rod with the computer keyboard until a tower is

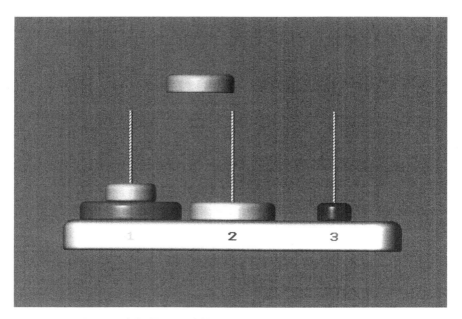

Figure 14.10 Screen of the Tower of Hanoi–Sevilla with five disks.

formed which is the same on the number 3 bar. Two kinds of administration are observed with the Sevilla version of the Tower of Hanoi, A and B, which are different from each other and allow or do not allow the subject to learn the principles or rules that govern the task. The A administration is that which better describes the means to solve the problems since the subject should discover the rules and principles of the test in order to solve it correctly.

A sample of 40 patients who had survived serious traumatic brain injury (GCS < 8), divided into two groups of 20 subjects each, were studied by León-Carrión and colleagues.[31] One group was composed of patients with frontal lesions and the other composed of patients having lesions other than frontal lobe. All of them were administered the Tower of Hanoi–Sevilla. Significant differences were found between the two groups in all the variables studied throughout this test. In the scores of total time ($p < 0.007$) and total movements ($p \leq 0.043$), the frontal group took more time than the non-frontal group. The frontal group also committed more errors of type 1 ($p < 0.000$) and type 2 ($p < 0.020$). The results showed that, as a group, the achievements of the non-frontal lesion group reach more sophisticated levels in their strategies. Subjects with frontal lesions have a limited capacity for using strategies. Their data confirms that the Tower of Hanoi–Sevilla is able to detect patients with frontal executive problems.

Neurologically-related Changes of Personality Inventory (NECHAPI)

The assessment of emotional aspects was not traditionally included as part of the neurological evaluation, but nowadays it has become essential in designing rehabilitation programs. For this reason, the battery includes a specific test to evaluate the emotional changes in brain injury patients.

NECHAPI is a clinical tool especially designed for observing the most frequent emotional changes found in patients with TBI, stroke, cerebral tumors, and other neurological disorders. This inventory consists of 40 items that a family member scores from 1 to 5, depending on how he or she thinks they define the patient: 5 indicates high frequency occurrence and 1 a minimum frequency. There are also intermediate scores. The family member has to score each item twice: the first score refers to the patient's condition before the neurological affectation, and the second refers to his or her present state. The 40 items on this test are grouped into five categories (Table 14.3) that family members must score with regard to the patient.

According to the study by Madrazo et al. in 1999, patients who had suffered severe TBI showed significant changes in emotional and behavioral aspects as seen in the reference values of NECHAPI.[2] In this study, emotional vulnerability was the factor that had the most frequent changes in this type of patient: 75% of them became more emotionally vulnerable. It also found that the irritability factor had changes in a high percentage of patients with a significance of 56.25%. The data indicated that sensation seeking

Table 14.3 NECHAPI test categories

1. *Irritability.*   High scores in this category indicate a tendency to be sensitive to offence and, therefore, interpreted as a threatening situation. It also indicates that the response to these apparently normal situations can be aggressive.
2. *Sensation seeking.*   When there are high scores in this category, it usually refers to people who want to experience new sensations and can also imply risks. This has often occurred in young people before suffering TBI.
3. *Emotional vulnerability.*   People with high scores in this area usually have very intense personal relationships, are easily influenced and have a tendency for depression and frustration.
4. *Sociability.*   This factor measures the quantity of social relations the patient has. If the scores are high, he or she normally has a facility for social relations and feels comfortable when surrounded by people.
5. *Emotional coldness.*   High scores in this area shows difficulty in feeling motivated by things. It also shows emotional coldness when faced with others' proposals and thoughts.

Table 14.4 Percentage of patients showing significant emotional changes after traumatic brain injury

Factors measured by NECHAPI	Percentage of patients showing significant change
Irritability	63
Sensation seeking	63
Emotional vulnerability	84
Sociability	42
Affective indifference	42

decreased an average of 23% in these patients and was significant in 50% of them. The changes which were observed and the percentage of patients with said changes are presented in Table 14.4. According to a study done by Vernè et al.,[32] patients who have suffered severe TBI showed significant changes in emotional and behavioral aspects according to the reference values of NECHAPI.[2] In this study, they observed that emotional vulnerability is a factor which most frequently showed changes in this type of patient: 75% become more emotionally vulnerable according to the reference values of the tests. It is also found that the irritability factor changed in a high percentage of the patients, being significant in 56.25%. Data indicated that the factor of sensation seeking decreased an average of 23% in these patients and was significant in 50% of them.

Conclusions

The Sevilla Neuropsychological Battery is an instrument to be used in the assessment of patients with neurological and acquired brain injury. The BNS offers a good level of reliability and validity for qualitative and quantitative diagnosis for classifying the severity of the injury and for following the evolution of the patients in a rehabilitation process. The battery also offers standardized normative data and makes neuropsychological evaluation more precise and reliable in order to design the rehabilitation program a given patient should follow afterwards.

References

1. León-Carrión, J. (1994). *Manual of human neuropsychology*. Madrid: Siglo XXI.
2. León-Carrión, J. (1998). Neurologically-related Changes in Personality Inventory (NECHAPI): a clinical tool addressed to neurorehabilitation planning and monitoring effects of personality treatment. *NeuroRehabilitation, 11*, 129–139.
3. Pérez-Gil, J. A., & Machuca Murga, F. (1999). Predictive validity of Sevilla Neuropsychological Battery (BNS) for traumatic brain injury. *Revist. Esp. Neuropsicol., 1*(1), 49–66.
4. Cohen, R. A. (1993). Attentional control: subcortical and frontal lobe influences. In R. A. Cohen (Ed.), *The neuropsychology of attention*. New York: Plenum.
5. Stuss, D. T., & Benson, D. F. (1984). Neuropsychological studies of the frontal lobes. *Psychol. Bull., 5*, 3–28.
6. Riccio, C. A., Reynolds, C., & Lowe, P. (2001). *Clinical applications of continuous performance tests: Measuring attention and impulsive responding in children and adults*. New York: Wiley.
7. Cohen, J. D., Barch, D. M., Carter, C. S., & Servan-Schreiber, D. (1999). Context-processing deficits in schizophrenia: converging evidence from three theoretically motivated cognitive tasks. *J. Abnorm. Psychol., 108*(1), 120–133.
8. León-Carrión, J., Rodriguez-Duarte, R., Barroso y Martín, J. M., Machuca, F., Domínguez-Morales, R., Murillo, F., et al. (1996). The attentional system in brain injury survivors. *Int. J. Neurosci., 85*, 231–236.
9. Gordon Systems Inc. (1986). *Technical manual for the Gordon diagnostic system*. New York: Dewitt.
10. León-Carrión, J., & Barroso y Martín, J. M. (1997). *Neurology of thinking: Executive control and frontal lobe*. Colección Neurociencias. Sevilla: Editorial Kronos.
11. Trobe J. (2001). *The neurology of vision*. Oxford: Oxford University Press [figure, p. 127].
12. Luria, A. R. (1966). *Higher cortical functions in man*. New York: Basic Books.
13. Christensen, A. L. (1974). *Luria's neuropsychological investigation: Text*. Copenhagen: Mungsgaard.
14. Baddeley, A. D., & Hitch, G. J. (1974). *Working memory*. In G. Bower (Ed.), *The psychology of learning and motivation* (pp. 47–89). New York: Academic Press.
15. Goldman-Rakic, P. S. (1987). Circuitry of primate prefrontal cortex and regulation of behaviour by representational memory. In F. Plum and U. Mouncastle (Eds.), *Handbook of physiology* (pp. 373–417). Washington, DC: American Physiological Society.
16. AWh, E., Smith, E., & Jonides, J. (1995). Human rehearsal processes and the frontal lobes: PET evidence. *Ann. N.Y. Acad. Sci., 769*, 97–117.
17. León-Carrión, J., & Domínguez Morales, R. (2000). Luria's Memory Words Test-

Revised: A study of regional cerebral blood flow in traumatic brain injury patients. *Revist. Esp. Neuropsicol., 2*, 92–103.

18. Zacks, R., & Hasher, L. (1994). Assessing frontal lobe function in children: views from developmental psychology. *Dev. Neuropsychol., 4*, 199–210.

19. Smith, E., & Jonides, J. (1999). Storage and executive processes in the frontal lobes. *Science, 283*, 1657–1661.

20. Ravnkilde, B., Videbech, P., Rosenberg, R., Gjedde, A., & Gade, A. (2002). Putative tests of frontal lobe function: a PET-study of brain activation during Stroop's test and verbal fluency. *J. Clin. Exp. Neuropsychol., 24*, 534–547.

21. MacDonald, A. W., Cohen, J. D., Stenger, Pérez-Santamaría,V. A., & Carter, C. S. (2000). Dissociating the role of the dorsolateral prefrontal and anterior cingulate cortex in cognitive control. *Science, 288*, 1835–1838.

22. Lezak, M. D. (1995). *Neuropsychological assessment.* Oxford: Oxford University Press.

23. Grant, P. B., & Berg, E. A. (1948). A behavioral analysis of degree of reinforcement and case of shifting to new response in a weigle-type card-sorting problem. *J. Exp. Psychol., 38*, 404–411.

24. Halstead, W. C. (1947). *Brain and intelligence. A quantitative study of the frontal lobes.* Chicago: University of Chicago Press.

25. Porteus, S. D. (1950). *The Porteus maze test and intelligence.* Palo Alto, CA: Pacific Books.

26. León-Carrión, J. (1995). *Manual de neuropsicología* [Handbook of Neuropsychology]. Madrid/México: Siglo XXI Editorial.

27. Gagné, R. M., & Smith, E. C. (1962). A study of the effects of verbalization on problem solving. *J. Exp. Psychol., 63*, 12–18.

28. León-Carrión, J., Morales, M., Forastero, P., Domínguez, M. R., Murillo, F., Jimenez-Baco, R., & Gordon, P. (1991). The computerized Tower of Hanoi: a new form of administration and suggestions for interpretation. *Percept. Motor Skills, 73*, 63–66.

29. León-Carrión, J. (1999). *Sevilla computerized neuropsychological test battery.* Madrid: TEA.

30. Madrazo, M., Machuca Murga, F., Barroso y Martín, J. M., Domínguez Morales, R., & León-Carrión, J. (1999). *Emotional changes after severe traumatic brain injury.* Congreso Virtual de Neuropsicología (Internet).

31. Barroso y Martín, J. M., León-Carrión, J., Murillo, F., Domínguez, J. M., & Muñoz, M. A. (1999). Executive functioning and capacity for problem solving in patients with traumatic brain injury. *Revist. Esp. Neuropsicol., 1*, 3–21.

32. Vernè, D., Mazzanato, T., Torrini, G., & Barettini, R. (2001). Functional outcome and instability of neurobehavioral factors in TBI subjects. In Abstract Book (p. 416), 4th World Congress on Brain Injury, Torino.

15 Methods and tools for the assessment of outcome after brain injury rehabilitation

José León-Carrión

Introduction

The evaluation of functional outcome after discharge from hospital in individuals with acquired brain injury (ABI) has become an important part of rehabilitation programs. Evaluation is the best way to corroborate the effectiveness of treatment as well as to justify the cost of rehabilitation services.[1,2] The quality of rehabilitation centers is directly related to the objectively measured outcome obtained after the patients' rehabilitation.

Many different factors influence outcome. Aside from the techniques and methods used during acute and post-acute rehabilitation, a patient's outcome is determined by such variables as the Glasgow Outcome Scale (GOS) score on hospital admission, length of coma (LOC), duration of post-traumatic amnesia (PTA), family support, and socio-economic level. The results of a rehabilitation program are also influenced by these same variables.

To measure outcome, we use behavior and motor scales. It is important to determine when outcome scales should be applied, or if the same scale can and should be administered at different points during a patient's recovery process. All scales are not equally useful at each different moment of a patient's recovery or rehabilitation. Some scales are valid during the acute phase, but not during the post-acute phase, and vice versa. When reporting a patient's outcome score, it should be clearly stated what scale was used, as well as in which stage of recovery it was applied. All scales should at the very least comply with acceptable prerequisites of reliability, construct validity, and ecological validity. Scales that depend exclusively on qualitative assessment should clearly specify the assessment procedure.

In this chapter we are going to review what we consider to be the most important and widely used instruments for measuring outcome after acquired brain injury: the Glasgow Outcome Scale (GOS), the Disability Rating Scale (DRS), the Barthel Index, the Functional Independence Measure (FIM), the Functional Assessment Measure (FAM), the Rancho Los Amigos Scale of Cognitive Functioning, the Portland Adaptability Inventory, the Community Integration Questionnaire, and the Neurologically-related Changes of Emotions and Personality Inventory (NECHAPI).

Scales to be used in the acute phase of traumatic brain injury

The Coma/Near Coma Scale

One of the main problems found in the acute phase is monitoring the patients coming out of coma spontaneously or from stimulation. The most common, widely used and accepted scale is the Glasgow Coma Scale. Recently, however, some behaviorally based scales for assessment and evaluation of minimally responsive patients have been developed. They are structured to monitor cognitive, behavioral, and pharmachological recovery. The best known are the Western NeuroSensory Stimulation profile, to be used with those patients who have slow recovery; the Sensory Stimulation Assessment Measure, which is an expansion of the Glasgow Coma Scale; the Coma Recovery Scale and the Coma/Near Coma Scale. In this section we are going to refer to the last one mentioned.

The Coma/Near Coma Scale (CNC) (Table 15.1) was developed by Rappaport et al. in 1992[3] with the aim of obtaining an instrument capable of detecting the most minimum clinical changes in minimally responsive patients. It is an expansion of the upper ranges of the Disability Rating Scale, including vegetative and extreme vegetative states. Scores are related to the responses to stimulation made by the patient based on 11 items, indicating severity of deficits: sensory, perceptual and primitive responses. Items grouping patients into one to five categories are: no coma, near coma, moderate coma, marked coma, and extreme coma. Rappaport found an interrrater reliability calculated at three time periods, OD 0.97. Alpha coefficients were 0.43, 0.65, and 0.65 at 1, 8, and 16 weeks post-injury. In our clinical experience, this is a good scale to be used in the intensive care unit when the patient is coming out of coma.

The Glasgow Outcome Scale (GOS)

The Glasgow Outcome Scale (Table 15.2) is one of the oldest scales used for measuring outcome after brain injury and was widely used prior to the development of new scales. The GOS was developed by Jennett and colleagues[4] in 1975 and an extended version was introduced in 1998 by Wilson et al.[5] The extended version (GOSE) is justified by the authors arguing that many of the main criticisms may be overcome by adopting a standard, well-specified format for the interview, and by being clear about the purposes and limitations of the GOS assessment. According to the authors:

> The GOS and GOSE were developed to allocate people who have suffered acute brain injury from head injury and non-traumatic brain injury into broad outcome categories. The scale reflects disability and handicaps rather than impairment; that is, it focuses on how the injury has affected functioning in major areas of life rather than on the particular deficits

Table 15.1 Rappaport Coma/Near-Coma Scale

RAPPAPORT COMA/NEAR-COMA SCALE

(For patients with a Disability Rating (DR) score ≥21, i.e., Vegetative State)[1]

(Complete form twice a day for 3 days then weekly for 3 weeks; every two weeks thereafter if DR score ≥21. If DR <21 follow monthly with DR scores.)

NAME _____ SEX _____ BIRTHDATE _____ TYPE OF INJURY: MVA _____ STROKE _____ DR _____

DATE OF INJURY/ILLNESS _____ DATE OF ADMISSION _____ HEAD INJURY _____ ANOXIA _____ DATE _____

FACILITY _____ RATER _____ OTHER (describe) _____ TIME _____

Parameter	Stimulus No.	Stimulus	No. of Trials	Response Measure	Score Options	Score Criteria								
AUDITORY*	1	Bell ringing 5 sec. at 10 sec. intervals	3▲	Eye opening, or orientation toward sound	0 2 4	≥3X 1 or 2X No response								
COMMAND RESPONSIVITY with priming**	2	Request patient to open or close eyes, mouth, or move finger, hand or leg	3	Response to command	0 2 4	Responds to command 2 or 3X Tentative or inconsistent 1X No response								
VISUAL with priming** Must be able to open eyes; if not, score 4 for each stimulus situation (scheme 3, 4, 5) and check here___ ***	3	Light flashes (1/sec. X5) in front; slightly left, right, and up and down each trial	5	Fixation or avoidance	0 2 4	Sustained fixation or avoidance 3X Partial fixation 1 or 2X None								
THREAT	4	Tell patient 'Look at me'; move face (20" away) from side to side	5	Fixation & tracking	0 2 4	Sustained tracking (at least 3X) Partial tracking 1 or 2X No tracking								
	5	Quickly move hand forward to within 1–3" of eyes	3	Eye blink	0 2 4	3 blinks 1 or 2 blinks No blinks								

					Score	Criteria															

OLFACTORY (block tracheostomy 3–5 seconds if present)	6	Ammonia capsule/ bottle 1" under nose for about 2 seconds	3	Withdrawal (w/d) or other response linked to stimulus	0 / 2 / 4	Responds 2 or 3X quickly (≤3 sec.) / Slowed/partial w/d; grimacing 1X / No w/d or grimacing
TACTILE	7	Shoulder tap – tap shoulder briskly 3X without speaking to patient; each side	3▲	Head or eye orientation or shoulder movement to tap	0 / 2 / 4	Orients toward tap 2 or 3X / Partially orients 1X / No orienting or response
	8	Nasal swab (each nostril entrance only – do not penetrate deeply)	3▲	Withdrawal or eye blink or mouth twitch	0 / 2 / 4	Clear, quick (w/in 2 sec.) 2 or 3X / Delayed or partial response 1X / No response
PAIN (Allow up to 10 sec. for response) If spinal cord injury check here ___ & go to stimulus 10	9	Firm pinch finger tip; pressure of wood of pencil across nail; each side	3▲	See Score Criteria	0 / 2 / 4	Withdrawal 2 or 3X / Gen. agitation/non-specific movement 1X / No response
	10	Robust ear pinch/pull X3; each side	3▲	Withdrawal or other response linked to stimulus	0 / 2 / 4	Responds 2 or 3X / Gen. agitation/non-specific movement 1X / No response
VOCALIZATION ▲▲ (assuming no tracheostomy) If trach. present do not score but check here ___	11	None. (Score best response)	**	See Score Criteria	0 / 2 / 4	Spontaneous words / Non-verbal vocaliz. (moan, groan) / No sounds

COMMENTS: (Include important changes in physical condition such as infection, pneumonia, hydrocephalus, seizures, further trauma, etc.)

Total CNC Score (add scores)	A
Number of items scored	B
Average CNC Score (A + B)	C
Coma/Near-Coma Level (0–4)†	D

[1] Rappaport et al. Disability Rating Scale for Severe Head Trauma Patients: Coma to Community. Arch Phys Med Rehabil. 63:118–123, 1982 (Revised Form 1987)

† See back for TRAINING NOTE and COMA/NEAR-COMA LEVELS.

* If possible use brain stem auditory evoked response (BAER) test at 80 db nHL to establish ability to hear in at least one ear.

** Whether or not patient appears receptive to speech, speak encouragingly and supportively for about 30 sec. to help establish awareness that another person is present and advise patient you will be asking him/her to make a simple response. Then request the patient to try to make the same response with brief priming before 2nd, 3rd and subsequent trials.

*** Make sure patient is not sleeping. Check with nursing staff on eye opening ability and arousability.

▲ Each side up to 3X if needed.

▲▲ Consult with nursing staff on arousability; do not judge solely on performance during testing. If patient is sleeping, repeat the assessment later. (Revised 8/90)

COMA/NEAR-COMA CATEGORIES

LEVEL	Range	Level of Awareness/Responsivity
0	0.00–0.89	NO COMA: consistently and readily responsive to at least 3 sensory stimulation tests* plus consistent responsivity to simple commands.
1	0.90–2.00	NEAR COMA; consistently responsive to stimulation presented to 2 sensory modalities and/or inconsistently or partially responsive to simple commands.
2	2.01–2.89	MODERATE COMA: inconsistently responsive to stimulation presented to 2 or 3 sensory modalities but not responsive to simple commands. May vocalize (in absence of tracheostomy) with moans, groans & grunts but no recognizable words.
3	2.90–3.49	MARKED COMA: inconsistently responsive to stimulation presented to one sensory modality and not responsive to simple commands. No vocalization.
4	3.50–4.00	EXTREME COMA; no responsivity to any sensory stimulation tests; no response to simple commands. No vocalization.

* Sensory stimulation tests are items 1, 2, 3, 4, 5, 6, 7, 8, 9, 10

TRAINING NOTE TO NEW RATERS:

While one person does the testing, 2, 3, or more observers rate each item *independently* (without discussion). Afterwards discuss ratings. If rating is changed, level initial rating but place changed rating in parenthesis next to it. Repeat this process on 5 to 10 patients or until raters train themselves to place patients at least in the same category range. Thereafter single ratings can be used but, for purposes of reliability, a minimum of two independent ratings per patient is encouraged. Ratings should be done at about the same time each day if possible. Under "Comments" record special information that may have had an extraordinary effect on the ratings on a given day – such as: Patient was severely ill with pneumonia; patient was vomiting; patient had known increase in intracranial pressure (viz., hydrocephalus); patient fell out of bed; etc.

ADDITIONAL COMMENTS:

Table 15.2 GOS Rating Scale

1. *Death*

2. *Vegetative state*
   There is no evidence of meaningful response. The patient is unable to communicate and interact with environment, no response to any stimuli.

3. *Severe disability*
   Patient is conscious but very dependent on other people, able to follow commands.

4. *Moderate disability*
   Patient is independent but disabled, unable to return to work or school due to physical and/or mental problems.

5. *Good recovery*
   Patient is able to come back to normal social and occupational activities, even if s/he has minor physical or mental deficits, and is able to return to work or school.

and symptoms caused by injury. It is not intended to provide detailed information about the specific difficulties faced by individual patients, but to give a general index of overall outcome.[5]

The GOS provides a gross measure of outcomes for large epidemiological studies, but provides inadequate detail for individual or program evaluation.[6] The low sensitivity of the GOS is counterbalanced by its ease of application.

The original scale is made up of five levels as follows: level 1 is death; level 2 is persistent vegetative state (absence of cortical function); level 3 is severe disability (conscious but disabled); level 4 is moderate disability (disabled but independent); level 5 is good recovery (back to normal life). These levels can also be grouped as poor outcome (GOS 1–3) and good outcome (GOS 4–5). The extended version divides each of the last three levels into two, resulting in eight levels. A patient is included in one of these eight levels after being discharged from the intensive care unit or from the hospital.

Because of its low sensitivity, the Glasgow Outcome Scale is not appropriate for measuring post-acute outcome, and both concurrent and ecological validity are poor.[7] We have found that this scale should only be used to evaluate the post-surgical outcome of a patient, which is the context for which it was developed, and not be used beyond the acute phase. It is our opinion that it has been a mistake to use the GOS as a scale for measuring post-acute outcome. Due to the low sensitivity and poor validity of the GOS, patients with severe cognitive and behavioral deficits have been mistakenly labeled as "good recovery". We could say that the GOS gives rise to many false positive outcomes when used outside of a surgical environment, which in turn gives rise to problems for these patients concerning access to post-acute treatment.

The Barthel Index

The Barthel Index (Table 15.3) is a simple index of independence used to score the actual physical activity of the patient. It was developed by Florence Mahoney and Dorothea W. Barthel in 1965.[8] It can be administered at different stages during the rehabilitation process. Every item of the scale is evaluated according to the amount of time and help needed by the patient for carrying out certain physical activities.

A clinimetric evaluation of the Barthel Index as a measure of limitations in daily activities and mobility was made by de De Haan et al.[9] in Amsterdam. Three different raters studied 35 patients from inpatient and 25 patients from outpatient departments using the Barthel Index in terms of score agreements, homogeneity and construct validity. They found that the Barthel Index was a highly homogeneous scale (Cronbach alpha, 0.96) and that there is excellent accordance of total scores and single items scores. All items contributed to reliability in a balanced way. Factor analysis showed that the items on the scale described one common underlying trait, explaining 81% of the score variance. They concluded that the Barthel Index is a sound instrument to measure disability in ADL and mobility, and that the scale is suitable for use in both patient care and research. Another study concerning reliability was carried out in 1991 by Wolfe et al.[10] They studied 50 patients with strokes of different severity identified by a community stroke register and interviewed by two or three different research nurses on two occasions that were 2–3 weeks apart. They found a very good kappa ($\kappa = 0.98$) and excellent agreement between raters (κ was equal to or greater than 0.88). They concluded that the Barthel scale is a more reliable and less subjective scale for assessing disability than other scales.

Wade and Collin[11] propose that the Barthel Index should be the standard index for clinical and research purposes. They found that this index is as good as any other single simple index of physical rehabilitation. They also recommended that it be adopted as the standard against which future indexes are compared. They concluded that the temptation to use variations of the standard Barthel Index should be resisted. In another study, Ranhoff and Laake[12] compared physicians' scores based on clinical interviews of elderly nursing-home patients with scoring by the nurses based on the reference method. Results showed that scores made by the doctors were higher than those by the nurses

An early rehabilitation-oriented extension of the Barthel Index was developed by Schönle.[13] He argued that patients with severe brain damage cannot be differentiated appropriately as floor effects show up with increasing severity of neurological impairment, as in comatose patients, or near or post-comatose patients in early rehabilitation. He developed the Early Rehabilitation Barthel Index (ERI), introducing states which require temporary intensive medical monitoring, tracheostome requiring special treatment (suctioning), intermittent artificial respiration, confusional state requiring

Table 15.3 The Barthel Index

Activity	Score

Feeding
  0 = unable
  5 = needs help cutting, spreading butter, etc., or requires modified diet
  10 = independent

Bathing
  0 = dependent
  5 = independent (or in shower)

Grooming
  0 = needs to help with personal care
  5 = independent face/hair/teeth/shaving (implements provided)

Dressing
  0 = dependent
  5 = needs help but can do about half unaided
  10 = independent (including buttons, zips, laces, etc.)

Bowels
  0 = incontinent (or needs to be given enemas)
  5 = occasional accident
  10 = continent

Bladder
  0 = incontinent, or catheterized and unable to manage alone
  5 = occasional accident
  10 = continent

Toilet use
  0 = dependent
  5 = needs some help, but can do something alone
  10 = independent (on and off, dressing, wiping)

Transfers (bed to chair and back)
  0 = unable, no sitting balance
  5 = major help (one or two people, physical), can sit
  10 = minor help (verbal or physical)
  15 = independent

Mobility (on level surfaces)
  0 = immobile or >50 yards
  5 = wheelchair independent, including corners, >50 yards
  10 = walks with help of one person (verbal or physical) >50 yards
  15 = independent (but may use any aid; for example, stick) >50 yards

Stairs
  0 = unable
  5 = needs help (verbal, physical, carrying aid)
  10 = independent

TOTAL (0–100)   —

Reproduced by permission from Mahoney and Barthel (1965).[8]

special care, behavioral disturbances requiring special care, swallowing disorders requiring special care and severe communication deficits. He studied 210 early rehabilitation patients and 312 patients with severe brain injury. He found that the extended scale permits differentiation of patients according to severity, avoids floor effects and allocates them to the appropriate phase of rehabilitation. He concluded that ERI is quick, economical, and reliable.

The Barthel Index was used by Stone et al.[14] for weekly monitoring of 102 patients diagnosed with stroke, fractured neck of femur and dementia. Their experience confirms that routine clinical use of the Barthel Index in this setting is feasible and responds to clinically important change, at least in group evaluation. It suggests that the Barthel may be useful in outcome measurement, case-mix adjustment and auditing discharge practices. To verify that the Barthel Index alone provides sufficient information about the long-term outcome of stroke, Wilkinson et al.[15] designed a cross-sectional follow-up study of people who had had their first stroke under 75 years of age. They compared and correlated the individual scores on the Barthel Index with the scores on other outcome measures. The mean interval between the stroke and the follow-up was 4.9 years. They found that the distinction of the Barthel Index as the standard outcome measure for populations of stroke patients is still justified for long-term follow-up, and may be a proxy for different outcome measures intended for the assessment of other domains. Verbally administered, the Barthel Index was found to be easy to use, reliable, sensitive to change and prognostically valuable by Brazil et al.[16] In another study, Kelly and Jessop[17] found the Barthel scores and FIM less useful in vocational rehabilitation where disabilities are less severe.

Rancho Los Amigos Scale

This scale (Table 15.4) was not originally designed[17] to measure outcome, but as an easy, useful tool to classify the cognitive functioning of patients with traumatic brain injury. It is widely used in the acute phase and is also currently used as an outcome measure following discharge. The Rancho Los Amigos Scale has eight levels to which a patient can be assigned as follows: I no response; II generalized response; III localized response; IV confused/agitated; V confused/inappropriate; VI confused/appropriate; VII automatic/appropriate.

A study made by Beauchamp et al.[18] estimated the reliability of the Rancho Los Amigos Cognitive Scale (LCFS) and found that the interrater reliability was 0.91. They also found that correlations between the scores of different pairs of observers were also high (mean rho values of 0.84). The authors concluded that this scale measures limited aspects of cognitive function, but it is simple to administer and did not take longer than the standard nursing neurological examination. Variability in scoring was related to the different degrees of stimulation used by examiners when assessing patients, not to differences in the interpretation of the responses of the patients. Zafonte and

Table 15.4 The Rancho Los Amigos Scale

Rancho Los Amigos Cognitive Scale

Level I. No response to pain, touch, or sight.

Level II. Generalized reflex response to pain

Level III. Localized response. Blinks to strong light, turns toward/away from sound, responds to physical discomfort, inconsistent response to commands.

Level IV. Confused/Agitated. Alert, very active, aggressive or bizarre behavior, performs motor activities but behavior is non-purposeful, extremely short attention span.

Level V. Confused/Non-agitated. Gross attention to environment, highly distractible, requires continual redirection, difficulty learning new tasks, agitated by too much stimulation. May engage in social conversation but with inappropriate verbalizations.

Level VI. Confused/Appropriate. Inconsistent orientation to time and place, retention span/recent memory impaired, begins to recall past, consistently follows simple directions, goal-directed behavior with assistance.

Level VII. Automatic/Appropriate. Performs daily routine in highly familiar environment in a non-confused but automatic robot-like manner. Skills noticeably deteriorate in unfamiliar environments. Lacks realistic planning for own future.

Level VIII. Purposeful/Appropriate.

---

colleagues[19] found a modest correlation between the Rancho Los Amigos Scale (at admission and at discharge) and the initial and lowest 24-hour Glasgow Coma Scale scores. The correlation coefficients are: Admission LCFS, 0.31 and 0.33; Discharge LCFS, 0.27 and 0.25.

We recommend the use of this scale due to its facility to place the patient at a certain level of cognitive state in the acute phase. We also recommend it because it is widely used and allows an easy understanding between clinicians when describing the clinical status of the patient.

Functional assessment measures for post-acute phase

The Disability Rating Scale (DRS)

The Disability Rating Scale was developed by Scranton et al. in 1970[20] as a measure of general functional status. In 1982, Rappaport et al.,[21] in an attempt to improve the GOS, used the DRS with people with traumatic brain injury. The DRS is easy to administer; it generally takes no more than 15 min. An important advantage of this scale is that scores can be used from the acute phase (baseline) up to the discharge of the patient, covering the different phases of recovery. The DRS provides a global measure of brain injury outcome, but lacks items that differentiate between more subtle disabilities.[6] A study by Fleming and Maas[22] concludes that Disability Rating Scores on admission to rehabilitation emerged as useful predictors of rehabilitation outcome. The predictive validity (length of hospital stay and discharge status) of Rappaport's Disability Rating Scale in people sustaining acute brain injury was studied by Eliason and Topp.[23] They found some evidence supporting predictive validity, but acurate prediction of length of hospitalization remains unclear. The DRS consists of eight categories (the first three categories are simple modifications of the Glasgow Coma Scale) and is scored through direct observation of the patient or through patient interviews, which can be carried out in person or by phone (Table 15.5).

A conference held in Houston to elaborate recommendations about outcome measures for clinical trials in Traumatic Brain Injury recommended the DRS as the primary outcome measure for patients with moderately severe brain injury (GCS = 9–12) 3 months after discharge. The DRS has good validity and is highly reliable,[22,23,24] although it has poor sensitivity when used on people with mild traumatic brain injury (DRS < 3) or on people with severe disability (DRS > 22). To increase sensitivity, Hall and colleagues[25] recommended adding a half-unit to items four to eight. This scale seems to have fewer ceiling effects than FIM or FIM+FAM. Interrater reliability was established by Rapaport et al.[21] The Pearson correlations were 0.97–0.98; test–retest reliability was 0.95[24] and concurrent validity as established by Rapaport et al.[21] ranged from $r = 0.35$ to 0.78. The predictive validity of the DRS at discharge is $r = 0.66$.[26] Results obtained by Gouvier et al.[24] show that the DRS possesses test–retest and interrater reliabilities, and concurrent and predictive validity. When the DRS is compared to the Levels of Cognitive Functioning Scale (LCFS), the DRS surpasses the LCFS in nearly every respect. The author concluded that these results offer psychometric justification for the use of the DRS for monitoring recovery from head injury.

Different studies have reported the use of the DRS in predicting employment in people with brain injury. Novack et al.[27] found that patients with scores above 15 upon admission to a rehabilitation program and above 7 on discharge were unable to return to work 1 to 2 years after the brain injury, while Cope et al.[28] found an 11% employment/school rate 1 year later in patients with a DRS of 7–20.

We also recommend the use of this scale when clinicians need to monitor the progress of the patient in rehabilitation, but they have to consider that this scale has difficulties in discriminating progress in some areas.

The Functional Independence Measure (FIM)

The Functional Independence Measure was developed by Keith et al. in 1987.[29] The FIM is composed of 18 items with a seven-point rating scale (a score of 1 for complete dependence, and 7 indicates complete independence). The FIM evaluates self-care (eating, washing oneself, showering/bathing, getting dressed, going to the toilet), sphincter control (vesical and anal sphincter), mobility (movement from the bed, chair and wheelchair, toilet, bath or

Table 15.5 Disability Rating Scale Form

DRS Rating Form **Name:** **Date:** **Rater:** **Total Score:**	**1. Eye opening** 0 Spontaneous 1 To speech 2 To pain 3 None Score:	**2. Communication ability** 0 Oriented 1 Confused 2 Inappropriate 3 Incomprehensible 4 None Score:
3. Motor response 0 Obeying 1 Localizing 2 Withdrawing 3 Flexing 4 Extending 5 None Score:	**4. Feeding (knows how and when)** 0.0 Complete 0.5 1.0 Partial 1.5 2.0 Minimal 2.5 3.0 None Score:	**5. Toileting (knows how and when)** 0.0 Complete 0.5 1.0 Partial 1.5 2.0 Minimal 2.5 3.0 None Score:
6. Grooming (knows how and when) 0.0 Complete 0.5 1.0 Partial 1.5 2.0 Minimal 2.5 3.0 None Score:	**7. Level of functioning (physical and cognitive disability)** 0.0 Complete independently 0.5 1.0 Independent in special environment 1.5 2.0 Mildly dependent-limited assistance (Non resident helper) 2.5 3.0 Moderately dependent-moderate assistance (person in home) 3.5 4.0 Markedly dependent (assistant with all major activities, at all times) 4.5 5.0 Totally dependent (24 hours nursing care) Score:	**Employability (as full-time worker, homemaker, or student)** 0.0 Not restricted 0.5 1.0 Selected jobs, competitive 1.5 2.0 Sheltered workshop, non-competitive 2.5 3.0 Not employable Score:

Summed scores suggesting the level of dysfunction are:
0 = None   1 = Mild   2–3 = Partial   4–6 = Moderate
7–11 = Moderately severe   12–16 = Severe   17–21 = Extremely severe
22–24 = Vegetative state   25–29 = Extreme vegetative state   30 = Death

shower), communication (comprehension, expression), psychosocial adjustment (social interaction, employability), and cognitive function (problem solving and memory). It is one of the most extensively used tools for evaluating the functional status of neurological patients, and has been widely used with patients with traumatic brain injury. Interrater reliability is between 0.86–0.97,[30,31] and it seems to show good face validity, internal consistency and discriminative capacity.[32]

The FIM mainly measures motor and self-care tasks which are common in everyday activities (13 items with a maximum possible score of 91), while cognitive deficits (50 items with a maximum possible score of 35) are underrepresented. One of the principal problems found with this scale is the ceiling effect. We prefer to use the FIM+FAM.

The Functional Assessment Measure (FAM) and the FIM+FAM/Revised

The FIM+FAM was designed recently as an instrument (Table 15.6) for evaluating functional outcome in patients with moderate or severe brain injury. The FAM was created in 1997 by Hall[33] to give more consistency to the FIM and thus eliminate the "ceiling effect" detected in the latter. It can be used at different stages of the rehabilitation process. The FAM contributed 12 new items which evaluate cognitive, behavioral, communication, and psychosocial information. The cognitive and emotional items added by the FAM are more complex than those requiring simple observation, and require that the person carrying out the observation be well trained. These items are related to orientation, attention, and emotions. As this may not always be the case, the reliability of interraters has not been well established, although Hall et al.[34] found a rater agreement of 89%. The validity of the instrument correlates significantly with clinical data of the acute phase, as well as the length of coma, post-traumatic amnesia, and the Glasgow Coma Scale.[34]

León-Carrión[35] has developed a new formula for the FIM+FAM, offering three new functional indexes: Maximum Recovery Percentage, Index of Functionality at Admission, and Index of Functionality at Discharge. The indexes can be applied to the complete scale or to each of the five categories of the scale. We have found this scale to be very useful in our clinical work.

Community Integration Questionnaire (CIQ)

The CIQ (Table 15.7) was specifically designed by Willer and colleagues[36] to evaluate the success of acquired brain injury patients' return to the community and to assess home integration, social integration, and productive activity in people with acquired brain injury. It is a 15-item questionnaire that can be completed as a self-report, or with the assistance of a family member or experienced caregiver. Questions refer to everyday independent activities such as shopping, household activities, food preparation, visiting friends, and

Table 15.6 FIM+FAM rating form

FIM+FAM	Scoring system	Self-care items score	
Name:	7 Complete independence (timely, safely)	1 Eating	1234567
Date:	6 Modified independence (extra time, devices)	2 Grooming	1234567
Rater:	5 Supervision (cuing, coaxing, prompting)	3 Bathing	1234567
Total score:	4 Minimal assistance (performs 75% or more of tasks)	4 Dressing upper body	1234567
	3 Moderate assistance (performs 50% to 74% of tasks)	5 Dressing lower body	1234567
	2 Maximal assistance (performs 25% to 49% of tasks	6 Toileting	1234567
	1 Total assistance (performs less than 25% of tasks	7 Swallowing*	1234567
		Score:	

Sphincter control		Mobility items		Locomotion	
8 Bladder management	1234567	10 Bed, chair, wheelchair	1234567	14 Walking/ wheelchair	1234567
9 Bowel management	234567	11 Toilet	1234567	15 Stairs	1234567
		12 Tub, shower	1234567	16 Community access*	1234567
		13 Car transfer*	1234567		
Score:		Score:		Score:	

Communication items		Psychosocial adjustment		Cognitive function	
17 Comprehension – Audio/visual	1234567	22 Social interaction	1234567	26 Problem solving	1234567
18 Expression – vocal, non-vocal	1234567	23 Emotional status*	1234567	27 Memory	1234567
19 Reading*	1234567	24 Adjustment to limitations*	1234567	28 Orientation*	1234567
20 Writing*	1234567	25 Employability*	1234567	29 Attention*	1234567
21 Speech intelligibility	1234567			30 Safety judgment	1234567
Score:		Score:		Score:	

so forth. Items are scored from 0 to 2 (except items 13–15), obtaining a total single score of community integration. The higher the score, the better the social integration. The test is easy to administer, completion time is 15 min, and can be self-administered or administered via a telephone interview.

A study by Dijkers found that the CIQ has problems of consistency, normative data, and ceiling effects. This author recommends the CIQ for population studies and program evaluation, but not for detailed evaluation of factors contributing to lack of community integration or changes in these factors over time in individual cases.[37] A comparison between patients'

Table 15.7 Community Integration Questionnaire (CIQ)

1. Who usually does the shopping for groceries or other necessities in your household?	2 Yourself alone 1 Yourself and someone else 0 Someone else
2. Who usually prepares meals in your household?	2 Yourself alone 1 Yourself and someone else 0 Someone else
3. In your home who usually does the everyday housework?	2 Yourself alone 1 Yourself and someone else 0 Someone else
4. Who usually cares for the children in your home?	2 Yourself alone 1 Yourself and someone else 0 Someone else * Not applicable, no children under 17 in the home
5. Who usually plans social arrangements such as get-togethers with family and friends?	2 Yourself alone 1 Yourself and someone else 0 Someone else
6. Who usually looks after your personal finances, such as banking or paying bills?	2 Yourself alone 1 Yourself and someone else 0 Someone else
7. Approximately how many times a month do you usually participate in shopping *outside* your home?	2 5 or more 1 1–4 times 0 Never
8. Approximately how many times a month do you usually participate in leisure activities such as movies, sports, restaurants, etc.?	2 5 or more 1 1–4 times 0 Never
9. Approximately how many times a month do you usually visit your friends or relatives?	2 5 or more 1 1–4 times 0 Never
10. When you participate in leisure activities do you usually do this alone or with others?	0 Mostly alone 1 Mostly with friends who have head injuries 1 Mostly with family members 2 Mostly with friends who do not have head injuries 2 With a combination of family and friends
11. Do you have a best friend with whom you confide?	2 Yes 1 No
12. How often do you travel outside the home?	2 Almost every day 1 Almost every week 0 Seldom/never (less than once per week)

13. Please choose the answer that best corresponds to your current (during the past month) work situation.	o Full-time (more than 20 hours/week) o Part-time (less than or equal to 20 hours/week) o Not working, but actively looking for work o Not working, not looking for work o Not applicable, retired due to age
14. Please choose the answer that best corresponds to your current (during the past month) school or training program situation.	o Full-time o Part-time o Not attending school, or training program o Not applicable, retired due to age
15. In the past month, how often did you engage in volunteer activities?	o Never o 1–4 times o 5 or more

reports with those of family members was made by Sander et al.[38] They found agreement levels for all 15 items when analyzing moderate to almost perfect kappa values. Almost perfect ratings were found for three out of four items on the Productive Activity scale. Patients' scores were higher than those reported by family members in the Home Integration scale, but differences were not considered clinically meaningfully. Patients showed higher levels of integration (total CIQ) in relation to their family members' estimation of them.

Psychometric characteristics of the CIQ determined by Willer et al.[39] indicated that the total scores are normally distributed for both people with and without traumatic brain injury. Significant differences were found between subjects with TBI and those without TBI for all three subscales and for total scores. Significant differences were also found among people with TBI living in three different settings: living independently; living in a supported community situation; living in an institution. According to the authors, intercorrelation between the three subscales demonstrated that the CIQ provides unique information in the assessment of community integration for persons with TBI. The need for normative data is investigated by Kaplan.[40] This author found that demographic variables mediated CIQ scores. Women were significantly higher on home integration. Older subjects had lower CIQ scores. Higher education levels were related to higher scores. There was a significant relationship between CIQ scores and both the Social Activity and Inactivity subscales of the Chronic Illness Problem inventory. The author concluded that CIQ norms for age, education, sex, and marital status are strongly recommended. A study to revise the factor structure and validity of the CIQ was carried out by Sander et al.[41] Their results provide further evidence for the validity of the CIQ. The factor structure is clinically and theoretically meaningful. The subscales and total scores show significant relationships with other widely used measures of outcome. We recommend the use of this scale to evaluate changes in community integration of people with brain injury who received post-acute rehabilitation.

Mayo–Portland Adaptability Inventory

The Portland Adaptability Inventory (PAI) was created by Muriel D. Lezak in 1987[42] to systematically evaluate the lack of behavioral and social adaptation that people with traumatic brain injury can exhibit. Items are rated from 0 to 3, except for alcohol and drug items. Ratings are based on the observation of the evaluators, family reports, medical records, clinical observations, and social history. The internal consistency coefficient is 0.938 for the complete inventory. Items are grouped into three different scales: Temperament and Emotionality (T/E); Activities and Social Behavior (ASB); Physical Capabilities (PC). Some authors found the PAI useful for predicting upon admission the vocational possibilities of patients after treatment, particularly in patients with mild or moderate brain injury.[37]

In 1994, Malec and Thompson from Mayo Medical Center developed the Mayo–Portland Adaptability Inventory (MPAI),[43] maintaining the PAI items and adding items for rating pain and other aspects of cognitive impairment. Although new versions of the MPAI have been developed, the MPAI-3 is currently the most frequently used. This version comes in three forms, one for staff, one for family, and one for the patient. Nine new items are included to better detect the moderate deficits that some people with mild brain injury suffer, such as fatigue, dizziness/imbalance, sensitivity to mild symptoms, and difficulties with financial and money management. The MPAI-3 consists of three subscales: the first two, the Physical/Cognitive Impairment scale and the Social Participation scale, examine physical and cognitive impairment separately from social participation; the third is the Pain/Emotional Disorder scale. Pearson reliability for the MPAI completed by survivors was 0.84 and item reliability was 0.99.[44]

This is a good instrument to be used when there is a need to monitor the progress made in behavioral and social adaptation of patients with acquired brain injury before, during, and after treatment.

Measure for emotional outcome after TBI

The Neurologically-related Changes in Emotions and Personality Inventory (NECHAPI).

It is important to ascertain emotional changes during and after rehabilitation of behavioral problems deriving from acquired brain injury. Although most outcome scales fail to measure emotional changes in the patient throughout the rehabilitation process and at discharge, the importance of measuring it cannot be denied and should be included in outcome measures. The NECHAPI[45] (Table 15.8) is a clinical tool specifically designed for measuring

Table 15.8 NECHAPI

NEUROLOGICALLY-RELATED CHANGES IN PERSONALITY INVENTORY (NECHAPI)
José León-Carrión

University of Seville, Spain

Center for Brain Injury Rehabilitation (C.RE.CER)

NAME:_____   DATE: _____/_____/_____

AGE:____ EDUCATIONAL LEVEL:____ SEX: ____MARITAL STATUS:____

	A	B	C	D	(1)
	LESS			MORE	
1. Is usually a hot blooded person	1	2	3	4	5
2. Usually experiences everything very intensely	1	2	3	4	5
3. Is difficult to calm down when he/she gets excited	1	2	3	4	5
4. Has very strong emotions	1	2	3	4	5
5. Sometimes behaves in a very cruel way	1	2	3	4	5
6. Gets upset easily	1	2	3	4	5
7. Is a violent person	1	2	3	4	5
8. Normally engages in dangerous behavior	1	2	3	4	5
9. Is usually in control of him/herself and his/her behavior	1	2	3	4	5
10. Is easily annoyed	1	2	3	4	5
11. Is a vulnerable person	1	2	3	4	5
12. Is a very sensitive person	1	2	3	4	5
13. Gets into a lot of trouble	1	2	3	4	5
14. Is not afraid of anything	1	2	3	4	5
15. Has a lot of friends	1	2	3	4	5
16. Is involved in a lot of social activities	1	2	3	4	5
17. In my opinion, drinks more than he/she should	1	2	3	4	5
18. Probably takes drugs sometimes	1	2	3	4	5
19. Likes to make other people suffer	1	2	3	4	5
20. Is always on the lookout for new emotional experiences	1	2	3	4	5
21. Is fickle	1	2	3	4	5
22. Doesn't offer explanations for what he/she does	1	2	3	4	5
23. Is definitely shy	1	2	3	4	5
24. Usually feels guilty about insignificant things	1	2	3	4	5

25. Could be described as being on the sadistic side	1 2 3 4 5
26. Does things as if he/she were fearless or unaware of danger	1 2 3 4 5
27. Is always open to new experiences	1 2 3 4 5
28. Is always looking for new sensations	1 2 3 4 5
29. Never takes into account how his/her actions may have made other people feel	1 2 3 4 5
30. Is not interested in very many things	1 2 3 4 5
31. Is a hostile person	1 2 3 4 5
32. Is a frustrated person	1 2 3 4 5
33. Is a very negative person	1 2 3 4 5
34. Is a depressive person	1 2 3 4 5
35. Is capable of committing suicide	1 2 3 4 5
36. Enjoys sex a lot	1 2 3 4 5
37. Probably wouldn't mind any kind of sexual experience, no matter how strange	1 2 3 4 5
38. Has a lot of sexual experience	1 2 3 4 5
39. Is easily angered	1 2 3 4 5
40. Has a strong desire to live	1 2 3 4 5

(1)

A: Family members that live with the patient

B: Girl/boyfriend; committed relationship

C: Close friends

D: Neighbors, acquaintances, other: please specify . . .

emotional changes presented by individuals after traumatic brain injury and cerebrovascular disorders, brain tumors and neurological disorders during and after neurorehabilitation. It contains 40 items which family members must rank from one to five, depending on how they feel it defines the patient, five being indicative of a high occurrence rate and one indicating minimum frequency. Family members score each item twice: the first time referring to the patient before the neurological disorder, and the second referring to him or her in their current neurological status. The 40 items of this inventory are grouped into five factors: anger, sensation seeking, emotional vulnerability, sociability, and emotional coldness. The reliability is 0.85. The NECHAPI can be repeated whenever necessary to monitor the emotional progress of a patient after neurorehabilitation. It is useful in registering the effects that neuropharmacotherapy may have on the emotional state of people with neurological disorders.

In a study conducted by Madrazo-Lazcano and colleagues,[46] comparing pre-TBI and post-TBI emotionality, it was found that patients with traumatic brain injury showed changes mainly in three factors of the NECHAPI. Their emotional vulnerability was seen to increase, while sociability and sensation seeking decreased. A deterioration was seen in which patients became more emotionally vulnerable and less emotionally stable. A change was noted in how patients perceive and manifest their emotions and feelings. Monitoring the changes throughout the course of rehabilitation and after discharge provides valuable information in regard to the effectiveness of the treatment and how to address it.

Concluding remarks

Outcome measurement constitutes part of the rehabilitation procedure in order to know the functional efficacy of the programs and methods used in the treatment of patients with acquired brain injury. Instruments to measure outcome have to complete the requirement of reliability and validity, and must be psychometrically acceptable. But they have to accomplish more than the psychometric criteria; they have to have ecological validity. That is to say, data should correspond to that which is observed in the patient's natural surroundings. It is recommended that the scales be used in the phases for which they were created (acute, post-acute, or social integration). The utilization of distinct scales in different phases from what they were created for can lead to making an inappropriate decision at a given moment.

References

1. Hall, K. M., Englander, J., & Wilmot, C. (1994). Commentary on model systems of care in neurotrauma: clinical perspectives and future directions. *NeuroRehabilitation, 4*, 76–83.
2. Cope, D., & O'Lear, J. A. (1993). Clinical and economic perspective on head injury rehabilitation. *J. Head Trauma Rehabil., 8*, 1–4.
3. Rappaport, M., Dougherty, A. M., & Kelting, D. L. (1992). Evaluation of coma vegetative states. *Arch. Phys. Med. Rehabil., 73*, 628–634.
4. Jennett, B., Snoek, J., Bond, M. R., & Brooks, N. (1981). Disability after severe head injury: observations on the use of the Glasgow Outcome Scale. *J. Neurol. Neurosurg. Psychiatry., 44*, 258–293.
5. Wilson, J. T. L., Pettigrew, L. E. L., & Teasdale, G. M. (1998). Structured interviews for the Glascow Outcome Scale: guidelines for their use. *J. Neurotrauma, 15*, 573–585.
6. Malec, J. F., Moessner, A. M., Kragness, M., & Lezak, M. D. (2000). Refining a measure of brain injury sequelae to predict postacute rehabilitation outcome: rating scale analysis of the Mayo–Portland Adaptability Inventory. *J. Head Trauma Rehabil., 15*, 670–682.
7. León-Carrión, J., Alarcon, J. C., Revuelta, M., et al. (1998). Executive functioning as outcome in patients after traumatic brain injury. *Int. J. Neurosci., 94*, 75–83.
8. Mahoney, F. I., & Barthel, D. (1965) Functional evaluation: the Barthel index. *Maryland State Med. J., 14*, 56–61.
9. De Haan, R., Limburg, M., Schuling, J., Broeshart, J., Jonkers, L., & Van Zuylen,

P. (1993). Clinimetric evaluation of the Barthel Index, a measure of limitations in daily activities. *Ned. Tijdschr. Geneeskd., 137*, 917–921.

10. Wolfe, C. D., Taub, N. A., Woodrow, E. J., & Burney, P. G. (1991). Assessment of scales of disability and handicap for stroke patients. *Stroke, 22*, 1242–1244.

11. Wade, D. T., & Collin, C. (1988). The Barthel ADL index: a standard measure of physical disability? *Int. Disabil. Stud., 10*, 64–67.

12. Ranhoff, A. H., & Laake, K. (1993). The Barthel ADL index: scoring by the physician from patient interview is not reliable. *Age Ageing, 22*, 171–174.

13. Schönle, P. G. (1995). The Early Rehabilitation Barthel Index – an early rehabilitation-oriented extension of the Barthel Index. *Rehabilitation (Stuttg.), 34*, 69–73.

14. Stone, S. P., Ali, B., Auberleek, I., Thompsell, A., & Young, A. (1994). The Barthel index in clinical practice: use on a rehabilitation ward for elderly people. *J. R. Coll. Physicians Lond., 28*, 419–423.

15. Wilkinson, P. R., Wolfe, C. D., Warburton, F. G., et al. (1997). Longer term quality of life and outcome in stroke patients: is the Barthel index alone an adequate measure of outcome? *Qual. Health Care, 6*, 125–130.

16. Brazil, L., Thomas, R., Laing, R., et al. (1997). Verbally administered Barthel Index as functional assessment in brain tumour patients. *J. Neurooncol., 34*, 187–192.

17. Kelly, S., & Jessop, E. G. (1996). A comparison of measures of disability and health status in people with physical disabilites undergoing vocational rehabilitation. *J. Publ. Health Med., 18*, 169–174.

18. Beauchamp, K., Baker, S., McDaniel, C., et al. (2001). Reliability of nurses' neurological assessments in the *cardiothoracic* surgical intensive care unit. *Am. J. Crit. Care, 10*(5), 298–305.

19. Zafonte, R. D., Hammond, F. M., Mann, N. R., Wood, D. L, Millis, S. R., & Black, K. L. (1996). Revised trauma score: an additive predictor of disability following traumatic brain injury? *Am. J. Phys. Med. Rehabil., 75*(64), 56–61.

20. Scranton, J., Fogel, M., & Erdman, W. I. (1970). Evaluation of functional levels of patients during and following rehabilitation. *Arch. Phys. Med. Rehabil., 51*, 1–21.

21. Rappaport, M., Hall, K. M., & Hopkins, H. K. (1982). Disability Rating Scale for severe head trauma: coma to community. *Arch. Phys. Med. Rehabil., 63*, 118–123.

22. Fleming, J., & Maas, F. (1994). Prognosis of rehabilitation outcome in head injury using the Disability Rating Scale. *Arch. Phys. Med. Rehabil., 75*, 156–163.

23. Eliason, M. R., & Topp, B. W. (1984). Predictive validity of Rappaport's Disability Rating Scale in subjects with acute brain dysfunction. *Phys. Ther., 64*, 1357–1360.

24. Gouvier, W. D., Blanton, P. D., LaPorte, K. K., & Nepomuceno, C. (1987). Reliability and validity of the Disability Rating Scale and the Levels of Cognitive Functioning Scale in monitoring recovery from severe head injury. *Arch. Phys. Med. Rehabil., 68*(2), 94–97.

25. Hall, K. M., Mann, N., High, W., Wright, J., Kreutzer, J., & Wood, D. (1996). Functional measures after traumatic brain injury: ceiling effects of FIM, FIM + FAM, DRS and CIQ. *J Head Trauma Rehabil., 11*(5), 27–39.

26. Eliason, M., & Topp, B. (1984). Predictive validity of Rappaport's Disability Rating Scale in subjects with acute brain dysfunction. *Phys. Ther., 64*, 1357–1359.

27. Novak, T. A., Bergquist, T. F., Bennett, G., & Gouvier, W. D. (1992). Primary

caregivers distress following severe head injury. *J. Head Trauma Rehabil., 6*(4), 69–77.

28. Cope, D. N., Cole, J. R., Hall, K. M., & Barkan, H. (1991). Brain injury: analysis of outcome in a post-acute rehabilitation system. *Brain Inj., 5*, 111–125, 127–139.

29. Keith, R. A., Granger, C. V., Hamilton, B. B., & Sherwin, F. S. (1987). The functional independence measure: a new tool for rehabilitation. *Adv. Clin. Rehabil., 1*, 6–18.

30. Hamilton, B. B., Laughlin, J. A., Granger, C. V., & Kayton, R. M., (1991). Interrater agreement of the seven-level Functional Independence Measure (FIM) [Abstr.] *Arch. Phys. Med. Rehabil., 72*, 790.

31. Linacre, J. M., Heinemann, A. W., Wright, B. D., Granger, C. V., & Hamilton, B. B. (1994). The structure and stability of the Functional Independence Measure. *Arch. Phys. Med. Rehabil., 75*, 127–132.

32. Dodds, T. A., Martin, D. P., Stolov, W. C., & Deyo, R. A. (1993). A validation of the functional independence measurement and its performance among rehabilitation inpatients. *Arch. Phys. Med. Rehabil., 74*(5), 531–536.

33. Hall, K. M. (1997). Establishing a national traumatic brain injury information system based upon a unified data set. *Arch. Phys. Med. Rehabil., 78*(4), S5–11.

34. Hall, K. M., Hamilton, B. B., Gordon, W. A., & Zasler, N. D. (1993). Characteristics and comparisons of functional assessment indexes. Disability Rating Scale, Functional Independence Measure and Functional Assessment Measure. *J. Head Trauma Rehabil., 8*, 60–74.

35. León-Carrión, J. (2001). The FIM + FAM revisited: the quantification of functional independence recovery. Sevilla: Center for Brain Injury Rehabilitation (CRECER) [Internal document].

36. Willer, B., Rosenthal, M., Kreutzer, J. S., Gordon, W. A., & Rempel, R. (1993). Assessment of community integration following rehabilitation for traumatic brain injury. *J. Head Trauma Rehabil., 8*, 75–87.

37. Malec, J. F., Smigielski, J. S., & DePompolo, R. W. (1991). Goal attainment scaling and outcome measurement in postacute brain injury rehabilitation. *Arch. Phys. Med. Rehabil., 72*(2), 138–143.

38. Sander, A. M., Seel, R. T., Kreutzer, J. S., Hall, K. M., High, W. M., & Rosenthal, M. (1997). Agreement between persons with traumatic brain injury and their relatives regarding psychosocial outcome using the Community Integration Questionnaire. *Arch. Phys. Med. Rehabil., 78*(4), 353–357.

39. Willer, B., Ottenbacher, K. J., & Coad, M. L. (1994). The community integration questionnaire. A comparative examination. *Am. J. Phys. Med. Rehabil., 73*(2), 103–111.

40. Kaplan, C. P. (2001). The community integration questionnaire with new scoring guidelines: concurrent validity and need for appropiate norms. *Brain Inj., 15*, 725–731.

41. Sander, A. M., Fuchs, K. L., High, W. M., Hall, K. M., Kreutzer, J. S., & Rosenthal, M. (1999). The Community Integration Questionnaire revisited: an assessment of factor structure and validity. *Arch. Phys. Med. Rehabil., 80*(10), 1303–1308.

42. Lezak, M. D. (1995). *Neuropsychological assessment* (3rd ed.). New York: Oxford University Press.

43. Malec, J. F., & Thompson, J. M. (1994). Relationship of the Mayo–Portland Adaptability Inventory (MPAI) to functional outcome and cognitive performance measures. *J. Head Trauma Rehab., 9*(4), 1–15.

44. Wright, B. D., & Masters, G. N. (1982). *Rating scale analysis*. Chicago, IL: Mesa Press.
45. León-Carrión, J. (1998). Neurologically-related changes in personality inventory (NECHAPI): A clinical tool addressed to neurorehabilitation planning and monitoring effects of personality treatments. *NeuroRehabilitation, 11*, 129–139.
46. Madrazo-Lazcano, M., Machuca-Murga, F., Barroso y Martín, J. M., Domínguez-Morales, M. R., & León-Carrión, J. (1999). Emotional changes following severe brain injury. *Revist. Esp. Neuropsicol., 1*, 75–82.

16 Assessment of response bias in impairment and disability examinations

Michael F. Martelli, Nathan D. Zasler, Shane S. Bush and Treven C. Pickett

Introduction

Evaluation of neurologic impairments and associated disability presents a significant diagnostic challenge. In cases of more catastrophic or functionally disabling injuries, the evaluations and opinions of different medical practitioners are often fairly consistent. In other cases, however, practitioners who specialize in brain injury assessment may express widely varying opinions.

Evaluation of impairment and disability following neurologic injury typically involves such contexts as social security disability application, personal injury litigation, worker's compensation claims, disability insurance policy application, other healthcare insurance policy coverage, and determination of competence to handle finances or other important life functions (e.g., parenting) or decisions. Traditionally, disability evaluations following injury have fallen within the purview of physiatrists, orthopedists, neurologists, neurosurgeons, psychiatrists, psychologists and neuropsychologists. However, in cases of less catastrophic impairment and disability, practitioners who specialize in neurological impairment and disability assessment are usually relied upon.

The area of impairment and disability evaluation may be one of the more misunderstood areas of work as it applies to treatment of persons with injury residua and/or functional limitations due to injury. The task of making determinations regarding impairment and disability in persons with neurologic impairment and injury is fraught with potential obstacles and confounding issues. This is due in part to the frequently subtle yet complex nature of the deficits involved, as well as the lack of formal, scientifically validated "rating systems" for most of the deficits associated with these disorders. Disentangling the multiple contributors to impairment and disability presents a diagnostic challenge and requires careful scrutiny.[1]

Persons with brain injury may present with some response bias to report or demonstrate impairment or related disability. Response bias, in this chapter, is defined as a class of behaviors that reflect less than fully truthful, accurate or valid symptom report and presentation. Importantly, response bias is a ubiquitous phenomenon affecting almost any domain of human self-report. However, in the context of impairment and disability evaluations, or insurance related evaluations, the importance of such bias becomes more acute.[2-4]

Given the frequent incentives to distort performance during impairment and disability examinations, assessment of examinee motivation to provide full effort during assessment becomes a necessary component of such evaluations. The importance of detecting response biases is critical with regard to providing accurate diagnosis. Accurate diagnosis is prerequisite to provision of appropriate and timely treatment, to obtaining optimal recovery, to prevention of iatrogenic impairment and disability reinforcement, and to appropriate legal compensation decisions. The impairment/disability context and other internal and environmental variables make ensuring accurate representation of a patient's functional status essential. In order to attempt to ensure such accuracy, a number of factors must be considered, including determination decisions regarding impairment and disability, examination displayed symptomatology, sensitivity and specificity of assessment measures, and ecological validity.

Blau[5] has expounded on the importance of determining response biases and measuring true levels of impairment in medicolegal situations. Essentially, in this arena, an alleged victim a of wrongful act or omission attempts to establish (a) causality in order to demonstrate entitlement to compensation for damages, which is awarded based on (b) level of damages suffered. In cases of less obvious, clear-cut and significant trauma with psychologic, neurologic or soft tissue damage, causality and level of current and future damages are more difficult to prove and expert evaluation and opinion are heavily relied upon for making legal determinations. In the parallel insurance situation, the insured attempts to access entitlements to healthcare treatment and disability benefits, and expert evaluation and opinion are relied upon for making policy determinations. In both cases, financial and other incentives clearly represent motivational factors that increase the likelihood of response bias in the form of exaggerated or feigned symptoms.

Examinee response biases

Examinee response bias can take several forms. Bias ranges from symptoms that may be minimized to those that are exaggerated or feigned. Such symptoms may be accurately or inaccurately attributed to different events. For instance, pre-existing symptoms may suddenly be attributed to an accident; symptoms previously not noticed may suddenly be given such prominence that attention and anxiety alone produce significant increases. Similarly, an accident may cause an aging person to do a self-inventory of health that reveals symptoms due to aging that were present but previously minimized. In addition, social realities also exert influence over response to injury and symptoms. For example, the vastly different consequences for diagnoses of cancer versus mild traumatic brain injury or back injury produce differential reinforcement. The former is clearly undesirable and negative, while the latter can result in highly desirable monetary compensation.

Martelli et al.[6] reviewed the literature and found that the following injury context variables were associated with poorer post-injury adaptation and recovery and increased likelihood of response bias:

- Anger, resentment, or perceived mistreatment.
- Fear of failure or rejection (e.g., damaged goods; fear of being fired after injury).
- Loss of self-confidence and self-efficacy associated with residual impairments.
- External (health, pain) locus of control.
- Irrational fear of injury extension, reinjury, or pain.
- Discrepancies between personality/coping style and injury consequences (e.g., highly physically active person with few intellectual resources who has a back injury).
- Insufficient residual coping resources and skills.
- Prolonged inactivity resulting in disuse atrophy.
- Fear of losing disability status, benefits, and safety net.
- Perceptions of high compensability for injury.
- Pre-injury job (task, work environment) dissatisfaction.
- Collateral injuries (especially if "silent").
- Inadequate and inaccurate medical information.
- Misdiagnosis, late diagnosis, or delays in instituting treatment.
- Insurance resistance to authorizing treatment or delays in paying bills.
- Retention of an attorney.
- Greater reinforcement for "illness" vs. "wellness" behavior.
- Dichotomous (organic vs. psychologic) conceptualizations of injury and symptoms.

These variables represent vulnerability factors, which can reduce effective coping with post-injury impairments and increase the likelihood of maladaptive coping and response bias. They are not mutually exclusive and, as with the variables presented below, more than one can contribute to symptom report and presentation

Additional review of the literature,[7,8] combined with clinical experience,[9] indicates the following significant sources of response bias that may be encountered during examinations:

1   *Cultural differences.* For example, many non-western cultures mix emotional and physical pain and symptoms at a conceptual and phenomenological level. Also, some cultures see failure to impose severe penalty/extract significant compensation for harm as a sign of weakness and disgrace in God's eyes.

2   *Reactive adversarial malingering (RAM).* RAM is based on fear, mistrust

of the opposing side's honesty, and mistreatment (e.g., from assumed "facts" in many work setting and cultures, including plaintiff attorney groups) and results in a deliberate pendulum-like overplaying of symptoms. RAM may be especially characteristic in persons or groups with tendencies toward suspiciousness, including immigrants, outcasts, outsiders, and those who feel chronically underprivileged, "slighted" or "short-changed".

3   *Conditioned avoidance pain-related disability (CAPRD)*. CAPRD represents phobic or extreme anxiety reactions wherein any competence (or ability or activity) is associated with excessive, overwhelming demands for pain exacerbation from external sources. Such demands may be expressed within and/or beyond conscious awareness. Kinesiophobia and cogniphobia are two types of CAPRD.

4   *Desperation-induced malingering (DIM) or Desperation-induced symptom exaggeration (DISE)*. Individuals that are particularly prone to these types of response bias may include the following: insecure immigrant workers, immigrants who tried introjection and feel resentful that they were not rewarded, aging workers, tired workers, workers insecure about work changes, workers fearing their own limited or declining abilities, persons whose premorbid coping was tenuous and who feel too overwhelmed and unable to cope with an additional stress, those with real or imagined abuse from others, such as employers, family, etc., immigrants who feel rejected by the culture and feel entitled, immigrants who feel disillusioned because the new land was not everything they had hoped (i.e., those who believe this to be a viable solution to a desperate situation). A second group of patients represented by this category are those making desperate pleas for help and those who, upon confronting tests that seem different and maybe easier than the real-life situations where they have problems, reduce effort to highlight their problems.

5   *Sociopathic, manipulative and opportunistic (SMO) personality traits*. These personality traits can be found in all groups, with estimated frequencies of generally between 5 and 10% in the chronic pain populations (approximately 20% in compensation situations).

6   *Passive aggressive, impatient, or rebellious (PAIR) personality traits*. Such individuals tend to resent others for not listening to them and believing them. They tend to resent imposed evaluations or doctors' visits, especially ones that examine psychological function or motivation. They may play games with doctors by withholding or undermining procedures or treatments, and may especially alter performance or play games on tests that seem non-challenging or not face valid.

7   *Psychological decompensation*. These individuals usually display conspicuous psychological distress and pathology that differentiates them from others.

8   *Skepticism*. Many individuals are very skeptical of doctors, examination

and examination procedures, and may be poorly motivated to comply with the conditions required for valid assessment.

9   *Iatrogenic bias.* A frequently overlooked form of bias is that which is iatrogenic to the nature of the insurance and adversarial legal system. In an effort to elucidate expectancy influences and bias for persons who have sustained injuries, Martelli et al.[6] collected survey attitudinal data from professionals who work with injured workers' compensation (WC) patients. A summary of the preliminary data is offered in Table 16.1, broken down by the four sample groups: (a) disability evaluators, comprising physicians, chiropractors, physical therapists and vocational evaluators; (b) staff from a rehabilitation neuropsychology service; (c) attendees at a case management conference, including over 50% WC case managers (d) rehabilitation/health psychologists. These data are quite compelling. Overall, approximately 25% of WC patients are believed to be exaggerating or malingering, with higher rates evidenced by WC case managers. This suggests a general skepticism and distrust faced by injured persons during evaluations. In contrast, the majority of professionals filling out the survey believed they would be treated unfairly by the WC system if they were injured, suggesting a general skepticism and distrust of the extant systems that fund evaluation and treatment of injury and disability.

Although these preliminary data are derived from small samples, and although generalizability across situations cannot be assumed, they nonetheless seem compatible with the levels of diffuse distrust observed by the authors in impairment and disability evaluation situations. These data highlight the importance of considering the apparently much different set of motivational factors that operate on examinees that present for disability evaluation. In addition, these data suggest a need for improving expectancies in independent examinations (e.g., perhaps via deliberate and thorough preparation of examinees prior to the examination).

In an interesting conceptualization of a major type of response bias in chronically disabled workers, Matheson[7,10–12] defined symptom magnification as a conscious or unconscious self-destructive and socially reinforced pattern of symptoms intended to control life circumstances of the sufferer, but which impede healthcare efforts. He further defined three major subtypes. The Type I "refugee" displays illness behavior, which provides escape or avoidance of life situations perceived as unsolvable. Somatization, conversion, psychogenic pain, and hypochondriacal disorders are conceptualized as extreme subcategories for this type. The Type II "game player" employs symptoms for positive gain. Although this type seems associated with the psychiatric diagnosis of malingering, Matheson argues that true malingering is a medicolegal concept, while Type II symptom magnifier is a treatable self-destructive syndrome. The Type III "identified patient" is motivated by maintenance of the patient role as a means of life survival. Associated psychiatric diagnoses include factitious disorder.

Table 16.1 Survey of attitudes regarding workers' compensation (WC)

Question	Respondent sample				
	Disability evaluating professionals (n = 19)	Rehabilitation psychology/ neuropsychology staff (n = 7)	Case managers (n = 17) including 8 WC case managers	Rehabilitation/ health psychologists/ neuropsychologists/ PMR MDs (n = 22)	Workers' compensation patients (n = 12)
1. Injured workers who fake, exaggerate, malinger (%)	19.2	24.7	28.5	19.2	35.0
2. Injured workers that WC treats unfairly (%)	49.2	62.5	23.2	42.6	74.2
3. Employers who treat injured workers unfairly (%)	53.5	41.2	32.7	35.6	65
4. Likelihood employer would treat you unfairly	43.75	54.2	46.4	23.6	70.8
5. Likelihood WC would treat you unfairly	60	65.9	48.9	40.44	77.75
Demographic data					
IV-1 Avg. Years_Employed	25.8	10.2	8.9	18.33	18.8
IV-2 Avg. Education	18.2	19.3	16.2	20+	14.2
IV-3 Sex	66% Female	57% Female	100% Female	76% Male	75% Male

Main and Spanswick[13] also examined simulated or exaggerated incapacity in persons claiming physical disability. They identified a list of features associated with simulated or exaggerated incapacity. These are included in Table 16.2.

Attribution and bias

A brief review of important sources of bias, or threats to objectivity, that require assessment during evaluation of physical, sensory and neurocognitive now impairments now follows.

Examinee attribution biases can confound accurate diagnosis. Examples include mistaking clinical entities like depression and sleep disturbance and their associated physical, cognitive, and motivation problems for physical or neurologic injury or sequelae. This can occur due to misattribution, over-attribution, retrospective attribution, illusory correlation, or to heightened awareness due to vigilance biases. Importantly, the previously mentioned conditions (e.g., depression, sleep disturbance) are reversible and may have been present prior to the injury without producing significant limitations. Furthermore, the emotional states or fatigue may be interacting with actual physical injury symptoms to increase impairment.

Examiner misattribution can similarly occur. Only methodical neuromedical assessment can differentiate sequelae secondary to brain injury from factors with overlapping symptoms, such as the following: cranial/cranial adnexal and cervical trauma impairments, chronic pain symptoms, psychological sequelae, motivational factors and/or other non-neurologic factors. When "abnormal" neurocognitive findings and/or non-specific somatic complaints are obtained, tendencies toward "over-diagnosis" of neurologic disorders, such as mild traumatic brain injury, can only be avoided through careful differential diagnosis. Brain injury specialists sensitized to neurologic symptoms have been observed by the authors to misdiagnose chronic pain

Table 16.2 Simulated or exaggerated incapacity in persons claiming physical disability[13]

Features identified as primarily suggestive of simulated or exaggerated incapacity
- Failure to comply with reasonable treatment
- Report of severe pain with no associated psychological effects
- Marked inconsistencies in effects of pain on general activities
- Poor work record
- Previous litigation

Features not primarily suggestive of response bias
- Mismatch between physical findings and reported symptoms
- Report of severe or continuous pain
- Anger
- Poor response to treatment
- Behavioral signs/symptoms

---

sequelae as post-concussive symptoms, which may result in an escalation of medical costs, prolongation of inappropriate treatment, and eventual treatment failure which may contribute to a sense of helplessness and chronic disability in the injured person. Conversely, similar observations have been made for psychiatrists and psychologists prone to infer psychiatric etiologies for all pathology, including brain injury or valid physical injury.

Response bias

Formal response bias assessment procedures, which are frequently lacking or only haphazardly attended to in clinical examinations, must be employed in order to increase the probability that clinical examination findings are accurate and valid reflections of impairment. Response bias exists on a continuum that extends from no bias through denial and unawareness of impairments, symptom minimization, and symptom magnification, to malingering. While we believe most examinees approach testing in a forthright and adequately motivated manner, it is necessary to examine the potential for response bias with each patient.

Denial and unawareness refer to neurologic phenomenon. These factors are usually more pronounced early after injury and are typically associated with more significant neurologic insults. They can lead to under-appreciation of deficits due to dysfunction in brain operations subserving awareness.

Symptom minimization, in contrast, is a consciously motivated phenomenon. It is usually motivated by either a desire to engage in activities that might otherwise be restricted, or as a defense against painful realizations about losses. Failure to detect such biases can lead to neglecting to identify important impairments and an overestimation of abilities that could potentially endanger the welfare of the examinee.

Symptom magnification, in contrast, refers to exaggeration of impairment. This can occur in relation to multiple factors and can serve a wide range of psychological needs. Some examples include efforts to: legitimize latent dependency needs; resolve pre-existing life conflicts; retaliate against employer or spouse or other; reduce anxiety; exert a "plea for help"; or solicit acknowledgment of perceived difficulties. Symptom exaggeration can also occur in patients with premorbid histories of psychiatric and psychoemotional problems who "latch on" to a specific diagnosis which not only becomes responsible for all life problems, but also promotes passivity, helplessness, and an external locus of control. When patients are assessed for claims of major disability following uncomplicated mild brain injury, non-neurologic contributors should be closely scrutinized. Depression, post-traumatic stress disorder and other anxiety conditions, and additional psychiatric syndromes generally have favorable psychological and functional prognosis given timely and appropriate assessment and treatment. Misdiagnosis of these conditions serves to promulgate misperceptions and amplify functional disability and healthcare costs.

Physicians should be familiar with examination strategies designed to evaluate non-organic musculoskeletal and neurologic disorders, including the use of specialized bedside examination techniques for physical and cognitive dissimulation. Examples include such strategies as Hoover's test for evaluation of malingered lower extremity weakness, sideways/backwards walking for assessment of feigned gait disturbance, and a positive Stenger's test on audiologic assessment for non-organic hearing loss. Other tests that might be of value in the context of response bias detection on the physical examination include: Mankopf's maneuver, strength reflex test, arm and/or wrist drop test, hip adductor test, axial loading test, Gordon-Welberry toe test, Bowlus and Currier test, Burns bench test, Magnuson's test, and others.[14]

Examination findings that suggest a non-neurologic basis for the observed impairments include patchy sensory loss, pain in a non-dermatomal distribution (such as a midline sensory demarcation), non-pronator drift, and/or astasia–abasia.[15] Motor and other impairment inconsistencies that fluctuate or disappear under hypnosis, drug-assisted interviews, or "presumed" non-observation may certainly increase the index of suspicion regarding non-organicity, although exceptions to this rule do exist. Faked hemiparesis is typically more common on the left side,[15,16] perhaps due to the fact that most persons are right hand dominant. Consistency regarding laterality of symptoms, particularly with neurologic impairment and/or referred pain, should be evaluated.

When of central (vs. peripheral) origin, pain complaints should be assessed, in part by concurrently assessing temperature perception, given that the same neural pathways mediate these sensations. When temperature sensation is preserved in the presence of a loss of pain sensation, after either brain or spinal cord injury, the deficit is not likely to reflect direct CNS impairment (the loss should occur contralateral to and below the level of the lesion). This point also reinforces the need to understand the neuropathology/pathology of the lesion based on imaging studies and to appreciate the implications that these findings have for anticipated clinical exam findings. Alleged pain imperception can be evaluated, as can nearly any reported neurological impairment for that matter, with appropriately designed forced choice testing. Additionally, examiners should realize that alleged pain imperception or loss of sensation is difficult to fake upon repeated bilateral stimulation. This is due to the fact that examinees that exaggerate rely on subjective strategies rather than truly responding to the strength of the stimuli. Therefore, assessments such as Von Frey hairs could be utilized in the aforementioned scenario to provide further objective evidence of feigned sensory deficits.

Defining pain and its possible deception is extremely challenging. The standard accepted definition of pain describes it as a physiologic and psychologic response to noxious stimuli, the latter being defined as a stimulus that may or does produce tissue damage.[17] One must, however, differentiate between psychic and physical pain in the context of performing an IME. Both factors are potentially inextricably intertwined with each other as well as with affective conditions such as depression and anxiety. Examiners must understand that multiple variables may impact on pain reporting and behavior and be totally valid yet potentially appear invalid. For example, arousal, stress, tension and anger all may exacerbate subjective reporting of pain and pain behavior, as may depression, through effect on physiologic function. Psychoemotional and psychosocial concomitants of chronic pain must also be appreciated, including loss of self-esteem, lowered frustration tolerance, depression, sexual dysfunction, including decreased libido, anger, and guilt.

Measures of response bias

Malingering is the deliberate symptom production for purposes of secondary gain. Malingering in the examination setting will often be reflected by response biased in the direction of poor performance. Measure of such response bias should always be administered in cases of medicolegal presentation, suspicion of any disincentive to exert full effort, or suspicion of sociopathic personality disorders. Any of several memory measures designed to assess atypical or worse than chance performance can be employed to assess response bias in cognitive performance.[18]

Evaluating clinicians should be familiar with psychological syndromes that may present as organic disorders, including, for example, factitious disorder, malingering, and somatoform disorders (conversion disorders including non-epileptic seizures (pseudo-seizures), somatoform pain disorder, somatization disorder, and undifferentiated somatoform disorder). Of course, the presence of a psychological syndrome and/or response bias does not necessarily exclude the diagnosis of an actual neurological syndrome. This certainly complicates the process of disentangling multiple clinical entities that sometimes coexist. Unfortunately, the science and art of methodical differential diagnosis is too often under-appreciated in the evaluation process.[1]

A relevant screening procedure that has frequently been used by physical therapists, physicians, and chiropractors for estimating when psychological factors are significantly influencing pain-related responses is the *assessment for Waddell's non-organic signs*.[19,20] Screening includes the following:

1 *Overreaction:* guarding/limping, bracing, rubbing affected area, grimacing, sighing.
2 *Tenderness:* widespread sensitivity to light touch of superficial tissue.
3 *Axial loading:* light pressure to skull of standing patient should not significantly increase low back symptoms.
4 *Rotation:* back pain is reported when shoulders and pelvis are passively rotated in the same plane.
5 *Straight leg raising:* marked difference between leg raising in the supine and seated position.
6 *Motor and sensory:* giving way or cog wheeling to motor testing or

regional sensory loss in a stocking or non-dermatomal distribution (rule out peripheral nerve dysfunction).

Additional non-organic signs include: lower extremity give-away; no pain-free spells in the past year; intolerance of treatments; emergency admissions to hospital with back trouble.[13,19]

Importantly, the presence of Waddell's or other non-organic signs does not exclude physical components as the cause of low back pain. Rather, they suggest only that psychological factors appear to be influencing the patient's responses and behavior. Physical and psychological findings are not mutually exclusive, and, psychological factors may more often be a result of low back pain than a cause.[21]

With regard to assessment of psychological and neuropsychological impairments and chronic pain, response bias represents an especially important threat to validity. Because these assessments usually begin with an interview about self-reported symptoms and subsequently rely heavily on standardized measures of performance on well-normed tests, the validity of the results requires the veracity, cooperation, and motivation of the patient. Recent evidence, however, suggests that patients seen for presumptive brain injury related impairments over-report pre-injury functional status.[22] This is especially true with post-concussive deficits since these symptoms often appear with similar frequency in the general population.[23] In addition, the demonstrated ability of neuropsychologists to accurately detect malingering in test protocols has been less than impressive.[24] Finally, the common practice of utilizing technicians to administer tests, as previously noted, has been called into question for reasons that include adequacy to detect and manage response bias issues.[25] Nonetheless, various instruments, techniques and strategies are available which have demonstrated at least some utility in detecting response bias, as a means of increasing confidence in the validity of assessment findings.

In Table 16.3, hallmark signs of response bias are presented. The signs can be applied to most aspects of a medical examination.

Notably, in the evaluation of response bias, as in evaluation of pre- and post-injury status, the following investigative tools may be used in conjunction with client interviews and testing: (a) school records; (b) medical records; (c) driver records; (d) military records; (e) criminal records; (f) employment records; (g) evaluations from other psychologists; (h) interviews with family members, friends, teachers, employers, etc.; (i) all materials available to the attorney through formal discovery or otherwise. Table 16.3 and these guidelines and strategies are presented as important indicators for interpreting patient examination data. Integration of contextual information, history, behavioral observation, interview data, collaborative data, and personality data, with measures of effort and neuropsychological test data provides the best information for estimating the degree to which a person was exerting full effort and the degree to which test results are reliable and valid and reflect actual abilities.

Table 16.3 Response bias: hallmark signs

I. *Inconsistencies within and between* (the potential contributions of significant psychiatric, attentional, comprehension, or other disorders that often involve inconsistent presentations should be considered)
1. Reported symptoms
2. Examination/test performance
3. Clinical presentation
4. Known diagnostic patterns
5. Observed behavior (in another setting)
6. Reported symptoms and examination/test performance
7. Measures of similar abilities (inter-test scatter)
8. Similar tasks or items within the same exam or test (intra-test scatter), especially when difficult tasks are performed more easily than easy ones
9. Different testing sessions

II. *Overly impaired performance (vs. expected)*
1. Very poor performance on easy tasks presented as difficult
2. Failing tasks that all but those with severe impairment perform easily
3. Poorer performance than normative data for similar injury/illness.
4. Below chance level performance

III. *Lack of specific diagnostic signs of impairment*

IV. *Specific signs of response bias on psychological or neuropsychological tests*
1. MMPI scale: F, F–K
2. MMPI-2 "fake bad"
3. Malingering detection tests
4. Actuarial formulas for clinical neuropsychological tests (e.g., WCST, CVLT)

V. *Interview evidence*
1. Atypical temporal relationship of symptoms to injury
2. Psychological symptoms, or symptoms that are improbable, absurd, overly specific or of unusual frequency or severity (e.g., triple vision)
3. Disparate examinee history or complaints across interviews or examiners
4. Disparate corroboratory interview data vs. examinee report

VI. *Physical examination findings*
1. Non-organic sensory findings
2. Non-organic motor findings
3. Pseudoneurologic findings in the absence of anticipated associated pathologic findings
4. Inconsistent examination findings
5. Failure on physical examination procedures designed to specifically assess malingering

---

The necessary recent increase in attention to response bias assessment has also been accompanied by frequently haphazard and overzealous application of poorly validated detection procedures and opinions regarding malingering. Further, some alarming trends have appeared that do not objectively or critically evaluate the weaknesses, as well as strengths, of these procedures. Based on a critical evaluation of the current state of the art, it appears that many common assumptions about response bias detection and malingering should be considered myths, for example, malingering: (a) should not be considered dichotomous, or *either/or* (i.e., present/not, malingering/not); (b) should not be considered something that clinicians can reliably or validly assess with any high degree of certainty, even when serious efforts are made; and (c) should not be considered a discrete entity that symptom validity tests (SVT) measure. Further, it should not be assumed that SVTs have a high degree of reliability and validity in predicting valid examination performance on other measures or functional ability in other settings, or that patients take the examination process as seriously as examiners do.

A summary of some of the major problems with current procedures is offered in Table 16.4.[26] This table is offered in order to: (a) emphasize the necessary caution with regard to over-interpretation of response bias procedures; and (b) emphasize the importance of employing multiple data sources and making thoughtful inferences only after integration of thorough historical information, interview, assessment, behavioral observations, collaborative interview and data sources, and so on.

In order to caution against simplistic and dichotomous conceptualizations with regard to diagnosis, Table 16.5 is presented, representing just 64 of the possibilities with regard to injury-related presentations. The represented possibilities range from persons with real, uncomplicated disorders with impairments on examination and in functional status and not exaggeration on

Table 16.4 General weaknesses of symptom validity tests (SVT)/measures

1. *Psychometric research inadequacies*: basic test construction issues such as reliability and validity.
2. *Limited generalizability of analogue research*: unknown differences between simulated and real malingerers.
3. *Variable group membership*: wide variability in samples for both simulators and symptom/disorder groups.
4. *Differential vulnerability to response bias*: some tests are more obvious while others are more subtle.
5. *Questionable Generalizability of findings*: from one SVT to other tests, to actual symptoms, or across time.
6. *Absence of mutual exclusivity*: poor effort can occur in presence of real disorders.
7. *Law of the instrument*: operational definitions wherein "malingering" becomes "what malingering tests measure". Specifically, the definitions of "effort", and validation studies to examine the construct, are often missing. Further "effort" cannot be assumed uniform for mild TBI, chronic pain, and depression, and for non-litigating and litigating situations.
8. *Questionable specificity*: the effects of fatigue, pain, disinterest, non-attended (computer) administration, mixing cognitive tests and SVTs in a battery with unknown validity, and other factors on response bias tests, are not understood and have not been addressed.
9. *Frequently high misclassification*: i.e., false positive or false negative rates.
10. *Use of most current SVT/indexes* with regard to diagnosis and decision making may violate APA ethics and *"APA Standards for Educational and Psychological Tests"*, given the aforementioned psychometric limitations.

Table 16.5 Diagnostic realities in asessment (e.g., ABI, chronic pain)

Physical disorder		Residual functional impairment		Residual testing impairments	
1. Yes		1. Yes, not exaggerated		1. Yes, not exaggerated	
2. Mixed	X	2. Yes, exaggerated	X	2. Yes, exaggerated	
3. Maybe		3. No, feigned		3. No, feigned	
4. No		4. No, not feigned		4. No, not feigned	
4		4		4	= 64

either (but possible minimization or denial) to persons with complicated, misattributed or non-existent disorders with only exaggerated impairments on examination or in functional status.

A cautious approach is indicated with regard to estimating the probabilities regarding presence or absence of physical impairment and response bias. In many, perhaps most, cases, integrating data from multiple sources and making inferences about which of the 64 possible combinations is most likely explanatory for the presenting condition is not sufficient. Subsequent delineation and descriptive characterization of the patient's effort and the validity of the results is often relevant. For instance, if a person has both actual symptoms and exaggeration, inferences must be generated not only about the degree of deliberateness and the degree of physical impairment, but also the degree of awareness of exaggeration on the part of the subject. Has the person adopted a sick role and talked themselves into believing they cannot perform certain tasks and lack certain abilities (e.g., somatoform disorder), with conscious withholding of effort due to intention of demonstrating what they believe to be true disabilities? Or, are they less conscious and aware, as in a conversion disorder? Or are they completely aware, but coping in a way that may be adaptive? An example is the case of an aging worker with a chronic history of back failures who has low self-esteem and a poor relationships with his/her employer. This employee may have a belief that another back injury is inevitable and will be cumulatively painful and disabling, will require uncomfortable interactions with others, that the company sometimes fires previously injured workers, that the company did not make obvious safety precautions to prevent their injury, and that no other job options are realistic.

Table 16.6 is included as summary of major response bias detection strategies that offer important information needed for interpreting the validity of medical examination and psychological test data.

Please note that a comprehensive review of existing literature was conducted in composing Table 16.6.[18,27–122] Multiple sources were used for most of the indicators. Special attention was given to reviews of specific empirical indicators such as those offered by Nies and Sweet[18] and Trueblood and Schmidt,[39] which served as a model for this effort. Notably, this

Table 16.6 Motivation assessment profile – neuropsychological assessment (MAP–NA)

Performance patterns on existing neuropsychological tests

Full-scale IQ	Low (vs. expected, estimated, etc.)
Digit span (floor effect)	**Age scale score < 7
Digit span: testing limits with "chunking"	Non-improvement with "chunking"
Arithmetic and orientation scale performance	"Near-miss" (Ganser errors)
WMS-R Malingering Index: Attention/ Concentration Index vs. Memory Index	Attention–Concentration Index score < General Memory Index (AC–GMI)
Paired Associate learning: Easy vs. Hard item performance	Hard Items ≥ Easy Items
General Neuropsych Deficit Scale (35)	**GNDS score < 44
Speech Sounds Perception Test performance	*> 17 errors (poor)
Seashore Rhythm Test performance	*> 8 errors (poor)
Finger Tapping Test	Unusually low without gross motor deficit
Tactual Stimulation Performance	Errors bilaterally vs. laterally
Finger Tip Number Writing – errors	**> 5
Finger Agnosia – errors	*> 3
Grip Strength	Unusually low without gross motor deficit
Categories Test performance	Rare or "spike three" errors; or > 1 error on Trials I or II
Wisconsin Card Sorting Test errors	Discrepant no. of perseverative vs. category errors
Recognition memory (RAVLT)	*< 6
Recognition memory (CVLT)	*< 13
List Learning Serial Order Effects	Abnormal patterns
Warrington Recognition Memory Test (RMT)	Score < 38 (RMW), < 26 (RMF)
Rey Complex Figure and Recognition Trial	Atypical Recognition errors (≥ 2); Recognition Failure error
Word Stem Priming Task performance	Poor or unusual performance

Instruments to specifically evaluate level of effort/response bias

Symptom Validity Testing (SVT)	< 50% chance level responding
Hiscock Forced Choice Procedure (HFCP)	< 50% chance level responding, < 66 correct
Victoria Symptom Validity Test (VSVT)	< 50% chance level responding, <16 on easy and/or hard items
Portland Digit Recognition Test (PDRT)	< 50%, chance responding
21-Item Test	< 5 on free recall, < 3 on free recall, < 13 on recognition, < 9 on recognition
Test of Memory Malingering (TOMM)	< 50% chance level responding
Forced Choice Test of Non-verbal Ability (61)	< 50% chance level responding
Dot Counting Test (DCT)	Correct/incorrect responses

Computer Assessment of Response Bias (CARB)	< 89% raises suspicion
Autobiographical Interview (36)	> 3 errors
Memorization of 16 Items Test (MSIT)	> 8 omissions, > 6 omissions, < 6 total correct
Rey Word Recognition List (WRL)	< 6 correct, < 5 (total correct minus false positives)
Rey Memory for 15 Items Test (MFIT)	< 3 complete sets, < 9 items [Lezak[38]]

Priming/implicit memory tests

Word completion memory test (WCMT)	$R < 9$ or inclusion < 15

Personality instruments with built-in detection designs

Personality Assessment Inventory (PAI) (104)	• Inconsistency (INC), Infrequency (INF), Positive Impression Management (PIM), and Negative Impression Management (NIM) scales • 8 score patterns thought to comprise a "Malingering Index" • > 2 patterns malingering suspected • > 4 patterns likely malingering
Minnesota Multiphasic Personality Inventory (MMPI-2)	• Validity indices (L, F, Fb, Fp, Ds, K, VRIN, TRIN), F-K(32) (103, 105) • The Fake Bad Scale (105) • Compare subtle to obvious items *Rogers (34) – cutoff scores:* *Liberal:* o *F-Scale raw score > 23* o *F-Scale T-Score > 81* o *F-K Index > 10* o *Obvious – subtle score > 83* *Conservative:* o *F-scale raw > 30* o *F-K index > 25* o *Obvious – subtle score > 190*

Qualitative variables in assessing response bias

Time/response latency comparisons across similar tasks	Inconsistencies across tasks
Performance on easy tasks presented as hard	Low scores or unusual errors
Remote memory report	Difficulties, especially if < recent memory, or severely impaired in absence of gross amnesia
Personal information	Very poor personal information in absence of gross amnesia
Comparison between test performance and behavioral observations	Discrepancies

Continued...

Table 16.6 Continued...

Inconsistencies in history and/or complaints, performance	Inconsistencies across time, interviewer, etc.
Comparisons for inconsistencies within testing session (quantitative and qualitative):	(A) Within tasks (e.g., easy vs. hard items)
	(B) Between tasks (e.g., easy vs. hard)
	(C) Across repetitions of same/parallel tasks (R/O fatigue)
	(D) Across similar tasks under different motivational sets
Comparisons across testing sessions (qualitative and quantitative)	Poorer/inconsistent performance on re-testing
Symptom self-report: complaints	High frequency of complaints; patient complaints > significant others'

Main & Spanswick indicators[13]
- Failure to comply with reasonable treatment
- Report of severe pain with no associated psychological effects
- Marked inconsistencies in effects of pain on general activities
- Poor work record and history of persistent appeals against awards
- Previous litigation

Symptom self-report: early vs. late symptom complaint	Early symptoms reported late

Neuromedical indicators

Hoover's Test	Test for malingered lower extremity weakness associated with normal crossed extensor response
Astasia abasia	"Drunken type" gait with near falls but no actual falls to ground
Non-organic sensory loss	Patchy sensory loss, midline sensory loss, large scotoma in visual field, tunnel vision
Non-organic upper extremity drift	Long tract involvement results in pronator type drift. Proximal shoulder girdle weakness and malingering typically present with downward drift while in supination
Stenger's Test	Test for malingered hearing loss during audiologic evaluation
Gait discrepancies when observed vs. not observed	If organic should be consistent regardless of whether observed or not
Gait discrepancies relative to direction of requested ambulation	Gait for a patient with hemiparesis should present similarly in all directions; malingerers do not as a rule practice a feigned gait in all directions

Forearm pronation, hand clasping and forearm supination test for digit/finger sensory loss	Malingered finger sensory loss is difficult to maintain in this perceptually confusing, intertwined hand/finger position
Pain vs. temperature discrepancies	Due to the fact that both sensory modalities run in the spinothalamic tract, they should be found to be commensurately impaired contralateral to the side of the CNS lesion
Lack of atrophy in a chronically paretic/paralytic limb	Lack of atrophy in a paralyzed/paretic limb suggests the limb is being used or is getting regular electrical stimulation to maintain mass
Impairment diminishes under influence of sodium amytal, hypnosis or lack of observation	All these observations are most consistent with non-organic presentations including consideration of malingering or conversion disorder
Incongruence between neuroanatomical imaging and neurologic examination	Lack of any static imaging findings on brain CT or MRI in the presence of a dense motor or sensory deficit suggests non-organicity
Arm drop test	An aware patient malingering profound alteration in consciousness or significant arm paresis will not let their own hand when held over their head, drop onto their face
Presence of ipsilateral findings when implied neuroanatomy would dictate contralateral findings	An examinee claiming severe right brain damage who claims right eye blindness and right-sided weakness and sensory loss
Tell me "when I'm not touching" responses	An examinee with claimed sensory loss who endorses that he does not feel you touch him when you ask him to tell you "if you do not feel this"
Lack of shoe wear in presence of gait disturbance	An examinee with claimed longer term gait deviation due to orthopedic or neurologic causes should demonstrate commensurate wear on shoes (if worn with any frequency)
Calluses on hands in "totally disabled" examinee	An examinee who is unable to work should not present with signs of ongoing evidence of physical labor

Continued...

Table 16.6 Continued...

Assistive device "wear and tear" signs	In any examinee using assistive devices for any period of time, e.g. cane, crutches, there should be commensurate wear on the device consistent with their claimed impairment and disability
Mankopf's Maneuver	Increase in heart rate commensurate with nociceptive stimulation during exam (there is some controversy on whether this always occurs)
Lack of atrophy in a limb that is claimed to be significantly impaired	If side-to-side measurements and/or inspection do not bear out atrophy, consider other causes aside from one being claimed
Sudden motor give-away or ratchetiness on manual strength testing	Considered to normally be a sign of incomplete effort or symptom exaggeration
Weakness on manual muscle testing without commensurate asymmetry of DTRs or muscle bulk	Suggests simulated muscle weakness if longstanding
Toe test for simulated low back pain	Flexion of hip and knee with movement only of toes should not produce an increase in low back pain
Magnuson's Test	Have examinee point to area several times over period of examination; inconsistencies suggest increased potential for non-organicity
Delayed response sign	Pain reaction temporally delayed relative to application of perceived nociceptive stimulus
Wrist drop test	In an examinee with claimed wrist extensor loss, have them pronate forearm, extend elbow and flex shoulder; if on making a fist in this position they also extend wrist, then non-organicity should be suspected
Object drop test	Examinee claims inability to bend down yet does so to pick up a light object "inadvertently" dropped by examiner

Hip adductor test	Test for claimed paralysis of lower extremity, similar to Hoover's test yet looks for crossed adductor response
Disparity between tested range of motion (ROM) and observed range of motion of any joint	When ROM under testing is significantly disparate (e.g., less) from observed, spontaneous ROM suspect functional contributors
Straight leg raise (SLR) disparities dependent on examinee positioning	Differences in SLR between sitting, standing and/or bending may suggest a functional overlay to low back complaints
Grip strength testing via dynamometer	Three repetitions at any given setting should not vary more than 20% and/or bell-shaped curve should be generated if all five positions are tested
Sensory "flip" test	Sensory findings should be the same if testing upper extremity in supination or pronation or lower extremity in internal vs. external rotation. Differences may suggest a functional overlay
Pinch test for low back pain	Pinching the lumbar fat pad should not reproduce pain due to axial structure involvement; if test is positive suspect a functional overlay.

table provides an illustrative summary of a constellation or profiling approach to response bias detection strategy use that relies on assessing relevant information for interpreting examination data. This multiaxial conceptual model is presented as a methodological approach for constructing a profile of motivation and response bias, which incorporates a wide array of findings from common instruments and procedures during evaluation. Empirical support exists indicating that each of these indicators has at least some utility in detecting suboptimal effort.[9,39] Importantly, review of original test manuals and studies should be conducted before employing any of these instruments. Also, as noted previously, numerous pitfalls and limitations of each of these procedures, both conceptual and methodological, exist. However, some increasing evidence exists for improved discrimination and increased reliability when multiple measures are employed.[40] The conceptual approach offered by the proposed motivation assessment profiling (MAP) is one where multiple factors are integrated as an optimal method for estimating the degree of effort and the degree to which examination findings are reliable and valid. This conceptual model and procedure (MAP) for estimating motivation economically incorporates currently available instruments and methods and the available published research for direct and indirect measurement of effort and response bias.

As can be seen in Table 16.6, most major objective personality measures and many neuropsychological measures have scales or indices that can be calculated,[41] such as the Memory Assessment Scales,[42] and the Rey Complex Figure Test and Recognition Trial,[43] that provide simulator performance data. The advantages inherent in such procedures include:

- reduced need for administering and charging for very long tests designed solely for detection of potential motivation problems (especially if negative), and for which numerous generalization difficulties exit
- limiting of protracted testing times which reduce the amount of proportionately available time for administering other relevant measures and conducting more comprehensive interview (examinee, collaborative others)
- potential enhancement of face validity of measures to examinees.

Importantly, the strategies in Table 16.6 are not offered individually and, again, are not intended to support a simple dualistic model that assumes examinees either try hard or malinger, or that evidence of less than full effort on any one test necessarily implies absence of impairment in other areas of examination or in real world abilities. Although they are also not offered with specific guidelines (e.g., failure on a specific number of indicators represents inadequate performance or response bias), the strategies are offered with the following suggestions:

- examination performance can be influenced by multiple factors that include desire to perform with full effort
- the degree of effort exerted on examinations exists on a continuum (vs. a dichotomy) and can be estimated by the extent to which indicators of poor effort are present
- reliability and validity of examination findings are dependent on relative assurances of full effort
- interpretation and diagnostic impressions are dependent upon reliable and valid examination results.

It should be emphasized that "failure" on one measure of response bias or malingering does not mean that the entire set of complaints is biased or invalid. Ethical guidelines caution against overzealous interpretation of limited test data. In fact, the only reasonable evidence of certain or definite malingering is confession or admission. A secondary form of evidence, although somewhat less than perfectly reliable, is when the person or examinee is detected, via surveillance, performing an act that they reported that they absolutely could not perform under any circumstance.

It should also be emphasized that a great disparity exists between the adversarial legal process where attorneys are advocates for their clients and the IME setting where the doctor must be dispassionate and objective. The danger of attorney "coaching" based on utilization of this material cannot be underestimated. This, of course, would then represent a form of "stealth" threat to the validity of examination data. This threat, or expected consequence of collision between the disparate legal and scientific ethics, has recently been documented in a publication noting a case of attorney client coaching.[123] However, compared to simpler models where only a couple of isolated response bias measures are used, it seems extremely unlikely that the multiple measures employed in the MAP approach could be understood and manipulated.

Finally, enhancing response bias detection as a means of optimizing interpretability of examination results, critical as it is, should not be considered the final step. Decreasing the potential for response is a more efficacious and economic approach to enhancing utility of neuropsychological assessment. The following explicit and comprehensive recommendations for enhancing motivation, assessing response bias, and increasing efficiency, utility and ecological validity of examination procedures are offered.

Conclusions: recommendations for enhancing validity in impairment and disability assessment findings

1   Utilize instruments with built-in symptom validity measures. Most major objective personality measures and many neuropsychological measures have scales or indices that can be calculated that provide simulator performance data. These instruments promote increased economy and efficiency of testing, probably enhance face validity of testing procedures, and afford a greater proportion of time for administration of other relevant measures and conducting interview.
2   Develop assessment procedures with built-in symptom validity measures.
3   Develop built-in symptom validity indicators for existing assessment procedures
4   Utilize comparisons with published patterns and indices indicating suboptimal test performance (e.g., serial position effects; Wechsler Memory Scale – Revised General Memory vs. Attention/ Concentration index).
5   Employ shorter symptom validity tests in order to minimize possibility of negative reactions owing to the nature of protracted participation in easy, boring tasks.
6   Employ more credible and less well-known symptom validity measures. For example, the Hiscock procedure looks easy and obvious and patients often comment, "Boy, this is easy . . . just remember the first number

from the list." The Rey 15 Item Test is also somewhat apparent, and it is even discussed in law journals.

7   Vary measures and procedures that are employed in order to prevent discrimination of real measures from symptom validity measures. Publicization of these tests has led to increased recognition by attorneys, clients, support groups, internet groups, and so on. Measure completion time for symptom checklists and psychological measures and compare with response times on cognitive measures for consistency.

8   Rely primarily on doctoral-level clinicians for all aspects of the examination, including interviewing and testing, with limited use and reliance on technicians. Experienced psychologists and physicians who test and interview are considerably more capable of the following: (a) integrating history, interview, and personality and emotional assessment data with more sophisticated clinical observations during examination; (b) adapting more creative modifications of testing procedures given suspicion of low motivation, as well as modifications to the testing process (e.g., provision of corrective feedback, instruction) to increase motivation and optimize effort; (c) benefiting from the probability that examinees will be less likely to believe they can mislead the "doctor"; (d) avoiding possible symptom exaggeration owing to fear that a non-doctoral testing technician will miss problems.

9   Increase administration of tests by clinicians who treat the types of patients they assess. This would likely help to assure more adequate clinical skills for detecting suboptimal performance, as well as collection of internalized tracking data to allow validation of previous inferences across time. Such tracking allows for continuous self-correction and increased internalized norms regarding ecological and predictive validity of psychological measures.

10   Ensure that emotional variables affecting motivation are adequately assessed during an interview that is conducted prior to testing. Specifically, assess the impact of anger or blame and feelings of resentment or victimization,[124] as well as the other variables shown in the literature to be associated with poor recovery and adaptation to impairment.[6]

11   Always assess interest/disinterest in the testing process and any obstacles or impediments to optimal effort and performance.

12   Prepare patients before beginning testing. Employ understanding, as well as education, in order that clients will be prepared to perform to the best of their ability. Emphasize that tests do not measure everything, but that they do assess effort. Emphasize interview data and corroborative data and functional abilities as important as testing.

13   Establish rapport and a basic working relationship with clients. Even in cases of independent examinations where the referral source and expectation is adversarially motivated, valid data collection requires a collaborative effort. The possibility of dissimulation might be reduced given

better rapport.[9] Address potential sources of bias directly, and provide feedback, education, and clarification.

14 Do not freely share information about symptom validity tests or known patterns of performance on neuropsychological instruments with non-psychologists. Other professionals adhere to a completely different set of professional ethics. Several recent law publications expose a practice of preparing clients for testing by counseling them with this information.[124]

15 Remain aware that, in science and medicine and neuropsychology, situations are rarely either/or, clear-cut, or unidimensional. Avoid simplistic conceptual models that are compatible with dichotomous approaches to assessing effort and response bias. Such approaches usually rely on a cutting score for one or two measures. Cutting scores, by their nature, always entail judgment,[125] inherently result in misclassification and impose an artificial dichotomy on an essentially continuous variables; and "true" cut scores do not exit.

16 Employ sophisticated, continuous conceptualizations of effort and response bias by using multiple independent measures of estimated effort. Employ a model that conceptualizes motivation and effort as continuous variables that can vary across tests, settings, and occasions. Performance data provides the best information for estimating the degree of effort exerted, and the degree to which test results are reliable and valid.

17 Spend time with patients and try to get to know them from a psychological perspective. If motivation seems poor, confront the person rather than proceed with a garbage in–garbage out (GIGO) approach. We cannot assume that everyone takes our tests seriously, is as honest or effortful on our tests as we would like, or that we will not have to work at getting them interested or invested in doing their best.

18 Utilize and devise models that measure the degree of apparent motivation and effort, using multiple data sources, and estimate confidence levels in inferences, given consideration of the multiple factors that contribute to test results. Employ similarly sophisticated models for assessing persistent impairments, adaptation to impairments, disability and so on. Probability statements based on multiple measures are probably best. Integration of contextual information, history, behavioral observations, interview and collaborative data, personality and coping data with multiple measures of effort or performance and current tests data and qualitative data provides the best information for estimating the degree of effort exerted, and the degree to which test results are reliable and valid.

References

1. Zasler, N. D., & Martelli, M. F. (1998). Assessing mild traumatic brain injury. *AMA Guides Newsletter*, November/December, 1–5.
2. Rohling, M. L., & Binder, L. M. (1995). Money matters: a meta-analytic review

of the association between financial compensation and the experience and treatment of chronic pain. *Health Psychol., 14,* 537–547.

3. Youngjohn, J. R., Burrows, L., & Erdal, K. (1995). Brain damage or compensation neurosis? The controversial post-concussion syndrome. *Clin. Neuropsychol., 2,* 112–123.

4. Binder, L. M., & Rohling, M. L. (1996). Money matters: a meta-analytic review of the effects of financial incentives on recovery after closed-head injury. *Am. J. Psychiat., 153,* 7–10.

5. Blau, T. (1984). *The psychologist as expert witness.* New York: Wiley.

6. Martelli, M. F., Zasler, N. D., Mancini, A., & MacMillan, P. J. (1999). Psychological assessment and applications in impairment and disability evaluations. In R. V. May and M. F. Martelli (Eds.), *Guide to functional capacity evaluation with impairment rating applications* (pp. 3–84). Richmond, VA: NADEP.

7. Matheson, L. (1990). Symptom magnification syndrome: a modern tragedy and its treatment – Part one: Description and definition. *Indust. Rehabil. Qu., 3,* 1–23.

8. Hayes, J. S., Hilsabeck, R. C., & Gouvier, W. D. (1999). Malingering traumatic brain injury: current issues and caveats in assessment and classification. In N. R. Varney and R. J. Roberts (Eds.), *The evaluation and treatment of mild traumatic brain injury* (pp. 240–290). Mahwah, NJ: Lawrence Erlbaum Associates Inc.

9. Martelli, M. F., Zasler, N. D., Nicholson, K., Pickett, T. C., & May, V. R. (2001). Assessing the veracity of pain complaints and associated disability. In R. B., Weiner (Ed.), *Pain management: A practical guide for clinicians* (6th ed., pp. 789–805). Boca Raton, FL: St. Lucie Press.

10. Matheson, L. (1988). Symptom magnification syndrome. In S. Isernhagen (Ed.), *Work injury* (pp. 48–91). Rockville, MD: Aspen.

11. Matheson, L. (1991). Symptom magnification syndrome: a modern tragedy and its treatment – Part two: Techniques of identification. *Indust. Rehabil. Qu., 4*(1), 1–17.

12. Matheson, L. (1991). Symptom magnification syndrome: a modern tragedy and its treatment – Part three: Techniques of treatment. *Indust. Rehabil. Qu., 4*(2), 1–24.

13. Main, C. J., & Spanswick, C. C. (1995). "Functional overlay", and illness behaviour in chronic pain: distress or malingering? Conceptual difficulties in medico-legal assessment of personal injury claims. *J. Psychosom. Res., 39,* 737–754.

14. Babitsky, S., Brigham, C. R., & Mangraviti, J. J. (2000). *Symptom magnification, deception and malingering: Identification through distraction and other tests and techniques.* VHS video. Falmouth, MA: SEAK.

15. Kaufman, D. M. (1995). *Clinical neurology for psychiatrists.* Philadelphia, PA: W. B. Saunders.

16. Hall, H. V., & Pritchard, D. A. (1996). *Detecting malingering and deception: Forensic distortion analysis.* Delray Beach, FL: St. Lucie Press.

17. Nicholson, K., Martelli, M. F., & Zasler, N. D. (2001). Myths and misconceptions about chronic pain: the problem of mind body dualism. In R. B. Weiner (Ed.), *Pain management: A practical guide for clinicians* (6th ed., pp. 465–474). Boca Raton, FL: St. Lucie Press.

18. Nies, K., & Sweet, J. (1994). Neuropsychological assessment and malingering: a critical review of past and present strategies. *Arch. Clin. Neuropsychol., 9,* 501–552.

19. Waddell, G., & Main, C. J. (1984). Assessment of severity in low back disorders. *Spine, 9*, 204–208.
20. Waddell, G., Main, C. J., Morris, E. W., Paola, M. D., & Gray, I. C. (1984). Chronic low back pain, psychologic distesss, and illness behavior. *Spine, 9*, 209–213.
21. Simmonds, M. J., Kumar, S., & Lechelt, E. (1998). Psychosocial factors in disabling low back pain: causes or consequences? *Disabil. Rehabil., 18*, 161–168.
22. Lees-Haley, P. R., Williams, C. W., Zasler, N. D., Margulies, S., English, L. T., & Steven, K. B. (1997). Response bias in plaintiff's histories. *Brain In., 11*, 791–799.
23. Lees-Haley, P., & Brown, R. S. (1993). Neuropsychological complaint base rates of 170 personal injury claimants. *Arch. Clin. Neuropsychol., 8*, 203–210.
24. Loring, D. W. (1995). Psychometric detection of malingering. Paper presented at the Annual Meeting of the American Academy of Neurology, Seattle, WA.
25. Cummings, J. L., et al. (1996). Report of the Therapeutics and Technology Assessment Subcommittee of the American Academy of Neurology. Assessment: neuropsychological testing of adults. *Neurology, 47*, 592–599.
26. Martell, M. F., Zasler, N. D., Nicholson, K., Hart, R. P., & Heilbronner, R. L. (2002). Masquerades of brain injury. Part III: Critical examination of symptom validity testing and diagnostic realities in assessment. *J. Controvers. Med. Claims, 9*, 19–21.
27. Martelli, M. F., & Zasler, N. D. (2002). Assessment of motivation and response bias following aquired brain injury (ABI). *J. Legal Nurse Consult., 13*, 7–14.
28. Bernard, L. C., McGrath, M. J., & Houston, O. (1993). Discriminating between simulated malingering and closed head injury on the Wechsler Memory Scale Revised. *Arch. Clin. Neuropsychol., 8*, 539–551.
29. Trueblood, W. (1994). Qualitative and quantitative characteristics of malingered and other invalid WAIS-R and clinical memory data. *J. Clin. Exp. Neuropsychol., 16*, 597–607.
30. Strauss, E., Spellacy, F., Hunter, M., & Berry, T. (1994). Assessing believable deficits on measures of attention and information processing capacity. *Arch. Clin. Neuropsychol., 9*, 483–490.
31. Rawlings, P., & Brooks, N. (1990). Simulation index: a method for detecting factitious errors on the WAIS-R and WMS. *Neuropsychology, 4*, 223–238.
32. Mittenberg, W., Theroux-Fichera, S., Zielinski, R. E., & Heilbronner, R. L. (1995). Identification of malingered head injury on the Wechsler Adult Intelligence Scale–Revised. *Prof. Psychol. Res. Pract., 26*, 491–498.
33. Mittenberg, W., Arzin, R., Millsaps, C., & Heilbronner, R. (1993). Identification of malingered head injury on the Wechsler Memory Scale. *Psychol. Assess., 5*, 34–40.
34. Rogers, R. (Ed.) (1997). *Clinical assessment of malingering and deception* (2nd ed.). New York: Guilford Press.
35. Reitan, R. M., & Wolfson, D. (1995). Influence of age and education on neuropsychological test results. *Clin. Neuropsychol., 9*, 151–158.
36. Millis, S. R., Putnam, S. H., Adams, K. M., & Ricker, J. H. (1995). The California verbal learning test in the detection of incomplete effort in neuropsychological evaluation. *Psychol. Assess., 7*, 463–471.
37. Wiggins, E. C., & Brandt, J. (1988). The detection of simulated amnesia. *Law Hum. Behav., 12*, 57–78.

38. Lezak, M. (1996). *Neuropsychological assessment* (3rd ed.). New York: Oxford University Press.
39. Trueblood, W., & Schmidt, M. (1993). Malingering and other validity considerations in the neuropsychological evaluation of mild head injury. *J. Clin. Exp. Neuropsychol., 15*, 578–590.
40. Vanderploeg, R. D., & Curtiss, G. (2001). Malingering assessment: evaluation of validity of performance. *NeuroRehabilitation, 4*, 245–251.
41. Goebel, R. A. (1983). Detection of faking on the Halstead–Reitan neuropsychological test battery. *J. Clin. Psychol., 39*, 731–742.
42. Williams, J. M. (1992). *The memory assessment scales.* Odessa, FL: Psychological Assessment Resources.
43. Meyers, J. E., & Meyers, K. R. (1995). *Rey complex figure and recognition trial.* Odessa, FL: Psychological Assessment Resources.
44. Beetar, J. T., & Williams, J. M. (1995). Malingering response styles on the Memory Assessment Scales and symptom validity tests. *Arch. Clin. Neuropsychol., 10*, 57–65.
45. Allen, L. M., & Cox, D. R. (1995). *Computerized assessment of response bias* (Revised ed.). Durham, NC: CogniSyst Inc.
46. Benton, A., & Spreen, O. (1961). Visual memory test: the simulation of mental incompetence. *Arch. Gen. Psychiat., 4*, 79–83.
47. Bernard, L. C. (1990). Prospects for faking believable memory deficits on neuropsychological tests and the use of incentives in simulation research. *J. Clin. Exp. Neuropsychol., 12*, 715–728.
48. Bernard, L. C. (1991). The detection of faked deficits on the Rey auditory verbal learning test: the effects of serial position. *Arch. Clin. Neuropsychol., 6*, 81–88.
49. Bernard, L. C., Houston, W., & Natoli, L. (1993). Malingering on neuropsychological memory tests: potential objective indicators. *J. Clin. Psychol., 49*, 45–53.
50. Delis, D. (1987). *The California verbal learning test.* San Antonio, TX: Psychological Corporation.
51. Arnett, P. A., Hammeke, T. A., & Schwartz, L. (1995). Quantitative and qualitative performance on Rey's 15-item test in neurological patients and dissimulators. *Clin. Neuropsychol., 9*, 17–22.
52. Green, P., Allen, L., & Astner, K. (1996). *The word memory test: A manual for the oral and computerized forms.* Durham, NC: CogniSyst Inc.
53. Green, P., Gervais, R., Astner, K., Kiss, I., & Allen, L. (1993). CARB malingering test results in 210 accident/compensation cases with and without head injury. Paper presented at the annual meeting of the National Academy of Neuropsychology, Phoenix, AZ.
54. Green, P., Iverson, G., & Allen, L. (1999). Detecting malingering in head injury litigation with the word memory test. *Brain Inj., 13*, 813–819.
55. Guilmette, T. J., Hart, K. J., & Giuliano, A. J. (1993). Malingering detection: the use of a forced-choice method in identifying organic versus simulated memory impairment. *Clin. Neuropsychol., 7*, 59–69.
56. Iverson, G. L. (1995). Qualitative aspects of malingered memory deficits. *Brain Inj., 9*, 35–40.
57. Iverson, G. L., & Franzen, M. D. (1994). The recognition memory test, digit span, and knox cube test as markers of malingered memory impairment. *Assessment, 1*, 323–334.

58. Iverson, G. L., Franzen, M. D., & McCracken, L. M. (1991). Evaluation of an objective assessment technique for the detection of malingered memory deficits. *Law Hum. Behav., 15*, 667–676.

59. Iverson, G. L., Franzen, M. D., & McCracken, L. M. (1994). Application of a forced-choice memory procedure designed to detect experimental malingering. *Arch. Clin. Neuropsychol., 9*, 437–450.

60. Iverson, G. L., Slick, D. J., & Franzen, M. D. (1996). Evaluation of a WMS-R malingering index in a non-litigating clinical sample. Paper presented at the annual meeting of the National Academy of Neuropsychology, New Orleans, LA.

61. Frederick, R. I., & Foster, H. G. (1991). Multiple measures of malingering on a forced-choice test of cognitive ability. *Psychol. Assess., 3*, 596–602.

62. Bigler, E. D. (1990). Neuropsychology and malingering: comment on Faust, Hart, and Guilmette (1988). *J. Consult. Clin. Psychol., 58*, 244–247.

63. Binder, L. M., & Pankratz, L. (1987). Neuropsychological evidence of a factitious memory complaint. *J. Clin. Exp. Neuropsychol., 9*, 167–171.

64. Binder, L. M., & Willis, S. C. (1991). Assessment of motivation after a financially compensable minor head trauma. *Psychol. Assess., 3*, 175–181.

65. Binder, L. M. (1992). Forced-choice testing provides evidence of malingering. *Arch. Phys. Med. Rehabil., 73*, 377–380.

66. Binder, L. M. (1993). Assessment of malingering after mild head trauma with the Portland Digit Recognition Test (published erratum appears in *J Clin Exp Neuropsychol 15*(6), 852). *J. Clin. & Exp. Neuropsychol., 15*, 170–182.

67. Cercy, S. P., Schretlen, D. J., & Brandt, J. (1997). Simulated amnesia and the pseudo-memory phenomena. In R. Rogers (Ed.), *Clinical assessment of malingering and deception* (2nd ed., pp. 108–129). NewYork: Guilford Press.

68. Brandt, J., Rubinsky, E., & Lassen, G. (1985). Uncovering malingered amnesia. *Ann. N Y Acad. Sci., 44*, 502–503.

69. Cliffe, M. J. (1992). Symptom-validity testing of feigned sensory or memory deficits: a further elaboration for subjects who understand the rationale. *Br. J. Clin. Psychol., 31*, 207–209.

70. Dalby, J. T. (1988). Detecting faking in the pretrial psychological assessment. *Am. J. Forensic Psychol., 6*, 49–55.

71. Daniel, A. E., & Resnick, P. J. (1987). Mutism, malingering, and competency to stand trial. *Bull. Am. Acad. Psychiatry Law, 15*, 301–308.

72. Dush, D. M., Simons, L. E., Platt, M., Nation, P. C., & Ayres, S. Y. (1994). Psychological profiles distinguishing litigating and nonlitigating pain patients: subtle, and not so subtle. *J. Pers. Assess., 62*, 299–313.

73. Ensalada, L. H. (1998). Illness behavior. *The AMA Guides Newsletter*, May/ June, 4–6.

74. Faust, D. (1995). The detection of deception. (Review). *Neurol. Clin., 13*, 255–265.

75. Faust, D., & Guilmette, T. J. (1990). To say it's not so doesn't prove that it isn't: research on the detection of malingering. Reply to Bigler, *J. Consult. Clin. Psychol., 58*, 248–250.

76. Cullum, C., Heaton, R., & Grant, I. (1991). Psychogenic factors influencing neuropsychological performance: somatoform disorders, factitious disorders and malingering. In H. O. Doerr and A. S. Carlin (Eds.), *Forensic neuropsychology*. New York: Guilford Press.

77. Braverman, M. (1978). Post-injury malingering is seldom a calculated ploy. *Occup. Health Saf., 47,* 36–40.
78. Franzen, M. D., Iverson, G. L., & McCracken, L. M. (1990). The detection of malingering in neuropsychological assessment. *Neuropsychol. Rev., 1,* 247–279.
79. Frederick, R. I., Sarfaty, S. D., Johnston, J. D., & Powel, J. (1994). Validation of a detector of response bias on a forced-choice test of nonverbal ability. *Neuropsychology 8,* 118–125.
80. Gilbertson, A. D., Torem, M., Cohen, R., & Newman, I. (1992). Susceptibility of common self-report measures of dissociation to malingering. *Dissociation: Progress in the Dissociative Disorders, 5,* 216–220.
81. Greiffenstein, M. F., Baker, W. J., & Gola, T. (1994). Validation of malingered amnesia measures with a large clinical sample. *Psychol. Assess., 6,* 218–224.
82. Heaton, R. K., Smith, H. H., Lehman, R. A., & Vogt, A. T. (1978). Prospects for faking believable deficits on neuropsychological testing. *J. Consul. Clin. Psychol., 46,* 892–900.
83. Hiscock M., & Hiscock, C. (1989). Redefining the forced choice method for the detection of malingering. *J. Clin. Exp. Neuropsychol, 11,* 967–974.
84. Hiscock, C. K., Branham, J. D., & Hiscock, M. (1994). Detection of feigned cognitive impairment: the two-alternative forced-choice method compared with selected conventional tests. *J. Psychopathol Behav Assess., 16,* 95–110.
85. Rose, F. E., Hall, S., Szalda, P., & Allen, D. (1995). Portland Digit Recognition Test – computerized: measuring response latency improves the detection of malingering. *Clin. Neuropsychol., 9,* 124–134.
86. Schretlen, D., Brandt, J., Krafft, L., & Van Gorp, W. (1991). Some caveats using the Rey 15-Item Memory Test to detect malingered amnesia. *Psychol. Assess., 3,* 667–672.
87. Slick, D., Hopp, G., Strauss, E., Hunter, M., & Pinch, D. (1994). Detecting dissimulation: profiles of simulated malingerers, traumatic brain-injury patients, and normal controls on a revised version of Hiscock and Hiscock's Forced-Choice Memory Test. *J. Clin. Exp. Neuropsychol., 16,* 472–481.
88. Meyers, J., & Volbrecht, M. (1999). Detection of malingerers using the Rey Complex Figure and Recognition Trial. *Appl. Neuropsychol., 6,* 201–207.
89. Meyers, J., Galinsky, A., & Volbrecht, M. (1999). Malingering and mild brain injury: how low is too low?, *App. Neuropsychol., 6,* 208–216.
90. Larrabee, G. J. (1992). On modifying recognition memory tests for detection of malingering. *Neuropsychol., 6,* 23–27.
91. Lee, G. P., Loring, D. W., & Martin, R. C. (1992). Rey's 15-item visual memory test for the detection of malingering: normative observations on patients with neurological disorders. *Psychol. Assess., 4,* 43–46.
92. Sbordone, R. J., Seyranian, G. D., & Ruff, R. M. (2000). The use of significant others to enhance the detection of malingerers from traumatically brain injured patients. *Arch. Clin. Neuropsychol., 15,* 465–477.
93. Schacter, D. L. (1986). On the relation between genuine and simulated amnesia. *Behav. Sci. Law., 4,* 47–64.
94. Horton, K. D., Smith, S. A., Barghout, N. K., & Connolly, D. A. (1992). The use of indirect memory tests to assess malingered amnesia: a study of metamemory. *J. Exp. Psychol.: Gen., 121,* 326–351.
95. Iverson, G., Green, P., & Gervais, R. (1999). Using the Word Memory Test to

detect biased responding in head injury litigation. *J. Cog. Rehab.*, March/April, 2–6.

96. Rogers, R. (1990). Development of a new classificatory model of malingering. *Bull. Am. Acad. Psych Law, 18*, 323–333.

97. Jacobsen, R. R. (1995). The post-concussional syndrome: physiogenesis, psychogenesis and malingering. An integrative model. *J. Psychosom. Res., 39*, 675–693.

98. Lees-Haley, P., & Brown, R. S. (1992). Biases in perception and reporting of following a perceived toxic exposure. *Percep. Mot. Skills, 75*, 533–544.

99. Pankratz, L., Fausti, S. A., & Peed, S. (1975). A forced-choice technique to evaluate deafness in the hysterical or malingering patient. *J. Consul. Clin. Psychol., 43*, 421–422.

100. Pankrantz, L. (1979). Symptom validity testing and symptom retraining: procedures for the assessment and treatment of functional sensory deficits. *J. Consul. Clin. Psychol., 47*, 409–410.

101. Lees-Haley, P., & Brown, R. S. (1993). Neuropsychological complaint base rates of 170 personal injury claimants. *Arch. Clin. Neuropsychol., 8*, 203–210.

102. Lees-Haley, P. R., & Brown, R. S. (1992). Biases in perception and reporting following a perceived toxic exposure. *Percep. Mot. Skills, 75*, 531–544.

103. Berry, D. T., Baer, R. A., & Harris, M. J. (1991). Detection of malingering on the MMPI: a meta-analysis. *Clin. Psychol. Rev., 11*, 585–591.

104. Morey, L. C. (1996). *Interpretive guide to the Personality Assessment Inventory (PAI)*. Odessa, FL: Psychological Assessment Resources.

105. Gough, H. G. (1954). Some common misperceptions about neuroticism. *J. Consul. Psychol., 18*, 287–292.

106. Lees-Haley, P. R., English, L. T., & Glenn, W. J. (1991). A fake bad scale on the MMPI-2 for personal injury claimants. *Psychol. Rep., 68*, 203–210.

107. Lees-Haley, P. (1997). Attorneys influence expert evidence in forensic psychological and neuropsychological cases. *Assessment, 4*, 321–324.

108. Hart, R. P., Martelli, M. F., & Zasler, N. D. (2000). Chronic pain and neuropsychological functioning. *Neuropsychol. Rev., 10*, 131–149.

109. Brady, J. P., & Lind, D. L. (1961). Experimental analysis of hysteria. *Arch. Gen. Psych., 4*, 331–339.

110. Brady, J. P. (1966). Hysteria versus malingering: a response to Grosz and Zimmerman. *Behav. Res. Ther., 4*, 321–322.

111. Martelli, M. F., Zasler, N. D., & Grayson, R. (2000). Ethics and medicolegal evaluation of impairment after brain injury. In M. Schiffman (Ed.), *Attorney's guide to ethics in forensic science and medicine*. Springield, IL: Charles C. Thomas.

112. May, R. V. (1998). Symptom magnification syndrome. In R. V. May and M. F. Martelli (Eds.), *Guide to functional capacity evaluation with impairment rating applications* (Vol. 2, pp. 1–22). Richmond, VA: NADEP.

113. Millis, S. (1992). Recognition Memory Test in the detection of malingered and exaggerated memory deficits. *Clin. Neuropsychol., 6*, 406–414.

114. Millis, S. R. (1994). Assessment of motivation and memory with the Recognition Memory Test after financially compensable mild head injury. *J. Clin. Psychol., 50*, 601–605.

115. Millis, S. R., & Kler, S. (1995). Limitations of the Rey Fifteen-Item Test in the detection of malingering. *Clin. Neuropsychol., 9*, 241–244.

116. Owens, R. G. (1995). The psychological signatures of malingering: assessing the legitimacy of claims. *Am. J. Forensic Psych., 13*, 61–75.
117. Palmer, B. W., Boone, K. B., Allman, L., & Castro, D. B. (1995). Co-occurrence of brain lesions and cognitive deficit exaggeration. *Clin. Neuropsychol., 9*, 68–73.
118. Perkins D., & Tebes, J. (1984). Genuine versus simulated responses on the Impact of Events Scale. *Psychol. Rep., 54*, 575–578.
119. Resnick, P. J. (1993). Defrocking the fraud: the detection of malingering. *Israel J. Psych. Rel. Sci., 2*, 93–99.
120. Babitsky, S., Brigham, C. R., & Mangraviti, J. J. (2000). *Symptom magnification, deception and malingering: Identification through distraction and other tests and techniques.* VHS video. Falmouth, MA: SEAK.
121. Rogers, R., Harrell, E. H., & Liff, C. D. (1993). Feigning neuropsychological impairment: a critical review of methodological and clinical considerations. *Clin. Psychol. Rev., 13*, 255–274.
122. Wedding, D., & Faust, D. (1998). Clinical judgement and decision-making in neuropsychology. *Arch. Clin. Neuropsychol., 6*, 233–265.
123. Youngjohn, J. R. (1995). Confirmed attorney coaching prior to neuro-psychological evaluation. *Assessment, 2*, 279–283.
124. Rutherford, W. H. (1989). Postconcussion symptoms: relationship to acute neurological indices, individual differences, and circumstances of injury. In H. S. Levin, H. M. Eisenberg, and A. L. Benton (Eds.), *Mild head injury* (pp. 229–244). New York: Oxford University Press.
125. Dwyer C. A. (1996). Cut scores & testing: statistics, judgment, truth, and error. *Psychol. Assess., 8*, 360–362.

17 Rehabilitation of cognitive disorders after acquired brain injury

The Combined Method (TCM)

José León-Carrión

Introduction

Cognitive disorders derived from traumatic brain injury occur frequently and affect most of the daily activities of the patients suffering from them. A study by Levin and colleagues[1] noted that 36% of the patients with severe brain injury had memory impairment. A more recent study by León-Carrión et al.[2] found a prevalence of 70% anterograde amnesia and 40% retrograde amnesia in a population of traumatic brain injury patients. These memory disorders limit the independence of those who have them and affect their family life as well as their social life. Recovery of diverse organic cognitive disorders has been pursued by psychologists and neuropsychologists for a long time.

There has traditionally been clearly evident pessimism about cognitive rehabilitation. The majority of articles published did not find that patients improved significantly after a "rehabilitation program". Those negative results were fundamentally based on three factors. The first was the excessively academic approach to these studies. That is to say, many academics who had no practical clinical knowledge designed programs for rehabilitation of cognitive functions which were theoretically well planned but had nothing to do with how an injured human brain functions nor with clinical reality. Neurocognitive reality was one thing and purely academic experiments another, as they only approached one limited part of the reality at best. In the second place, there was the investigators' lack of knowledge about the dynamic of interrelations that exist in the deterioration of cognitive functions after brain injury. An injured brain does not function the same as a brain which is intact. Likewise, a diffuse axonal lesion affecting the functioning of memory is not the same as a focal lesion affecting memory: neurofunctional cognitive systems are the basis of rehabilitation. Third, not everything done with patients is rehabilitation or can be called a "rehabilitation program". Many rehabilitation centers do not have permanent neuropsychologists on their staff constantly working with patients every day. The majority of them do not have their activities carried out by specialists, which makes it difficult to compare the efficacy of specific rehabilitation programs.

Current clinical data indicate that it is possible to improve and rehabilitate organic cognitive deficits with new techniques and methods of rehabilitation. In our clinical experience, we have found that successful treatment and recovery of cognitive disorders derived from traumatic brain injury are related to the locus and magnitude of the lesion, and to the pharmacological and neuropsychological strategies used.

The existing pessimism about cognitive rehabilitation has led to the development of prosthetic procedures directed at including patients in the community. Due to the strong, predominant influence in journals and publications that prosthetic rehabilitation is the only rehabilitation possibility, the rehabilitative approach to treatment and research on neurocognitive deficits and disorders following brain injury has almost been ignored for decades. The goal of this chapter is to reveal the existence of two clearly distinct models of rehabilitation of memory and other cognitive functions: the prosthetic model and the Combined Method. They differ in both methodology and in the results obtained.

The prosthetic method of cognitive rehabilitation

During the 1970s and 1980s there was a strong belief that restoring organic memory disorders was an impossible goal.[3-5] Although some rehabilitation techniques were experimented with, the majority of them were based on the knowledge of a cognitive psychology of the memory with little or no cerebral basis. In the early 1990s, Leng and Copello[6] tried to discover if any of these cognitive techniques were effective in memory recovery. They reviewed some of the approaches used for memory rehabilitation in patients with brain injury: Rote Learning, Elaborative Encoding Strategies, Visual Mnemonics, External Memory Aids, and the Method of Vanishing Cues. Results showed that Rote Learning was not useful, Elaborative Encoding Strategies were not popular with patients and the Method of Vanishing Cues has serious limitations. They found that only Visual Mnemonics may be useful for patients with memory disorders, and that External Memory Aids were useful for forgetful patients. These results were not very encouraging for the professionals dedicated to the recovery of organic memory disorders. This pessimism together with the difficulties found in rehabilitation gave rise to strengthening the prosthetic method of cognitive rehabilitation.

At the end of the last century, the efficiency of treatment for cognitive disorders still continued to be controversial. Carney et al.[7] evaluated evidence of the effectiveness of cognitive rehabilitation methods for improving outcomes in people with traumatic brain injury (TBI). After analyzing 600 potential references, 32 studies met predetermined inclusion criteria. They found that two randomized controlled trials and one observational study provided evidence that specific forms of cognitive rehabilitation reduce memory failures and anxiety, and improve self-concept and interpersonal relationships for people with TBI. The durability and clinical relevance of these findings is not established. Based on this evidence, they recommend the application of compensatory cognitive strategies, adapted to groups of patients and to individuals, to improve the functional ability of people with TBI. For them, intervention of this type must be delivered within a broader program that accounts for individual needs and utilizes various cognitive remediation technologies traditionally labelled restorative and/or compensatory. They conclude:

> In absence of strong evidence for the effectiveness of other cognitive rehabilitation methods and in light of the strong possibility that traditional distinctions for therapies (restorative versus compensatory) are simplistic and not clinically useful, we see no good reason why they should not be abandoned. In nearly all the studies in this review, patients improved. Although group differences were rarely observed, recovery across group occurred. Until we have done the necessary work to be able to demonstrate how improvement has come about, we are obligated to provide the services and care at our disposal for these people.[7]

Prigatano[8] has argued that the review by Carney and colleagues is "a good example of what I call scientism – that is, the practice of focusing on the statistical and research design properties of a study without understanding the phenomena under investigation". But reviews like that reinforce the use of the prosthetic method in the rehabilitation of people with acquired brain injury.

A cognitive orthotic could be defined as the use of devices that provide support for those impaired cognitive functions as a consequence of a brain or neurological condition. The prosthetic method of cognitive rehabilitation is based on the belief that neurocognitive functions (memory, reasoning, attention, executive functions, etc.) are not recuperable, or that recuperation is so limited that the patient cannot lead an independent life, so the best solution is training the patient to use external aids in carrying out daily activities and those which allow an independent life. According to Gorman,[9] "assistive technology devices enhance strengths in order to counterbalance the effects of the person's disability and provide alternative ways to perform tasks, thus promoting disability compensation". For others, this method is ideal and the one to choose for those patients who live in isolated areas with impossible or difficult access to rehabilitation centers, but the new techniques of teleneurorehabilitation are now competing with the use of the prosthetic method in these cases.

Different authors work within the prosthetic system. Thus, Wilson et al.[10] and Wilson et al.[11] promoted the use of NeuroPage, a simple and portable paging system developed in California by an engineer (his son had brain injury) who worked with a neuropsychologist. The NeuroPage was designed to help neurologically impaired patients who had significant everyday problems through a paging system. McGhee Pierce et al.[12] suggest the use of a computer-assisted exercise system, and others propose the use of micro-computers as external memory aids for memory problems[13] or palmtop computers.[14,15] Other authors recommend the use of diary training alone or a diary and self-instructional training.[16] As mobile phones have spread worldside, Wade and Troy[17] recommend them as new memory aids. Programmable Personal Digital Assistants (PDAs) are recommended by Pergami[18] as excellent tools in medical practice (www.palmspot.com/software/detail/ps7303a_9888.htlm;www.lcs.mgh.harvard.edu/dxplain.html; www.-pdacentral.com/palm/reference_ default.html). Telerehabilitation is also proposed by Ricker et al.[19] and by Tam et al.[20] to assist with problems in memory. The use of a portable voice organizer to remember therapy goals is proposed by Hart and colleagues.[21] The ISAAC cognitive prosthetic system has been introduced by Diamond et al.[22] as a small, individualized, wearable cognitive prosthetic assistive technology system to assist patients in their home environments and improve the patient's functional independence.

The major goals of cognitive orthotic have been described by Bergman,[23] always under the condition that effective cognitive orthotic design required understanding of the resources and limitations of the brain-injured person for whom the system is intended:

1   Support performance of live activities that the individual cannot execute independently as a result of cognitive deficits.
2   Provide people with brain dysfunction the necessary support for executive function deficiencies and specific cortical impairment.
3   Provide cues for activities of planning and scheduling, particularly for mobile individuals with brain damage.
4   Promote effective self-management to the fullest extent possible, given the individual's abilities and motivation, and the state of current technology.
5   Promote meaningful self-sufficiency in daily living through a selection of ecologically relevant tasks.
6   Increase self-confidence and self-esteem in individuals with cognitive impairment following their successful experiences with the computer.

As Diamond et al.[22] report, the orthotic method or assistive technology can be effective for a limited group of patients and circumstances. The devices described have significant shortcomings that reduce their appropriateness and effectiveness for many patients, especially those with more severe cognitive impairment. The authors consider one shortcoming is their unsuitability for delivering complex or lengthy procedural guidance. Recording devices can typically accommodate only a relatively small number of simple information elements.

The goal of this chapter is to introduce the Combined Method of neurorehabilitation, but we have also considered it important to briefly introduce the prosthetic method of neurorehabilitation for cognitve disorders as an optional treatment.

The Combined Method (TCM) of cognitive rehabilitation

Evidence of the worthiness of cognitive rehabilitation has been documented. Having reviewed 23 class I articles, Cicerone[24] observed that 17 provided positive evidence for the effectiveness of cognitive rehabilitation, and 7 of them provided evidence of generalized improvement of functional abilities. Among the six studies with negative results, several compared different kinds of remediation with improvement from both treatments, and one demonstrated a treatment effect when patients with milder residual impairments were re-examined. According to this author, the available evidence of the effectiveness of cognitive rehabilitation should enable clinicians to advocate the most effective and realistic treatments for individuals who require neurocognitive rehabilitation.

Further work by León-Carrión et al.[2] evaluated the effectiveness of an integral and holistic rehabilitation treatment program for patients with neurocognitive and neurobehavioral disorders after traumatic brain injury, using medico legal values. They studied ten consecutive patients with severe TBI aged between 19 and 39. All of them underwent a holistic, intensive, and multidisciplinary program for six months. All subjects were assessed at the beginning and at the end of the treatment using a broad neuropsychological test battery and the legal criteria of classification. Results showed a high level of the program's efficiency in the majority of the patients. Reductions of more than 70% in emotional deficits were obtained, and more than 60% in the global recovery of the patients who took part in the programs. The best outcomes were in orientation and attention, and 60% of the patients managed to completely eliminate the post-traumatic depressive syndrome.

There was another study by Balmaseda and colleagues[25] to assess the functional recovery in people who had suffered a stroke. They studied seven patients aged around 43 years old (SD = 13.20) seeking treatment for cognitive, behavioral and motor deficits after 2 years of onset; they received treatment during a mean period of 7.57 months (SD = 2.99). Results show an overall recovery after treatment with the combined method of 64.74%, showing recovery in all areas: cognitive, behavioral, and motor. The highest percentage of recovery was obtained in cognitive functioning; mean cognitive functionality at the end of treatment was 86.91%. The motor and physical functionality was 84.41% and some patients obtained 100% functionality by the end of the treatment in some areas. These two studies were used in the Combined Method of neurorehabilitation.

The Combined Method[26] is the use of both pharmacological and neuropsychological strategies together in the design of rehabilitation programs for acquired brain injury patients. TCM is a methodological engineering process, combining knowledge about the intact and non-intact functional brain with cognition, emotion, behavior, and neuropharmacology, resulting in a new functional cerebral reorganization which allows the patient to have psychological and social coherence. With the Combined Method, it is important to know the pharmacodynamics of cognition as well as rehabilitation strategies.

Neuropharmacology for neurocognitive disorders

The Combined Method for cognitive rehabilitation is based on the following pharmacological principles:

1   Neurotransmitters play a crucial role in cognitive processes, including the storage of new information, the retrieval mechanisms, parallel processing, speed processing or timing, and also in executive functioning. It has also been suggested that they play a role in the modulation of plasticity.
2   Neurons basically need some drugs to synthesize certain neurotransmitters.
3   When traumatic brain injury occurs and causes a lack of neurotransmitters, there is a reduction in the number of neurotransmitters reaching the brain. Then a process occurs where the neuron itself consumes the cellular deposit of the neurotransmitter, producing a decrease or lack in that neurotransmitter, which alters anatomical functioning and interferes with its functional properties.
4   In some cases, as in the case of choline, the alteration of the components of the membranes and the action of proteases end up destroying the membranes, freeing the zone where the receptors are. In this case, receptors that are made up of a precursor protein and a polypeptide B-amyloid will probably end up forming amyloid deposits.[27]
5   Any therapeutic action should begin with the administration of the appropriated drugs or substances to avoid the cascade of biochemical and molecular reactions caused by that alteration.

The Combined Method requires knowledge of the neuropharmacology of cognitive processes and mechanisms. Unfortunately, not many placebo-controlled trials exist for guiding neurocognitive treatments, and those that exist still require more discussion and replication. Table 17.1 shows agents recommended in different trials to enhance attention, memory and language in patients with brain injury. But in any case, prescription of these agents has to be carefully studied to know if they are suitable for the patient's present situation and in regard to side-effects and possible negative effects.

The cholinergic hypothesis of memory

From the pharmacological point of view, much research has been done,[28–30] originating with the cholinergic memory hypothesis introduced in the 1960s which indicates that organic memory disorders can be associated with lesions of the cholinergic neurons of the basal forebrain and with disruption of cholinergic functioning in the hippocampus. Injury to these neurons

Table 17.1 Some drugs used to enhance different aspects of attention, language and memory

Attention	Memory	Language
Amantadine	Bromocriptine	Amphetamine
Amitriptyline	Choline	Bromocriptine
Amphetamine	Clonidine	Carbidopa/levodopa
Clonidine	Citicholine	Tricyclic antidepressants
Desipramine	D-Amphetamine	
Methylphenidate	*Ginkgo biloba*	
Pemoline	Nimodipine	
Protriptyline	Selegiline	

diminishes their capacity to modulate neural activity through the release of acetylcholine (ACh). Others[31,32] deem it unlikely that ACh is primarily involved in encoding new memories because ACh is not fast acting and appears to play a more modulatory role in most synapses.

The cholinergic system in the central nervous system consists of several neural components which are localized throughout the rostrocaudal extent of the brain and spinal cord. Approximately 70% of the cholinergic innervations of the neocortex, hippocampus, amygdala, and olfactory bulb arise from neurons in the basal forebrain, through which cholinergic transmission may modulate the activity of cortical areas. Lamour et al.[33] reported that 30% of neocortical neurons are cholinoceptive, and the rate of firing is increased for most ACh applications. It seems that ACh released from cholinergic fibers of the basalocortical pathway influences the morphological development of the cerebral cortex and exerts a facilitatory, permissive role in processes of synaptic plasticity during the critical postnatal period and during adulthood. While there is ample evidence for the role ACh plays in the control of the cerebral blood flow, it appears that the cortical cholinergic afferents originating in the basal forebrain are not involved in such an event. It is presumed that ACh released from intrinsic cortical cholinergic cells may mediate the cerebrovascular action.[34]

Effects of anticonvulsants on cognition

Different drugs appear to exercise negative effects on human cognition and should be carefully monitored when recommended to brain injury patients. Phenytoin, carbamazepine and valproic acid are often prescribed for patients with traumatic brain injury due to the risk of post-traumatic epilepsy. All three drugs appear to exert some effect on cognitive and motor functions in epileptic patients, and these impairments worsen at increasing serum levels. The varied length of experience with each drug makes it difficult to assign relative weight to the evidence for or against each.[35] In a double-blind, placebo-controlled study,[36] 40 patients receiving phenytoin and 42 receiving carbamazepine from 6 to 44 months for seizure prophylaxis after brain injury were assigned to continue or discontinue treatment. Results showed that no significant differences were found in the performance of patients in medication and placebo groups for either drug at the end of the placebo phase. Patients in the combined group showed significant improvement on several measures of motor and speed performance following cessation of drug treatment. The authors concluded that both phenytoin and carbamazepine seem to have negative effects on cognitive performance, particularly on tasks with significant motor and speed components.

Effects of antipsychotic agents

An important number of traumatic brain injury patients receive treatment with antipsychotic agents because of their behavior and cognitive state, often confused with a clinical picture of post-traumatic psychotic or demented state.[37] However, antipsychotic medication for brain injury patients has many cognitive risks which should be contemplated for the rehabilitation program and the cost/benefit relationship should be evaluated even for those with psychotic symptoms, agitation, aggressivity and other maladaptive behavior. Some studies have demonstrated that select areas of cognition improve after antipsychotic agent discontinuation in subjects with traumatic brain injury.[38] Thus, it is important to know the pharmacodynamics of each one of the cognitive processes to be rehabilitated and, at the same time, know which medications taken by brain injury patients for prophylactic or medical purposes affect their cognitive functioning. In this section of the chapter we have pointed out the most up-to-date, relevant aspects.

The neuropsychological principles of the combined method

1　In order for the brain to work, it needs to consume oxygen and sugar. The supply of oxygen and sugar is via blood flow. When a cognitive process starts, the cerebral zones involved in that process are more active than the others requiring oxygen and glucose. If the brain injury impedes blood from reaching those brain zones, the different cognitive processes cannot be carried out. The brain has not got reserves of sugar and oxygen, signifying that the brain needs a continuous supply of blood.

2　Cognition is a broad concept and even a specific cognitive function can be expressed as a network of related functional subsets. Cognitive disorders after brain injury can be varied and different memory disorders can be found in the same person.

3　Each memory disorder after brain injury should be approached with its specific techniques, preferably in a general context of rehabilitation.

4　Memory rehabilitation should be appropriate for each patient, i.e., tailor-made for each individual. The program of rehabilitation should take into consideration the characteristics and idiosyncrasies of specific kinds of memory disorders and other cognitive and motor deficiencies that each patient has.

5   The patient's effort in performing cognitive exercises is a fundamental part of the rehabilitation process in the combined method. If no effort is used, there is not enough cerebral activity to revitalize the physiology and neuronal activity necessary in the areas of the brain associated with memory.

6   Compensatory methods (diaries, programmed watches, etc.) are neither rehabilitators nor can they be considered facilitators for the recuperation of the cognition of the patients. They are actually impediments to rehabilitation because they prevent the patient from using his/her own resources and necessary efforts for memory recovery, indispensable for recuperation. They should be used if all other treatments fail, in emergencies or in cases where rehabilitation is impossible. Compensatory methods are cognitive orthopedic.

7   The rehabilitation of memory via the Combined Method is based on the same principles as physical therapy: to recover functionality, first resolve the physical injury and then neuropsychological training should be applied to exercise the impaired cognitive functions.

8   Cognitive rehabilitation is a complex process that requires neuropsychologists to be well trained in the evaluation and rehabilitation of the different cognitive disorders.

Testing the Combined Method

We originally tested our hypothesis by choosing a homogeneous group of patients with the same lesion site, a brain site associated with memory functions. All patients had severe memory deficits which had been clinically and psychometrically tested. We had to demonstrate that the cholinergic drug administered to the patients has affinity for the lesional site associated with memory. The hypothesis is that this drug restores blood flow in the lesioned area and that, once blood flow is restored and maintained in the hypoperfused areas, it is then possible to improve memory functions and that is when neuropsychological treatment can be most successful.[39]

Two studies were carried out. The first study measured the regional cerebral blood flow (rCBF) of seven patients with TBI with very severe memory deficits, once while resting and once 1 h after the administration of citicholine (CDPc). In the second study, two groups of five patients of the same characteristics underwent an ecological neuropsychological memory rehabilitation program; during which time, one group was administered a placebo (Group A) and the other received CDPc (1 g/d v.o.) (Group B). The results of the first study showed a hypoperfusion of the inferior left temporal cerebral blood flow during rest state while an induced normalization was observed after administration of the drug. Results of the second study showed that in all of the areas explored, patients who underwent concurrent neuropsychological and CDPc treatment showed significant improvement in memory volume and verbal fluency. Members of the group that received neuropsychological treatment + placebo failed to show significant improvement in any of the neuropsychological areas explored after completing the abbreviated memory rehabilitation program. We would state that persistent organic memory disorders can be treated successfully only if one is able to first normalize and then maintain blood flow in the injured areas of the left temporo-basal zone at the same time an ecological program of neuropsychological rehabilitation is applied.

We can conclude that CDP-choline seems to be a drug with special affinity for cerebral areas associated with memory acting just where needed, normalizing blood flow in the hypoperfused left temporo-basal region, and making neuropsychological training effective. In general, data seem to point out that cognitive rehabilitation would follow the principle of first restoring and maintaining cerebral blood flow in the lesional site and then exercising function. In this study on memory rehabilitation, memory recuperation was made possible by first normalizing blood flow at the lesional site and simultaneously doing neuropsychological training.

The scientific logic of the Combined Method

The most relevant finding in that study, with the greatest implications in regard to treatment and rehabilitation of organic memory problems, is the significant difference found in the rCBF patterns between the rest state and the state of CDPc activation and learning. The results showed that CDPc restores diminished blood flow, specifically in the clinically significant hypoperfused zone responsible for memory processes at a cortical level. Our data indicates that CDPc acts just where it is needed: the blood flow level normalizes, increasing in the left infero-posterio-temporo-basal area. This can be due to the cholinergic mechanisms involved in the control of the cerebral arterial system[40] and cerebral microvasculature.[41] According to other authors, when CDPc is systematically administered, the cholinomimetic agents and the acetylcholine itself induce an increase in cerebral blood flow.[33,34] In our patients, this increase of blood flow was registered as a normalization of the blood in the left temporo-basal region.

To understand the meaning of this normalization, one must consider the functioning of the cerebral cortex in relation to regional blood flow. The brain self-regulates its blood flow levels according to the specific needs of oxygen and glucose. The most active cortical areas at any given moment are those that are consuming more oxygen and glucose. Functional cerebral activity is dependent on being able to metabolize these nutrients. Therefore, at the cortical level, in order to have normal cognitive functioning, the cerebral areas responsible for these functions – in the case of memory, the temporo-basal area – must be able to metabolize more oxygen and glucose as these processes are carried out. This implies that if, due to a traumatic lesion, cerebral areas corresponding to the cognitive processes do not receive the proper nutrients, these processes cannot be completed. Thus, patients will show a cognitive deficit; in our case study, a severe memory disorder.

Therefore, the observations made in our study are especially important concerning the treatment and rehabilitation of memory processes. Our data show that the levels of cerebral blood flow in patients treated with CDPc are brought to normal in temporal zones, especially in the basal zone. This enables them to normalize their functions, thus facilitating memory processes. This is done through a restructuring of the cerebral regional levels of blood flow. Clinical experience demonstrates that administration of CDPc alone is not enough for all patients to improve memory. Our hypothesis was that CDPc-induced normalization of blood flow levels facilitates memory processes, but that it should be maintained while patients undergo specific neuropsychological rehabilitation programs for memory. Establishing and maintaining normal blood flow and then exercising cognitive functioning through neuropsychological rehabilitation will improve the cognitive functions.

This indicates that cognitive therapy could follow the same principles as physical therapy: when there is a physical injury in the brain, there is a subsequent functional impairment. To recover functionality, first you have to resolve the underlying basis of this functional impairment, which is the physical injury. Once this is done, you have to exercise the function in order to recover it. Therefore, in cognitive therapy, first brain tissue would have to recover and maintain its metabolic activity with a normalization of blood flow in the specific areas related to cognition and, then, neuropsychological training would be applied to exercise the impaired cognitive functions.

Prognosis and course of cognitive deficits using the Combined Method

To determine the course and efficacy of the Combined Method for the rehabilitation of cognitive disorders, León-Carrión et al.[42] studied 19 TBI patients during a 6-month neurorehabilitation program at the Center for Brain Injury Rehabilitation (CRECER) in Seville, Spain. Of these patients, 84% were males aged 14–39 years and had a Glasgow Coma Scale less than 8 and a CT or MRI demonstrating severe brain injury. Everyday cognitive functioning was clinically scored with the COSS[43] on a scale of 1–10 by the same therapist that conducted the session with the patient. Results from neuropsychological assessment at admission were taken as baseline. Scores of 1–2 were assigned to subjects with severe impairment (almost no response, normalcy at 10–20%); a score of 7 was given to subjects exhibiting good response, but still too scarce to be considered totally normal (normalcy at 70%); scores of 7 indicate patients at near or almost normalcy. A score of 10 was assigned for statistical or clinical normalcy (normalcy at 100%).

Table 17.2 Mean scores on a scale of 1–10 from admission to discharge (beginning of month 7) for rehabilitation of cognitive disorders and number of hours needed to achieve goal of placing patient at 70% of normalcy

Disorders	Admission	Discharge	Hours/sessions
Long-term memory	4.20	7.70	67.1
Short-term memory	3.80	7.40	68.2
Orientation	7.50	9.40	80.2
Calculation	4.30	6.80	58.6
Attention	4.50	7.00	65.2
Automatisms	4.50	7.00	70.9
Mental control	3.20	7.20	47.2
Planning	4.30	7.50	79.2

Table 17.2 displays the mean scores obtained by the patients at admission and discharge, as well as the number of hours needed for each cognitive function to recover up to 70% of normalcy.

The results of this study show that cognitive disorders can be treated and that it is possible to place the patients near normalcy and even at normalcy. In other words, the results show that patients who took part in the neuro-psychological rehabilitation program entering, for example, with a level of short-term functional memory of 38% in comparison to normalcy were discharged with a level of about 74%. They gained a 58% mnestic capacity. The patients who entered the rehabilitation program with an average level of long-term functional memory at 42% left with 77%, gaining a 56% mnestic capacity. Results show that patients with serious memory deterioration severely affecting their daily activities find that their memory functions closer to normal and less dysfunctional after treatment, which gives them more independence and personal autonomy. Those entering with a 43% planning capacity were discharged after 6 months with 75% of their functional planning capacity. As we have previously indicated, patients usually present more than one cognitive problem, which means we must add the times together for both/all of them. TBI patients with diffuse axonal damage usually have at least two or three cognitive deficits. We can say that a combined intensive, holistic and multidisciplinary treatment needs at least 150 hours of cognitive rehabilitation, to be added to the hours the patient needs for rehabilitation of speech, and physical and emotional rehabilitation.

Timing for recovery using the Combined Method

Cognitive rehabilitation needs time and continuity in the treatment. The effectiveness of the Combined Method depends on time continuity and the intensity of the sessions dedicated to cognitive training. The number of specific memory rehabilitation sessions undergone by each of the 19 patients in our study sustaining cognitive problems and participating in a CRECER neurorehabilitation program for 6 months can be observed in Table 17.2. Therefore, in order to situate our patients at levels of over 70% of their memory, 68.2 sessions of 1 h each were needed to treat specific short-term memory deficiencies, 67.1 1 h sessions for those of long-term memory, and 79.2 h were needed for planning. Results also point out another important factor for rehabilitation of organic cognitive disorders: the process of recovery is not regular, there are ups and downs. Sometimes the treatment does not appear to advance; in fact, it seems to recede (not more than 15% of the time). This can be temporary, and a month later recuperation continues. If the downtrend is over 15%, the underlying cause must be found immediately. For this reason, a patient should not be discharged when there is rapid progress. Our data indicate that the process of rehabilitation has to be continued until consolidation of all progress is achieved.

Conclusion

There are two main approaches to treating cognitive disorders of patients with acquired brain injury, the prosthetic method and the Combined Method. This chapter has introduced briefly the first and explained more in detail the second.

Rehabilitation of cognitive disorders is a possible goal when the appropriate methods of detecting, assessing, evaluating and rehabilitating are used. Planning of the timing and intensity of rehabilitation is required. The process of recovery is complex, with ups and downs during the whole process, and discharge or leaving the rehabilitation program is not recommended until the progress obtained is consolidated. Up until now, the Combined Method, in our experience, seems to be the method of choice for obtaining the best results in placing the patients at the closest level possible to cognitive normalcy.

References

1. Levin, H. S., Grossman, R. G., Rose, J. E., & Teasdale, G. (1979). Long-term neuropsychological outcome of closed head injury. *J Neurosurg., 50*, 412–422.
2. León-Carrión, J., Machuca, F., Murga-Sierra, M., Domínguez-Morales, R. (2001). Outcome after an intensive, holistic and multidisciplinary rehabilitation program after traumatic brain injury. Medico legal values. *Rev. Neurol., 33*, 377–383.
3. Miller, E. (1978). Is amnesia remediable? In M. M. Gruneberg, P. E. Morris, and R. N. Sykes (Eds.), *Practical aspects of memory*. New York: Academic Press.
4. Wilson, B. A., & Moffat, N. (1984). Rehabilitation of memory for everyday life. In J. E. Harris and P. Morrid (Eds.), *Everyday memory: Actions and absent-mindedness*. London: Academic Press.
5. Schacter, D. L., & Glisky, E. L. (1986). Memory remediation: restoration, alleviation and the acquisition of domain-specific knowledge. In B. Uzzell and Y. Gross (Eds.), *Clinical neuropsychology of intervention*. Boston: Martinus Nijhoff.

6. Leng, N. R. C., & Copello, A. G. (1990). Rehabilitation of memory after brain injury: is there an effective technique? *Clin. Rehab., 4*, 63–69.

7. Carney, N., Chesnut, R. M., Maynard, H., Mann, N. C., Patterson, P., & Helfand, N. (1999). Effect of cognitive rehabilitation on outcomes for people with traumatic brain injury: a systematic review. *J. Head Trauma Rehabil.*, 277–321.

8. Prigatano, G. P. (1999). Commentary: beyond statistics and research design. *J. Head Trauma Rehabil., 14*, 308–311.

9. Gorman, P., Dayle, R., Hood, C. A., & Rumrell, L. (2003). Effectiveness of the ISAAC cognitive prosthetic system for improving rehabilitation outcomes with neurofunctional impairment. *NeuroRehabilitation 18*(1), 57–67.

10. Wilson, B. A., Evans, J. J., Emslie, H., & Malinek, V. (1997). Evaluation of NeuroPage: a new memory aid. *J. Neurol. Neurosurg. Psychiatry, 63*, 113–115.

11. Wilson, B. A., Emslie, H. C., Quirk, K., & Evans, J. J. (2001). Reducing everyday memory and planning problems by means of a paging system: a randomised control crossover study. *J. Neurol. Neurosurg. Psychiatry, 70*, 477–482.

12. McGhee Pierce, S., Mayer, N. H., & Whyte, J. (2001). Computer-assisted exercise systems in traumatic brain injury: cases and commentary. *J. Head Trauma Rehabil., 16*, 406–413.

13. Kim, H. J., Burke, D. T., Dowds, M. M., & George, J. (1999). Utility of a microcomputer as an external memory aid for a memory-impaired head injury patient during in-patient rehabilitation. *Brain Inj., 13*, 147–150.

14. Kim, H. J., Burke, D. T., Dowdes, M. M., Boone, K. A., & Park, G. J. (2000). Electronic memory aids for outpatient brain injury: follow-up findings. *Brain Inj., 14*, 187–196.

15. Wright, P., Rogers, N., Hall, C., Wilson, B., Evans, J., & Emslie, H. (2001). Enhancing an appointment diary on a pocket computer for use by people after brain injury. *Int. J. Rehabil. Res., 24*, 299–308.

16. Ownsworth, T. L., & Mcfarland, K. (1999). Memory remediation in long-term acquired brain injury: two approaches in diary training. *Brain Inj., 13*, 605–626.

17. Wade, T. K., & Troy, J. C. (2001). Mobile phones as a new memory aid: a preliminary investigation using case studies. *Brain Inj., 15*, 305–320.

18. Pergami, P. (2003). PDAs in clinical practice: having a database in your hand but keeping the decision in your brain. *Neuroinformatics, 5*, 207–209.

19. Ricker, J. H., Rosenthal, M., Garay, E., DeLuca, J., Germain, A., and Abraham-Fuchs, K., et al. (2002). Telerehabilitation needs: a survey of persons with acquired brain injury. *J. Head Trauma Rehabil., 17*, 242–250.

20. Tam, S. F., Man, W. K., Hui-Chan, C. W., Lau, A., Yip, B., & Cheung, W. (2003). Evaluating the efficacy of tele-cognitive rehabilitation for functional performance in three case studies. *Occup. Ther. Int., 10*, 200–311.

21. Hart, T., Hawkey, K., & Whyte, J. (2002). Use of a portable voice organizer to remember therapy goals in traumatic brain injury rehabilitation: a within-subjects trial. *J. Head Trauma Rehabil., 17*, 556–557.

22. Diamond, B. J., Shreve, G. M., Bonilla, J. M., Johnston, M. V., Morodan, J., & Branneck, R. (2003). Telerehabilitation, cognition and user-accessibility. *NeuroRehabilitation, 18*, 171–177.

23. Bergman, M. M. (2003). The essential steps cognitive orthotic. *NeuroRehabilitation, 18*, 31–46.

24. Cicerone, K. D. (1999). Commentary: the validity of cognitive rehabilitation. *J. Head Trauma Rehabil., 14*, 316–321.

25. Balmaseda, R., Domínguez-Morales, M. del R. León-Carrión, J., & García-Bernal, I. (2000). Rehabilitation of the consequences affecting independent functioning in patients with cerebrovascular disorders. Paper presented at the First Spanish–Portuguese Congress of Psychology, Santiago de Compostela, Spain.

26. León-Carrión, J. (1997). *Neuropsychological rehabilitation, fundamentals, directions and innovations.* Delray Beach, FL: St. Lucie Press.

27. Lozano, R. (1991). CDP-choline in the treatment of cranealencephalic trauma. *J. Neurol. Sci., 103,* S31–S41.

28. Bierdman, G. B. (1970). Forgetting of an operant response: physostigmine produced increases in scape latency in rats as a function of time of injection. *Quar. J. Exp. Psychol., 22,* 384.

29. Squire, L. R., Glick, S. D., & Goldfarb, J. (1971). Relearning at different times after training as affected centrally and peripherally acting cholinergic drugs in mice. *J. Comp. Physiol. Psychol., 74,* 41.

30. Stanes, M. D., Brown, C. P., & Singer, G. (1976). Effect of physostigmine on Y maze discrimination retention in rats. *Psychopharmacologia, 46,* 269.

31. Duckless, S. P. (1986). Cholinegeric intervention of cerebral arteries. In C. Owman and J. E. Hardebo (Eds.), *Neural regulation of brain circulation* (pp. 235–243). Amsterdam: Elsevier.

32. Azneric, S. P., Honig, M. A., Milner, T. A., Greco, S., Iadecola, C., & Reis, O. J. (1998). Neural and endothelial sites of acetylcholine synthesis and release associated with microvessels in rat cerebral cortex: ultrastructural and neurochemical studies. *Brain Research, 454,* 11–30.

33. Lamour, Y., Dutar, P., & Jobert, A. (1982). Excitatory effect of acetylcholine on different types of neurons in the first somatosensory neocortex of the rat, laminar distribution and pharmachologic characteristics. *Neuroscience, 7,* 1483.

34. Martinez-Murillo, R., & Rodrigo, J. (1995). The localization of cholinergic neurons and markers in the CNS. In T. W. Stone (Ed.), *CNS neurotransmitters and neuromodulators: Acetylcholine.* Boca Raton, FL: CRC Press.

35. Massagli, T. (1992). Prophylaxis and treatment of posttraumatic epilepsy with phenytoin. *West. J. Med., 157,* 663–664.

36. Smith, K. R., Goulding, P. M., Wilderman, D., Goldfader, P. R., Holterman Hommes, P., & Wei, F. (1994). Neurobehavioral effects of phenytoin and carbamazepine in patients recovering from brain trauma: a comparative study. *Arch. Neurol., 51,* 653–660.

37. León-Carrión, J. (2002). Dementia due to head trauma: an obscure name for a clear neurocognitive syndrome. *NeuroRehabilitation, 17,* 115–122.

38. Stanislav, S. W. (1997). Cognitive effects of antipsychotic agents in persons with traumatic brain injury. *Brain Inj., 11,* 335–341.

39. León-Carrión, J., Domínguez-Roldán, J. M., Murillo-Cabezas, F., Domínguez-Morales, M. R., & Muñoz-Sanchez, M. A. (2000). The role of citicholine in neuropsychological training after traumatic brain injury. *Neurorehabilitation, 14,* 33–40.

40. Wishaw, I. Q. (1985). Cholinergic receptor blockade in rats impairs local but not taxonomic strategies for place navigation in a swimming pool. *Beh. Neurosci., 99,* 979.

41. Wishaw, I. Q. (1989). Dissociating performance and learning deficits on spaital navigation tasks in rats subjected to cholinergic muscarinic blockade. *Brain Res. Bull., 23,* 247.

42. León-Carríon, J., et al. (2003). Time and course of recovery of post-TBI cognitive disorders after neurorehabilitation. Submitted to *Neuroreport*.

43. León-Carríon J. (2001). *Crecer Outcome Scoring Scale*. Center for Brain Injury Rehabilitation Crecer. (Internal document).

18 Neuropsychological recovery in children and adolescents following traumatic brain injury

Peter D. Patrick, Sean T. Patrick, and Erin Duncan

Introduction

The purpose of this chapter is to review the state of neuropsychological recovery of children following traumatic brain injury. To understand the restoration of mental life in the child is to journey through many areas of study and scientific investigation. It is the hope of the authors that this chapter accomplishes the following:

- An appreciation and increased knowledge of the various disciplines that must interface when addressing pediatric neuropsychological recovery.
- That the reader gains a general knowledge background ranging from severe acute medical recovery to the return home and psychosocial factors involved in recovery.
- That the reader specifically reviews the effects of injury at the basic biologic levels onto the ever challenging level of psychological, social levels of recovery.
- That the reader comes to understand the dynamic and significant role development plays in our understanding, measurement and application of clinical skills when assisting the child to recover from traumatic brain injury.

It is the dynamic neurodevelopmental and psychosocial context of the study, evaluation, and treatment of childhood traumatic brain injury (TBI) that presents the clinician with both challenge and opportunity. The clinician must address several unique issues when assisting the injured child not only to recapture his lost abilities, but also gain the foundation for continued maturation across all areas of life. The child's brain is an evolving group of systems whose degree of function will allow or prevent the child from acquiring the skills necessary to manage the demands of everyday living with a satisfactory amount of safety and success. The therapeutic emphasis during the child and adolescent's recovery is not solely to regain pre-injury functional abilities, but to resume, as near as possible, the developmental trajectory that the child was progressing upon.

The child's recovery is most similar to that of the adult counterpart during the acute phase, where there is a shared emphasis on medical stability. Once medically stable the different developmental needs of the child and the adult become important. Simple deficits may prevent the child from acquiring experiences that in the healthy child are the basis for more crucial development and growth. The potential exists for a severe social deficit to arise, for example, secondary to the missed opportunity to participate consistently in group activities. This difficulty in addition to the impact of the primary deficit serves to complicate and lengthen the course of childhood rehabilitation. The child's developmental environment is also of distinct importance, requiring the clinician to project further out in time and consequence when evaluating and treating.

One of the most difficult challenges to rehabilitating the child is addressing the complex behavioral limitations and deficits in executive function that may result. While the ability to regain high-level skills will determine much of the child's ultimate success, a complete program also embraces the interdependent functioning of the child's social systems, namely, family and school. The clinician can mobilize, coordinate and interrelate strict medical technology with social sciences and social engineering to assist the individual's recovery. For those children who were considered "at risk" prior to the TBI, this same consideration can be focused on normalizing development where possible.

While the literature continues to expand rapidly, there exists much that is undetermined or nonstandardized. Few guidelines or standards exist and further research is a universal call from most published sources. Integrating the ongoing research with the existing treatment approaches, that in some cases have survived intact for 30 years or more, provides an additional challenge and opportunity. "Best-evidence" reviews form the basis for much of this writing as all interested parties continue to expand the knowledge base from which childhood rehabilitation programs can be designed and delivered.

Incidence, prevalence and cause

A historical review of the study of childhood and adolescent TBI yields several results. Even in those study segments where quantifiable data has yet to be fully developed, the following themes are evident:

- TBI in children and adolescents accounts for significant morbidity and mortality, and is a source of long-term deficit from both unintentional and inflicted causes.
- The times of childhood and adolescence contain particular risks that influence the incidence and prevalence of TBI.
- The results of mild, moderate, and severe TBI greatly influence the total number of years of disability.
- There appear to be specific risk factors that may help predict the

occurrence of TBI in children and teenagers and these pre-injury factors set childhood TBI apart from those found in an adult population.

Important studies have been completed that uncover the true impact of TBI on our youth. A 1990 report concluded: "traumatic brain injuries (TBI) are the leading causes of death and permanent disability in children and adolescents".[1] This conclusion was supported by works in 1992 that stated that accidents were the leading cause of death in children and that traumatic brain injury "accounts for a large proportion of these deaths".[2] Useful in scaling the magnitude for the impact of TBI was the separate 1990 determination that an alarming number of children, approximately 5%, suffer a fatal injury according to Kraus et al.[3] TBI was reported as early as 1987 by Kraus at an incidence of 132/100,000 in females 15 years old and younger, with their male counterparts affected at a rate of 185/100,000.[4]

The severity of these injuries is well addressed in studies concluding that the majority of injuries, some 93%, are mild in nature.[4] Age-specific data has also been collected that begins to demonstrate the societal consequences of TBI. Early in life, aged 0–5 years, males and females approximate one another with comparable rates of injury. This younger age bracket, for both sexes, is a high-risk period for TBI where falls, other accidents and inflicted injuries appear as primary causes. An additional high-risk period exists for children during the teenage interval. During the mid to late adolescent years, it appears that the mechanism of injury (e.g., automobile accidents) and individual decision making (e.g., increased risk taking and experimenting behaviors) interact to elevate the incidence of all injuries for males as compared to their female cohorts. Males during the school age and teenage years suffer TBI at a 2:1 ratio versus females. The role of accidents and violence in all age groups should be noted as a primary cause of childhood and adolescent TBI.

According to DiScala and Savage, who monitored a total of 27,036 children through the National Pediatric Trauma Registry, data indicates that childhood and adolescent TBI is very real and has long-term consequences. Of all children 26.2% suffer a head injury at some point in their lives. The impact from TBI is shown in that more than half of these children are left with clinically measurable deficits: 11.2% have 1 to 3 functional limitations including limited activities of daily living (ADLs) such as bathing, dressing, walking, and feeding. Of the affected children 34.3% had 4 to 10 limitations including ADLs, and of these children with more involved injuries, 64.3% suffered cognitive changes, and 63.3% behavioral alterations. Of those children with 1 to 3 limitations 94.5% were discharged to the home, while in the group with > 4 limitations, the resulting deficits were severe enough to prevent 60.3% from being discharged to the home. In fact 50.5% were discharged to structured rehabilitation settings.[5-7]

A developmental perspective

An understanding of the underlying processes of biological, psychological, and psychosocial development enhances the understanding of the complexities surrounding the rehabilitation of the child after TBI. The developmental influences at the time of injury and during the protracted period of recovery are significant technical and clinical factors. In particular, two elements of development become important in understanding the care of TBI in children.

- The direct consequences of injury on the developing brain and how this may affect the eventual level of neurologic maturity achieved
- The psychosocial phases of development, in particular the child's experience as a family and community member, and the effect experience has on the developing brain.

Both can be significantly altered and as circular in their influence during recovery as they are during normal development. Unlike in the adult, however, where development is largely complete, the child has yet to mature biologically or psychosocially.

At birth the infant brain is roughly 50% of the volume of the adult brain.[8] It will show nonlinear development with cell development varying over time and from location to location. Brain development can be divided into eight stages:

- neuroplate development
- cell localization and proliferation
- cell migration from point of origin to point of function
- cell clustering that will lead to identifiable subparts of the overall brain
- continued differentiation/specialization of the immature neuron
- the proliferation of connections amongst cells
- selective cell death or apoptosis, reducing the numbers according to the need and development of function
- "pruning" or the selective reduction in initial connections providing alternative connectivity.[9]

During the first 2 months of life the number of neurons will reach a maximum, first in the posterior cortex. Frontal areas, however, will increase for approximately 2 years.[10] A period of slowing occurs until about 6 years of age, followed by a prolonged steady state until the eventual decline begins in the fourth or fifth decade.[11] Frontal areas will also demonstrate different growth patterns when compared to posterior areas. Frontal area growth spurts are noted early, within the first year, as well as to a lesser degree between the ages of 7–9 years. Rapid growth is again seen during late adolescence and young adulthood.[12]

The manner in which brain injury affects the maturing brain has been studied clinically and experimentally in human subjects and animal models.[11–13] The human brain, known as an altricial brain, continues to develop following birth. The mostly embryonic activities of cell development, division, and migration are followed by periods of proliferation and pruning that continue beyond birth.[11] In addition to pruning, the myelination of cells and the intricate emerging relationships between neurons and glial support cells proceed throughout childhood.

The work of Rakic[14] and colleagues has greatly contributed to our understanding of this process. The earlier post-natal period of proliferation is focused on increasing the numbers of neurons. More importantly, however, may be the continued refinement, cell development, and specialization of cell connectivity. This refinement focuses on the growing complexities of synaptic development and the increasing number of dendrites and their connections. The additional numbers of cells and the refinement of end-organ neuronal development allow for more intricate and numerous connections.

The ongoing proliferation of cells and pathways from region to region is followed by a period of shaping and segregation known as "pruning". Pruning allows for a modification in neuronal connections, according to need, stimulation and experience. It is the process that "downsizes" and refines the connectivity in the brain. Apoptosis is the genetically programmed dying off of neurons that drives the process. Apoptosis is active in early life and then, except in disease processes, goes dormant until later adult life.[15] The extent of apoptosis in humans is unique among mammalian brains, where it occurs to a greater degree than in other species.[16]

Through the childhood years the developing brain continues to experience maturational influences which center around the myelinization of tracks and the ongoing relationship between neuronal tracks and support glial cells. The regional development of neuronal tracks and more complex circuitry results in the more established configuration of the adult brain.

As different sections of the cortex develop they connect with the frontal organizing cortex and activate a new need for frontal maturation. Frontal maturity appears to be interwoven with the development of the posterior region and its connection. This feed-forward process initiates new growth in frontal regions as necessary. It appears that the frontal area and its nonlinear development is somehow cued by the posterior development and their growth connections with the anterior frontal regions. This same phenomenon would likely be true with limbic and subcortical connections to the frontal lobes. Their role in spurring frontal development and activation leads to the orchestrating systems that eventually serve the executive function.[12]

The widespread connectivity in the infant brain differs from the adult brain that has developed a refined and systematic connectivity. The plasticity of the brain decreases as it becomes more defined. We see that this plasticity may allow the child's brain a more promising opportunity for recovery than the adult's, by capitalizing on its ability to construct new connections and associations. Our understanding of the recovery of brain function after injury has advanced. However, the intricacies of cell survival and re-engagement remain unclear. Bach-y-Rita comments on the recovery potential of the human brain and explores the "unmasking of" inactive pathways following injury.[17] It is suggested that undamaged areas are usurped for older function, and that "neuronal group selection" is a potential mechanism of restoration.

The protracted period of active development and modification that drives the dynamic changes extending through the early years of life is crucial in considering the childhood TBI. Injuries at different points along the developmental trajectory may produce extensive deficits that become evident only in time, or alternatively, may produce modest deficits that are well compensated for by the brain's ability to re-establish functional connectivity. It is speculated that the brain's ability to shape itself and be shaped by the environment results from the evolutionary survival pressures that rewarded this adaptability to change. Understanding and, if possible, using this capability in the modern rehabilitation effort is advantageous.

Cortical architecture and function

The cortex contains the most advanced abilities to process information and, as described above, undergoes an integrated developmental process. The four lobes of the cortex (e.g., occipital, parietal, temporal and frontal lobes) differ in terms of their maturational timing. The primary projection areas for visual, auditory and tactile/proprioceptive skills, mature first with the sensory-motor strips. Secondary and large overlapping tertiary areas of the brain follow. Receiving input from thalamic and subcortical structures, which mature in advance of the cortex, the higher brain structures are positioned to receive, store and combine information in intricate patterns and combinations. The unique behaviors and expressions of the child arise from the intricate combination of information, projected through complex white track structures below the surface to the frontal cortex. When combined with emotional and motivational elements, fed through the limbic connections, intentions and developed action plans are created.[18,19]

In part it is the unique cell architecture of the cortex that supports and allows the development of cognitive, perceptual, and emotional/motivational skills. The cell fields' uniqueness supports and allows the types of information acquisition and processing termed learning. The cortex is composed of six distinctive layers of cell development. These layers differ in the size and branching of each cell. Layer I has been called a "synaptic field" of interfacing dendrites and axons that originate in thalamic, deeper cortical layers and even from elsewhere (e.g., contralateral hemisphere) in the cortex. Layer II is an external granular layer that contains many small pyramidal cells and interneurons well adapted to support integrating activities. Layer III, an external pyramidal layer, is dominated by the interconnecting abilities of small and abundant pyramidal cells, while Layer IV, another granular layer, is composed of stellate cells with lesser combinations of smaller interneurons and pyramidal cells. The internal pyramidal layer, Layer V, is composed of large Betz and pyramidal cells characteristic of the motor areas and frontal lobes. Layer VI comprised of "fusiform cells" allows for complex interconnections and the use of interneurons and pyramidal cells. These layers are not uniformly represented in the cortex. Each cross-section of the cortex has its own unique distribution of layers dependent upon its location and function.

If self-control and executive development are to be achieved or re-established, the child needs to fully develop the skills of information acquisition and processing. This is accomplished through the complex systems of the brain that are directed by the frontal cortex.[20] These systems have developmental milestones and must ultimately work in concert if complex learning and behavior are to flourish. Functioning systems will allow for the development of internal models and guiding processes, both cognitive and emotional. The most advanced forms of language, cognitive, emotional and motivational skills are possible because of the intricate manner in which the cerebral cortex can take in, combine, and use information. Internalizing knowledge and then creating guiding models, which stand separate and independent from the environment, provides the individual the opportunity to envision solutions, consider consequences, and experience creativity in the course of serving self-care, self-protection, social discourse and group membership needs. Table 18.1 has Barkley's[105] list of elements as it relates to the evolution of executive skills in the child.

Luria, in his writings on *Higher Cortical Functions in Man* and *The Working Brain*, takes great efforts to relate the architecture of the cortex to the appearance and emergence of the sophisticated skills that serve and promote the survival and success of children and adults.[18,19] Luria reviews the nature in which the cortical architecture supports mental development. For example, initial reception by the visual processing unit of the occipital lobe relies on densely packed cells of Layer IV, and requires a somatotopical representation paralleling the distribution of the retinal fields. The secondary projection areas that integrate like sensory input into patterns rely more on the reticulum and broadly integrating cells of Layers II and III. The difference in the layers' distribution between primary and secondary projection areas is

Table 18.1 The hybrid model of executive functions

Developmental elements
Behavioral inhibition
Non-verbal working memory
Internalized speech (verbal working memory)
Self-regulation of affect/motivation/arousal
Ability to reconstitute
Motor control/fluency/syntax

Reproduced by permission from Barkley (1997).

apparent on histologic review. Clearly evident is the manner in which layers are preferentially represented to correlate with the function of the given projection areas. Furthermore, the large "overlapping" areas (tertiary projections) of the parietal–temporal–occipital interface that are responsible for some of the most complex integrations of information show yet another cellular composition, relying instead on multiform layers that mature later.

The brain has been described as "a self-organizing system" which requires the interplay of maturing brain structures and neurotransmitter systems.[20] It is important to understand that the neuronal architecture is complemented by neurotransmitter systems uniquely developed to process information in a manner that will eventually support complex reasoning and social conduct. For example, it would appear that noradrenergic projections from the locus ceruleus and cholinergic projections from the basal forebrain depend on "activity dependent changes" that in turn influence "neuronal interconnections". These structures and systems rely on learning to achieve cognitive function, and in turn are reliant on experience to "optimize genetically determined blueprints of connectivity". Following birth, much of higher cortical development is "experience-dependent".

Of key importance to the pediatric and adolescent neuropsychologist is the idea that these areas and layers mature at different times. Since the cortical apparatus serving the evolution of higher mental skills changes over time post-natally, additional diagnostic and prognostic obstacles face the clinician. Anticipating the effects of a lesion on mature, maturing and yet-to-mature sites remains a challenging area of research and practice.

Psychological and psychosocial development

No less important than biological development in the understanding of childhood TBI is the impact that psychological and psychosocial factors have. Traditional theorists have fully developed these themes to provide a rich context within which the stages of development and the effects of TBI are better understood. The level of psychological development and the psychosocial experiences that have previously occurred also influence the state of the brain. The theoretical works of Piaget and Erikson[21,22] exemplify the cognitive and psychosocial tasks of development, which are dependent upon and influence the state of the brain (see Table 18.2).

In Cockrell's chapter, "Pediatric Brain Injury Rehabilitation", the author reports on psychological and psychosocial elements that predispose children to TBI such as "high aggression scores".[23] Drawing from the works of others the writing concludes that high aggression increased with low socio-economic status, instability in the home including frequent moves, and parent factors such as single parenthood, distress and unhappiness. Cockrell also states that problems with discipline, encopresis, and feelings of fear correlate with pediatric injury rates in general.

The stage of psychological development at the time of injury is crucially

Table 18.2 The theoretical context of psychosocial development

Piaget[21] Cognitive stages	Age	Erikson[22] psychosocial stages
Sensory-motor intelligence	Birth–2 years	Trust vs. mistrust
Object permanence		
Distinguishes self from others		Autonomy vs. shame/ doubt
Develops perception of cause and effect		
Entirely present-oriented		
Preoperational stage	2–7 years	Initiative vs. guilt
Language		
Initial symbolic thought		Industry vs. inferiority
Egocentric		
Concrete operations	7–11 years	
Logical thought		
Recognizes consistent properties		
Formal operations	12 years and older	Identity vs. identity confusion
Abstract reasoning		
Deductive: hypothesis testing		
Future-oriented	Young adulthood	Intimacy vs. isolation
	Middle Age	Generativity vs. stagnation
	Old Age	Integrity vs. despair

Data from Piaget,[21] Erikson.[22]

important when considering the lasting effects of that injury. The psychological status combines with the biological stage of development, the influences of family, environment and even culture, to specify a unique profile for a child at a point in time. The attitudes and resources of the family, the nature of the parent–child attachment and the quality of family and peer relationships all contribute to defining a child's resource pool from which he or she can draw in the attempt to experience, endure and eventually recover from injury. Bach-y-Rita[17] reiterates that much as in the initial developmental periods when learning and the brain shape each other, there appears a similar relationship where the "role of early and late rehabilitation, with attention to psychosocial and environmental factors, appears to be critical to recovery". Recovery is a product of the interactive type, location and severity of injury during a particular developmental period.

Traumatic brain injury

Mild head injury in children

As epidemiologists report, the majority of head injuries are categorized as mild TBI (mTBI).[3-7] They have a range of causes from auto accidents to sports-related injuries, to falls and violence. The most common complaints are headache, fatigue, dizziness, sleep disturbance, concentration problems, and memory difficulties. The Aspen Concensus Work Group defines mTBI according to the American Congress of Rehabilitation Medicine 1991 criteria:

- Any period of loss of consciousness.
- Any loss of memory for events before or after the accident.
- Any alteration in mental state at the time of the accident.
- Focal neurological deficits without post-traumatic amnesia > 24 h, Glasgow Coma Score 13–15 after 30 min, LOC 30 min or less.[24]

According to the work group, mTBI is accompanied by pathophysiological changes noted in animal model studies. The work group concludes that there can be focal changes in the blood–brain barrier which correlate with CT/MRI changes in humans. There can be an excitotoxic storm, and/or increased glucose metabolism followed by hypo-metabolism. The group concludes that there is "insufficient data regarding the predictive value of symptoms and diagnosis of post concussive syndrome". Also, the work group recognizes "complicated" mTBI, which persists beyond the expected point of spontaneous recovery. According to O'Shanick and Rosenberg's[24] presentation at the Third World Congress in 1999:

- CT should be used to define or exclude surgical lesions in mTBI with abnormal GCS, mental status, or neurological exam, or a history of LOC or amnesia.
- Option: MRI may be used in the acute evaluation to identify and define surgical lesions.
- Option: MRI may be used to evaluate persistent mTBI symptoms even with negative CT imaging.
- A neurocognitive assessment after mTBI should include the evaluation of attention, choice reaction time and information processing.
- Impairments in complicated mTBI should be evaluated via standardized psychometric assessment.
- Standardized assessment is useful in persistent post-concussive assessment.

Moderate and severe TBI

Moderate and severe injuries leave ongoing disturbances to cognitive performance, educational experience, and school and community re-entry. Although the child's resilience to injury and ability to withstand injury may vary from the adult equivalence there is ample evidence to suggest that the long-term consequences of injury are measurable and significant.

Alberico and colleagues[26] in a consecutive series study at the Medical College of Virginia compared 100 pediatric injuries (age 0–19) to 230 adult injuries (age 20–80). Accounting for the standardization of care, measurements were obtained that suggested pediatric patients attain a favorable outcome more often than adult patients, in 43% of the study cases vs. 28%. Follow up at 1 year showed good outcomes in 55% of the children and 21% of the adults, with the trend in recovery evident as early as 3 months postinjury. Children also had a lower mortality rate, 24%, compared to adults at 45%.

Additional findings from the Alberico group demonstrated a much higher incidence of surgical mass lesions in the adult group (46%) than in the children (24%). A relatively low mass lesion and a higher incidence of cerebral swelling were reported earlier in a 1978 article by Bruce et al.[27] They concluded that this difference may in fact suggest a "different pathophysiological response" in children. Such comparison helps us to appreciate the uniqueness of the childhood injury from yet another perspective.

Despite the improvements seen versus an adult population, there is little doubt that the consequences of early TBI persist through the developmental years. As early as 1979, Levin reported on the neuropsychological sequelae of closed head injury in children and teens.[28]

Ewing-Cobbs in 1987[25,29] found the long-term effects on language and these results were validated more recently by Fennell and Mickle[30] in 1992. In 1997, again Ewing-Cobbs et al. using a prospective, longitudinal follow-up study[31] concluded that children aged 4 months to 7 years with moderate and severe TBI suffered deficits in all areas studied: composite IQ, receptive and expressive language, and verbal and performance IQ. Severe TBI also resulted in lower motor scores when compared to IQ scores. Both receptive and expressive language scores were reduced after severe TBI, with expressive language scores falling further than receptive. The age of onset did not seem to effect this sample. All neuropsychological measures improved over 6 months and remained stable from 6 to 24 months. The article concluded that the ongoing failure to improve in individual areas resulted in a reduction in learning rate and impaired the acquisition of new learning over time. This placed the children further behind their age groups.

Emanuelson led researchers in Gothenburg, Sweden to publish articles on follow-up with children suffering severe TBI.[32] In 1996 25 patients with severe TBI were followed: 2–6 years after trauma, 23/25 reported at least one sequela and 21/25 had multiple sequelae. Behavioral disturbances were so significant that none of the patients were able to return to normal functioning. In 1998 the Emanuelson group re-examined 18 children at a mean of over 7 years post-injury to examine their extended outcomes. Only 28% of the group of adolescent victims functioned within "normal limits".[33] They found that poor social integration was the most significant disability. While the research design was less than robust, there appeared reasonable evidence to show children suffering ongoing limitations in complex social behaviors.

A Washington University group, Jaffe et al., in the first of several articles in the 1990s reported a prospective cohort study on the "Severity of Pediatric Traumatic Brain Injury and Early Neurobehavioral Outcome".[34] The study focused on pre-injury academic, personality and psychosocial abilities of 98 children aged 6–15 years, with mild to severe closed head injury. Importantly, the authors used a research design to capture the relative changes rather than the population comparison changes. A cohort-matched design reinforced the finding that traumatic brain injury is a major cause of ongoing pediatric disability. When compared to controls, the authors found:

> The pattern of decline in performance (even though standard scores at times were within normal limits) when compared to the cohort matching increased with severity of brain injury and was consistent for measures assessing intelligence, memory, speed of motor performance, adaptive problem solving and academic performance.[34]

These children were described as at risk to experience problems in the acquisition of academic skill, new learning and "higher-order cognitive abilities".

Another paper in 1995[35] reinforced these findings while focusing on neurobehavioral sequelae, while other works demonstrated significant, sustained impairment, and a link between the rate of change of improvement and the severity of injury.[34,35] The authors also commented on the predictive value of the time to reach a GCS of 15 for those children initially registering a 6 or greater, and went on to report that limitations were greatly "underestimated" when scores and performance were compared to population norms instead of matched cohorts.

The ability to predict functioning and recovery is highly sought and a target of much research. The predictive value of several standard indices was the focus for 1996 work from the University of Washington. The authors compared the effectiveness of the GCS and Children's Orientation and Amnesia Test. Academic performance (COAT) and memory performance were also measured. They found that the days to 75% performance on the COAT and the days to reach a GCS score of 15, along with the initial GCS, were significant predictors of immediate and 1-year status. One-year academic and memory performances were most accurately inferred by considering multiple instruments and measures. The overall results supported the use of COAT measures of post-traumatic amnesia to indicate the child's neurobehavioral and functional levels.[36]

Levin et al.[37] studied the complex behavioral manifestations of closed head injury by turning their attention to the effects of injury on self-control and "executive skills" in children. Using the Wisconsin Card Sorting Task, Design Fluency, Verbal Fluency, 20 questions, the California Verbal Learning Task, and the Tower of London task, the authors studied 102 children and adolescents. The study identified five significant factors affecting executive skills:

1 Poor mental fluency.
2 Reduced ability for planning.
3 Reduced ability to "hold information in thought" while working a problem.
4 Inability to "internalize" or make private the use of language and thought.
5 Inability to remain focused and avoid impulsiveness.

In outlining the deficits that the child or adolescent encounters after moderate or severe TBI, it is clear that skills at all levels, from rote learning to higher cognitive integrations may be damaged. Research continues to clarify not only the mechanisms and physiology of injury but also the behavioral and developmental impact. Understanding the conclusions, the ambiguities and the manner in which the research is conducted can be important tools in practice.

Complex neuropsychological disturbances following brain injury

The fund of experience, the repertoire of developed behaviors and emotional skills, and the learning profile each child possesses before injury are important. During the assessment and evaluation, knowing the pre-injury profiles of the strengths and limitations within each domain becomes important to understanding the specific child's foundation of psychological skills. Also, the necessary level of habilitation vs. rehabilitation is determined by the pre-injury constellation of skills once attained. The motivational style and emotional management skills that each child possessed prior to injury help to delineate the potential for change and development during the rehabilitation. A pre-injury psychological and behavioral profile will be important with any type, nature or severity of lesion.

Acute care

The early stages of recovery are characterized by medically stabilizing the child and reintroducing skills once possessed. This phase of "restoration rehabilitation" differs from the adult in that the child will be attempting to learn many skills for the first time. As the child is medically able to tolerate the introduction of various stimuli, the focus is on orientation, mental endurance, basic problem-solving skills, and memory function. Restoring language and communications and sensory-motor skills are of equal importance. Complex disturbances in cognition, conduct, emotional management and group membership are initially addressed during the hospital stay but receive more attention in the post-acute environment.

An article by Sakzewski and Ziviani of Queensland, Australia[38] finds three factors emerging as important indicators of the length of hospital stay for children with TBI. These factors are the severity of injury, the complicating medical factors, and the effects of interventional procedures. The depth and length of coma and the duration of post-traumatic amnesia correlate closely to the length of stay in the hospital. Secondary complications such as subdural hematoma, infection and multiple injuries also positively correlate with length of stay. They comment on the negative relationship between "wait days" and rehabilitation status, when the child is "waiting" to move from acute medical care. The authors cite an article by Blackerby who concluded that the timely onset and adequate intensity of rehabilitation are "two main intervention strategies that have been cited in current literature as important in preventing excessively long hospital stays".[39]

Increasing the traditional treatments, such as occupational, physical and speech therapy, was seen to reduce the number of days in the hospital for children. Discharge planning also received mention as its influence on interventions and the length of stay can be quite profound, especially in areas such as the USA where additional pressures to reduce treatment costs resonate. The article points out that discharge planning in children does differ when compared to adults. For example, the influence of functional development and the efforts to continue the growth process after the accident introduce a significant variable. The type, variety and availability of community services differ and present an organizational challenge secondary to coordinating multiple agencies. Yet, these community services, including school and childcare, can be crucial in the retraining of the emotional management, social discourse, group membership and age appropriate executive skills that have increasingly been identified as important determinants of long-term success.[40]

A comprehensive investigation sought to look further into the practice of interventional techniques. The Evidence Report/Technology Assessment: Rehabilitation for Traumatic Brain Injury in Children and Adolescents of 1999 considered the question "Does the application of early, intensive medical rehabilitation in the acute care hospital improve outcomes for children with traumatic brain injury?".[41,42] An exhaustive, evidence-based literature review found that most of the literature addressing this question was characterized by sample and design limitations, restricting the generalization of the findings. The authors found "no randomized controlled trials" and "no comparative studies" addressing the question. Noting these limitations the authors presented three "observational studies". One was specific to the question of 38 severely injured children and adolescents. The children received "intense, multidisciplinary neurorehabilitation" and were evaluated using the

Glasgow Outcome Scale and a "vigilance score" designed by the investigators: 74% were "minimally responsive" on admission. At 12 weeks only 21% were classified similarly. Noting the attrition in the sample size, the status at discharge using the GOS included 3 patients in a vegetative state, 13 severely disabled, and 7 and 8 experiencing moderate and good recovery, respectively. A 6-month follow-up identified a similar distribution.[42] This report suggests a graded improvement over time for those children undergoing rehabilitation, with greater changes initially and a slowing response over time.

The low response child: vegetative and minimally conscious states

In considering the treatment effort, there is no more fundamental problem of recovery than that of regaining consciousness. Many children will suffer the experience of coma but will naturally emerge and follow expected (e.g. Rancho Los Amigos Scale) stages of emergence and recovery. Another smaller group of children will leave coma and fail to spontaneously awake. These children enter a condition between coma and wakefulness. A recent interest in this condition resulted in the formation of the expert groups, the Multi-Society Task Force on Persistent Vegetative State 1994[43] and the Aspen Consensus Conference 1996.[44] These work groups addressed several complicated issues, the first of which being the confusion surrounding the use of adequate and consistent terminology. The Multi-Society Task Force came to define the vegetative state as "a clinical condition of complete unawareness of self and the environment, accompanied by sleep–wake cycles, with either complete or partial preservation of hypothalamic and brain-stem autonomic functions". The task force went on to emphasize that these individuals demonstrate "no evidence of sustained, reproducible, purposeful, or voluntary behavioral responses . . . and show no evidence of language comprehension or expression". There exists a varying degree of preservation of the cranial nerve and spinal reflexes.[43]

The vegetative state is considered present after 1 month of no awareness with poor to incomplete arousal. Such a state becomes "persistent" when present 1 year following TBI or lasting 3 months in persons with degenerative and metabolic disorders or developmental malformation. The Multi-Society Task Force concluded that cause dictates clinical course, and that recovery of consciousness following 12 months in a vegetative state caused by a traumatic injury is "unlikely in adults and children". According to Whyte et al.[45] children with traumatic vegetative state have 62% chance of regaining some level of consciousness at the end of 1 year. The same determination for a nontraumatic injury population was not found. However, the Aspen Neurobehavioral Work Group concluded that recovery from a "nontraumatic, persistent vegetative state" after three months is "exceedingly rare in both adults and children".[44]

An additional classification between coma and wakefulness has been identified as "minimally conscious". Giacino et al.[46] recommended a "uniform nomenclature" which included the grade of minimally conscious states that were to be differentiated from coma and vegetative state (Table 18.3). According to the authors these individuals would have arousal (poor to weak) with awareness of self and environment (continuous or intermittent) and the basics of communication (elementary ability for yes/no responses). Additional work by Giacino and Kalamar, and the Aspen Neurobehavioral Work Group refined the definitions and comparisons of the various low response states.[47]

Treatment and prognostication for children in these states remains a challenge. The accuracy of diagnosis confounds both the clinical intervention and a review of the existing literature. A 1993 article by Childs et al.[48] describes the problem. The authors found that from a sample of 193 children, 49 were more than 1 month post-injury in either a coma or vegetative state. Of the 49, 18 (37%) were inaccurately diagnosed as remaining in coma. The authors concluded that the difficulties faced during diagnosis may have resulted from a "confusion in terminology, lack of extended observation of the patients, and lack of skill or training in the assessment of neurologically devastated patients".

Other work, by Ashwal et al. in 1992 surveyed members of the Child Neurology Society regarding the aspects of diagnosis and the management of the persistent vegetative state in children.[49] They found that 93% of those surveyed (26% of the society membership) believed that the diagnosis of PVS

Table 18.3 The coma, vegetative and minimally conscious states

	Arousal	*Awareness*	*Communication*
Coma	Eyes do not open spontaneously, no sleep–wake cycle, no arousal to stimulation	No evidence of awareness of self or environment, no gestures, purposeful motor movement, or perception	No evidence of verbalization or no yes/no response
Vegetative state	Eyes open spontaneously; sleep–wake cycle resumes; arousal often sluggish and poorly sustained	No evidence of perception, no communication or purposeful motor movement	No evidence of verbalization or gesture, no yes/no response
Minimally conscious state	Eyes open spontaneously; normal to abnormal sleep–wake cycle; arousal level is inconsistently poor	Reproducible but inconsistent evidence of perception, communication ability, or purposeful motor activity; visual tracking often intact	Ranges from none to unreliable and inconsistent yes/no response with verbalization and gestures

Modified from Giacino et al.[46]

could be made in children: 84%, however, did not believe the diagnosis applied to children younger then 2 months and 30% did not believe the diagnosis could be made between the ages of 2 months and 2 years. Those sampled believed that 3–6 months was the "minimum observation period" to reach a conclusion about PVS, and a large majority (86%) believed that age affected the length of time needed to make the diagnosis: 75% of those surveyed believed neurodiagnostic studies would be of value and supportive of the clinical diagnosis.

Therapeutic considerations included that 75% "never" withhold fluid and nutrition from infants and children in PVS and 28% "always" give medication for pain and suffering. However, only 20% believed that children experience "pain and suffering". Respondents' opinions regarding life expectancy ranged by age group from 4.1 years to 7.4 years for children less than 2 months and older than 7 years respectively. Separate work by Ashwal et al.[50] with 847 children in a persistent vegetative state supported the expectation of increasing longevity with age. Etiology did not appear to differentiate survivors as the age of event did (see Table 18.4).

The place of care and residence was surveyed (Table 18.5) with the survival duration also found to vary with the type of facility.

The treatment for such children has not been differentiated from adult recommendations. The Multi-Society Task Force[43] concluded in their "Clinical Management" recommendations:

> The main functions of the clinical management program are to: improve and maintain the clinical state of the patient; prevent secondary complications; provide the clinical physical environment for optimal recovery;

Table 18.4 The relationship of age at the time of injury to survival

Age (years)	Length of survival (years)
< 1	2.6
1–2	4.2
2–6	5.2
7–18	9.9
>19	9.9

Table 18.5 The relationship between place of care and survival

Residence	Length of survival (years)
Own home	4.5
Institution	5.2
Skilled nursing or private hospital	3.2
Other community care facility	3.7

provide support for the family; assist reintegration into the community; and where recovery is unlikely, provide a disability management program aimed at preventing unnecessary complications and minimizing the long-term care needs of the patient.

The Task Force goes on to include the following:

The main avoidable complications requiring careful monitoring and appropriate preventative and treatment programs are: increased muscle tone leading to contractures; bladder and renal tract complications; constipation or diarrhea; under nutrition; respiratory infections; stress ulceration; deep vein thrombophlebitis; decubitus ulceration; heterotopic ossification; complications of medications and disruption of family dynamics.

The majority of current efforts are focused on the medical management and preservation of medical stability. Stimulation techniques and medication interventions remain "optional" recommendations.

The literature on the use of stimulation techniques has resulted in mixed conclusions and recommendations. A 1993 work by Wilson and McMillan[51] and again in 1996[52] determined that sensory stimulation could alter the unconscious patients' behavior and may reduce the duration of acute coma. The authors, however, cautioned that there is a need for further research. This sentiment was echoed by others, Zasler and Horn[53] and Vanier et al.,[54] cautioning against generalizations, and those that after a more recent literature review concluded there was too little information available to effectively evaluate these types of programs.

However, the state of art for stimulation activities appears to have the potential for "individual change" while not as yet finding any consistent "group effect". For example the study by Wilson and colleagues in 1996[52] reports a meta-analysis on data from 24 "single case experimental studies" evaluating the immediate effects following traumatic brain injury. The authors concluded that "multimodal stimulation produced greater behavioral changes than unimodal stimulation, and the use of personally salient stimuli in multimodal stimulation the greatest changes of all". The authors felt age and gender both influenced the magnitude of change but that the time from injury did not. Yet, the authors indicated that emergence from the vegetative state was not predicted by the magnitude of behavior change resulting from the sensory stimulation.

The Multi-Society Task Force suggests that the term "sensory regulation" may be a more relevant concept than that of "sensory stimulation". They also agree on caution when considering broader application of these findings. Everything should be done, however, to provide an "optimal environment" for emergence from the vegetative state. The group position with regards to stimulation is as follows:

1 Unregulated stimulation is destructive and counterproductive.
2 The windows of potential responsiveness are short.
3 Stimulation should be simple, consistent, and repeated.
4 There is "no evidence to demonstrate whether enjoyable, or familiar sensations are more effective".
5 Rest should precede specific controlled sensory input.
6 Family information about pre-injury likes and dislikes may be helpful in sensory selection.
7 A baseline should be obtained before initiating sensory regulation.

The use of psychostimulants and dopamine agonists dates back to at least 1970, with DiRocco[55] and 1980 with Van Workem.[56] The task force cautions that there are no reliable and randomized studies to look at medication efficacy on a group level and goes on to caution that some medication may impede emergence. They list the possible iatrogenic effects of antiseizure medications, and those used for controlling spasticity. Once medical co-morbid conditions and iatrogenic influences have been ruled out the international work group holds out medication as an "option".

Most recently, the minimally conscious and vegetative child has been addressed through an empirically driven protocol at the University of Virginia.[57] The clinical decision making of the Kluge Children's Rehabilitation Center Low Response Evaluation and Treatment Protocol includes:

• Medical assessment and monitoring.
• Nursing evaluation and management.
• Serial neurobehavioral status examination.
• Arousal/awareness therapies.
• Determination of pharmacologic intervention.

Importance is given to the differential diagnosis and a determination of the child's pathway of emergence. It is recognized that the majority of children emerge in an uncomplicated manner and follow expected changes as listed in the Rancho Los Amigos Scale. However, there is a smaller group of children who experience complicated and non-traditional emergence from coma. This group of low-response children can remain so due to medical conditions, both co-morbid and iatrogenic, as well as for neuropathic reasons. This differentiation is important for its effect on decision making, prognosticating and resource mobilization. The complicated emergence due to medical causes is treated first, by eliminating those interfering conditions. The child who remains either in a vegetative or minimally conscious state is then understood to be in a neuropathic state of complex emergence from coma. It is this group that then is considered for optional treatments (see Figure 18.1). No strong trends have been experienced in the treatment of the group that follows a complicated emergence for medical reasons. Once appropriately treated some join the ranks of the uncomplicated children and resume their progress

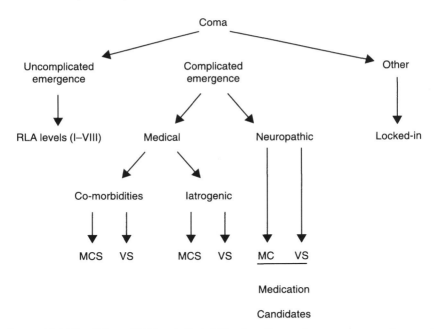

Figure 18.1 The Kluge Children's Rehabilitation Center low response pathway of emergence

through the Rancho Los Amigos levels, while others remain low response and as neuropathic designates are candidates for optional treatments. The selection of treatments, in addition to medical and environmental management strategies, is determined by pathway analysis. Also, the use of time determinants for intervention is based on evidenced-based and best practice guidelines from the Multi-Society Task Force[43] and the works of Giacino and Zasler.[46,47] Developed to be literature based, peer reviewed, and professionally recognizable, the resulting protocol is systematic, empirically driven, clinically monitored and measured, and provides for the establishment of a standardized database.

Post acute and community re-entry

According to Patrick[58] it is the move to the "applied phase" of recovery when many of the dynamic issues of rehabilitation emerge. The need to belong again in the family and community places great strains on complex behavioral skills. Often, difficulties become evident only after the patient is outside the traditional medical setting and back into everyday living. This applied rehabilitation phase builds beyond the strict use of medical technologies and is characterized by the introduction and prominence of other treatment team members. The mental health caregiver and educators can now become important components of the treatment team. A shift in the use of technology typically accompanies this stage of rehabilitation. Applied rehabilitation utilizes instructional technologies and systems engineering, as opposed to the medically oriented procedures of the restorational phase that focused on symptom reduction and skill acquisition. The post-acute, applied phase will expand its focus on skill utilization and how well the child is able to apply learning. Developmental trajectories, family systems, community resources and status dictate, along with the neuropsychological sequelae, each child's unique need.

The cognitive and behavioral sequelae that persist beyond the traditional period of rehabilitation present some of the most difficult and challenging problems for children and their families. Complex behavioral disturbances such as limits in self-control, poor emotional management, dysexecutive states and limited social discourse can prove to be the most disqualifying of problems. Even after successful restoration and application of sensory motor skills, basic cognitive abilities and the ability to communicate, the child may be disqualified for opportunities at home, in the community and at school. It is the decline in group membership skills and the impairments to social interactions that can be so costly to success and require extended attention.

Efforts to address the individual's ability to control and direct their own behaviors through behavior supports has included behavioral analysis which uses among other techniques, shaping programs, behavioral contingencies and extinction paradigms.[59,60] However, the social learning and collaborative model of intervention appears to be gaining support and appears to address not only the individual cognitive needs of the child but the need to support transaction skills and build social discourse competencies.

Ylvisaker and Feeney[61] demonstrate a particular sensitivity towards the development of cognitive and communication skills, and have developed important writings. The authors' 1995 work "Traumatic Brain Injury in Adolescence: Assessment and Reintegration" points out the need for the restoration of communication skills within the context of psychosocial development. In addition, the authors point out that restoring executive skills for self-determination and self-direction takes on added importance. Ylvisaker and Feeney attempt to address such complex deficits as impaired self-awareness and the child's inability to self-evaluate. For example, to address a lack of awareness in a "less confrontational" manner the authors suggests: (a) negotiating assessment tasks; (b) facilitating "product monitoring" tasks (encouraging comparing and contrasting of problem-solving approaches); (c) establishing "self-monitoring systems" (establishing logs, encouraging self-assessment of performance); (d) using natural consequences to teach; (e) increasing engagement in planning interventions and activities, positive future planning.

According to Ylvisaker and Feeney these efforts stand in contrast to more confrontational experiences, such as peer confrontation, verbal recitation of limitations (leading to verbal awareness alone), observation of self on video or direct presentation of low test results, all of which may be provocative and inflammatory. Ylvisaker states in other work[62] that "the most likely communication challenges relate to the socially skilled application of available speech and language skills, not their possession".

Ylvisaker and Feeney develop their ideas and approach further in a 1998 publication on *Collaborative Brain Injury Intervention: Positive Everyday Routine*,[63] an approach that weaves the knowledge of behavioral scheduling, communication skills, social discourse training and psychosocial development. The authors guide, recommend and demonstrate methods of restoring positive daily routines and interactions. They suggest enlisting the child and adolescent to participate in shaping the assessment, establishing "behavioral momentum", and focusing the child and caregiver interactions on establishing productive and positive routines. Relying on Luria and Vygotsky's principals that cognition (especially complex cognition) develops first during interactions between the child and a more "mature thinker" and is then internalized, Ylvisaker and Feeney approach communication, cognitive development and executive functions as interrelated activities. The use of "antecedent control" vs. the reliance on consequences and contingencies offers a proactive manner of addressing complex cognitive and neurobehavioral limitations.

The return to school

Other than the return home, the child's resumption of his educational experience stands as the most important milestone to recovery. For it is within the context of returning to school that the child's cognitive, behavioral and psychosocial needs are addressed. However important this would appear to be, it has not been an easy transition to make from hospital to school. The special needs of the child and family are still not recognized in many communities. It is the return to school that greatly accelerates the child's need to regain the developmental momentum so significantly affected by brain injury.

In a 1997 article by DiScala et al.,[7] the authors report on a large sample of children followed through the National Pediatric Trauma Registry numbering 24,021 as they return to the school and home environment. The authors indicate that of the children with functional limitations only 23.7% were referred for physical therapy, 13.2% for occupational therapy, and 10.1% for speech services. The neuropsychological status of the school age children demonstrated that while 18.7% had cognitive limitations, only 1.8% were referred to special education programs, only 2% were referred for psychological help, and only 2.8% received family counseling. Rehabilitation beyond the traditional medical center appears wanting and in need of attention. The authors conclude: "the majority of children with traumatic brain injury and functional limitations due to the injury return home at time of discharge from acute care with limited referral to potentially beneficial services".

Related work calls for a better interface between medical and educational services.[65] It is reported that families are often forced to serve as the liaison between the two systems. Within the educational system alone there appears a need to formalize and improve the communications between "regular education, special education and related services". Early school models of "separate-and-distinct" contributed to isolation and communication breakdowns. A "school re-entry model" has begun, however, to merge the information and services of the educational and medical systems. For example, acute rehabilitation hospitals have begun to recognize the increasing use of their hospital-based school systems with TBI children at early phases of intervention. Hospitals like Kennedy Krieger Institute in Maryland, Alfred I. DuPont Institute in Delaware and the Kluge Children's Rehabilitation Hospital at the University of Virginia include the participation of hospital-based teachers in their severe and early stage treatment programs.

The "continuum-of-care services model" has evolved where, as Savage states: "Professionals in both rehabilitation and education have recognized that simply returning the child to school, exchanging information between systems, and completing specialized training do not necessarily ensure long-term success in the transition and reintegration of the child." The enduring nature and complexity of the cognitive and neurobehavioral sequelae brought about the need for a new type of intervention beyond what the public school-based programs could provide. These took the form of residential, campus-based programs for students with behavioral and psychological needs. They combine the post-acute rehabilitation needs of the child with ongoing educational placement and instruction.

Savage[64,65] in his role as Program Director at the May Institute developed the May Center for Education and Neurorehabilitation in Massachusetts. More recently with his work with Barcroft NeuroHealth he continues his work in a community-based school for brain injured students suffering neurobehavioral limitations. Savage institutionalizes the interactions and cooperative efforts of families, local schools, funding sources and medical personnel, including primary care physicians, neuropsychologists, community agencies and allied therapies. This new model, along with advances in the development of critical care pathways and classification and regressions trees (CARTS), extends the ability to deliver functional, outcome-driven interventions for children and their families.

The development of comprehensive and well integrated programs follows the earlier work of Savage,[64] Blosser and DePompei,[66] and Ylvisaker and Feeney.[61] Their combined efforts have greatly advanced the identification, classification and understanding of the needs for children with brain injury as they approach community, family and school intervention. The 1991 paper by Savage[65] addresses the confusions in the medical and educational interface, the terminology and the classifications that contributed to less than satisfactory rehabilitation solutions. He states that placement decisions involve three key issues: the transition between the hospital and school; the classification and initial student placement; and educational programming.

The breadth of professional training, the school resources, and the availability of programming in the community affected these decisions. To cultivate more successful transitions, it is recommended that the following four steps are taken:

1   Involve the school-based special education team in the hospital or rehabilitation setting.
2   Train all school-based staff who will have contact with the student.
3   Plan for the short- and long-term support service needs of the student.
4   Continue follow-up by the rehabilitation professionals.

Parents and advocates are advised to consider:

1   Does the school know the definition of TBI and neurologic sequelae?
2   Does the school know what the child can do now?
3   Does the school know what the child needs to do next?
4   What environmental or program changes does the child need in school?
5   Who will be responsible for the child's educational program?
6   How will the family know that the educational program is working for the child?

More recent writings by Blosser and DePompei[66] consider the educational needs of children from a global reference point. Using the Royal Alexandra Hospital for Children, Brain Injury Rehabilitation Service model, the authors identify the need for consistent data collection regarding the injury and the outcome. The treatment and educational teams must be fully informed of the medical, neurodevelopmental and neuropsychological profile of the child and the implications for his or her needs and recovery while moving through the continuum of care. There is also a need to initiate the school reintegration planning immediately upon the child's admission to the healthcare facility. As with others, these authors recognize the need for a "sensitivity to developmental issues".

Growth is a series of transitional experiences that takes the child across interactions, environments and evolving challenges. Each teacher or therapist typically captures a smaller piece of the overall process when a greater perspective and appreciation for the whole would be valuable. The teacher needs awareness of early care and the acute care therapist needs to know about school and home environments. Among the group's recommendations is an emphasis on maintaining objective creativity in addressing the previously described circumstances that define each child's unique needs. Beyond the similarities that are likely found between cases, it is, in fact, more likely that the unique interaction of biophysical, psychological and socio-cultural needs will determine the outcome rather than the strict neurology of the injury.

The Carney group at Oregon State University addressed the question of children and school education in their evidenced-based literature review.[41,42]

The work group asked "Do children with brain injuries who are provided with special education that is designed to accommodate the needs of TBI have better outcomes than (a) those provided with special education that is not so designed and (b) those who do not receive special education?" The Carney group found no randomized, controlled investigations addressing this multi-part question. The literature provides descriptions of programmatic interventions without the rigor of Class I methodology.

One comparison group study by Light et al.[67] examined the effects of participation in a neurocognitive education project with a comparison group of TBI children who were not able to enroll due to distance. The duration of participation varied from 3 to 7 months with from 19 to 68 hours of tutoring. The comparison group and treatment groups all appeared to improve when comparing pre-test and post-test measures of neuropsychological functioning, intelligence, educational, and adaptive behaviors.

A survey study by Parkin et al. in 1996[68] asked parents what they could identify as contributing to the successful return to school for their children. The sample of 53 identified four factors as important and contributing to outcomes: the presence of a school aide that supported reintegration; the attitude of the school program about the importance of reintegration; the home medical aide; and the "pre-trauma medical and behavioral condition" of the patient.

According to the Carney group[41,42] the remaining literature related to their evidenced-based question consisted of case studies wherein the children repeatedly demonstrated improvement with intervention. The reviewers were quick to caution that design limitations restrict the generalization of findings. Among the case studies, however, improvements were noted during the testing period and declines to baseline were repeatedly reported once the interventions were suspended. The variety of interventions included the "enhancement of social networks" in the school environment, and the introduction of cognitive and behavioral training within a special education program for TBI children.[67] Another report by Ylvisaker and Feeney in 1995[61] commented on improved verbal memory testing following cognitive intervention, while an additional study used photographic cues and verbal rehearsal techniques to improve participation. Glang and colleagues[69] in 1997 investigated the effects of "individualized direct instruction" for reading, language and math and found improved academic performance.

Telzrow[70] in her article "Management of Academic and Educational Problems in Head Injury" also emphasizes the need for educators to have a level of clinical familiarity that provides an appreciation of the complex interactions of the pre- and post-injury experiences and environments as neuropsychological variables in recovery. She identifies the conflict between medical and educational agencies and the lack of appropriate adjustment programs as deterrents to successful re-entry. Telzrow mentions that such things as the "inadequate school calendar", the 9-month year that includes numerous breaks, all demand transitional abilities from the children least able to manage them. Such a calendar limits the consistency and comprehensiveness of interventions for TBI children. She also mentions the complications of school schedules and the "non-instructional practices" that interfere with re-entry (e.g., the typical environmental stimulation encountered outside of the learning during the school day). She offers ten "characteristics of quality educational delivery systems":

1   Maximally controlled environments.
2   Intensive and repetitive.
3   Behavioral programming.
4   Simulation experiences.
5   Readjustment counseling.
6   Low pupil: teacher ratio.
7   Emphasis on process.
8   Integrated instructional therapies.
9   Cueing, fading and shadowing learning.
10 Home–school liaison.

The ability of the school system to greatly impact the child with TBI cannot be overemphasized. While facing hurdles and inconsistencies, this system is progressing internally and in its ability to integrate with other components of the entire treatment continuum. New models are developing and old ideas being revisited as study knowledge and practical experience confirm the value of the focused school re-entry program.

Life-span perspective

The review by Carney et al.[41] illuminates the importance of developmental psychology and especially life-span psychology, which "focuses on the study of stability and change in human behaviors throughout the entire life course". Life-span psychology attempts to model the relationships between individual change and the interaction of factors influencing such change.[71-72] These authors suggest that intra-individual changes can be plotted on a growth curve so as to produce a trajectory, which is descriptive of the child or adult's path. The emphasis is on the trajectory as a function of the continuous interaction of biological features (Heredity), past environmental influences (Pa) and present environmental (Pr) influences:

$$B_{age} = f(H, E_{pa}, E_{pr})$$

Since the child with brain injury suffers an altered trajectory and pathway, the introduction of life-span psychology hopes to determine "predictors of individual growth curves". As stated by Carney[41] both stability and change could be described by recovery curves "as a function of an intervention, spontaneous recovery, and short- and long term outcomes". This philosophy for conceptualizing the child's behaviors following brain injury has at its roots the potential for changing the research methodology and quantification of change.[73] Supporting the use of longitudinal research designs, life-span measures for "growth curve models" would be valuable. Such efforts have been developed under the headings "general linear mixed models, multilevel models or hierarchical linear models".[74]

According to the Carney group, software applications currently exist. These models allow the development of mathematical formulas that compare inter-individual changes with intra-individual changes, an element at the heart of understanding the complexities of recovery from brain injury. Carney sites the research of Thompson et al.[75] and all who applied such quantification techniques to the study of the Glasgow Coma Scale, the duration of impaired consciousness and age. With a 5-year longitudinal window the authors were able to relate initial measures to individual results that were summarized in an individual growth curve.

The report by Carney[41] continues on to explore the use of cluster analysis in quantification designs. She states that "clustering algorithms are used to classify children based upon repeated measures of outcomes of interest". The time series is another technique to capture causal links between interventions and outcome. Presently, though, there are no pediatric studies using this technique. This approach is established to make comparisons that relate influences on performance factors over time. In general the Carney group review of growth curve analysis introduces new ways to approach the multi-factorial nature of recovery across the extended periods known to be relevant. The inter- and intra-individual comparisons necessary are in need of newer methods that can accurately capture the child's recovery.

The impact of neurobehavioral changes on the family

Although changes in cognitive and neurobehavioral skills are increasingly more recognizable in some survivors, we are just beginning to understand their affect on family members (Table 18.6). Importantly, it can be the after effect on family that reveals the limitations and impairments of the individual.

Table 18.6 Most frequent concerns expressed by family members

1. Fatigue
2. Impulsivity
3. Frustration leading to anger
4. Tendency to interrupt other's conversation
5. Social isolation
6. Labile mood
7. Problems with decision making
8. Memory impairment
9. Difficulty following directions

Reproduced by permission from Willer et al.[77]

Jacobs revealed that 48% of those injured were living at home with family.[76] Discharge to the family is all too often considered the most desirable outcome and, in some instances, serves as the default option for housing, supervision, and attendant or direct care. Therefore, the impact on family membership and participation can be considerable. Family members, who are still navigating their own catastrophic reaction, frequently find themselves responsible and alone to care for, monitor, manage and direct their loved one's treatment, daily routine and re-entry to the greater world. This situation can have multiple affects.

In their chapter, "The Family System: Impact, Assessment, and Intervention", Kay and Cavallo[78] speak of the family's attempt to "right itself" and to "re-establish a homeostasis". The authors list distinguishing features between TBI and other catastrophic illnesses. They mention first the impact of cognitive, emotional, and behavioral sequelae and the alterations of personality. Second is the chronic nature of these deficits and the ongoing nature of the changes in personhood. Third, due to demographics, these alterations "generally affect the young and those in the early stages of their development". Kay and Cavallo review the findings of Glasgow Research on Subjective Burden establishing a graphic context for understanding the challenge before most families (Table 18.7).

Survivor-specific factors

Kreutzer et al.[82] also examined family stressors. Their research indicates that the recovering individual's level of emotional and personality disturbances is predictive of levels of family disturbances. The changes in emotion and personality, in contrast to changes in physical abilities, more often account for family disturbance. In a later study, Kreutzer et al.[83] reported that 50% of caregivers reported distress. Family members displayed "greater levels of unhealthy functioning" when compared to non-patient and medical normative scores, and there appeared to be a positive correlation between stress and role changes with the onset of health problems. Similarly, Hall et al.[84] found that changes in psychosocial disability persist and prove to be among the

Table 18.7 Family subjective burden research

1. Behavioral, affective, and personality changes cause most burden; cognitive changes cause intermediate burden, and physical changes cause least burden

2. Patient and family members agree most rating physical problems; intermediate when rating cognitive problems, and least about emotional–behavioral problems

3. Over time, family burden increases, becoming more linked to personality changes, moreover, less to neurological severity

4. There is no one-to-one correspondence between degree of deficits and degree of burden

Data from Brooks and McKinlay;[79] Brooks et al.;[80] Livingston.[81]

most challenging to families. Complaints voiced by family members included the lack of involvement in leisure activities, fatigue, slowness, and forgetfulness. Hall's study emphasized the importance of "increasingly severe" temper outbursts, anxiety, and self-centeredness. Aggression was reported in 31% of the cases studied.

At a 2-year follow-up stress was considerably higher for those families with an "at risk" psychosocial history and insufficient funding for care. Accompanying this, according to Hall, were increased uses of medication, increased substance abuse, decreased employment, and depleted financial resources. Reinforcing the socio-economic features of this impact, the study indicates that at 1 year post-injury 47% of caregivers had altered or relinquished their jobs, and at 2 years 33% still confronted income limitations. Similar to many studies, the caregivers, spouses and parents reported greater difficulty with behavior problems than did the survivor.

Mintz et al.[85] report on the families' ability to assess psychosocial maturity within their survivor and the correlation with distress. Using developmental psychosocial cognition methods (negotiation strategies, Selman's model of social perspective-taking and Damon and Hart's multidimensional model of self-understanding), the authors found that the survivors, within a sample of 21, consistently responded at psychosocially immature levels. Of note, family members were consistent in their ability to accurately rate the survivor at their level of functioning. The study points out that as the family members increasingly rated their child as socially immature, their own scores for depression and anxiety increased.

Family-specific factors

In addition to the survivor-specific factors that correlate with distress and burden, there is an increased recognition of family and symptom specific factors as well. Wade et al.[86] report that poor pre-injury functioning of parents and the presence of parental psychological disorders place families at higher risk for long-term disruption. Livingston[87] found that the pre-injury psychiatric and physical health history of relatives accounted for 30% of the variance when rating the sense of burden.

Ravara et al.[88] studied families within a pediatric population. Included in their sample of 81 were mildly, moderately, and severely injured patients whose families were assessed at 3 months, 1 year and 3 years post-injury. The authors concluded, "pre-injury functioning was the best predictor of three year outcomes". One-third to one-half of the parents with moderately to severely injured survivors reported medium to high strain in multiple areas. Low levels of family control and high levels of expressiveness predicted positive outcomes in the severe group. The pre-injury family characteristics that correlated with positive outcomes were higher levels of communication, expressiveness, and problem-solving efforts, utilization of resources, role flexibility, and greater orientation toward activities. Characteristics of the positive outcome families also included lowered levels of conflict, control, and stress.

Other research regarding the increased responsibility placed on family members suggests that overall family isolation negatively related to outcomes. A 1995 study by Finset et al.[89] found that 57.4% of the families interviewed reported a decline in social networks. Other work by Kozloff[90] identified that in addition to declines in social networks, the family members' "multiplex relationships" increased. Interestingly, Kozloff also points out that families with higher socio-economic status were able to maintain existing roles.

Another family-specific dynamic is the ability to manage loss. Unlike finite losses (e.g., death of a member), traumatic brain injury can cause infinite loss for the survivor and family. The families of survivors have been described as having "chronic sorrow" (or "episodic loss", where repetitious remembrances and continuous navigation of milestones place the family member back into a state of grief.[91] The dynamic, open-ended grief process challenges the family skills and strength to maintain health and perspective.

Each family recovers in relationship to their survivor's changes, advances, and setbacks (Table 18.8). Over time, there have been many efforts to describe the states of family recovery and progression. Perhaps the most well-known study of the stages of grief is Kubler-Ross.[92] Although lacking scientific validation and reliability studies, Rape et al.[93] and Lezak's[94] stages are also frequently referenced.

In a broad survey by McMordie et al.[95] of adjustment after head injury, families were asked to comment on their satisfaction with "professional health care services". The authors explored ratings on topics including quality, education, helpfulness, referrals and prognosis. Of great concern was the lack of post-hospitalization resources and education about outcomes. The highest scoring rate for "helpfulness" was for those who provided "hands-on" services, while social services professions were rated significantly lower. Limited contact with the psychologist or neuropsychologist was a focus of concern.

Table 18.8 Stages of family recovery

Acute stage	On return to community
1. Initial shock	1. Happiness with survival, expect full recovery
2. Emotional relief, denial, unrealistic expectations	2. Bewilderment and anxiety
3. Acknowledgement of permanent deficits, emotional turmoil	3. Discouragement and guilt
4. Bargaining	4. Depression, despair
5. Mourning or working through	5. Grieving
6. Acceptance and restructuring	6. Reorganization and emotional disengagement

Data from Rape, Bush, and Slavin,[93] and Lezak.[94]

Sharon Hostler has taken the focus on the family to a new level. Her book *Family Centered Care: An Approach to Implementation*[96] focuses on how to have families "meaningfully participate in medical decision making" and how to develop an institutional culture flexible enough to respond to the ongoing collaboration between families and practitioners (Table 18.9).

In an environment so compellingly important to the welfare of the child with TBI, it is of direct benefit to that child to address specific family needs. Constraints on resources and access will continue to test the ability of the treatment team to successfully address family needs directly, but with an appreciation for the integrated nature of the patient's condition and its influence on the family, consideration can be provided where possible. Again recognizing the circular relation between these elements, advances in one aspect of the scenario can spur progress in another to the ultimate benefit of the whole.

Outcomes

The goal of rehabilitation in the child is clearly to restore pre-injury functioning and the ability to progress appropriately through new growth challenges. The measure for any treatment outcome should be as unique as the program designed to achieve it. The literature base may in the future reliably predict probable outcomes or at a minimum set the level of expectations. Even the most rigorous of work will face the challenge of developing conclusions consistent enough to apply across a meaningful cross-section of the intensely unique and specific cases that exist in practice. The value of today's information is that it describes the complexities between outcome and the type or severity of injury, and documents those situations where predisposing factors and other influences were shown to relate to outcomes. This information, towards which all other efforts truly point, remains outside our full understanding, but is useful as both guide and goal.

Table 18.9 The elements of family-centered care

1. The family is the constant in the child's life, while the healthcare service systems and personnel within those systems are transient and fluctuate
2. Family and professional collaboration is facilitated at all levels of care, from the individual patient to the program and policy level
3. The racial, ethnic, cultural, and socio-economic diversity of the family is honored
4. Family strengths and individuality are recognized, and the family's different coping mechanisms are respected
5. Complete and unbiased information is shared with families on a continuing basis and in a supportive manner
6. Family-to-family support is encouraged and facilitated
7. The developmental needs of the infants, children, adolescents and their families are understood and incorporated into healthcare programs
8. Policies and programs are implemented that provide emotional and financial support to meet the needs of families

The age and type of insult appear to affect the magnitude of injury as well as the length and type of the recovery curve. A review article by Chugani, et al.[11] in *Brain Development* concluded that the brain's ability to tolerate and rebound from focal injury depends on these factors in addition to the level of brain maturity, the integrity of surrounding and contralateral areas, as well as epilepsy and medication. These conclusions are, however, tempered by the following comment:

> Although evidence of functional brain reorganization can be demonstrated in these (clinical and experimental models) it is emphasized that the neurobiological rules that govern intrahemispheric vs. interhemispheric reorganization of function in the brain are, at present, poorly understood. There is a great need and promise that advancement in the neurosciences will allow the clinician to more directly understand and treat the essential disorder and not the sequelae.[11]

Long-term measures of participation were conducted by Marjaleena and colleagues[97] who reported on preschool age children with severe brain injury between January 1959 and December 1969. A final evaluation was completed when the children reached adult age. They found that only 23% (9/39) of the children were employed and another 26% (10/39) were working in sheltered workplaces; 36% (14/39) lived independently and 6 (15%) required mental health treatments. The study concluded that "after the severe brain injury, the sense of identity was the best indicator of final outcome".

As mentioned above, there is a continual search for those markers that will provide insight on future recovery. In an article entitled "Predicting of Neurobehavorial Outcome 1–5 years Post-Pediatric Traumatic Head Injury", Woodward et al.[98] suggest that the interaction of premorbid characteristics and acute medical effects best predict long-term sequelae. The authors list the absence of pre-injury learning problems and older age at the time of injury as likely influences for more favorable recoveries. It is also stated that acute medical measures of normal pupil reactions and higher cerebral perfusion pressure during critical care prognosticate better outcomes.

Ponsford et al.[99] continue by looking at the behavioral outcome for children following mild head injury, finding also the influence of pre-injury characteristics. They state that children with previous head injury, pre-existing learning difficulties, neurologic disease or psychiatric disease of "family problems" were more "at risk" for ongoing difficulties. The authors suggest that early detection, identification and education of these children and their families potentially affect the ongoing nature of their complaints.

An article by Yeates et al.[100] supported the theme of pre-injury factors by pointing out that although the majority of children with mild head injury do not report ongoing post-concussive symptoms, of those who do there is a higher incidence of premorbid neurological and psychosocial "vulnerability". Post-injury decrements in neuropsychological and neurobehavioral functioning are seen.

Changing focus to look at post-injury factors, the Carney group[41,42] reported on outcomes of children with anoxic brain injury and TBI studied by Vander Schaff et al.[101] A sample size of 98 was tracked during varying lengths of rehabilitation and different times of introduction. The study concluded that earlier admission to rehabilitation suggested more functional mobility. Once adjusting the group sample for artifact of severity on the length of stay, the study concluded that the duration of unconsciousness correlated with the return of functional mobility. There appeared no relationship between mobility and the length of time from injury. Here again design and sample development influence the generalization of response and limits of interpretation.

In attempting to grasp the issue, research examines many aspects of the injury and recovery including the biological, social, and treatment variables. Beyond the knowledge supplied by these and other studies, their scope serves as reinforcement to the theme that as the problem is multifaceted so too must be the solutions.

Quality of life as outcome measures

The measure of success during recovery from brain injury is complex. One certainty however, is that the definition of success changes over the course of recovery (Table 18.10). What was once acceptable during acute care and trauma intervention is no longer satisfying during the recovery stage. And again, what was a useful measure of improvement during medical rehabilitation does not apply to the post-acute, community-based recovery. Continuing on in this manner across the different phases of recovery, it must then be determined what relevant measures of success are during each of the various phases.

In September 1999 under the leadership of Prof. Dr. E. Neugebauer, Universitat zu Koln, an international study group, the conference on "Quality of Life after Multiple Trauma", was convened to review the state of the art for measuring the quality of life.[102] A pediatric subcommittee was to look

Table 18.10 "Success" during the phases of recovery

Stage of recovery	Definition of success
Acute medical and trauma	Survival, maintaining life
Hospital-based rehabilitation, acquisition/relearning	Medical stability, skill
Post-acute, community rehabilitation	Skill utilization/application
	Freedom of movement/independence
Long-term living	Life-style management, quality of life

at the status of quality of life measurement in children following traumatic brain injury, and a consensus was reached that the quality of life measures could be considered outcome measures for short, intermediate and long-term recovery.

An evidenced-based literature review by Braga and Sollaci identified 43 articles on the subject of quality of life and pediatrics.[103] Only four were identified that then satisfied the inclusion criteria and definition; only one of which by Melchers et al.[104] was Class I research. This project "An Early Onset Rehabilitation Program for Children and Adolescents after Traumatic Brain Injury: Methods and First Results" was published in 1999. Given the importance of quality of life measures, the need is great for further study.

The pediatric subcommittee concluded that although there exist a number of generic quality of life measures (e.g., Child Health Questionnaire, SF-36), instruments with specific norms or items for children with TBI do not. Until such time as one is available it was recommended that generic instruments be used with supplemented domain specific questions. The committee believes the unique domains involved with treatment, cognitive, perceptual and physical recovery would be important. Also, such issues as school and family reactions and assessment would be essential. The use of both the child's response and that of the guardian would allow a look at the overall system. Unique clinical features such as the child's estrangement from staff, location and family were special to the TBI child as determined by the committee, as were the changes in personality and temperament that can occur but remain uncaptured in generic instruments. In addition the special nature of the child's confrontation with the community and the recognition of deficits, as well as coping with the school, family and community, required special attention given the nature of TBI. For it is in the self-assessment of lifestyle and sense of well being that the final definition of success is to be found. A sense of quality as can only be determined by the individual child and family members is the ultimate definition of success.

Lessons learned

There are a great many efforts being made to improve the lives of children and adolescents with traumatic brain injury. Leading organizations (Brain Injury Association of America, International Brain Injury Association) have dedicated significant energy and resources to education, advocacy and integration of efforts in the USA and throughout the world. Work groups for practice guidelines and experts from many fields have been supported and encouraged to advance and persist in their efforts to improve the course of injured children and their families. The current state of practice is complex but progressing. Many realize the need to advance to more sophisticated levels of research, using Class I and Class II efforts to yield evidence on cause and response and create more broad-based standards of care. For now, some of the many lessons learned include:

1   Appreciate the extent and prevalence of TBI in children and adolescents.
2   Understand the immediate and extended consequences of moderate and severe injury, with recognition that complex mTBI requires special monitoring, evaluation and intervention.
3   Understand that there are children at risk and these children should be considered not only in the rehabilitation effort, but in our first line prevention efforts as well.
4   The brain's neuronal architecture and its neurochemical transmitters evolve post-natally in a structure developed to process information in a manner that allows for complex problem solving and social behaviors and membership. Consequently, injury at early stages disrupts the neurological basis for these complex functions and dependent upon the specifics, may determine the child's long-term success.
5   The final expression of each TBI is the product of neurologic injury, within a developing brain as it interacts with pre-injury psychosocial development and the family context that surrounds each child.
6   Recovery does not stop with restoration of medical well-being and the relearning of skills; the child must be able to apply himself to the environments of everyday life.
7   Families must be addressed and at-risk factors for the family and child must be a focus of care; family-centered care is a necessity, not a luxury.
8   The measurement of success is not complete until quality of life data is determined and collected.

References

1. Guyer, B., & Eller, B. (1990). Childhood injuries in the United States. *American Journal of Diseases of Children, 144*, 649–652.
2. Silver, J. M., Hales, R. E., & Yudofsky, S. C. (1996). Neuropsychiatric aspects of traumatic brain injury. In R. E. Hales and S. C. Yudofsky (Eds.),*The American Psychiatric Press Textbook of Neuropsychiatry* (2nd ed.). Washington, DC: American Psychiatric Press.
3. Kraus, J. F., Rock, A., & Hemyari, P. (1990). Brain injuries among infants, children adolescents and young adults. *Am. J. Dis. Child., 144*, 684–691.
4. Kraus, J. F. (1987). Epidemiology of head injury. In P. R. Cooper (Ed.), *Head Injury*, 1–19.
5. DiScala, C., Savage, R., et al. (1996). *Children and adolescents with disability due to traumatic injury: A data book.* National Pediatric Trauma Registry from the Research and Training Center at Tufts University School of Medicine, New England Medical Center.
6. DiScala, C., et al. (1999). The National Pediatric Trauma Registry from the Research and Training Center at Tufts University School of Medicine, New England Medical Center, April.
7. DiScala, C., Osberg, J. S., & Savage, R. C. (1997). Children hospitalized for traumatic brain injury: transition to postacute care. *J. Head Trauma Rehabil., 12*, 1–10.
8. Epstein, H. T. (1980). Stages in human brain development. *Dev. Brain Res., 30*, 114–119.

9. Finger, S. (1978). *Recovery from brain damage: Research and theory*. New York: Plenum Press.

10. Huttenlocher, R. R. (1984). Synapse elimination and plasticity in developing human cerebral cortex. *Am. J. Ment. Dis., 88*, 488–496.

11. Chugani, H. T., Muller, R. A., & Chugani, D. C. (1996). Functional brain reorganization in children. *Brain Development, 18*, 347–356.

12. Thatcher, R. W. (1991). Maturation of the human frontal lobes: physiological evidence for staging. *Dev. Neuropsychol., 7*, 397–419.

13. Hudspeth, W. J., & Pribram, K. H. (1990). Stages of brain and cognitive maturation. *J. Ed. Psychol., 82*, 881–884.

14. Rakic, P. (1988). Specification of cerebral cortical areas. *Science, 241*, 170–176.

15. Povlishock, J. T. (1999). Cutting edge research in traumatic brain injury. Paper presented at Third World Congress on Brain Injury, Quebec City, June 12–17.

16. Baron, I. S., Fennell, E., & Voeller, K. (1995). *Pediatric neuropsychology in a medical setting*. Oxford: Oxford University Press.

17. Bach-y-Rita, P. (1990). Brain plasticity as a basis for recovery of function in humans. *Neuropsychologia, 28*, 547–554.

18. Luria, A. (1968). *Higher cortical functions in man*. New York: Basic Books.

19. Luria, A. (1973). *The working brain: An introduction to neuropsychology*. New York: Basic Books.

20. Singer, W. (1986). The brain as a self-organizing system. *Eur. Arch. Psychiatry Neurol. Sci., 236*, 4–9.

21. Piaget, J. (1952). *The origins of intelligence*. New York: International Universities Press.

22. Erikson, E. (1963). *Childhood and society* (2nd ed.). New York: Norton.

23. Cockrell, J. (1996). Pediatric brain injury rehabilitation. In R. E. Hales and S. C. Yudofsky (Eds.), *The American Psychiatric Press Textbook of Neuropsychiatry* (2nd ed.). Washington, DC: American Psychiatric Press.

24. O'Shanick, G. J., & Rosenberg, J. (1999). Mild traumatic brain injury guideline development, Paper presented at Third World Congress on Brain Injury, Quebec City, June 12–17.

25. Ewing-Cobbs, L. E., Levin, H. S., Eisenberg, H. M., & Fletcher, J. M. (1987). Language functions following closed head injury in children and adolescents. *J. Clin. Exp. Neuropsychol.*, 167–178.

26. Alberico, A. M., Ward, J. D., Choi, S. C., Marmarou, A., & Young, H. F. (1987). Outcome after severe head injury. Relationship to mass lesions, diffuse injury, and ICP course in pediatric and adult patients. *J. Neurosurg., 67*, 648–656.

27. Bruce, D. A., Schut, L., Bruno, L. A., Wood, J. H., & Sutton, L. N. (1978). Outcome following severe head injuries in children. *J. Neurosurg., 48*, 679–688.

28. Levin, H. S., & Eisenberg, H. M. (1979). Neuropsychological outcome of closed head injury in children and adolescents. *Childs Brain, 5*, 281–292.

29. Ewing-Cobbs, L. E., Levin, H. S., Eisenberg, H. M., & Fletcher, J. M. (1987). Language functions following closed head injury in children and adolescents. *J. Clin. Exp. Neuropsychol.*, 167–178.

30. Fennell, E. B., and Mickle, J. P. (1992). Behavioral effects of head truma in children and adolescents. In M. B. Tramontana & S. R. Hooper (Eds.), *Advances in child neuropsychology* (Vol. 1, pp. 24–49). New York: Springer-Verlag.

31. Ewing-Cobbs, L., Fletcher, J. M., Levin, H. S., Francis, D. J., Davidson, K., & Miner, M. E. (1997). Longitudinal neuropsychological outcome in infants

and preschoolers with traumatic brain injury. *J. Int. Neuropsychol Soc., 3*, 581–591.

32. Emanuelson, I., von Wendt, L., Lundalv, E., & Larsson, J. (1996). Rehabilitation and follow up of children with severe traumatic brain injury. *Childs Nerv. Syst., 12*, 460–465.

33. Emanuelson, I., von Wendt, L., Beckung, E., & Hagberg, I. (1998). Late outcome after severe traumatic brain injury in children and adolescents. *Ped. Rehab., 2*, 65–70.

34. Jaffe, K. M., Fay, G. C., Polissar, N. L. et al. (1992). Severity of pediatric traumatic brain injury and early neurobehavioral outcome: a cohort study. *Arch. Phys. Med. Rehabil., 73*, 540–547.

35. Jaffe, K. M., Polissar, N. L., Fay, G. C., & Liao, S. (1995). Recovery trends over three years following pediatric traumatic brain injury. *Arch. Phys. Med. Rehabil., 76*, 17–26.

36. Massagli, T. L. T., Jaffe, K. M., Fay, G. C., Polissar, N. L., Liao, S., & Rivara, J. B. (1996). Neurobehavioral sequelae of severe pediatric traumatic brain injury: a cohort study. *Arch. Phys. Med. Rehabil., 77*, 223–231.

37. Levin, H. S., Fletcher, J. M., Kufera, J. A. et al. (1996). Dimensions of cognition measured by the Tower of London and other cognitive tasks in head-injured children and adolescents. *Dev. Neuropsychol., 12*, 17–34.

38. Sakzewski, L., & Ziviani, J. (1996). Factors affecting length of hospital stay for children with acquired brain injuries: a review of the literature. *Aus. Occ. Ther. J., 43*, 113–124.

39. Blackerby, W. F. (1990). Intensity of rehabilitation and length of stay. *Brain Inj., 42*, 167–173.

40. Davidson, L. L., Hughes, S. J., & O'Connor, P. A. (1988). Preschool behavior problems and subsequent risk of injury. *Pediatrics, 82*, 644–651.

41. Carney, N., et al. (1999). *Rehabilitation for traumatic brain injury in children and adolescents* (AHCPR publication No. 00-E001). Portland, OR: Oregon Health Sciences University, September.

42. Carney, N., Chesnut, R. M., Maynard, H., Mann, N. C., Patterson, P., & Helfand, M. (1999). Effect of cognitive rehabilitation on outcomes for persons with traumatic brain injury: a systematic review. *J. Head Trauma Rehabil., 14*, 277–307.

43. The Multi-Society Task Force on PVS (1994). Medical aspects of the persistent vegetative state. *N. Engl. J. Med., 330*, 1499–1508.

44. Aspen Concensus Group (1996). Workgroup on the vegetative and minimally conscious states. Paper presented at the Biomedical Institute, Aspen Colorado, March 19–23.

45. Whyte, J., Laborde, A., & DiPasquale, M. C. Assessment and treatment of the vegetative and minimally conscious patient. In M. Rosenthal, E. R. Griffith, J. S. Kreutzer, and B. Pentland (Eds.), *Rehabilitation of the adult and child with traumatic brain Injury* (3rd ed.). Philadelphia, PA: F. A. Davis.

46. Giacino, J. T., Zasler, N. D., Whyte, J., Kate, D. I., Glenn, M., & Andary, M. (1995). Recommendations for the use of uniform nomenclature pertinent to patients with severe alterations in consciousness. *Arch. Phys. Med. Rehabil., 76*, 203–207.

47. Giacino, J. T., & Kalamar, K. (1997). The vegetative and minimally conscious states: a comparison of clinical features and functional outcome. *J. Head Trauma Rehabil., 12*, 36–51.

48. Childs, N. L., Mercer, W. N., & Childs, H. W. (1993). Accuracy of diagnosis of persistent vegetative state. *Neurology, 43*, 465–467.
49. Ashwal, S., Bale, J. F. Jr, Coulter, D. L., et al. (1992). The persistent vegetative state in children: report of the Child Neurology Society Ethics Committee. *Ann. Neurol., 32*, 570–576.
50. Ashwal, S., Eyman, R. K., & Call, T. L. (1994). Life expectancy of children in persistent vegetative state. *Ped. Neurol., 10*, 27–33.
51. Wilson, S. L., & McMillan, T. M. (1993). A review of the evidence for the effectiveness of sensory stimulation treatment for coma and vegetative states. *Neuropsychol. Rehabil., 3*, 149–160.
52. Wilson, S. L., Powell, G. E., Brock, D., & Thwaites, H. (1996). Vegetative state and responses to sensory stimulation: an analysis of 24 cases. *Brain Inj., 10*, 807–818.
53. Zasler, N. D., & Horn, L. J. (1996). *Medical rehabilitation of traumatic brain injury*. Philadelphia, PA: Hanly and Belfus.
54. Vanier, M., Lamoureux, J., & Dutil, E. (1999). Clinical efficiency of stimulation interventions for patients in coma or vegetative states after head injury. Paper presented at Third World Congress on Brain Injury, Quebec, Canada, June 12–17.
55. DiRocco, C., Maira, G., Meglio, M., & Rossi, G. F. (1974). L-Dopa treatment of comatose states due to cerebral lesions: preliminary findings. *J. Neurosurg. Sci., 18*, 169–176.
56. Van Workem, T. C., Minderhound, J. M., & Gottschalt, N. G. (1982). Neurotransmitters in the treatment of patients with severe head injuries. *Eur. Neurol., 21*, 227–234.
57. Patrick, P., Patrick, T., Poole, J., & Hostler, S. (2000). Evaluation and treatment of the vegetative and minimally conscious child: a single subject design. *Behav. Interventions, 15*, 225–242.
58. Patrick, P. (1994). Applied rehabilitation. *ReLearning Times: Newsletter of Learning Services*.
59. Jacobs, H. E. (1993). *Behavior analysis guidelines and brain injury rehabilitation*. Gaithersburg, MD: Aspen Publications.
60. Kazdin, A. E., & Weisz, J. R. (1998). Identifying and developing empirically supported child and adolescent treatments. *J. Consult. Clin. Psychol., 66*, 19–36.
61. Ylvisaker, M., & Feeney, T. J. (1995). Traumatic brain injury in adolescence: assessment and reintegration, *Semin. Speech Lang., 16*, 32–44.
62. Ylvisaker, M. (1993). Communication outcome in children and adolescents with traumatic brain injury. *Neuropsychol. Rehabil., 3*, 367–387.
63. Ylvisaker, M., & Feeney, T. J. (1998). *Collaborative brain injury intervention: Positive everyday routines*. San Diego, CA: Singular Publishing Group.
64. Savage, R. C. (1997). Integrating rehabilitation and education services for school-age children with brain injuries. *J. of Head Trauma Rehabil., 12*, 11–20.
65. Savage, R. C. (1991). Identification, classification, and placement issues for students with traumatic brain injuries. *J. Head Trauma Rehabil., 6*, 1–9.
66. Blosser, J., & DePompei, R. (1994). *Pediatric traumatic brain injury: Proactive interventions*. San Diego, CA: Singular Publishing Group.
67. Light, R., Neurmann, E., Lewis, R., et al. (1987). An evaluation of neuropsychological based reeducation project for the head injured child. *J. Head Trauma Rehabil., 2*, 11–25.
68. Parkin, A. E., Maas, F., & Rodger, S. (1996). Factors contributing to successful

return to school for students with acquired brain injury: parent perspective. *Aust. Occup. Ther. J., 43*, 133–141.
69. Glang, A., Todis, B., Cooley, E. et al. (1997). Building social networks for children and adolescents with traumatic brain injury: a school-based intervention. *J. Head Trauma Rehabil., 12*, 32–47.
70. Telzrow, C. R. (1987). Management of academic and educational problems in head injury. *J. Learning Disabil., 20*, 536–545.
71. Baltes, P. (1987). Theoretical propositions of life-span development psychology: on dynamics of growth and decline. *Dev. Psychol., 23*, 611–626.
72. Baltes, P., Reese, H., & Nesselroade, J. (1977). *Life-span development psychology: Introduction to research methods.* Monterey, CA: Brooks/Cole.
73. Montado, L., & Schmitt, M. (1982). Issues in applied developmental psychology: a life-span perspective. In P. Baltes and O. Brim (Eds.), *Life-span development and behavior.* New York: Academic Press.
74. Bailey, D. J., Burchinal, M., & McWilliam, R. (1993). Age of peers and early childhood development. *Child Devel., 63*, 287–309.
75. Thompson, N. M., Francis, D. J., Stuebing, K. K. et al. (1994). Motor, visual-spatial, somatosensory skills after closed head injury in children and adolescents: a study of change. *Neuropsychology, 8*, 333–342.
76. Jacobs, H. E. (1988). The Los Angeles head injury survey: procedures and initial findings. *Arch. Phys. Med. Rehabil., 69*, 425–431.
77. Willer, B., Rosenthal, M., Kreutzer, J., & Rempel, R. (1993). Assessment of community integration following rehabilitation for traumatic brain injury. *J. Head Trauma Rehabil., 8*, 75–87.
78. Kay, T., & Cavallo, M. (1994). The family system: impact, assessment, and intervention. In J. M. Silver, S. C. Yudofsky, and R. E. Hales (Eds.), *Neuropsychiatry of traumatic brain injury.* Washington, DC: American Psychiatric Press.
79. Brooks, D. N., & McKinlay, W. (1983). Personality and behavioural change after severe blunt head injury – a relative's view. *J Neurol. Neurosurg. Psychiatry, 46*, 336–344.
80. Brooks, N., Campsie, L., Symington, C. et al. (1987). The effects of severe head injury upon patient and relative within several years of injury. *J. Head Trauma Rehabil., 2*, 1–13.
81. Livingston, M. G. (1987). Head injury: the relative's response. *Brain Inj., 1*, 33–39.
82. Kreutzer, J. S., Marwitz, J. H., & Kepler, K. (1992). Traumatic brain injury: family response and outcome. *Arch. Phys. Med. Rehabil., 73*, 771–778.
83. Kreutzer, J. S., Gervasio, A. H., & Campliar, P. S. (1994). Primary caregivers' psychological status and family functioning after traumatic brain injury. *Brain Inj., 8*, 197–210.
84. Hall, K. M., Karzmark, P., Stevens, M., Englander, J., O'Hare, P., & Wright, J. (1994). Family stressors in traumatic brain injury: a two-year follow-up. *Arch. Phys. Med. Rehabil., 75*, 876–884.
85. Mintz, M. C., van Horn, K. R., & Levine, M. J. (1995). Developmental models of social cognition in assessing the role of family stress in relatives' predictions following traumatic brain injury. *Brain Inj., 9*, 173–186.
86. Wade, S., Drotar, D., Taylor, H. G., & Stancin, T. (1995). Assessing the effects of traumatic brain injury on family functioning: conceptual and methodological issues. *J. Ped. Psychol., 20*, 737–752.

87. Livingston, M. G. (1987). Head injury: the relative's response. *Brain Inj., 1,* 33–39.

88. Ravara, J. M., Jaffe, K. M., Polissar, N. L., Fay, G. C., Liao, S., & Martin, K. M. (1996). Predictors of family functioning and change three years after traumatic brain injury in children. *Arch. Phys. Med. Rehabil., 77,* 754–764.

89. Finset, A., Dyrnes, S., Krogstad, J. M., & Berstad, J. (1995). Self-reported social networks and interpersonal support two years after severe traumatic brain injury. *Brain Inj., 9,* 141–150.

90. Kozloff, R. (1987). Networks of social support and the outcome from severe head injury. *J. Head Trauma Rehabil., 2,* 1423.

91. Olshansky, S. (1962). Chronic sorrow: a response to having a mentally defective child. *Social Casework, 43,* 190–193.

92. Kubler-Ross, E. (1969). *On death and dying.* New York: Macmillan.

93. Rape, R. N., Bush, J. P., & Slavin, L. A. (1992). Toward a conceptualization of the family's adaptation to a member's head injury: a critique of developmental stage models. *Rehabil. Psychol., 37,* 3–22.

94. Lezak, M. D. (1988). Brain damage is a family affair. *J. Clin. Exp. Neuropsychol., 10,* 111–123.

95. McMordie, W. R., Rogers, K. F., & Barker, S. L. (1991). Consumer satisfaction with services provided to head-injured patients and their families. *Brain Inj., 5,* 43–51.

96. Hostler, S. L. (1994). *Family-centered care: An approach to implementation* (pp. 464–478). Charlottesville, VA: University of Virginia, Children's Medical Center, Kluge Children's Rehabilitation Center.

97. Marjaleena, K., Kyykaa, T., Nybo, T., & Jarho, L. (1995). Long-term outcome after severe brain injury in preschoolers is worse than expected. *Arch. Ped. Adoles. Med., 149,* 249–254.

98. Woodward, H., Winterhalter, K., et al. (1999). Prediction of neurobehavioral outcome 1–5 years post pediatric traumatic head injury. *J. Head Trauma Rehabil., 14,* 351–359.

99. Ponsford, J., Willmott, C., Rothwell, A., et al. (1999). Cognitive and behavioral outcome following mild traumatic head injury in children. *J. Head Trauma Rehabil., 14,* 360–372.

100. Yeates, K. O., Luria, J., Bartkowski, H., Rusin, J., Martin, L., & Bigler, E. D. (1999). Postconcussive symptoms in children with mild closed head injuries. *J. Head Trauma Rehabil., 14,* 337–350.

101. Vander Schaff, P. J., Kriel, R. L., Krach, L. E., et al. (1997). Late improvement in mobility after acquired brain injury in children. *Ped. Neurol., 16,* 306–310.

102. Neugebauer, E. (1999). *BMBF Conference on Quality of Life after Multiple Trauma,* Wermelskirchen, Germany, September 29–October 2.

103. Braga, L. W., & Sollaci, L. B. (1999). Instruments for the evaluation of quality of life in children and adolescents with brain injury: a systematic review of the literature. Paper presented at the BMBF Conference, Germany, September 29–October 2.

104. Melchers, P., Maluck, A., Suhr, L., et al. (1999). An early onset rehabilitation program for children and adolescents after traumatic brain injury (TBI): methods and first results. *Restorative Neurol. Neurosci., 14,* 153–160.

105. Barkley, R. A. (1977). The effects of methylphenidate on various types of activity level and attention in hyperkinetic children. *Journal of Abnormal Child Psychology,* 5 (4): 351–369.

19 Medical rehabilitation of TBI after intensive care

*Claudio Perino, Paolo Pietrapiana,
Enrico Fiorio, Andrea Maestri, and
Roberto Rago*

Introduction

This chapter examines, from a multidisciplinary medical standpoint, some of the early problems that occur in the acute rehabilitation setting after the occurrence of severe traumatic brain injury. The first part is about the rationale and necessity of adopting proper transfer criteria from intensive care (IC) or neurosurgical units to the rehabilitation ward. Not all patients necessarily need to follow a common path, as individual and general criteria must be taken into account. A safe transfer from an IC unit requires continuity of treatment, appropriate referral and timing, stabilized medical conditions, and patient's initial collaboration. The second part deals with the necessity to gather an appropriate database to classify patient's initial status, rehabilitation procedures and intervention, discharge planning, and outcome. The third part deals with a number of relevant associated medical factors which may influence speed and quality of recovery: prevention of venous thromboembolism, nutrition and swallowing, tracheotomy management, treatment of visual disorders and impairments, and subacute neuro-orthopedic and heterotopic ossification treatment.

Optimal rehabilitation of severe TBI sequelae requires specialized facilities which can provide integrated long-term care. In our experience, it is not usually advisable to transfer patients from intensive units to general rehabilitation wards, as the level of treatment quality and intensity that is needed may be markedly different from other types of neurological disorders (e.g., stroke in the elderly).

In Italy, there has been a trend to identify regional facilities which would address this issue within the framework of a national health system, incorporating public and private hospitals. The main characteristics of these regional centers are:

- Serving a regional population of approximately 2 million people.
- Treating 200–300 severely brain-injured subjects (inpatients and outpatients) annually.
- Providing comfortable logistics to patients and families.

- Providing intensive nursing rehabilitation.
- Incorporating multidisciplinary diagnostic and treatment protocols.
- Addressing family issues.
- Conducting research and providing education to involved professionals.

Regarding inpatient accomodation, we prefer ample single rooms, with the possibility to comfortably host a family relative over a 24 hour period if necessary. Room furnishings include a clock, a wall calendar, a bulletin board, TV and VCR sets, and the possibility of bringing small personal belongings of emotional relevance to patient and family. Quiet individual treatment rooms are necessary for all therapies (physical, occupational, language, cognitive, etc.), while larger common rooms are reserved for group sessions, staff and family meetings.[1]

Specialized nursing is of paramount importance for these patients.[2,3] Nursing care includes specific attention to management of excretory functions, skin care, positioning, wound medication, respiratory and nutritional care. The nursing staff also needs to be supported in terms of training, motivation and prevention of burn-out. They are a vital part of any rehabilitation program, they participate in treatment planning, follow its implementation, and play a major role in instructing and monitoring family members on the ward.[4]

For every subject, accurate evaluation of pathologial findings, impairments and disabilities is a prerequisite for rehabilitation planning and adequate treatment procedures. Professionals from different backgrounds need to integrate in a team structure, coordinating short-, medium- and long-term projects. In our experience, due to multiple consequences of trauma, medical specialties most commonly involved during acute rehabilitation are: physiatry, neurology, neurosurgery, orthopedic surgery, ophthalmology, radiology and otolaryngology. Priorities and multiple-step interventions need to be identified in order to provide a logical and sequential therapeutical approach. Consultations may also frequently include internal medicine specialists.

Other essential contributors are physical, occupational and speech/language therapists, nutritionists, psychologists, social workers and education specialists. There is also need for a team coordinator and supervisor, usually a physician, and a case manager or primary therapist, responsible for every subject's rehabilitation program, therapeutic implementation, quality control and verification.

Team meetings and formal and informal contacts among professionals constitute the base for discussion and clinical problem solving. Finally, family needs, patient's psychosocial background, cost/benefit evaluation and economic constraints should be taken into clear and explicit consideration.[5]

In Italy, funding in severe TBI cases is mostly through the public national health system, and the rehabilitation length of stay is not limited by law or health insurance coverage at the moment, but is left to the best clinical judgment of the hospital medical directors.[6]

Transfer criteria from intensive care to acute rehabilitation

Transfer procedures from neurointensive care to a specialized acute rehabilitation facility need to follow regulations and a set of clinical criteria. In general, it is necessary to guarantee some basic objectives:

1 *Safety*, which means the least possible risk when moving from full-time to partial vital functions monitoring.
2 *Continuity* of treatment and care.
3 *Appropriate timing*, or in other words, no patient should be stationed in intensive care any longer or any shorter than needed.
4 *Appropriate referral*, as not all subjects are ready to benefit and respond to an intensive and comprehensive rehabilitation treatment.

As alternatives, some patients may be transferred to hospital-based, skilled nursing facilities or to non-hospital-based residential facilities for long-term care. Naturally, the characteristics and services offered by these structures will depend on the type of healthcare provided by that particular country, its health organization and resource limitations.

A comprehensive brain injury inpatient facility should provide at least continuous medical assistance, clinical monitoring and emergency intervention, daily consultations with a physiatrist or other pertinent medical specialist, adequate skilled nursing, a minimum of 3 h of diversified therapies 5 days a week, and training/education of patient and family. It is advisable that the receiving rehabilitation facility be provided with a detailed summary of history, past and present clinical conditions and all important records by the intensive care medical director. If possible, it is sound medical practice that the physiatrist or neurologist from the rehabilitation facility pay a visit to the patient before transfer, to verify conditions and prognostic potentials.

Written information should include at minimum all personal relevant data, medical history, accident circumstances, principal and accessory diagnoses, acute gravity indices, lesions at brain imaging, description of neuromuscular consequences, level of cognitive functioning, medical complications, level of impairment and disability, vital functions parameters and their relative degree of instability, surgical procedures and needed medications. As a complement, some information on family and psychosocial situation is usually helpful.

The Italian Society of Rehabilitation Medicine has established some clinical transfer criteria to inpatient acute rehabilitation facilties. Not all of them should always be literally and strictly followed, but at least they constitute a set of good practice guidelines on which to develop a clinical decision. Seven parameters have been identified, and general indications apply to each of them:

1 *Level of assistance*
   • No need for 24-h vital functions monitoring.

- No need for skilled nursing for more than 6 h/day.
2 *Level of consciousness*
- At least 3 or more, as measured by the LCF Rancho Scale.
3 *Surgery*
- No need for surgical procedures in the short-term period.
4 *Metabolic condition*
- Maintainance of adequate parameters with enteral nutrition (NGT or PEG allowed).
- No severe gastro-intestinal, hepatic or renal complications.
5 *Respiratory condition*
- Spontaneous breathing (no mechanical assistance).
- Unassisted arterial oxygen saturation of at least 95%.
- Resting respiratory frequence of less than 25/min.
- Negative radiography for severe pulmonary infection.
- No infection or complication of tracheostomy (tube allowed).
6 *Cardiovascular condition*
- No severe cardiac complications or cardiac failure.
- Hypertension allowed, if pharmacologically controllable.
- Adequate renal perfusion (diuresis of more than 50 ml/h).
7 *Infectious condition*
- Controllable infections allowed.
- Severe multisystemic infections not allowed.

When the patient is transferred to our rehabilitation center, he or she is usually accompanied by one or more family members. Early contacts with families are essential to start a process of education and cooperation.[7-11] A first formal family meeting is organized as soon as possible by the attending physiatrist and clinical psychologist. There are a number of objectives attached to this procedure:

- *Verify the level of family information* in terms of understanding the injury, forseeable consequences and implications. Contact with professionals in the intensive care phase have frequently not been adequate or sufficient to clearly and realistically inform involved family members.
- *Evaluate expectations* and in general get a sense of the family psychological attitudes, hopes and degree of cooperation or opposition.[12]
- *Understand psychosocial background*, patient's premorbid situation and accident circumstances.
- *Identify a primary family member* to preferably relate to for communication and education.
- *Inform about rehabilitation ward rules and regulations* (this part may also be fulfilled by the chief nurse).[13]
- *Inform about daily organization* of rehabilitation schedule, nursing procedures and further contacts with attending physician and other professionals.[14,15]

Subsequent family meetings are scheduled usually every 2 weeks to discuss intervening problems, to refer to progress or setbacks, to initiate personal psychological family counseling and to prepare patient's home discharge if possible and advisable.

Practice guidelines for database collection

The Italian Society of Rehabilitation Medicine, through its active TBI group section, has indicated a number of recommendations for the physiatric evaluation of TBI patients.[16] These include:

1 A detailed evaluation of the subject's condition, performed by trained rehabilitation professionals, is essential before and during all stages of the recovery process.
2 The evaluation model should follow the standards set by the ICIDH-2 of the World Health Organization.
3 A complete physiatric evaluation should have the following objectives:
   • diagnostic definition in relation to its severity
   • functional prognosis and provisional psychosocial prognosis
   • estimate of rehabilitation needs (qualitative and quantitative) of patient and family
   • planning and implementation of treatment interventions
   • outcome evaluation and quality control.
4 Data collection should include at least the following:
   • detailed evaluation of acute clinical pathological parameters, referring to both the brain injury and all other injuries and complications
   • pre-traumatic information on social, vocational and lifestyle parameters
   • significant pre-traumatic medical history
   • complete evaluation of impaiments, disabilities and handicaps
   • forseeable quality of life and general health issues.
5 Standardized, well-known scales, tests and procedures should be utilized.
6 Data should be communicable to all rehabilitation professionals involved.
7 Data should be collected longitudinally for a period of no less than 1 year and, if possible, up to 3 years.

Based on these general recommendations, a "minimum database protocol" has been established for use in all Italian specialized TBI rehabilitation facilities. The document has a first part to be completed at rehabilitation admission, and a second part to be filled out at discharge or at subsequent follow-ups. It was designed to be realistically completed, and thus does not include all possible significant data. However, any kind of additional material may be used in any facilities for special purposes. The ultimate goal is to build an Italian national rehabilitation database, different in some aspects but somewhat comparable to the TBI model database in the USA.[17,18]

The Opening Protocol includes:

1 *Demographic and social data.*
2 *Premorbid medical history* (traumatic, psychiatric, neurological, physical, substance abuse, legal).
3 *Accident circumstances.*
4 *Acute care hospital information.*
5 *Global severity of TBI* (worst Glasgow Coma Score of first 24 h).
6 *Evaluation of primary damage* (brain injury as classified by ICD-9 CM; CT scan as classified by Marshall et al.:[19] associated traumatic damage as of ICD-9).

This is followed by the Admission and Outcome Protocol, including:

1 *Acute length of stay information and provenance.*
2 *Evaluation of secondary pathology* (yes/no on infectious, respiratory, cardiovascular, cutaneous, orthopedic, neuromuscular and secondary neurological problems).
3 *Impairment evaluation* (LOC duration, GCS on rehab. admission, LCF Rancho Scale, PTA as measured by GOAT; respiratory, nutritional, excretory, neurovegetative, seizure impairments; motor impairment as classified by Griffith and Mayer).[20]
4 *Disability evaluation* (Glasgow Outcome Scale extended, Disability Rating Scale).[21]
5 *Handicap evaluation* (as measured by the Community Integration Questionnaire, Italian version).[22]
6 *Quality of life evaluation* (global subjective scale for subject and accompanying relative).[23]

It is possible (and recommended) to add standardized measures for more detailed movement evaluation, cognitive and behavioral disabilities, speech and language impairments, attention, memory and executive function disorders.

Each facility may have sets of additional data and special tests designed for their own treatment or research purposes. In our center we also regularly use the Functional Independence Measure and the Functional Assessment Measure,[24,25] have standardized neuropsychological testing, and have developed our own scales for swallowing, movement, speech and language disorders. Some of these will be illustrated later in this chapter. As a general rule, both the minimum database protocol and other measures are designed to fit computer software format. Studies are underway to produce a complete computerized day-to-day physiatric medical flow chart.

Prevention and treatment of venous thromboembolism

It is well beyond the scope of this chapter to review all possible medical complications after severe TBI and polytrauma. Among these, however, we have chosen venous thrombosis and subsequent pulmonary embolism, for its implications in terms of frequency (third cause of late death after sepsis and multiple organ failure), prevention and treatment.[26] Necroscopy studies establish a high incidence of post-traumatic deep vein thrombosis (up to 65%), while approximately a 20% rate of pulmonary embolism can be found in deceased acute trauma subjects. Considering the lowered early mortality rate due to improvements in acute care, this incidence may have increased recently, becoming a leading cause of death after primary survival.[27,28]

In examining the pathogenesis of venous thromboembolism, it is important to remember that it is most frequently associated to pelvic, hip, femur or tibia fractures, to spinal cord injury, to surgical procedures, old age, heart failure, and to prolonged bed immobilization.[29] Most of the severe TBI cases have at least one of these associated conditions, and their risk is certainly much increased. Moreover, clinical characteristics suggestive of thrombosis only minimally correlate with venographic studies: in other words, clinical detection of this problem greatly underestimates its incidence.[30]

Pathophysiologically, favoring factors include local venous endothelial damage, decreased venous flow associated with inactivity and bedrest, and hypercoagulable states due to the post-trauma release of circulating thromboplastin, activated procoagulants and platelets. Age over 40 and blood transfusions were also identified as aggravating risk factors.[29]

In contrast, with post-surgery patients, the effectiveness and safety of prophylactic measures is not precisely defined in patients with major multiple trauma.[31] Available studies mainly apply to blunt trauma patients; very seldom are TBI patients randomized because of their multiple risks and concurring problems. On the other hand, it must be remembered that there may still be a high thrombotic incidence even when potent antithrombotic drugs are used. However, prevention is still the most reliable method to reduce incidence of life-threatening complications. There are a number of options that can also be partially combined: mechanical methods, oral anticoagulation, antiaggregant drugs, heparin derivates, dermatan sulfate, dextran, and vena cava filter placement.

Most of the different mechanical approaches (elastic stocking compression, intermittent pneumatic compression, electrical stimulation of triceps muscles, passive mobilization) have an effect of partially preventing deep vein thrombosis in neurotrauma patients.[32] These methods are substituting inactive lower extremity muscle pumps. If not carefully monitored, pneumatic compression may also cause temporary venous occlusion and release of plasminogen activating factor and, as electrical stimulation is labor intensive and uncomfortable, the best clinical practice option is still the use of graded-compression stockings.

Oral anticoagulation, with warfarin or analogues, is theoretically applicable, but poses the risk of bleeding complications, and thus there is little enthusiasm in this direction for the TBI patient. As an antiplatelet–antiaggregant agent, aspirin has been shown to be effective in reducing the risk of pulmonary embolism after hip fracture, but due to limited information, its use is not recommended at present in major trauma patients.[33]

Low-dose subcutaneous unfractioned heparin has been used in the past in controlled trials of spinal cord patients, with venography as an endpoint.[34] Its use had to be prolonged over a 2 month period to be effective, with a high incidence of bleeding (24%). More recently, low molecular weight (LMW) heparin is more advantageous in terms of both efficacy and safety.[35,36] Thus, the best pharmachological prophylactic option is, at present, LMW heparin given subcutaneously every 12 h for at least 1 month.

Dermatan sulfate (thrombin inhibitor) and dextran (plasminogen activator) may be both effective and safe in trauma patients (no bleeding side-effects), but their reduction of thrombotic risk is much lower than that of LMW heparin.

Inferior vena cava filter insertion is warranted only in those patients with objectively confirmed proximal vein lower extremity thrombosis, but with strong contraindications, complications or failure of pharmacological agents. TBI subjects are, however, considered high risk patients for this procedure. On the other hand, it should be remembered that filters reduce the risk of severe pulmonary embolism, but have no influence on deep vein thrombus formation.[37]

The best practical approach to prophylaxis is thus a combination of mechanical approaches (stockings and mobilization) with pharmacological options (LMW heparin and/or antiaggregants). A recent study has been applied to neurosurgical patients, with a significant reduction of embolic complications.[38] At present, however, there is not a first-class study which demonstrates prevention efficacy in very severe TBI patients.

Finally, in regard to treatment of established and documented deep vein thrombosis,[39] the standard therapeutic approach in general trauma patients is initial intravenous heparinization with concomitant oral anticoagulants. Heparin dosage is adjusted according to close laboratory monitoring of activated partial thromboplastin time (1.5–2.5-fold over baseline measures), it is administered for at least 5 days to allow time for warfarin anticoagulation to occur, and then discontinued. At present, there is the option to use LMW heparin subcutaneously, three times a day from the beginning and without need for close laboratory monitoring.

Oral anticoagulation is usually continued for 4–6 months after major thromboembolic episodes, with the prothrombin time prolonged to an INR of 2.0–3.0.[40] In TBI patients there are no current studies to support this standing, and timing and safety are uncertain.

Nutrition and swallowing rehabilitation

Nutrition and swallowing are closely related in survivors of severe traumatic brain injury, and their status should be monitored to avoid inappropriate weight loss or other complications. As the physiological swallowing mechanism is usually impaired, parenteral or enteral feeding is established as soon as possible to avoid malnutrition.[41,42]

Naso-gastric (NG) or percutaneous endoscopic gastrostomy (PEG) tubes may be placed to allow bolus or continuous feeding, and to compensate for the increased catabolism and energy expenditures associated with brain injury itself.[43] However, it should be remembered that there might be a reduction of the lower esophageal sphincter tone and that gastric feeding may cause airway aspiration. In these cases, enteral jejunal feeding is preferred.[44]

There are many complications associated with malnutrition: for example, hypercatabolic protein depletion can lead to peripheral edema, skin breakdown, delayed wound healing, decreased immunocompetence, respiratory surfactant reduction, higher risk of infections and muscle wasting. Gastrointestinal effects of inadequate dietary intake include intestinal enzyme loss, malabsorption syndromes due to microvilli functional alterations and subsequent diarrhea. Therefore, adequate calories and protein supplies must be started no later than the second day after injury.[45]

The use of initial total parenteral nutrition (TPN) may also be considered an alternative to enteral feeding, as it was suggested that more calories are provided this way.[46] Another approach has been proposed, with initial use of TPN, slow addition of enteral feeding and gradual switch to providing all nutrition through the gastrointestinal system.[47] The main indications for TPN include:

1 Forseeable short-term acute phase.
2 Generalized sepsis.
3 Gastrointestinal lesions or complications.
4 Oro-facial lesions and fractures.
5 Pulmonary aspiration.
6 Severe malabsorption and intractable diarrhea.

The disadvantages of TPN may be unrecognized hyperglycemia, lactate accumulation, excessive fluid intake with cardiovascular consequences, or the possibility of iatrogenic pneumothorax and septic contamination of the intravenous lines.

If relevant dysphagia persists after the patient is transferred from the intensive care unit to an acute rehabilitation ward, enteral nutrition is used by us, in most cases, for a number of reasons: it is closer to physiologic feeding; it has a lower complication rate; it provides adequate calorific, amino acid, vitamins and other nutrients intake; it is easier to mantain and less expensive.[48] However, as already mentioned, there are some contraindications: gastrointestinal infections or trauma-related lesions, intestinal occlusion; intractable vomiting; airway aspiration; severe malabsorption with diarrhea; NG or PEG-related complications.

Naturally, partial or total oral feeding is the goal to be reached as soon as possible. A combination of swallowing mechanism recovery and adequate level of cognitive functioning is required to make improvements in this direction. When dysphagia is present, it is necessary to address this rehabilitative issue with specific intervention protocols.[49]

Patients with swallowing disfunctions (neurogenic dysphagia) have much longer rehabilitation lengths of stay than patients who rapidly recover normal swallowing.[50] Neurogenic dysphagia is a syndrome which has different and multiple components: cognitive and attentional disfunctions; swallowing reflex alterations due to brainstem damage; sensorimotor cranial nerve lesions; peripheral receptor sensory damage and deafferentation.[51,52]

Swallowing assessment should be focused mainly on cognitive control over eating circumstances and neuromuscular control of the swallowing sequence. A reduction in cognitive integrity may limit the patient's attention, cooperation and action sequencing, while motor discoordination, muscle weakness or spasticity pose high risk of dysphagia and aspiration of food in airway passages.

The act of swallowing can be divided into four separate phases that smoothly combine to produce coordinated bolus ingestion: oral intake and preparation (partly voluntary), oral (mostly reflex), pharyngeal and esophageal (totally reflex). In severe TBI cases any combination of disfunctions can be observed.

The first approach to the patient is bedside examination. Medical charts must be thoroughly reviewed. Subsequently, there are indications for clinical evaluations of the respiratory function, including tracheostomy and endotracheal tubes if present, oral and pharyngeal inspection, cranial nerve function evaluation, observation of spontaneous saliva swallowing, level of cognitive status, and, if possible, language, voice, oral praxis examination, reflex and voluntary swallowing and coughing. A skilled clinician is usually able to predict from a complete exam the likelihood and degree of swallowing pathology.[53]

A number of instrumental techniques may consequently be considered. Most commonly used are fiberoptic endoscopic evaluation of swallowing (FEES), and videofluorography. The latter consists of a modified barium swallow study with solid, semisolid and liquid boluses, performed in the radiology department with the assistance of a physician and a skilled speech pathologist. Images are electronically recorded, memorized and digitally elaborated for further study. They can be viewed later as single frame, slow motion or normal speed pictures.

Swallowing abnormalities have been classified into eight categories:[50]

1   Swallowing reflex prolonged over 1 s (up to 5 s).

2   Swallowing reflex very delayed or absent.
3   Bolus entering hypopharynx before initiation of swallowing reflex.
4   Pooling in the valleculae.
5   Swallowing mechanism triggered at the piriform sinus.
6   Pooling in the piriform sinus.
7   Aspiration of bolus in airway below true vocal folds.
8   Reduced hypopharyngeal peristalsis or pharyngeal paralysis.

Obviously, it is common to assess multiple abnormalities, as they are mostly interconnected and interdependent. If a subject receives a pathological rating in at least three of these categories, he or she is labeled as severely dysphagic.

Rehabilitation of dysphagia in these cases becomes complex and challenging. Therapeutical procedures require that the subject use an NG or PEG tube for the necessary time before making physiological swallowing improvements. Weaning from enteral lines can be achieved when it is possible to feed the patient orally with an adequate amount of necessary calories, nutrients and fluids. Usually an NG tube is mantained with more collaborative subjects, in milder dysphagia and for shorter periods of time (up to 1 month). On the other hand, a PEG procedure is preferable if longer rehabilitation periods are foreseen, or if the patient is only minimally conscious and with alternating degrees of collaboration.

During this period it is recommended to continue with hypercalorific dietary intake (2000–2500 calories/day and 1.5–2.0 g protein/kg body weight). In fact, if continuing hyperadrenergic metabolic activity persists, this causes carbohydrate and fat mobilization from body storage tissues and a consequent protein hypercatabolic state with abundant amino acid release and waste.

In our experience, PEG advantages include reduced aspiration risk (vs. NG), fewer iatrogenic endothelial lesions, higher subjective tolerability and less discomfort (agitated patients tend to pull NG tubes frequently and risk lesions), and a global improvement of rehabilitation management.

PEG complications may be immediate (during or after positioning), early (within a few days) or late (after weeks). Major problems in TBI patients include death risk (1%), gastric or esophageal perforation, massive gastric bleeding, and generalized sepsis. The most common less severe complications are fever, localized infections, tube migration, dislocation or mulfunction, and localized hemorrhage.

To facilitate maximum recovery from dysphagia, most acute rehabilitation programs use an interdisciplinary team approach. Our team members include a physiatrist, otolaryngologist, speech therapist, nurse, dietician, and occupational therapist. The patient and the referral caregiver are also integral members of the treatment team. At our center, these are the respective tasks:

1   *Physiatrist*: prescribes medication, coordinates and verifies team activity, is responsible for intervention planning, invasive medical procedures and outcome.
2   *Otolaryngologist*: evaluates airway condition and swallowing functions, performs bedside examination, fiberoptic laryngeal endoscopy, videofluorography and participates in treatment planning.
3   *Speech therapist*: evaluates swallowing, voice, language, communication and praxis, performs dysphagia treatment sessions, verifies progress and outcome, educates nurses and family members.
4   *Nurse*: assists physicians during medical invasive procedures, controls protocol execution and patient's responses, supervises family members and participates in treatment planning meetings.
5   *Dietician*: regulates dietary prescriptions, participates in planning and patient supervision.
6   *Occupational therapist*: treats patient, educates family and elaborates best personalized compensatory strategies.

Regarding videofluoroscopic evaluation, we have modified the original *impairment classification*, reducing the eight abnormalities described by Field[50] to five categories:

1   Prolonged or delayed oral phase.
2   Bolus entering hypopharynx before reflex initiation.
3   Delayed or absent swallowing reflex.
4   Reduced pharyngeal peristalsis or paralysis.
5   Airway aspiration.

Furthermore, we grade aspiration from 4 (100% of bolus in airways) to 0 (no aspiration), with intermediate degrees of 3, 2 and 1, (75%, 50% and 25% of aspiration, respectively). Coughing reflex during videofluorography, in case of aspiration, is graded 0 (absent), 1 (partial) and 2 (present and valid). Swallowing reflex is scored as 0 (absent), 1 (delayed) and 2 (within limits). Barium bolus dripping in hypopharynx is scored 4–0, as in aspiration. This scaling allows us to document improvements at follow-up videofluoroscopies.

We have also developed a *global swallowing and nutritional function evaluation scale*:

- *Grade 0*: Total enteral or parenteral nutrition. Videofluorography is unsafe or impossible.
- *Grade 1*: Total enteral nutrition. Possible indirect therapy (oropharyngeal sensory stimulation) after videofluorography.
- *Grade 2*: Combined enteral nutrition and some modified oral food intake (< 50%). No oral liquids. Possible direct active dysphagia rehabilitation therapy.

- *Grade 3*: Oral nutrition prevails over enteral nutrition. Some oral liquids. Modified food quality and consistency. Rehabilitation continues.
- *Grade 4*: Total oral nutrition. Need of modified food, compensatory strategies and prolonged feeding time. Occasional dysphagia for liquids may persist.
- *Grade 5*: Normal physiological feeding.

Swallowing rehabilitation therapy is defined as a number of facilitating and compensating techniques to improve safe consumption of food and liquids without jeopardizing airway integrity. We have divided our approach into five different sectors:

1 *Generalized treatment*: includes respiratory and postural training, enhancement of oral praxis, voluntary apnea control, phonation and vigilance/attention training.
2 *Indirect reflex treatment*: consists of multiple sensory stimulation of lips, oral cavity, tongue, velopendulum and pharynx with light mechanical, thermal and taste stimuli applications.
3 *Direct specific treatment*: involves active patient collaboration and includes a number of voluntary and compensatory strategies (controlled breathing, modified head and neck postures, chewing exercises, controlled voluntary swallowing, and voluntary coughing activation).
4 *Special techniques*: includes muscle reflex re-education, swallowing fractioning, especially adapted feeding devices, supraglottic swallow, Mendelsohn maneuver, liquid and food consistency adaptations and diet modification.
5 *Family intervention*: involves thorough family education and training, with clear explanations of goals and techniques, practical feeding sessions, maintenance of daily feeding and drinking records, and supervision of progress and outcome.

Enteral nutrition (NG or PEG) can be withdrawn when there is clear evidence of:

1 No airway aspiration.
2 Good recovery of patient's attention and feeding cooperation.
3 Adequate oral dietary intake (including fluids) at a reasonable eating speed.
4 Slight occasional liquid dysphagia tolerated if reflex and active coughing are present.
5 Adequate family members' education.

Tracheostomy management

As far as problems related to airway management are concerned, the use of tracheostomy and mechanical ventilation has become standard during

ICU interventions in severe TBI cases with prolonged coma. This is most important for providing adequate oxygenation and hyperventilation, managing respiratory secretions, and as a protection against aspiration risks. When the patient is transferred to an acute rehabilitation ward, he or she is often still using an endotracheal tube. There are a number of medical rehabilitation issues directly connected to this condition:

1   *Hygiene of tracheostomy and endotracheal tube.* It is necessary to maintain optimal cleaning of stoma and breathing apparatus to prevent any infection.

2   *Airway humidification.* Upper airways are excluded from ventilation and tend to dry up rapidly. It is important to use devices that provide moisture to nasopharyngeal and laryngeal cavities. Oral hygiene is also mandatory.

3   *Secretion management.* Periodic aspirations may be required to clear airway passages. Posture modifications should also be used to drain different pulmonary lobes bilaterally. When operating a surgical aspirator, it is recommended that a procedure of antiseptic rules and atraumatic maneuvers be followed. Suction pressure should not exceed 120 mm/Hg, catheters should be properly and professionally handled to avoid unecessary unpleasant stimulations and procedure should not last more than 15 s. Monitoring of peripheral oxygen saturation, heart and respiratory rates is important to avoid or to promptly recognize vagal reactions and oxygen desaturation. Cardiovascular problems due to arrhythmias may be a possible complication of aspiration maneuvers.

4   *Tube substitution.* For hygiene and cleaning it is necessary to change endotracheal tubes periodically (depending on individual conditions, every 3–7 days). Decannulation and recannulation should be performed skillfully and carefully. Stoma tends to retract and even to close rapidly.

5   *Phonation.* Windowed endotracheal tubes allow recovery of speech if patient is conscious. Special plugs are used to close tracheostomy, test autonomous ventilation and possibly initiate speaking.

6   *Decannulation.* There is no standardized, universally accepted protocol. Usually uncuffed windowed tubes are downsized, then plugging is used to ascertain unaided respiration, secretion control, effective coughing and aspiration risk. Before final removal, constant plugging must be tolerated, reflex and voluntary coughing must be valid, and arterial oxygen saturation should be kept to adequate levels. Some complications can be expected after decannulation: tracheal granulomas (50%), tracheal malacia (20%), tracheal stenosis (10%), and laryngeal pathologies (dysphonia, breathy voice, vocal cord paralysis).[54] For these reasons, a laryngoscopy is always recommended after prolonged use of endotracheal tubes. Decannulation is not to be considered trivial due to the potential risk of airway obstruction, pneumonia and death, mostly with low-level cognitive functioning subjects.[55,56]

7   *Outcome*. Even with significant residual pathology, some TBI survivors may not show symptoms of residual airway obstruction or tracheal stenosis, mostly because they do not exercise hard enough to elicit dyspnea and exertion intolerance. Subjects who are motorically intact may experience difficulties with subsequent aerobic retraining, and thus remain partially impaired.

Rehabilitation of visual disorders

Recovery of visual functions is one of the main goals to be attained by the rehabilitation team. Vision is involved in all therapeutical and daily life activities, and its impairment weighs heavily on long-term global outcome. Epidemiologically, in our central database series of 250 treated subjects, the incidence of visual problems is 49% in very severe TBI cases (mean GCS, 6.3; mean LOC, 25.7 days). Of these, 4% of subjects had monocular vision before trauma, 12% have post-traumatic peripheral paralysis of one or more oculomotor nerves (third, fourth or sixth cranial nerves), 15% have partial or complete post-traumatic optic nerve atrophy (usually monolateral), and 69% have complex ocular sensorimotor disturbances, due to brainstem internuclear and supranuclear pathway dysfunctions leading to functional dyplopia, loss of binocular vision, strabismus, visual confusion and accommodation difficulties. Some authors have defined this clinical picture as "post-trauma vision syndrome" (PTVS), which may also include symptoms of chronic headache, focusing, staring, reading and writing difficulties, vertigo and proprioceptive postural disorders.[57,58]

Therefore, in our experience, it is essential for an effective rehabilitation team to include a neurophthalmologist and an orthoptist or optometrist as qualified specialists for visual rehabilitation problems.[59–61] The ophthalmologist's evaluation begins with the intensive care phase, and it includes orbit, adnexa and anterior segment (cornea and iris) inspections, pupillary reflexes and intrinsic eye motility, direct ophthalmoscopic fundus and, if partial patient collaboration is possible, coarse evaluation of extrinsic ocular motility and visual acuity.[62] The neurophthalmologist cooperates at this stage with the intensive care specialist, the neurosurgeon, the maxillofacial and the plastic surgeons in diagnosing and treating anatomical damage to the visual system.

When the subject is transferred to a rehabilitation setting and at least partial cooperation is possible, rehabilitation efforts must be focused on the integrated visual sensory and motor functions, and the visual therapist comes into play. At this point, a thorough ophthalmological evaluation is recommended. It is necessary that the subject be able to sit upright, communicate verbally, and respond to commands, requests and testing procedures. Attention may still be shifting or transient, and the examiner must take fatigue, behavioral disturbances or incomplete cooperation into account, and realize that the time-consuming examination needs patience.[63] Neurophthalmologic testing includes:

1   *Adnexa and anterior segment biomicroscopic evaluation.*
2   *Far and near visual acuity*, eventually with cycloplegic refraction and lens correction.
3   *Contrast sensitivity testing.*
4   *Ocular tonometry.*
5   *Indirect ophthalmoscopic or biomicroscopic fundus.*
6   *Kinetic perimetry and visual evoked potentials* (VEP) if necessary.

An orthoptic evaluation is usually indicated following the neurophthalmologist's visit. The main tasks of the orthoptist are to test eye motility and sensory visual functions, to discuss recovery potential, to organize treatment sessions and therapeutic procedures. The orthoptist also needs to take into account vigilance, attention, memory, speech and spatial representation problems. The first approach may not be easy. It includes an understanding of the global clinical picture, and should promote patient's motivation and enhance response reliability. Orthoptic evaluation, usually performed in two or three separate sessions, includes:

1   *Head posturing observation.* An asymmetrical compensatory head and neck positioning may be indirect evidence of ocular paralysis. As a general rule, it is observed that head positioning tries to eliminate dyplopia by excluding functional involvment of the paretic muscle. Most common abnormal postures are: face slightly turned left or right, chin raised or lowered, head tilted over either shoulder. Other neurological or orthopedic abnormal postural components should be considered.
2   *Duction examination.* Ductions are rotation movements involving one eye at a time. Testing consists of alternatively covering one eye, while the other moves according to specific commands in the eight main spatial directions: right, left, up, down, downwards left and right, upwards left and right. The purpose is to detect abnormal single-eye motility and direction.
3   *Version or binocular movement examination.* Hering's law states that reciprocal innervation to functionally connected eye muscles permits smooth, coordinated eyeball movements. To examine versions, the subject is asked at this point to move both eyes following specific commands. With the head in primary frontal steady position, he or she is required to fixate a moving light target in the eight main glancing directions, as mentioned above. The purpose is to detect bilateral oculomotor imbalance.
4   *Cover test.* This is the most common test for detecting eye deviations. It is performed at long and short distance, asking the subject to stare at a given target and using an eye cover. Either eye is covered for a few seconds and then uncovered.

5 *Subject interview*. When adequate communication is resumed, direct patient questioning is a fundamental instrument to elicit information about visual problems and to start a therapeutic relationship. Working together is essential for obtaining results in visual rehabilitation.

6 *Visual acuity testing*. This is performed by looking at letters on a screen at a distance of 10 ft. Single eye acuity is measured with necessary lens correction if appropriate. Testing requires patience, enough time to elicit best responses and subject's maximum attention and collaboration. Close sight is measured at reading distance with a Jaeger reading table. Visual acuity may change over time during the recovery period and repeated measures are recommended.

7 *Worth test*. This is a method to rapidly determine if the patient has single binocular vision, diplopia or one-eye suppression (amblyopia). The subject wears glasses with red and green filters and then looks at a device with four crossed lights (left and right are green, upper is red and lower is white) from a distance of 15 ft. There is also an instrument for short distance testing. Patient is requested to say how many lights he or she sees. Long or short distance discrepancies should be recorded.

8 *Bielschowsky test*. This is the most reliable clinical method to detect deficits of the fourth cranial nerve.

9 *Long and short distance fusion measurement*. Sensory fusion is defined as the capacity of the visual cortex to integrate binocular sensory information in one tridimensional, single image. Motor fusion, on the other hand, deals with the capacity to coordinate both eyes to lead equivalent images to corresponding retinal points, when eyes or objects move in space. The two functions are separate but correlated. A special decreasing prismatic device is used to measure fusion amplitude while the subject stares at a light target from a distance of 1 and 12 ft.

10 *Deviation angle measurement*. The procedure uses prismatic corrections to quantify angular deviations at different glancing positions and at different fixation distances.

The obvious purpose of an accurate evaluation is an exact diagnosis and the best possible treatment planning for the individual subject. Unfortunately, therapy does not follow precise protocols and absolute rules, and it may be left to clinical judgment and personal experience. Timing of intervention, however, requires that the patient's visual problems be approached as soon as possible: there is no rationale to wait for "spontaneous recovery" of visual functions, as it often happens that natural compensation may render subsequent therapy more difficult and longer. Second, it is essential for the visual therapist to be accepted and to promote subject's early collaboration, as vision recovery is a requisite for all other treatment sessions. Some patients might refuse or oppose treatment due to unawareness of their visual problems, their aggressive attitude or the high attentional demands that rapidly cause fatigue. Other subjects, with evident clinical eye deviation, do not report diplopia, mostly because central suppression of second images intervenes as a compensatory mechanism. Furthermore, the neurological and behavioral conditions can vary rapidly, and a week-old evaluation may not reflect the current situation.

There are also some conditions that exclude patients from binocular therapy visual training: among these are severe eyeball damage, optic nerve atrophy, extensive visual pathway or occipital cortex lesions (central cortical blindness). Other pathologies may have surgical indications: corneal leucomas, post-traumatic cataracts, retinal detachments, subretineal post-traumatic neovascularizations, orbital fractures and dislocations.[64] The primary goal of visual therapy is elimination of diplopia and recovery of binocular single vision if possible. Partial or total correction of diplopia helps the subject in everyday life and represents substantial support to the successful development of all other rehabilitation activities. A detailed description of rehabilitation techniques is not possible unless accurate single-case reports are used.[65] However, it can be stated that available therapeutic orthoptic means include use of combined strategies: correction glasses, sectored partial occlusion, prismatic lenses and continuous therapy with orthoptic fusion exercises.[66-68]

In regard to surgical therapy for paralytic squint, we have never recommended it until 1 year after the event, and we generally believe that "less is best". Sometimes late surgical corrections are indicated for cosmetic reasons only. We think that the traditional nosographic treatment scheme for paralytic strabismus is inadequate for most TBI subjects, particularly in the period from coma exit to neurological stability, requiring at least a few months in severe cases. Follow-up of patients with individualized visual function recovery protocols is usually maintained for a period of 12–24 months, even if the drop-out rate is as high as 15%.

Although widely accepted, standardized protocols are still to be designed, as in many other rehabilitation procedures. From our clinical experience we think that early intervention contributes to limiting and correcting sensorimotor visual impairments, and that the so-called spontaneous recovery of diplopia often leads to monocular vision due to neuronal mechanism economy. Thus, absence of treatment, or a "wait-and-see" attitude for natural recovery to happen, are inappropriate and should be avoided.

Subacute neuro-orthopedic treatment of complications

Germane to TBI direct consequences, there are a number of accessory subacute and post-acute orthopedic pathologies which may be directly related to the intervening primary polytrauma, or to subsequent musculoskeletal complications.[69,70] Schematically, they are divided as follows:

1   Contractures linked to spastic central neurological paralysis.
2   Deformity linked to peripheral nerve lesions.

3   Heterotopic ossifications in periarticular and muscle tissues.
4   Unrecognized or improperly treated primary orthopedic lesions.

Spastic contractures

They are considered the most common secondary complication of upper motoneuronal damage after TBI, and a partial failure of early rehabilitation intervention. Sometimes, in spite of optimal primary care, they are a consequence of intractable muscle imbalance in the extremities. They are defined as any articular range of motion loss with functional consequences. A similar concept is that a muscle or group of muscles has shortened or retracted as to prevent full motion of any joint that it crosses. Multiple interventions are possible: antispasticity drugs, phenol nerve blocks, botulinum toxin injections, intrathecal baclofen administration, splinting, multiple casting, manual stretching, passive motion exercises, etc.[71]

Functional neurorthopedic surgery is usually considered when every other intervention has been tried with partial or no success. It should naturally be integrated in the global rehabilitation program and timed with a multiple-step strategy if necessary, to obtain best functional results with a minimum of post-surgery immobilization.[72] Before surgery, it is also necessary to evaluate clinical patterns of motor dysfunction, voluntary muscle control, stiffness, contractures, deformities and practical intractability of muscle–tendon retractions with other available means. Testing includes dynamic EMGs, simultaneous measurement of joint motion, kinematic three-dimensional movement data, and, if lower extremities are involved, standing and gait analysis.

Orthopedic surgery may involve both musculotendon and bone structures. Tenotomies or tendon release are indicated to balance muscular groups with preinsertional tendon sections, while tendon lengthening is preferably obtained with aponeuromyotenotomies or Z-lengthening. Tendon transfer is considered to be controversial after upper motorneuron lesions, as it could lead to somewhat unpredictable results due to late motor recovery (risk of hypercorrection) or residual activity of inconsistent muscle–tendon transfer. Skeletal surgery may consist of capsulotomies (joint release), orthopedic joint stabilization and fusion (arthrodesis) or joint movement limitation (arthroresis).

In most instances, late orthopedic functional surgery is reserved for lower extremities, as standing and walking can be more frequently improved by this approach. Upper extremity intervention, generally speaking, is proposed mostly for hygiene or cosmetic reasons, although certain cases may benefit in terms of arm–hand functions. Here is a list of possible surgical options in the following dysfunctional patterns:

1   *Adducted/internally rotated shoulder* (release of pectoralis major, teres major, subscapularis and latissimus dorsi may be considered; shoulder joint capsulotomy is not indicated).

2 *Abducted/externally rotated shoulder* (release of supraspinatus).

3 *Bent elbow* (biceps tendon and brachioradialis muscle release, in conjunction with its fractional myotendinous lengthening).

4 *Pronated forearm* (pronator teres and/or pronator quadratus release).

5 *Bent wrist* (release of extrinsic wrist and finger flexors; transfer of tendon wrist flexors into wrist extensors; radiocarpal arthrodesis).

6 *Clenched fist* (lengthening of flexors digitorum, flexor tendon release, superficialis to profundus tendon transfer).

7 *Thumb-in-palm* (flexor pollicis longus and adductor pollicis release, Z-lengthening of flexor pollicis longus, interphalangeal or intermetacarpal arthrodesis).

8 *Adducted hip/scissoring thigh* (controlled adductor tenotomy, obturator neurectomy is controversial).

9 *Flexed hip* (release of hip flexors, iliopsoas lengthening).

10 *Flexed knee* (fractional lengthening of biceps femoris, gracilis and semimembranous, Z-lengthening of semitendinosus).

11 *Equinous foot* (lengthening of triceps surae).

12 *Equinovarus foot* (tendo Achillis lengthening + peroneus brevis tenodesis + os calcis arthrodesis, or tibialis anterior transposition into third metatarsal bone and toe flexor release, or lateral transposition of tibialis posterior).

13 *Equinovalgus foot* (triceps lengthening and double ankle arthrodesis).

14 *Great toe extension* (release of extensors hallucis).

Deformity in peripheral nerve lesions

Peripheral nerve injuries (PNI) can go undetected after major politrauma, and may be later underreported or underestimated. The diagnostic delay is usually between 1 week and 3 months. PNI incidence after severe, high-velocity motor vehicle accidents varies from 11% up to 34%.[73,74] Lesions can be directly caused by the primary trauma, or secondarily attributable to compression/traction on extremities (heterotopic ossification, improper positioning, incorrect casting or other iatrogenic causes).

Accurate clinical examination is crucial in detecting abnormalities. It may be challenging because of poor cooperation, associated upper motorneuron weakness syndrome or orthopedic limb immobilization. A peripheral injury is suspected when there is muscle tone discrepancy (spasticity/flacidity) in the same limb, sensory deficit, abnormal movement patterns, areflexia, muscular atrophy and fasciculations. A flail extremity due to peripheral injury should be considered until disproven. Electrodiagnostic studies (EMG and nerve conduction studies) should be performed to confirm clinical suspicion, though they may be somewhat limited due to low pain tolerance, altered mental status and other concomitant CNS lesions.

Three degrees of nerve injury are usually described: neuropraxia (only functional disruption), axonotmesis (interruption of axonal continuity) and neurotmesis (transection of axon and neural tubule). The degree of spontaneous recovery is mostly related to site and severity of anatomical damage. Lesions can be schematically devided into:

1   *Brachial plexus* (it is important to distinguish between pre- and post-ganglionic damage; a mechanism usually linked to tearing/avulsion of nerve roots, and/or neck–shoulder girdle complex trauma).
2   *Circumflex nerve* (concomitant to shoulder trauma or luxation).
3   *Radial nerve* (injured after fracture of midshaft humerus, hypertrophic callus formation or unstable upper arm fracture).
4   *Ulnar nerve* (may result from elbow trauma, forearm fractures, cast compression, heterotopic ossification or arm and wrist spasticity).
5   *Median nerve* (most frequent in wrist compression for increased flexion or repetitive use).
6   *Sciatic nerve* (due to hip fracture with dislocation, or hip heterotopic ossification).
7   *Peroneal nerve* (traumatic knee dislocation, compression by improper casting, incorrect orthopedic traction).

Therapeutic interventions need sound clinical judgment and depend on severity/site of lesion, age, time after trauma, signs of spontaneous recovery, concomitant central neurological damage and levels of residual functioning. Clinical experience favors acute repair neurosurgery after clean, sharp neural laceration. The intervention on blunt PNI is often delayed up to 1 month. Results are better in upper extremity radial or medial nerve lesions.[75]

Success in peripheral nerve grafting depends not only on technical and anatomical considerations, but also on correct postoperative limb positioning, vascularization and residual sensori-motor functioning. Reconstructive functional surgery can also be used to overcome peripheral muscle paralysis: e.g., a latissimus dorsi transfer, or a pectoralis major-to-biceps transfer may restore elbow flexion in a paralyzed arm.

Dynamic splinting is another treatment option (e.g. ankle–foot or hand–wrist orthosis), with the additional advantage of providing proprioceptive sensory feedback during rehabilitation exercises.

Orthopedic surgery may finally consist of arthrodesis/arthroxesis interventions for stabilization of joints which have lost any functional activity. In these cases, the coexistence of spastic contractures may indicate a need for tendon release or lengthening.

Heterotopic ossification (HO)

This has been defined as the formation of mature lamellar bone in soft tissues, most frequently in periarticular and muscular tissues. The process involves osteoblastic activity and deposition of calcium salts without the proper structural organization of real bone. It has been reported in a number of neurological and immobilization-related conditions, including consequences of severe TBI. HO has been described as *neurogenic* (after neurologic injury), *post-traumatic* (after direct trauma to muscle/other soft tissue or after surgery), and *progressive* (rare genetic autosomal dominant disease).[76] After severe TBI, the incidence of this condition may be as high as 20% and, if surgical treatment of fractures is associated, this estimate may greatly increase.[77,78]

The specific pathophysiological cause of HO is still unclear. Most likely it is due to a combination of local factors, with final osteoblastic activation and an unknown systemic or genetic predisposition. Other factors involved seem to be prolonged bed immobilization and coma. The final consequence is the rapid differentiation of mesenchymal fibroblasts into bone-forming cells. An inflammatory mechanism is also involved, as the initial calcification foci mature into extensive ossification, with a metabolic rate and local blood flow of two to three times higher than regular bone tissue.

Localization is frequent around the hip, elbow, shoulder and knee, in decreasing order of incidence. Concomitant spasticity increases frequency, and pediatric or younger age may decrease it. HOs tend to mature around large joints, interosseal membranes and peritendineal or preinsertional muscle areas. Once developed, this may lead to decreased range of motion, pain, local temperature increase, and limb swelling. Complications may lead to peripheral nerve or vascular compressions, and final joint rigidity/ankylosis.

Diagnostic tools range from clinical examination to radiographs with different angular projections, levels of fractioned alkaline phosphatase and bone scintigraphy with ^{91}Tc. Differential diagnosis includes thrombophlebitis, septic arthritis, unrecognized fracture or hematoma. Prophylaxis and early treatment have been tried with nonsteroidal anti-inflammatory drugs (indomethacin, salicylates and ibuprofen), etidronate disodium and with multiple dose or single-dose radiation to reduce inflammatory mechanisms, calcium deposition and to prevent fibroblast conversion into bone precursor cells.[79,80]

The role of physical therapy in patients with HO is controversial. The major goal is to preserve function and maintain range of motion, but an aggressive exercise regimen might actually increase ossification: literature generally supports active motion or gentle passive joint mobilization. Spasticity treatment is naturally a major component in this direction.

Surgical treatment, consisting of partial or total removal of HO, is indicated when there is significant practical, functional limitation due to its presence. Timing of surgery is not totally defined. Preference for late intervention and waiting until new bone formation (documented by scintigraphy) has completely stopped used to be the common approach.[81] Now, earlier and more aggressive surgery is becoming prevalent, considering that:

1 Earlier surgical intervention has not proven to cause an increase in HO recurrence.
2 Smaller HO masses may pose fewer technical problems during surgery.
3 Earlier intervention facilitates rehabilitation and functional recovery.
4 Larger HO predispose to bleeding and complex issues in reconstructive surgery.

Surgical techniques need to consider the easiest access route and the risk of massive postoperative bleeding due to the high level of vascularization in the ossified mass. Other complications include infection, peripheral nerve lesions, and recurrence. At the elbow it is usually advisable to use a posterior access, with particular care dedicated to the integrity of the ulnar nerve. At the hip, a technically more challanging anterior surgical approach, with attention to the femoral artery and nerve, is often necessary. It is advisable to remove the largest possible portion of the ectopic bone formation; if too little is removed, there is a much higher recurrence risk. Intra-operatory problems may arise if peripheral nerve or vascular parts are embedded into the bone mass, and it may be necessary to use microsurgical or vascular surgical competence.

In the early postoperative phase, various treatment recommendations are given: low-dose radiation, etidronate and/or non-steroidal anti-inflammatory agents and an active and passive range of motion exercises, all intended to promote better functional recovery and to prevent recurrence.

Unrecognized lesions

It is not uncommon for some orthopedic lesions to go undetected or be poorly treated in the acute phase due to the multiple neurological and systemic consequences of a severe trauma, to general critical conditions, to the necessity of delaying surgery until the patient is medically stable, or the possibilty of simply missing a complete early diagnosis of all traumatic implications.[74] For these reasons, in a later phase, it is necessary to revise the global orthopedic situation. What might be found are *fracture non-unions/ mal-unions* (both diaphysary or meta-epiphysary), *joint subluxations* and *joint capsule or ligament lesions*.[82]

Mal-union risk can be increased by spasticity, patient's agitation or incorrect fracture stabilization, and may cause a number of limb deformities: shortening, varus or valgus axial deviations or rotational or complex deformities. Clinical detection is easily confirmed by radiographic examination. Joint lesions can also be clinically diagnosed and confirmed by MRI or echography.

In the subacute and chronic phase of severe TBI, post-traumatic orthopedic deformities should be considered in terms of functional consequences. Late surgical treatment is indicated only when there is a substantial functional alteration in the osteoarticular segment, and it should be planned as a facilitation and not as an obstacle in the rehabilitation treatment. Surgical tecniques should be as simple and non-invasive as possible: callostomies, corrective focal osteotomies and simple, stable osteosynthesis.

Synostosis of the interosseous membrane between radius and ulna is often a complication of forearm fractures and may lead to a loss of functional prono-supination; its surgical correction is not always preferable to a more conservative tutorization.[83]

Particular problems may be posed by the need for prosthetic joint substitution in a young patient, as this is a contraindication to joint replacement. Moreover, surgical intervention should be guided by the neurological condition of the affected limb, as it would be useless to optimally treat a paralyzed segment. Finally, joint reconstructive surgery should be postponed until functional improvement is evident, and if the segment remains symptomatic.

Summary

The sequelae of TBI form a multifaceted condition, which involves interventions from a number of medical specialists and non-medical professionals. Some of the problems could be the results of the trauma itself, others are related to the brain injury and its evolution. Prolonged immobilization, premorbid pathology and, possibly, iatrogenic causes may play a role in this complex clinical picture.

During the acute phase, diagnosis and treatment of some of these aspects might be undetected or postponed. When medically stabilized, the patient is transferred to a specialized rehabilitation facility. It is at this point that a thorough re-evaluation of all conditions is mandatory. A complete examination is often possible only if the subject can at least partially collaborate and comprehend language. The clinician needs to be specially trained to deal with cases of uncooperation, and requires special clinical expertise to avoid mistakes. For example, testing vision can be particularly difficult and time consuming. This same concept may apply to all clinical fields where subjective information is required. Moreover, serial evaluations are often required to follow the course of the recovery process.

The use of technology is helpful in those instances where it is possible to produce objective data. The goal of the rehabilitation team is to obtain optimal management, improve global outcome and reduce complications, long-term costs and disability.

References

1. Pietrapiana, P., Bronzino, M. P., Perino, C., & Rago, R. (1997). Acquired brain injury physical rehabilitation. In J. León-Carrión (Ed.), *Neuropsychological rehabilitation: Fundamentals, innovations and directions* (p. 227). Delray Beach, FL: St. Lucie Press.
2. Henderson, E. J., Morrison, J. A., et al. (1990). The nurse in rehabilitation after severe brain injury. *Clin. Rehabil., 1*, 167.

3. Grzankowski, J. A. (1997). Altered thought processes related to traumatic brain injury and their nursing implications. *Rehabil. Nurs., 22*, 24–31.

4. Antoinette, T. (1996). Rehabilitation nursing management of persons in low-level neurologic states. *Neurorehabilitation, 6*, 33.

5. Ashley, M. J., Krych, D. K., & Lehr, R. P. (1992). Cost–benefit analysis for post-acute rehabilitation of traumatically brain-injured patient. *J. Insur. Med., 24*, 186.

6. High, W. M. Jr, Hall, K. M., Rosenthal, M., Mann, N., Zafonte, R., Cifu, D. X., et al. (1996). Factors affecting hospital length of stay and charges following traumatic brain injury. *J. Head Trauma Rehabil., 11*, 85.

7. McLaughlin, A. M., & Carey, J. L. (1993). The adversarial alliance: developing therapeutic relationships between families and the team in brain injury rehabilitation. *Brain Injury, 7*, 45.

8. Hall, K. M., Karzmark, P., Stevens, M., Englander, J., O'Hare, P., & Wright, J. (1994). Family stressors in traumatic brain injury: a two-year follow-up. *Arch. Phys. Med. Rehabil., 75*, 876.

9. Witol, A. D., Sander, A. M., & Kreutzer, J. S. (1996). A longitudinal analysis of family needs following traumatic brain injury. *Neurorehabilitation, 7*, 175.

10. Serio, C. D., Kreutzer, J. S., & Gervasio, A. H. (1995). Predicting family needs after brain injury: implications for intervention. *J. Head Trauma Rehabil., 10*, 32.

11. Serio, C. D., Kreutzer, J. S., & Witol, A. D. (1997). Family needs after TBI: a factor analytic study of the Family Needs Questionnaire. *Brain Inj., 11*, 1.

12. Springer, J. A., Farmer, J. E., & Bouman, D. E. (1997). Common misconceptions about TBI among family members of rehabilitation patients. *J. Head Trauma Rehabil., 12*, 41.

13. Shaw, L. R., & McMahon, B. T. (1990). Family–staff conflict in the rehabilitation setting: causes, consequences, and implications. *Brain Inj., 4*, 87.

14. Eisner, J., & Kreutzer, J. S. (1989). A family information system for education following traumatic brain injury. *Brain Inj., 3*, 79.

15. Kreutzer, J. S., Sander, A. M., & Fernandez, C. C. (1997). Misperceptions, mishaps, and pitfalls in working with families after TBI. *J. Head Trauma Rehabil., 12*, 63.

16. Boldrini, P., et al. (1998). Progetto per un database sulla valutazione [Evaluation database project]. *Giorn. It. Med. Riabil., 12*, 5.

17. Dahmer, E. R., Shilling, M. A., Hamilton, B. B., et al. (1993). A model system database for traumatic brain injury. *J. Head Trauma Rehabil., 8*, 12.

18. Hall, K. M. (1997). Establishing a national TBI information system based upon a unified data set. *Arch. Phys. Med. Rehabil., 78*, 5.

19. Marshall, L. F., Marshall, S. B., Klauber, M. R., et al. (1992). The diagnosis of head injury requires a classification based on computed axial tomography. *J. Neurotrauma, 9*, 287.

20. Griffith, E. R., & Mayer, N. H. (1990). Hypertonicity and movement disorders. In M. Rosenthal et al. (Eds.), *Rehabilitation of the adult and child with traumatic brain injury* (2nd ed., p. 652). Philadelphia, PA: F. A. Davis.

21. Hall, K. M., Cope, D. N., & Rappaport, M. (1985). Glasgow Outcome Scale and Disability Rating Scale: comparative usefulness in following recovery in traumatic head injury. *Arch. Phys. Med. Rehabil., 66*, 35.

22. Lombardi, F., et al. (1997). Validità del CIQ e sistema nomativo italiano [CIQ validity and Italian normative system]. *Giorn. Ital. Med. Riabil., 11*, 23.

23. Gill, T. M., & Feinstein, A. R. (1994). Critical appraisal of the quality of quality of life measurements. *JAMA, 272*, 619.

24. Hall, K. M., Hamilton, B. B., Gordon, W. A., et al. (1993). Characteristics and comparisons of functional assessment indices: DRS, FIM and FAM. *J. Head Trauma Rehabil., 8*, 60.

25. Hall, K. M., Mann, N., High, W. M., et al. (1996). Functional measures after TBI: ceiling effects of FIM, FIM-FAM, DRS and CIQ. *J. Head Trauma Rehabil., 11*, 27.

26. Clagett, G. P., Anderson, F. A., et al. (1995). Prevention of venous thromboembolism. *Chest, 108*, 3125.

27. Rubinstein, I., Murray, D., & Hoffstein, V. (1988). Fatal pulmonary embolism in hospitalized patients. *Arch. Intern. Med., 148*, 1425.

28. O'Malley, K. F., & Ross, S. E. (1990). Pulmonary embolism in major trauma patients. *J. Trauma, 30*, 748.

29. Geerts, W. H., Code, K. I., et al. (1994). A prospective study of venous thromboembolism after major trauma. *N. Engl. J. Med., 331*, 1601.

30. Montgomery, K. D., Geerts, W. H., et al. (1996). Thromboembolic complications in patients with pelvic trauma. *Clin. Orthop., 329*, 68.

31. Verstraete, M. (1999). Prevention and treatment of venous thromboembolism after major trauma. *Trauma, 1*, 39.

32. Knudson, M. M., Lewis, F. R., et al. (1994). Prevention of venous thromboembolism in trauma patients. *J. Trauma, 37*, 480.

33. Antiplatelet Trialists Collaboration (1994). Overview of randomized trials. *Brit. Med. J., 308*, 235.

34. Merli, G., Herbison, G., et al. (1988). Deep vein thrombosis in acute SCI patients. *Arch. Physic. Med. Rehabil., 69*, 661.

35. Geerts, W. H., Jay, R., et al. (1996). A comparison of low-dose heparin with LMW heparin as prophylaxis against venous thromboembolism after major trauma. *N. Engl. J. Med., 335*, 701.

36. Agnelli, G., & Sonaglia, F. (1997). Prevention of venous thromboembolism in high-risk patients. *Haematologia, 82*, 496.

37. Gosin, T. S., Graham, A. M., et al. (1997). Efficacy of prophylactic vena cava filters in high risk trauma patients. *Ann. Vasc. Surg., 11*, 100.

38. Nurmohammed, M. T., van Riel, A. M., et al. (1996). LMW heparin and compression stockings in the prevention of VT in neurosurgery. *Thromb. Haem., 75*, 233.

39. Hirsh, J. (1990). Diagnosis of VT and pulmonary embolism. *Am. J. Cardiol., 65*, 45.

40. Hyers, T., Hull R., & Weg, J. (1995). Antithrombotic therapy for venous thromboembolic disease. *Chest, 108*, 225.

41. Borzotta, A. P., et al. (1994). Enteral versus parenteral nutrition after severe closed head injury. *J. Trauma, 37*, 459.

42. Wilson, R. F., & Tyburski, J. G. (1998). Metabolic responses and nutritional therapy in patients with severe head injuries. *J. Head Trauma Rehabil., 13*, 11.

43. Sunderland, P. M., & Heibrun, M. P. (1992). Estimating energy expenditure in TBI: comparison of indirect calorimetry with predictive formulas. *Neurosurgery, 31*, 246.

44. Saxe, J. M., et al. (1994). Lower esophageal sphincter dysfunction precludes safe gastric feeding after head injury. *J. Trauma, 37*, 581.

45. Bloomfield, E. L. (1986). Extracranial complications of head injury. *Neurol. Crit. Care Clin., 5*, 881.

46. Young, B., Ott, L., Twyman, D., et al. (1987). The effect of nutritional support on outcome from severe head injury. *J. Neurosurg., 67*, 668.

47. Fitzpatrick, B. C., & Harrington, T. R. (1992). Nutrition in head injured patients. *J. Neurosurg., 76*, 170.
48. Hadley, M. N., Grahm, T. W., & Harrington, T. (1986). Nutritional support and neurotrauma: a critical review of early nutrition in 45 acute HI patients. *Neurosurgery, 19*, 367.
49. Logeman, J. A., Pepe, J., & Mackay, L. E. (1994). Disorders of nutrition and swallowing: intervention strategies in the trauma center. *J. Head Trauma Rehabil., 9*, 43.
50. Field, L. H., & Weiss, C. J. (1989). Dysphagia with head injury. *Brain Inj., 3*, 19.
51. Lazarus, C. L. (1989). Swallowing disorders after traumatic brain injury. *J. Head Trauma Rehabil., 4*, 34.
52. Cherney, L. R., & Halper, A. S. (1996). Swallowing problems in adults with traumatic brain injury. *Semin. Neurol., 16*, 349.
53. Lazarus, C. L., & Logemann, J. A. (1987). Swallowing disorders in closed head trauma patients. *Arch. Phys. Med. Rehabil., 68*, 79.
54. Law, J. H., et al. (1993). Increased frequency of obstructive airway abnormalities with long-term tracheostomy. *Chest, 104*, 136.
55. Nowak, P., Cohn, A., et al. (1987). Airway complications in patients with closed head injuries. *Am. J. Otolaryngol., 8*, 91.
56. Klingbeil, G. (1988). Airway problems in patients with TBI. *Arch. Phys. Med. Rehabil., 69*, 493.
57. Padula, W. F., Argyris, S., & Ray, J. (1994). Visual evoked potentials (VEP) evaluating treatment for post-trauma vision syndrome (PTVS) in patients with traumatic brain injuries. *Brain Inj., 8*, 125.
58. Morton, R. L. (1995). Visual dysfunction following TBI. In M. J. Ashley and D. K. Krych (Eds.), *TBI rehabilitation* (p. 171). Boca Raton, FL: CRC Press.
59. Gianutsos, R., Ramsey, G., & Perlin, R. R. (1988). Rehabilitative optometric services for survivors of acquired brain injury. *Arch. Phys. Med. Rehabil., 69*, 573.
60. Cohen, A. H., & Rein, L. D. (1992). The effect of head trauma on the visual system: the doctor of optometry as a member of the rehabilitation team. *J. Am. Optom. Assoc., 63*, 530.
61. Lepore, F. E. (1995). Disorders of ocular motility following head trauma. *Arch. Neurol., 52*, 924.
62. Sabates, N. R., Gonce, M. A., & Farris, B. K. (1991). Neuro-ophthalmological findings in closed head trauma. *J. Clin. Neuroophthalmol., 11*, 273.
63. Baker, R. S., & Epstein, A. D. (1991). Ocular motor abnormalities from head trauma. *Surv. Ophthalmol., 35*, 245.
64. Schlageter, K., Gray, B., Hall, K., Shaw, R., & Sammet, R. (1993). Incidence and treatment of visual dysfunction in traumatic brain injury. *Brain Inj., 7*, 439.
65. Cohen, A. H. (1992). Optometric management of binocular dysfunctions secondary to head trauma: case reports. *J. Am. Optom. Assoc., 63*, 569.
66. Suter, P. S. (1995). Rehabilitation and management of visual dysfunction following traumatic brain injury. In M. J. Ashley and D. K. Krych (Eds.), *TBI rehabilitation* (p. 87). Boca Raton, FL: CRC Press.
67. Freeman, P. B., & Jose, R. T. (1996). Enhancing decreased sight of patients with traumatic brain injury. *Neurorehabilitation, 6*, 203.
68. Raymond, M. J., Bennett, T. L., Malia, K. B., & Bewick, K. C. (1996). Rehabilitation of visual processing deficits following brain injury. *Neurorehabilitation, 6*, 229.

69. Groswasser, Z., Coehn, M., & Blandstein, E. (1990). Polytrauma associated with TBI: incidence, nature and impact on rehabilitation outcome. *Brain Inj., 4*, 161.
70. Yarkony, G., Sahgal, V. (1987). Contractures: a major complication of craniocerebral trauma. *Clin. Orthop. Rel. Res., 219*, 93.
71. Djergaian, R. S. (1996). Management of muscoloskeletal complications. In L. J. Horn and N. D. Zasler (Eds.), *Medical rehabilitation of TBI* (p. 459). Philadelphia, PA: Hanley-Belfus.
72. Mayer, N. H., Esquenazi, A., & Keenan, M. A. E. (1996). Analysis and management of spasticity, contractures and impaired motor control. In L. J. Horn and N. D. Zasler (Eds.), *Medical rehabilitation of TBI* (p. 411). Philadelphia, PA: Hanley-Belfus.
73. Garland, D., & Bailey, S. (1981). Undetected injuries in head injured adults. *Clin. Orthop. Rel. Res., 155*, 162.
74. Stone, L., & Keenan, M. (1988). Peripheral nerve injuries in the adult with TBI. *Clin. Orthop. Rel. Res., 233*, 136.
75. Dubuisson, A., & Kline, D. (1992). Indications for peripheral nerve and brachial plexus surgery. *Neurol. Clin. North Amer., 10*, 935.
76. Garland, D. (1991). A clinical perspective on common forms of HO. *Clin. Orthop., 263*, 13.
77. Varghese, G. (1992). Heterotopic ossification. *Phys. Rehabil. Clin. North Amer., 3*, 407.
78. Garland, D. (1988). Clinical observations on fractures and heterotopic ossification in the SCI and TBI populations. *Clin. Orthop. Rel. Res., 233*, 86.
79. Glenn, M. (1988). Update on pharmacological treatment of heterotopic ossification. *J. Head Trauma Rehabil., 3*, 86.
80. Coventry, M., & Scanlon, P. (1981). The use of radiation to discourage ectopic bone. *J. Bone Joint Surg., 63*, 201.
81. Garland, D., & Hanscom, D., et al. (1985). Resection of HO in the adult with head trauma. *J. Bone Joint Surg., 67A*, 1261.
82. Botte, M., & Moore, T. (1987). The orthopedic management of extremity injury in head trauma. *J. Head Trauma Rehabil., 2*, 13.
83. Garland, D., & Dowling, V. (1983). Forearm fractures in the head injured adults. *Clin. Orthop. Rel. Res., 176*, 190.

20 The holistic, multidisciplinary, and intensive approach of treatment

The CRECER method

José León-Carrión and María del Rosario Domínguez-Morales

Introduction

The treatment and rehabilitation of individuals with acquired brain injury are not homogeneous, even in rehabilitation centers within the same country. There are different brain injury rehabilitation centers offering different kinds of services and providing different degrees of efficiency. This chapter focuses on one of the models of rehabilitation of the multiple consequences that acquired brain injury can produce in an individual. To situate and understand models of rehabilitation, we are going to briefly review the main approaches to rehabilitation. There are three different models which focus on the treatment of people with brain injury: care programs, traditional programs, and holistic programs, as illustrated in Figure 20.1.[1] Our model (CRECER) corresponds to the last one.

Care programs are defined as those in which neither the staff nor the

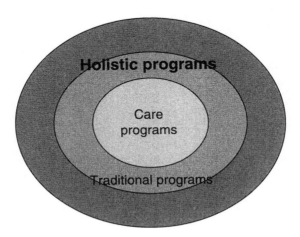

Figure 20.1 Models of brain injury programs.

organizational structure are specialized or deeply knowledgeable about what brain injury is or what it means. The care professionals are not highly specialized and auxiliary personnel provide most of the care, not rehabilitation, with little to no specific training or certification. They offer care; they do not offer treatment programs. A treatment program is that which tends towards a progressive improvement in the individual through the use of techniques and procedures. Care programs often maintain the individual in the center for years, given that the goal is neither the recuperation of the individual nor the achievement of the highest possible degree of independence. Their objective is dignified care and comfort for the individual.

Traditional programs or *face-specialization programs* treat the individual from within a health system, as though he or she were just another individual whose pathology responds to the interventions and prescriptions of traditional medicine. In other words, these programs do not consider that the TBI patient suffers disorders requiring specialized intervention from professionals specialized in brain injury. This means that if he or she needs psychological attention, it will be the regular staff clinical psychologist who will assist them. This same psychologist could be treating a patient suffering from depression, a gambling addict, or a child with family problems. If a psychiatrist is needed, they will call upon the regular staff psychiatrist, who could be treating a hypochondriac one minute, and the next an individual with a panic attack. This same scenario can continue with all the specialized care that the TBI patient needs. These are apparently specialized, quality programs. However, this is not really so, given that this is a pseudo-specialization or a "face specialization". The specialization is apparent, not real. The specialty of these professionals is not brain injury.

Interdisciplinary holistic programs are those which are composed of teams of brain damage specialists from different fields: neuropsychologists, speech therapists, neurologists, psychiatrists, neurosurgeons, physiatrists, physical therapists, and so forth. Each member of such a team has acquired knowledge and credentials as specialists in brain injury. This is the most commonly followed organizational model for Centers of Brain Injury Rehabilitation in Europe as can be seen in the European centers pioneering in this type of program in Copenhagen, Denmark,[2] Turin, Italy[3] and Seville, Spain,[4] to mention a few. In these centers, the professionals directly involved in the care and treatment of the individual must be specialized. The auxiliary personnel are not in direct contact with the patient and have no direct responsibilities in either care or treatment.

Different studies have demonstrated different outcomes depending on the type of program in which the patient is included. In a comparison study of acute programs and custodial nursing home care, it was found that stroke patients' functional outcomes improved in acute programs.[5,6] In a review on stroke patients, Stewart et al.[7] found that the available research indicates that, although subacute rehabilitation services are effective, the greater intensity of rehabilitation services offered by acute rehabilitation – when tolerated – showed improved short- and long-term outcome. León-Carrión et al.[8] found a 70% recovery from emotional problems in patients after an intensive, holistic and multidisciplinary program, and a recovery of more than 60% from the global deficits patients presented before entering the rehabilitation program.

The CRECER integral, intensive and multidisciplinary model of rehabilitation for people with acquired brain injury

The main characteristic of the CRECER programs is that they are multidisciplinary, integral and intensive. Traumatic brain injury causes multiple disorders and impairments that affect different cerebral areas and systems, resulting in muscular, motor, cognitive, behavioral, sensitivity, emotional and social disorders, among other things. Each system has to be rehabilitated by professionals specializing in them, as well as in brain injury. Rehabilitation of brain injury sequelae cannot be nor should be carried out by personnel who are not specialized in brain injury: not all physicians are specialized in brain injury rehabilitation, nor are all psychologists, speech therapists or physical therapists. Successful rehabilitation depends very much on the experience each professional has had in rehabilitating patients, and also on the specific techniques and programs used. The CRECER method of rehabilitation is carried out by a multidisciplinary team in accordance with an individually designed treatment program for each patient.

In contrast to other rehabilitation approaches, integral treatment provides the brain injury patient with an adequate framework for his or her recuperation as it broaches the cases from all angles. All deficits of the patient are treated simultaneously with perfectly studied and synchronized timing. Treatment of acquired brain injury sequelae should not involve isolating one from another. It is necessary to understand and rehabilitate the whole person with an integral approach in order to obtain results that are truly useful for patients and their family members. Holistic rehabilitation programs are characterized by being carried out by specialized professionals, they are interdisciplinary, ecologically valid, and divided into phases in which all of the aims, methods and professionals are perfectly synchronized. In addition, these rehabilitation programs make use of quantitative as well as qualitative evaluation.[1] The programs are intensive in that each of the patient's deficits is allotted the necessary time and dedication: distribution of time is one of the central aspects of CRECER treatment.

We will describe the characteristics of the CRECER neurorehabilitation program based on six points from an operational point of view:

1   It is necessary to have specialized personnel in each of the areas in which the patient needs treatment.
2   All patients follow a rehabilitation treatment which has been designed by

specialized personnel and adapted specifically to his or her particular needs.

3   The patient/specialist ratio in brain injury should always be at least one specialist for every two patients.

4   Adequate and dignified installations. This means that there should be no architectural barriers which impede some patients from having free access to places they need to go to. There should be rooms for individual rehabilitation and group experiences, as well as whatever is necessary to facilitate intimacy. Hygiene and cleanliness of installations are of course essential, as well as renovation and repair of any part of the building that needs it.

5   The center must have the necessary apparatus and rehabilitation techniques for carrying out the work in an efficient manner. Equipment and knowledge must be up to date.

6   Our center mainly treats patients with severe brain injury (minimal response status and severe and moderate neurocognitive disorders).

A broad description of the structure of CRECER multidisciplinary, integral and intensive programs is now presented, and also data about the published results attained after application of the programs.

Neuropsychological rehabilitation

Neuropsychological rehabilitation is a discipline which has changed in the last few decades, becoming a required instrument in neurological and neuropsychiatric rehabilitation programs. Holistic neuropsychological rehabilitation is related to all intellectual, emotional, behavioral, vocational, and social aspects of the life of an individual who has suffered brain injury. It is carried out in a multidisciplinary area and neuropsychologists work closely together with other brain injury professionals to rehabilitate individuals with neurological disorders. Neuropsychological rehabilitation is one of the strong points of CRECER.

The first step in a neuropsychological rehabilitation program is a thorough evaluation of the cognitive capacities and emotional state of the patient. In order to be able to rehabilitate, a patient's profile must first be known to be able to design an individualized program of treatment (starting from the capacities which have been preserved or affected less). These evaluations are made by a team of multidisciplinary professionals specializing in brain injury including neuropsychologists, neurologists, rehabilitators, physical therapists and speech therapists, as well as any other professional who might be needed in a particular case.

Goals are set for each patient based on the conclusions reached in the evaluation process. The main goal is to attain a maximum degree of independence, help him or her to assimilate the traumatic event that happened and foment the full potential of the patient's capacities via cognitive and physical rehabilitation, cognitive-behavioral treatment, pharmacology, psychotherapy, group treatments and occupational, vocational and family therapy.

In the rehabilitation process of the CRECER models of rehabilitation, the neuropsychologist plays a fundamental part in designing the rehabilitation program, striving to coordinate the different levels of intervention (physiotherapy, speech therapy, occupational therapy, etc.) with the patient so that work sessions can be fully taken advantage of. Cognitive areas most frequently worked on are spatial–temporal orientation, attention, memory, planning, executive functions, calculation, writing and language. Individual (Figure 20.2) and group cognitive ecological rehabilitation sessions are held daily for this purpose, as well as exercises performed on the computer and cognitive ecological rehabilitation which activate skills acquired in these rehabilitation sessions.[9] Thus the patient little by little confronts daily activities in his or her life with the aim of obtaining maximum independence and functioning. Bearing this in mind, sessions of occupational therapy are coordinated with the area of physical rehabilitation and physiotherapy with the purpose of trying to coordinate the patient's abilities with his or her motor, cognitive and functional limitations. The level of functioning reached with these types of activities will not only benefit the patient's gaining

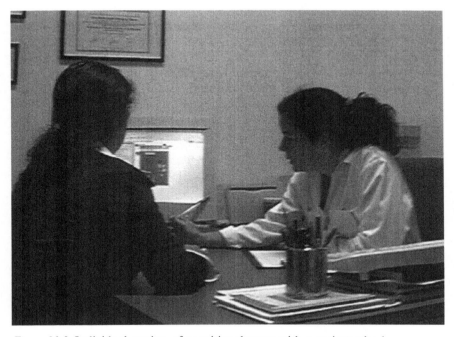

Figure 20.2 Individual session of cognitive therapy with a patient who has a severe cognitive disorder after traumatic brain injury.

independence, but also emotional development, basically in those aspects related to self-esteem, and this leads to a better adherence to treatment.

Behavioral and emotional disorders are treated with special combined strategies. Thus, problems of aggression, lack of sexual inhibitions, depression, mood changes, etc. require rigorous planning of all details for adequate treatment.[10] Treatment also includes sessions of individual psychotherapy in which personal conflicts arising from the accident are approached and, according to León-Carrión,[1] are normally related to changes in self-image, decrease of self-esteem, loss of independence, frustration of projects, loss of friends, etc. As well as individual psychotherapy sessions, there are group sessions in which subjects of interest to the patients are approached, such as aspects related to the accidents and problems that have to be faced, etc. Also, family therapy is carried out in order to achieve rehabilitation tasks that can be continued when the patient goes home.

Speech rehabilitation

The majority of traumatic brain injuries (TBI), as well as cerebro-vascular disorders, evolve with alterations in language and speech that directly affect the patient's ability to communicate. Dysarthria and aphasia are the most characteristic disorders following brain injury.[11,12]

Approximately 34% of the patients who survive severe TBI have dysarthria.[13-15] There are different types of dysarthria with varying degrees of severity of language and communication deficits, resulting in a long, complicated rehabilitation. It is difficult to find a uniform protocol for rehabilitation of post-traumatic brain injury patients with dysarthria. Treatment for these patients should be especially designed for each one of them. All rehabilitation programs for dysarthria patients should begin with neurological, neuropsychological and phoniatric examinations and, lastly, an exploration of the motor processes of speech. Based on this thorough examination process, patients can be classified according to their symptoms in four types of mixed dysarthrias: spastic–ataxic, spastic–hypokinetic, spastic–flaccid, and flaccid–ataxic. However, the most common one following brain injury is mixed spastic dysarthria, resulting from bilateral lesions of the upper motor neurons. To offer satisfactory results in the rehabilitation of this type of dysarthria, CRECER has developed methods (Figure 20.3) of treatment of:

- Respiratory dysfunction.
- Articulatory and praxic dysfunction.
- Laryngeal and velopharyngeal dysfunctions: voice.
- Prosodic dysfunction.

The other large group of language disturbances frequently brought on by brain injury is aphasia. The etiology of this disturbance has different causes: vascular, tumoral, and traumatic. In a revision of patients treated at

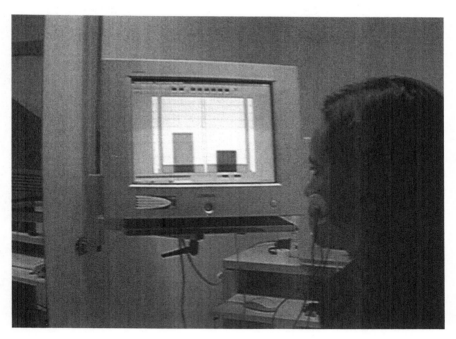

Figure 20.3 Using the NeuroBird system for rehabilitation of facial movements in a patient with spastic dysarthria.

CRECER, the distribution – according to the etiology of the aphasia – is 62% vascular, 32% traumatic, and 6% tumoral. The aphasic disorder can affect verbal language by altering comprehension and/or expression, and written language by affecting reading and/or writing. Most of the aphasic patients have one feature in common – difficulties in naming tasks – but, depending on the type of aphasia, there are different associated disorders: anomia, alexia, agraphia, etc. In order to carry out an effective rehabilitation program, it is fundamental to evaluate the following areas thoroughly: fluidity, auditory comprehension, denomination, reading, writing, repeating, automatic mechanisms, comprehension of written language and presence of paraphasic errors. Once the evaluation is completed, and depending on the affected area, rehabilitation is started. In the area of fluency, aspects such as articulatory agility, length of phrases, verbal agility, etc. are taken into consideration. For auditory comprehension, tasks in differentiating, identifying and obeying orders, etc. are carried out. Denomination is approached by visual confrontation, free association, etc. and deficits appearing in the reading/writing process are retaught.

Physical rehabilitation

Physical rehabilitation plays an important part in CRECER rehabilitation programs for those who require it. The majority of the patients with brain injury and serious cerebrovascular disorders have difficulties with balance and posture that seriously limit their possibilities of recovering independent mobility and autonomy, as well as hemiplegia or hemiparesia. Spasticity is one of the big challenges to physical rehabilitation in these patients since intervention possibilities are limited.

Balance retraining is a basic part of recovering numerous pathologies in these patients. Various techniques with acceptable results have been used systematically up to the present time in the recovery process of balance problems.[16,17] CRECER uses a unique computerized system for the sole purpose of balance training and it is one of the most effective systems for neurological patients. This type of training consists of recuperating the ability to control the projection of one's center of gravity in the vertical position, developing automatic control mechanisms via biofeedback and executing them in static, as well as dynamic, forms of posture.

Several kinds of treatments are considered which are alluded to as sensory-motor re-education of patients with hemiplegia or hemiparesis, and different combinations of techniques are used according to the patient's particular problem. In general, what have been referred to as *traditional physiotherapy techniques* are no longer used when treating this type of patient, consisting of analytical treatment directed at peripheral musculoskeletal disorders from brain lesions initiated a few weeks after observation of the clinical picture.

An effective complement to rehabilitation programs has been used for these patients: electromyographic biofeedback (EMG). It is a specific application of biofeedback techniques for solving neuromuscular problems. The term biofeedback applied to neuromuscular rehabilitation is based on the possibility of voluntary control and modification of certain biological processes when information about them is supplied at the same time. In this way, the person learns to control unintentional physiological responses whose regulation has been interrupted or altered by the brain lesion produced. Its theoretical development is in the field of clinical psychology and specifically in techniques of instrumental conditioning, utilizing the information administered to the patient as an immediate contingent of the execution of a movement to increase/decrease the frequency of its appearance, informing the patient about the consequences of this movement and thus helping his or her voluntary control.

At the CRECER Center of Rehabilitation for Brain Injury, we use a system of computerized muscular training, NeuroBird, as well as other physiotherapy techniques, for physical rehabilitation. It is based on the utilization of complex programs of electromyographic biofeedback.

The NeuroBird system of muscular training for spasticity, posture control, balance, trembling and emotional reactivity

The NeuroBird computerized system of total functional muscular training consists of the following elements: a two-channel EMG amplifier with multiple peripheral electrodes, an interface connected to a personal computer and a monitor that receives signals from a screen. The system is complemented with an installation of additional peripheral electrodes, such as an indicator for control of shaking, a stabilizing platform (used for rehabilitation of balance and posture control), a myotonometer MYOTONUS-02 connected to the computerized system that allows a numerical collection of information about muscular tone, storage and comparison of different sessions for a posterior presentation in graphic form of this evolutionary information. Measuring muscular tone is done via the application of transcutaneous pressure of certain strength to a chosen muscle, producing the resulting measurement of deformation in it. In the second phase, that of muscle tone training, sensors are used to pick up the electromyographic signal that is placed on the skin with elastic bands. We can objectively see the exact level of the patient's progress every moment with this system.

The process of treatment consists of two clearly differentiated parts. The first is *measuring the muscle tone* to be trained in states of activity and relaxation in order to evaluate its state. The second part is self-healing muscular training, using electromyographic information of the movements made by the patient. The patient knows at the time of movement the degree of precision it has, which allows him or her to learn how to make movements correctly. Before starting, it is necessary to do several trial movements that permit the computerized system to obtain a threshold which adjusts to the parameters of work for each of the individual muscles, thus personalizing the training according to the needs of each patient.

The sessions for rehabilitation of spasticity are designed to decrease exaggerated reactions when stretching groups of spastic muscles, thus achieving more activity in the agonist muscle of the impaired movement and, therefore, increasing its muscle tone and better quality of movement due to a more adequate relationship between agonist and antagonist muscles. These two parameters – the relation between agonist–antagonist and muscle tone – are controlled every minute by the NeuroBird and MYOTONUS-02 systems, respectively (Figure 20.4).

Physical and motor rehabilitation via the NeuroBird system offer the following advantages:

- Individualized treatment, allowing specific program designing for each patient according to his or her muscular necessities and adapting the type of training to the actual needs of each patient.
- Greater precision than in traditional techniques since one muscle at a time can be chosen, isolated and treated.

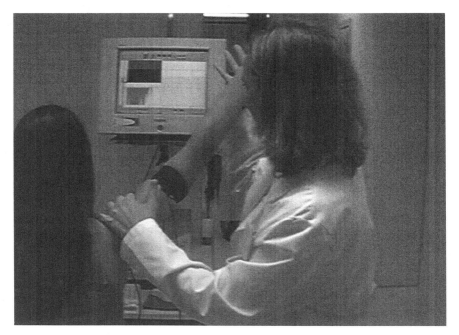

Figure 20.4 A session of rehabilitation with the NeuroBird system for movement and spasticity disorders in the triceps muscle.

- The characteristics of the system permit obtaining values from the work carried out in real time and instantaneously, so that the observation of the results permits the establishment of pertinent modifications and corrections for better functioning of muscular work in the rehabilitation program.
- The system allows modification of parameters such as length, intensity, threshold of work, repetitions of muscular response during training, etc., thus establishing more accuracy in this type of muscle training and its results.

Occupational therapy/functional therapy

The CRECER model of occupational/functional therapy is based on the patient, centering on his or her outlook, values, needs and life-style. It is a process of mutual respect based on building up the patient's independence. The therapists are specifically trained in knowledge of the patient's deficits affecting independence and how to go about his or her rehabilitation. Occupational/functional therapy is based on rehabilitating all those skills related to the patient's self-care, productivity/work and leisure. The vocational rehabilitation program is a dynamic process directed towards returning to work or one's studies, or retraining for other types of work.

To carry out this program, the therapists take note of the environment the patient moves in, his or her interests and motivation, culture, values, beliefs and the role the patient plays in his or her surroundings. In the same way, the CRECER program of functional therapy does not simply adapt to the patient's limitations, but rather tries to overcome them, first neurologically and then functionally, until the point where the objective of maximum independence can be achieved. The program has a format of application, timing and style of execution.

Efficiency in specialized treatments

All CRECER programs are subject to daily control of the progress made in each patient so that the neurofunctional state of the patient and efficacy of the methods applied are clear at any given moment. Evaluation of physiotherapy as well as neuropsychological therapy, speech therapy and communication, and occupational/functional therapy is carried out via instruments of control and evaluation specifically designed for them. Global data obtained has been published in scientific journals and presented at national and international congresses.[18–20]

León-Carrión et al. presented a study in 1999 analyzing the results obtained for a group of 10 patients with brain injury who received integral treatment (Figure 20.5) via the CRECER intensive program for 6 months. The percentage of recovery obtained by the patients was studied at the end of treatment in different areas of deficits in every one of the patients.

"Space–time disorientation" after 6 months of integral, multidisciplinary and intensive treatment obtains a global reduction of over 85% (86.12%). Rehabilitation of attentional deficits has a similar level of efficacy; this type of deficit is the most common in patients who were studied (90%). Data shows an 80% reduction of the intensity of these deficits in the patients who were treated.

Another of the areas of cognitive functioning that is frequently affected in brain injury patients is the *memory*: "retrograde amnesia", "anterograde amnesia" and problems of memory in "post-commotional syndrome". Rehabilitation of these types of deficits has resulted in a reduction of 45% of their intensity in 6 months. The bulk of the scores assigned to deficits is determined by anterograde amnesia, the deficit receiving the highest scores in the sequelae reported in the study. Such an intense deficit is difficult to completely restore in a period of 6 months, thus that which is achieved is a decrease of intensity in the majority of the cases, and an extension of the time of treatment. Those who wish to study rehabilitation of memory in depth can review the work of León-Carrión,[24] where the original CRECER model is described, and the work of León-Carrión and colleagues (2000) about the Combined Method of cognitive rehabilitation via simultaneous pharmacological and neuropsychological therapy (see Chapter 17).

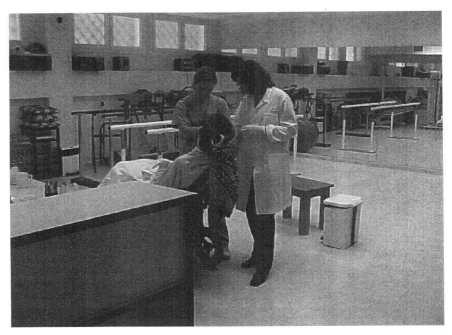

Figure 20.5 Speech and physical therapy joint session with a patient in a state of minimum response (see León-Carrión, Van Eeckout, Domínguez-Morales & Pérez Santamaria, 2002a; León-Carrión, Van Eeckout, Domínguez-Morales & Pérez Santamaria, 2002b; León-Carrión, Domínguez-Roldán, & Domínguez-Morales, 2001, for more details of intervention in these types of patients)[21–23].

Executive functions deserve special mention,[25] i.e., those deficits related to capacities of planning, problem solving, cognitive and prospective flexibility, etc. The results show a reduction of 30.77% of intensity of the symptoms the patients had in executive function capacities and in Moria syndrome. New techniques currently applied increase this percentage considerably, but the data has not yet been published.

In another study of these types of patients by Madrazo et al. in 1999,[26] emotional changes observed in patients with traumatic brain injury have made important advances, as well as neurocognitive deficits derived from the lesions, and will be the main areas of work for neuropsychological rehabilitation programs. There are various ways these changes affect patients, depending a great deal on the type of lesion involved. The most important percentage of changes are those produced by a lesion affecting the frontal area related to control of behavior and executive functioning. Excitability, irritability and annoyance or syndromes of apathy and disinterest are the emotional changes observed in patients with frontal lesions.[27] Other changes refer to affectivity, humor and behavior which can be altered by moods, initiative and aggressivity. Treatment of emotional sequelae for this group of patients offers excellent results, showing a reduction of over 70% of the sequelae. Post-commotional syndrome and excitability–aggressivity obtain results of a 71.67% reduction of symptoms and one point less, 70%, for organic syndrome of personality. Finally, results are obtained for post-traumatic depression syndrome with a 75.61% reduction of intensity of symptoms, achieving a total elimination of symptoms in 60% of the cases.[10]

When comparing the general state of the patients who were studied at the beginning and end of the treatment, we can observe a 62.7% reduction of the deficits they had upon admission to hospital. This implies a high rate of efficiency in CRECER rehabilitation programs.

Conclusions

This chapter introduces the CRECER model of holistic, integral, intensive and multidisciplinary methods of rehabilitation of patients with acquired brain injury. These models need the cooperation of a team of different professionals specialized in brain injury. All of them have to work in a coordinated manner to pursue the goal: maximum independence of the patient. Several conclusions can be made from the data presented in the chapter. First, the CRECER model of integral, intensive and multidisciplinary treatments seems to achieve a 62.7% reduction of the sequelae presented by severe traumatic brain injury patients 6 months after commencement of the rehabilitation program. Second, as far as neurosensory–motor rehabilitation is concerned, computerized systems are used (as well as traditional physiotherapy) in the treatment of physical sequelae of brain injury. The NeuroBird computerized EMG system allows individualized treatment, more accuracy, real-time data of the state of the patient, personalized work parameters and immediate feedback on the patient's execution of movements, among other things. Finally, treatment of brain injury deficits and sequelae should be approached with more optimism than in past decades since the results of the patients who undergo adequate treatment attest to functional results, facilitating greater independence in these patients.

References

1. León-Carrión, J. (1998). Rehabilitation models for neurobehavioral disorders after brain injury. *Brain Inj. Source, 22*, 16–32.
2. Caetano, C., & Christensen, A. L. (1997). The design of neuropsychological rehabilitation: the role of neuropsychological assessment. In J. León-Carrión (Ed.), *Neuropsychological rehabilitation: Fundamentals, innovations and directions* (p. 63). Delray Beach, FL: St. Lucie Press.
3. Pietrapiana, P., et al. (1997). Acquired brain injury physical rehabilitation. In J. León-Carrión (Ed.), *Neuropsychological Rehabilitation: Fundamentals, Innovations and Directions* (p. 227). Delray Beach, FL: St. Lucie Press.

4. León-Carrión, J. (1998). Traumatic brain injury in Spain. *Anuario de Noticias Médicas, 3686*, 32–34.
5. Kramer, A. M., et al. (1997). Outcome and costs after hip fracture and stroke: a comparison of rehabilitation settings, *J. AR. Med. Assoc., 277*, 396.
6. Keith, R. O., et al. (1995). Rehabilitation for stroke: a comparison. *Arch. Phys. Med. Rehabil., 76*, 495.
7. Stewart. D. C., Miller, M. A., & Cifu, D. X. (1998). The role of subacute rehabilitation services after brain injury. *Neurorehabilitation, 10*, 13.
8. León-Carrión, J., et al. (1999). Outcome after an intensive, holistic and multidisciplinary rehabilitation program after traumatic brain injury. *Revist. Española Neuropsicol., 1*, 2–3, 49.
9. León-Carrión, J. (1997). An approach to the treatment of affective disorders and suicide tendencies after TBI. In J. León-Carrión (Ed.), *Neuropsychological rehabilitation. Fundamentals, innovations and directions.* Delray Beach, Fl: St. Lucie Press.
10. León-Carrión, J., de Serdio Arias, M. L., Cabezas, F. M., Domínguez-Roldán, J. M., Domínguez-Morales, R., & Sánchez, M. A. (2001). Neurobehavioural and cognitive profile of traumatic brain injury patients at risk for depression and suicide. *Brain Inj., 15*, 175–181.
11. León-Carrión, J., Viñals, F., Vega, O., & Domínguez-Morales, R. (2001). Spastic dysarthria: phonation disorder rehabilitation after traumatic brain injury. *Revist. Española Neuropsicol., 3*, 34–45.
12. León-Carrión, J., & Viñals, F. (2000). Evolution of the recovery in a cerebrovascular patient with anomic aphasia. *Revist. Española Neuropsicol., 2*, 21–29.
13. Rusk, H., Block, J., & Lowman, E. (1969). Rehabilitation of the brain-injured patient: a report of 157 cases with long term follow up of 118. In E. Walker, W. Caveness, and M. Critchley (Eds.), *The late effects of head injury* (pp. 327–332). Springfield, MA: Charles S. Thomas.
14. Olser, J. H., Ponsford, J. L., & Curran, C. A. (1996). Outcome following traumatic brain injury: a comparison between 2 and 5 years after injury. *Brain Inj., 10*, 841–848.
15. Sarno, M. T., Buonaguro, A., & Levita, E. (1986). Characteristics of verbal impairment in closed head injured patients. *Arch. Phys. Med. Rehabil., 67*, 400–405.
16. Barroso y Martín, J. M., García-Bernal, M. I., Domínguez-Morales, R., Mikhailenok, E., & Voronina, O. (1999). Total functional recovery in hemiparetic left post-brain injury patient through a neuromuscular bio-feedback computerized program Remiocor-02. *Revist. Española Neuropsicol., 1*, 69–88.
17. Domínguez-Morales, R., Mikhailenok, E., Voronina, O., & García-Bernal, M. I. (2000). Higher functional recovery through computerized neuromuscular biofeedback program Remiocor-2. *Brain Inj. Source, 4*, 22–25.
18. León-Carrión, J. (2000). Timing for cognitive recovery. Paper presented at 4th World Congress on Brain Injury, Torino, Italy, May.
19. León-Carrión, J., Machuca Murga, F., Murga Sierra, M., & Domínguez-Morales, R. (1999). Outcome after an intensive, holistic and multidisciplinary rehabilitation program after traumatic brain injury: medico-legal values. *Revist. Española Neuropsicol., 1*, 49–68.
20. Domínguez-Morales, R., & León-Carrión, J. (2001). Impact of intensive, holistic and multidisciplinary treatment (CRECER) in the economical compensation of

brain injury patients as a consequence of traffic accident. *Monografías de la Revist. Española Neuropsicol.; Neuropsicología legal y forense del daño cerebral, 3*, 77–84.
21. León-Carrión, J., Van Eeckout, P., Domínguez-Morales, R., & Pérez Santamaría, F. J. (2002a). The locked-in syndrome: a syndrome looking for a therapy. *Brain Inj., 16*, 571–582.
22. León-Carrión, J., Van Eeckout, P., Domínguez-Morales, R., & Pérez Santamaría, F. J. (2002b). The locked-in syndrome: a syndrome looking for a therapy. *Brain Inj., 16*, 555–569.
23. León-Carrión, J., Domínguez-Roldán, J. M., & Domínguez-Morales, R. (2001). Coma and vegetative state: medico-legal aspects. *Revist. Española Neuropsicol., 3*, 63–76.
24. León-Carrión, J. (1997). *Neuropsychological rehabilitation. Fundamentals, directions and innovations*. Delray Beach, FL: St. Lucie Press.
25. León-Carrión, J., & Barroso y Martín, J. M. (1997). *Neuropsychology of thought process. Executive control and frontal lobe*. Sevilla: Kronos.
26. Madrazo, M., Machuca Murga, F., Barroso-Martín, J. M., Domínguez-Morales, R., & León-Carrión, J. (1999). Emotional changes following severe brain injury. *Revist. Española Neuropsicol., 1*, 75–82.
27. Lezak, M. D. (1999). *Neuropsychological assessment*. New York: Oxford University Press.

21 The role of stem cells in the rehabilitation of brain injury*

José León-Carrión

Introduction

This chapter is an approximation to stem cells and therapeutic brain repair for acquired brain injury. Repairing brain injury and its consequences is one of the main objectives of brainstem cell research. In the next pages we focus on the use of stem cells for the remediation of cognitive and behavioral problems associated with different lesional brain sites. Stem cell investigation is also producing an interesting scientific as well as social debate about the possibilities of its use in controlling and curing illnesses; the scientific debate is also occurring in basic sciences which we will introduce below.

It is well established that some organs in the human body are able to regenerate themselves – the skin or the liver – while others, for example, the brain and heart, are not able to.[1] The apparent resistance of the human brain to regenerate its neural components contrasts with the high level of neurogenesis observed in nonmammal vertebrates such as fish, amphibians, reptiles and birds,[2-4] although neurogenesis is not always the same, even within the same species. Neurogenesis depends a great deal on the genetic component. The brain is built by multipotent cells that are able to self-renew for an extended period of time.

In the field of neurology and brain injury, stem cells without doubt play an important role given the high incidence of disorders derived from acquired brain injury. One of the approaches to cellular replacement is to transplant multipotential cell populations, which can generate any required cell population, regardless of the specific need. The most important advantage of multipotent stem cells is their capacity to generate large number of cells required for transplantation. Their major two shortcomings are the efficiency of differentiation and, consequently, the efficiency of the transplant, and that multipotential cells rather than other kinds of cells could be influenced by the host environment.[5] Repairing brain injury is not fully possible without basic and clinical research in neuroscience where neurobiologists, pharmacologists,

* This chapter has been possible thanks to an agreement of collaboration between the University of Sevilla Neuropsychology Laboratory and the Center for Rehabilitación of Brain Injury (CRECER), Sevilla, Spain. Part of the chapter was published by *Revista Español de Neuropsicología*, 5(1), 1–13.

geneticists, neuropsychologists, neurosurgeons and others have to work together. The aim is very ambitious, but success in this endeavor would be a paradigmatic leap in confronting health and life, as well as professionally. The following pages try to introduce this debate in the field of human brain injury rehabilitation.

Neural stem cells in mammals

All cells in the nervous system are generated by a simple layer of neuroepithelial cells and are derived from the ectodermis of the embryo. Via a process of molecular and morphological changes, they become the nervous system. Stem cells are embryonic cells, that is to say cells whose destinies have not been decided. They are cells that are transformed through a process of differentiation and proliferation in distinct types of cells. These embryonic cells are different from all other types of cells found in the organism. Thus, theoretically, when a stem cell transplant is carried out from an embryo to an injured area of the brain, there is regeneration of the damaged tissue since these cells are potentially capable of differentiating at this time, once they have been transplanted in the brain, into the same type of brain cells that were injured.

Neural stem cells are defined as those which are able to generate neuronal tissue or which come from the nervous system, are capable of self-renewal and can generate other types of cells different from themselves through a process of symmetric cell division. It seems that neural stem cells change their competence during development to respond to environmental cues. In the same way, some adult stem cells present new characteristics in comparison to fetal ones, which means that neural stem cells change their biological behavior throughout life.[6] Neuronal stem cells can also be defined by their original tissue or by their multipotential. There are totipotential stem cells which are those that can be implanted in a live animal's uterus and produce a complete living organism, with complete central and peripheral nervous systems. Pluripotential stem cells are those capable of producing all types of cells of an organism, including nervous system cells, with the exception of trophoblasts of the placenta. When out of context, these cells are not able to create a form and structure of an organism. These pluripotential cells are the same as embryonic stem cells and are presently used for creating transgenic animals, and their commercial and clinical use is being considered.

Recent studies have expressed the possibility that stem cells from one tissue are able to produce cells of another different tissue. This has to do with the cellular lineage that all cells have since the differentiation of cells usually depends on the lineage of each cell. Stem cell studies are challenging the changes produced in these lineages once the stem cells have been exposed to a new environment. In any case, it must be taken into account that cellular neurogenesis, the differentiation and proliferation of stem cells, depends on autonomous cellular regulators modulated by external signs. Among these regulators are the proteins responsible for producing symmetrical cell division, nuclear factors that control genetic expression and chromosome modifications that are produced in daughter cells and non-stem cells, like watches that set and control the number of revolutions during division. This aspect is important to review because it makes the role that genetics plays apparent in stem cell research.

At the present time new sources of stem cells, distinct from embryonic, are being sought. It has been found that adult bone marrow might be a source of stem cells since it has been observed to be capable of differentiating in a variety of red globules, producing cells in bone marrow, and at present trying to produce brain cells. This is not a difficult task; there are around a trillion cells in the human brain with the distinction that between 10 and 100 million neuronal cells represent more than 50 phenotypes of distinct neurotransmittors and every one of these neurons can receive an average of over 1000 efferent synapses. Another important distinction is that axonal projections of a specific neuron (e.g., those of the cortico-spinal tract) can travel the length of the body to innervate objectives that can be over one meter's distance from a cell body of the neuron.

The nervous system of adult mammals has a limited capacity for self-regeneration. However, there are a few exceptions of capacity for neurogenesis in the brain. One important fact for neuropsychology is that neural stem cells exist in adult mammals which are constantly generating new neurons: the subventrical zone of the lateral ventricle and the subgranular layers of the hippocampal dentate gyrus.[7-10] Adult neurogenesis of regenerative capacity seems to be regulated by interaction with the environment; thus the dependence of neurogenesis on neuropsychological aspects is of primary importance. Practically no studies have reported adult cortical neurogenesis other than those described above. According to Magavi and Macklis,[11] it is unclear whether neurogenesis normally occurs in the neocortex of any mammals, but further examination of potential constitutively occurring neurogenesis in the classically non-neurogenic regions will be required to definitively assess the potential existence of perhaps extremely low-level neurogenesis.

We also have to mention that different researchers have explored the use of animal tissue for brain repair (xenobiotic sources) but xenografted neural tissue itself generates a number of practical, ethical, safety, and immunological issues that have to be addressed prior to a clinical xenotransplant program. Perhaps the single biggest unsolved problem is the immune response. The brain does not seem to be an immunologically privileged site. Grafts placed in the brain survive longer than elsewhere, but are ultimately rejected.[12]

Substitution of neural cells by stem cells

Cell therapy in the brain needs to consider the purity of the cells, the quantity of the cells available, the ability of the cells to migrate, their ability to differentiate appropriately, and whether cues exist at the implantation site to direct differentiation *in vivo*. Although at the moment no stem cell type fulfills the following requisites, the substitution of neuronal cells by stem cells with the aim of restoring brain-injured tissue is a task to be carried out in certain circumstances:

1 Determine and identify the specific cluster of cells which need to be regenerated.
2 Isolate and/or propagate a source of tissue capable of utilizing replacement strategies.
3 Characterize and determine the identity of the selected cell cluster with genetic and biochemical markers.
4 Identify the immediate precursors that generate new living neurons.
5 Integrate stem cells in the host brain without risking the individual's health.
6 Ascertain the survival capacity of the neurons once they are transplanted, and their capacity for forming connections to the patient's brain.
7 Determine if the subject's brain is able to integrate and use the implanted neurons.

For the neuronal repair to be successful, it is necessary to determine the temporization and sequence of the neurons during the development of the brain. Rakic[12] has carried out various studies about the neurocortex to determine the temporization and sequence of neurogenesis in different cytoarchitectonic areas. His results show that corticogenesis begins almost simultaneously around 30–40 days' development of the embryo in all areas they studied. On the other hand, these authors have found that the cessation time of neurogenesis is more variable, ranging from day 70 of the embryo's limbic system to day 102 in the visual cortex (Figure 21.1). According to these authors, the majority of the kinds of neurons in the central nervous system of monkeys are generated during a specific and highly restricted gestational period. The only exceptions are the granulated cells of the olfactory bulb, cerebellum and hippocampus in which genesis continues after birth. The duration of the neurogenetic period of a certain brain structure does not depend on its size or final number of centers. The final number of neurons depends on the species and on the initial size of the founder cell clusters in proliferating zones until they are exhausted at a certain point. The conclusion reached is that the most identifiable neurons of a species are generated during periods of development preceding birth.

Memory and hippocampus

The hippocampus is a crucial zone of the brain for memory processes and emotional control, but at the same time has a special trait which is not shared with other cerebral zones, except the olfactory bulb. Neurogenesis continues in human adults (also in rodents and other primates) throughout life in the

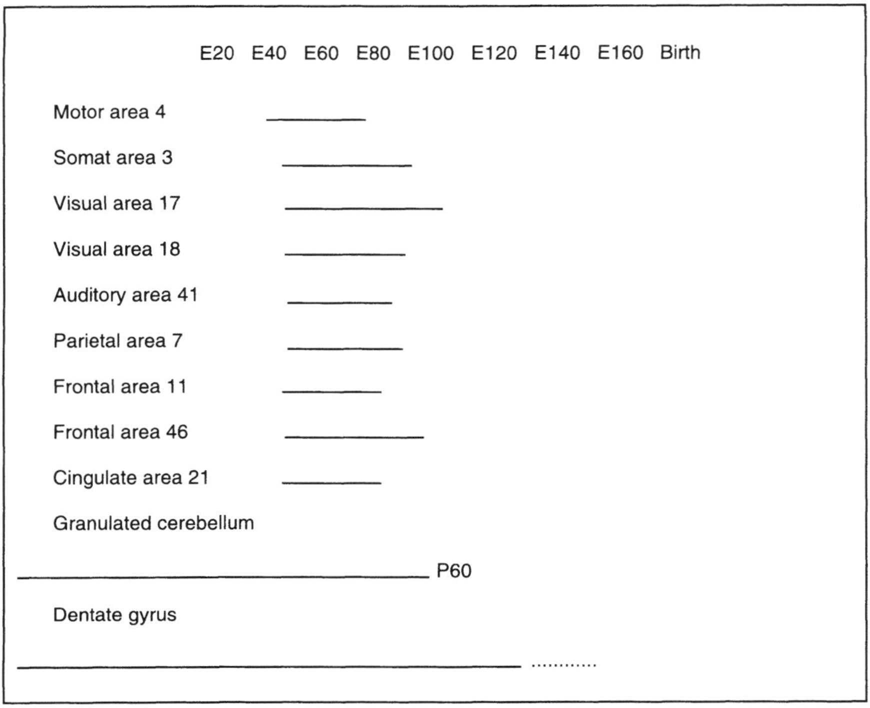

Figure 21.1 Neuron formation time in principal kinds of neocortical neurons in the central nervous system of macaque monkey. The age of the embryo is represented in post-conception days (E = embryo; P = postnatal) on the horizontal line. Modified from Rakic.[12]

dentate gyrus of the hippocampus, as it was already confirmed by Bayer, Yackel and Puri in 1982.[24] For this reason, basic knowledge is fundamental for the efficacy of brain regeneration procedures in processes of memory and recuperation. The existence of neurogenesis in the hippocampus, from an evolutionary point of view, means that it is essential for the continuation of life. Thus we can say that the basic functions associated with the hippocampus, memory and emotions are necessary for survival.

From the neuropsychological point of view, hippocampal neurogenesis is affected, and/or modulated, by physiological and behavioral aspects. Aging affects neurogenesis adversely. This could be due to at least two factors: first, a depletion of multipotent precursors occurs; second, a change in the levels of the molecular factors which influence neurogenesis,[13] although for Cameron and McKay,[14] at least in the hippocampus, there is a survival of multipotent precursors in elderly people. Other studies have demonstrated that behavior and environment play an important role in neurogenesis of the hippocampus. A study by Kempermann and colleagues[15] showed that when animals who have lived in a rich and stimulating environment were compared to those who lived in a normal laboratory environment, the first had a greater number of new cells in the hippocampus. However, stress reduces neurogenesis in rodents as well as primates.[16,17] Some authors have asked if the hippocampus plays a relevant role in depression. Jacobs et al.[18] propose that the underlying cause of depression is an insufficiency of neurogenesis in the hippocampus. In fact, antidepressants are associated with an increase of neurogenesis.[19]

The possibility of manipulating or influencing neurogenesis using neuropsychological and pharmacological techniques in the subgranular zone of the hippocampus dentate gyrus is the objective of much important present research. However, as Eisch and Nestler[20] point out: "the principal limitation in the field today is the lack of direct evidence of the important role of newborn neurons in hippocampus functions." For this reason, neuropsychologists are essential in this field of research. They are the ones who best know the functions of brain zones and how to recover those functions.[21] Table 21.1 shows a partial list of live manipulations that increase or decrease neurogenesis (number of surviving neurons 2 or more weeks after the mitotic marking injection) in adult rodents compared to other control groups. This shows the clearly defined role of neuropsychologists and basic neuropsychological research in neurogenesis of brain tissue.

Ethical and social aspects

The great social and ethical debate taking place at the present time is about the legitimacy of using human embryos for research and the foreseeable development of the use of embryonic stem cells. Embryonic stem cells

Table 21.1 Facilitation or inhibition of neurogenesis through neuropsychological intervention, showing that adult neurogenesis is regulated by an important quantity of environmental, behavioral and physiological factors

Stress	−
Corticosterone	−
ADX	+
Growth factors	+
Antidepressant medication	+
Electroconvulsive crisis	+
Opiates	−
Rich environment	+
Voluntary physical exercise (running)	+
Hippocampus-dependent learning	+
Advanced age	−
Glutamate	−
Serotonin	+
Estrogens	+
Ischemia	+
Dietary restriction	+

which can be used generally come from embryos, those "in reserve", which are frozen in clinics for fertilization and infertility treatment. Infertility treatment requires that different eggs be created for implantation in the mother. Excess eggs are frozen again in case it is necessary to re-implant if the former are not successful. It is even more polemical when the creation of embryos is carried out for the purpose of being a stem cell source. Blood from the placenta is another source of stem cells. At this stage, no ethical problems have been raised about it. In fact, there are companies that offer to collect and store the blood from the umbilical cord in case the newborn might need his or her own stem cells in the future, or to use for another family member or another person. Another more controversial source of stem cells is cloning (substituting the DNA of a woman's egg with a cell from the donor). The idea is that the created embryo contains the complete composition of another person, for example, the one who needs the transplant. Once this embryo is implanted in the woman's uterus it could theoretically be a source of stem cells which would contribute to cellular regeneration.

The search for and production of scientific knowledge via scientific research offers enormous intellectual compensation as well as being an important social function As Frankel[22] says, stem cell research promises to fulfill these requisites. For this author, as for us, it must be accepted that public policy in a pluralistic society cannot resolve all the differences in respect to socially sensitive issues. Controversy is inevitable between what can be done and what should be done. One solution is to agree upon the criteria used for establishing a policy regarding research and use of stem cells, but it is not easy to do in a pluralistic society with individuals and groups with such distinct personal, social, political, and religious interests. Frankel points out that there should be a balance between the promotion of scientific research and clear explanations to the public, demanding straightforward expectations and requirements from scientists for stem cell research. This should all be in proportion to the seriousness of the expectations raised and not create arbitrary barriers which paralyze potential benefits.

The European Group on Ethics in Science and New Technologies (EGE), as the assessing committee of the European Commision, has decided that, "due to the lack of consensus in respect to the status of human embryons, it appears to be inappropriate to impose a moral code . . . It is crucial to settle human embryo research, in countries where permitted, under strict public control as well as assuring a maximum transparency whether carried out in private or public sectors." According to Lenoir,[23] this is due to the fact that stem cell research in Europe will finally depend on the values of European citizens. Europeans uphold the point of view that public authorities should establish principles in accordance with how research is carried out. On the other hand, they continue, due to the fact that Europe has an excessive number of scientists, there is consensus that the scientific agenda should be congruent with basic social values. For Lenoir, the solution for the European Union is going to depend on two factors. First, in Europe the principle of human dignity is stronger than the principle of non-restricted freedom to investigate. Second, in order to avoid irreversible harm, there is a strong emphasis on the principle of adequate precaution in pursuing economic interests because of the implications that stem cell research has for society as a whole.

In any case, the world and society have changed sufficiently for allowing advances that will change the way of living, illness and cures. An effort towards achieving consensus and looking at the positive side is necessary, as well as the necessary controls.

Conclusions

Stem cells are natural units of embryonic generation, and also adult regeneration, of a variety of tissues in an organism. Stem cell research presents a new challenge to brain injury rehabilitation. Researchers in all areas of the neurosciences are trying to find the mechanisms underlying neurogenesis. For neuropsychologists, as well as neuroscientists, our participation corresponds to the role of being experts in human brain functioning as there is no point investigating neuronal stem cells if their function is not known. Research is just beginning and all substantial contributions signify advances on this path. Ethical and social aspects deriving from embryonic research must still be defined, however.

References

1. National Research Council. National Council Report (2001). *Stem cells and the future of regenerative medicine.* Washington, DC: National Academy Press.
2. Rakic, P. (2002). Adult corticogenesis: an evaluation of the evidence. *Nat. Rev. Neurosci., 3*, 65–71.
3. Meyer, R. L. (1978). Evidence from thymidine labeling for continuing growth of retina and tectum in juvenile goldfish. *Exp. Neurol., 59*, 99–111.
4. Goldman, S. A., & Nottebohm, F. (1983). Neuronal production, migration and differentiation in a vocal control nucleus of the adult female canary brain. *Proc. Natl. Acad. Sci. USA, 80*, 2390–2394.
5. Carpinter, M. K., Mattson, M., & Rao, M. S. (2003). Sources of cells for CNS therapy. In T. Zigova, E. Y. Snyder, and P. Sanberg (Eds.), *Neural stem cells for brain and spinal cord repair.* Totowa, NJ: Humana Press.
6. Arsenijevic, Y. (2003). Mammalian neural stem-cell renewal. Nature versus nurture. *Mol. Neurobiol., 27*, 73–98.
7. Tanapat, P., Hastings, N. B., Reeves, A. J., & Gould, E. (1999). Estrogen stimulates a transient increase in the number of new neurons in the dentate gyrus of the adult female rat. *J. Neurosc., 19*, 5792–580.
8. Lois, C., & Alvarez-Buylla, A. (1994). Long-distance neuronal migration in the adult mammalian brain. *Science, 264*, 1145–1148.
9. Kosaka, T., & Hama, K. (1986). Three-dimensional structure of astrocytes in the rat dentate gyrus. *J. Comp. Neurol., 249*, 242–2609.

10. Cameron, H. A., Woolley, C. S., McEwen, B. S., & Gould, E. (1993). Differentiation of newly born neurons and glia in the dentate gyrus of the adult rat. *Neuroscience, 56*, 337–344.

11. Magavi, S. S., & Macklis, J. D. (2003). Induction of adult neurogenesis: molecular manipulation of neural precursors in situ. *Ann. NY Acad. Sci., 991*, 229–236.

12. Rakic, P. (2002). Neurogenesis in adult primate neocortex: an evaluation of the evidence. *Nat. Rev. Neurosci., 3*, 65–71

13. Kuhn, H. G., Dickinson-Anson. H., & Gage, F. H. (1996). Neurogenesis in the dentate gyrus of the adult rat: age-related decrease of neuronal progenitor proliferation. *J. Neurosci., 16*, 2027–2033.

14. Cameron, H. A., & McKay, R. D. (1999). Restoring production of hippocampal neurons in old age. *Nat. Neurosci., 2*, 894–897.

15. Kempermann, G., Kuhn, H. G., & Gage, F. H. (1997). More hippocampal neurons in adult mice living in an enriched environment. *Nature, 386*, 493–495.

16. Gould, E., McEwen, B. S., Tanapat, P., Galea, L. A., & Fuchs, E. (1997). Neurogenesis in the dentate gyrus of the adult tree shrew is regulated by psycho-social stress and NMDA receptor activation. *J. Neurosci., 17*, 2492–2498.

17. Pixley, S. K., Dangoria, N. S., Odoms, K. K., & Hastings, L. (1998). Effects of insulin-like growth factor 1 on olfactory neurogenesis in vivo and in vitro. *Ann. NY Acad. Sci., 855*, 244–247.

18. Jacobs, B. L., Praag, H., & Gage, F. H. (2000). Adult brain neurogenesis and psychiatry: a novel theory of depressions. *Mol. Psychiatry, 5*, 262–269.

19. Malberg, J. E., Eisch, A. J., Nestler, E. J., & Duman, R. S. (2000). Chronic antidepressant treatment increases neurogenesis in adult rat hippocampus. *J. Neurosci., 20*, 9104–9110.

20. Eisch, A. J., & Nestler, E. J. (2002). To be or not to be: adult neurogenesis and psychiatry. *Clin. Neurosci. Research, 1–2*, 93–108.

21. León-Carrión, J., Domínguez-Roldán, J. M., Murillo-Cabezas, F., Domínguez-Morales, M. R., & Muñoz-Sanchez, M. (2000). The role of citicholine in neuropsychological training after traumatic brain injury. *Neurorehabilitation, 14*, 33–40.

22. Frankel, M. S. (2000) In search of stem cell policy. *Am. Assoc. Adv. Sci., 287*, 1397.

23. Lenoir, N. (2000). Europe confronts the embryonic stem cell research challenge. *Science, 287*, 1425–1427.

24. Bayer, S. A., Yackel, J. W., & Puri, P. S. (1982). Neurons in the rat dentate gyrus granular layer substantially increase during juvenile and adult life. *Science*, May 21; 216 (4548): 890–892.

22 Complementary medicine and TBI

George A. Zitnay

Introduction

"First do no harm" is the best-known passage from the writings of Hippocrates, the father of medicine, which he wrote as advice to practicing physicians. The statement asks physicians to consider safe healing methods before resorting to potentially more dangerous therapies for the treatment of acute and chronic ailments.

Our western society and, specifically, our medical and scientific community have focused their attention on treating symptoms and diseases. While this allopathic approach is rational and logical, it is not the only approach to healing. This chapter will focus on complementary medicines. These practices are not alternatives but complementary to traditional western medicine. Complementary techniques in the post-acute treatment of brain injury are used in many places around the world. These techniques include such practices as T'ai Chi, acupuncture, hippotherapy, yoga/meditation, massage therapy, music therapy, etc. These practices will be discussed later in the chapter. Since Hippocratic times, there have been two distinct schools of thought in medicine. One school of medical thought sought to understand the physiochemical working of the human body and created ever-changing theories about the cause of illness and disease. It defined health as the absence of symptoms and defined disease as an entity and as a localized condition. People with similar conditions were considered to have a specific disease. Physicians sought to get rid of the disease or intervene between the physiochemical cause and its effect. The practitioners of this school of thought called themselves Rationalists, and this approach developed into the modern biochemical model.

The other school of thought, whose practitioners called themselves Empiricists, was less interested in explaining why a specific treatment worked and, more importantly, sought to observe what actually worked to heal people. According to Empiricists, health was not simply the absence of symptoms but a high level of physical and psychological vitality. Diseases were not simply entities that were localized to an unhealthy body part, but rather represented a response to an imbalance of the entire body and mind. It was not enough to treat a diseased part without treating the whole individual. Empiricists applied natural methods to augment the body's own defenses so that it could heal itself. This school of thought developed into the modern natural medicine model.

By the age of 6, the brain has almost reached its full size, and the changes begin to come more slowly. Traditionally, it has been thought that by adulthood the brain was "hard wired", its neural connections as fixed as the circuits of a computer. Thus the damage caused by a traumatic brain injury, stroke, or brain tumor was believed to be basically irreversible. Over the past decade, neuroscientists have come to realize that this viewpoint is incorrect. An adult brain may not have the same level of flexibility as a child's brain, but it does change. With this realization has come the hope that scientists may eventually be able to assist the brain to heal – repairing damage from TBI, stroke, etc.

To this end, researchers are following two lines of investigation. Some seek to understand how the brain responds to injuries, with the goal of aiding its repair efforts. Others are studying the normal growth and development of the young brain, since we now know that similar activity takes place in the mature brain but at a greatly reduced level. If they can understand this developmental process, doctors and neuroscientists believe they will find ways to induce the brain to heal itself.

Dr. Richard Frackowiak at Hammersmith Hospital in London is investigating the brain's response to injury. He focuses on patients who have lost some control of their muscles because of damage to the major system areas to the brain. Almost all such patients, he reports, show some amount of spontaneous recovery. "It may be minor, it may be major," he says, but the question remains, why does this happen and what happens in the brain that results in recovery? If he can learn the mechanism of recovery, it may be possible to help the recovery along, to promote full recovery in patients who would normally regain only part of their abilities, and to create partial recovery in patients who would normally not recover at all. Frackowiak says he has found three mechanisms by which the damaged brain rewires itself to recover from injury. In some cases, adjacent areas of the brain take over the function of a damaged area. A second type of injury response can occur in cases of damage to sections of the brain that operate in tandem with other areas – after the injury, those partners work harder to take up the slack. If neither of those strategies works, he says, the brain can tediously relearn how to do various movements that it could perform with ease before the injury. In short, Frackowiak says, "There is a lot of remodeling that goes on as the brain responds to injury." Although he only studies motor areas of the brain, he says that a similar pattern holds in other sections of the brain, including those areas responsible for language and memory.

By understanding how the brain responds to injury it should be possible to tailor therapies that work hand in hand with this response. By studying the developing brain, researchers have found that the picture is much different than one thought. Dr. Story Landis[1] from Case Western Reserve University School of Medicine says that the brain is surprisingly flexible in its development, and this flexibility may hold the key to finding ways to heal the brain. According to Dr. Landis, "One of the most important advances in the past decade has been the recognition that the formation of the nervous system is not intrinsically programmed." She says, "There is not a specific genetic program that makes out a stereotyped sequence of events which must occur. In fact, rather the developing nervous system is shaped by sets of cell–cell interactions." It is that cell–cell interaction which may offer scientists a way to intervene in the mature brain and help it recover from injury. This has led to a dramatic surge of information about the nature of molecules that can support the survival of motor neurons. These factors are so-called trophic factors. All of this has led to experimental work with fetal tissue, new pharmaceuticals which prevent the brain from continuing to hurt itself by developing, neuroprotector drugs, free radical scavengers and pharmacological blockers that could intercept neurotransmitters or interrupt them lingering in a cell after injury.

Perhaps one of the most exciting things to come out of the last decade is the growing understanding of how the brain works and how it responds to its environment. This has allowed neuroscientists to lay to rest one of the longest running debates in science – the nature–nurture question. For centuries people have argued about what determines human nature and behavior. Is it all in the genes, so that an individual's nature is relatively fixed when he or she is born? Or are we products of our environment, little more than blank slates waiting to be written upon by the society in which we are raised? The answer to the debate is neither. The more scientists learn about the brain, the clearer it becomes that the structure of an individual's brain is the result of a complex interplay between nature and nurture, with the two forces working together and modifying each other's messages to an extent that it becomes almost meaningless to talk about the individual contribution of one or the other. Take, for example, the development of the visual cortex, the area of the brain responsible for vision and one of the best understood brain systems. The way that the neurons of the visual systems develop is specified by a person's genes, but those genetic instructions do not amount to a blueprint that specifies where each neuron will go and what other neurons it will connect with. Instead, the development that is still going on in the months after birth relies on input from the environment to help direct the neurons. If an infant develops a cataract in one eye that prevents him or her from seeing out of that eye during the critical development period, the part of the visual system responsible for that eye does not develop properly and he or she will never see normally from that eye. In other words, the genes directing the development of the eye do not operate in a vacuum – they are designed so that their actions are responsive to signals from the outside. Just as the environment influences the expression of a person's genes, those genes influence what environment a person experiences.

These discoveries are good news for professionals, therapists, family members, and others who work with people with brain injury. The doors are wide open for a broad range of options: pharmaceuticals, gene therapy, traditional therapy and especially complementary medicine, since complementary medicine serves as an assist or complement to traditional medicine. This is important because neuroscientists are telling us that the brain is not hard wired, that it is plastic and capable of new learning. Complementary medicine then can play a significant role in helping the brain heal. Complementary medicine can work on the neuronal level or on the environmental level.

What is complementary medicine? A complement means something that completes, makes up a whole or brings to perfection. Complementary, according to the *Oxford Dictionary*, means "forming or serving as a complement; completing, supplying mutual needs or offsetting mutual lacks". How is complementary medicine being used to heal the brain of persons with brain injury? In many countries treating sickness and injury with acupuncture, massage, T'ai Chi, guided imagery or herbal remedies was considered irrelevant. Not so any longer. When the US National Institutes of Health established the Office for Alternative Medicine (OAM) professionals began to take notice. Now in most countries complementary medicine is seen as an important tool or resource along with traditional medicine. Complementary medicine then serves as a complement and makes up the whole of traditional medicine. To better understand what traditional medicine is, we need to learn a little history. The basic tenets of Chinese or eastern medicine were in place over 3000 years ago. Practitioners of traditional Chinese medicine have for centuries looked at the "chi" (energy) in treating people with a wide range of conditions. In ancient Greece, while the followers of the Greek God Asklepios focused on treatment, the followers of his daughter Hygeia focused on healing. Western medicine relies more heavily on the "matter" of the body, its cells, and its chemicals. This century's technological advances in imaging, genetics, pharmacology, nuclear medicine and computerization have increased western medicine's proficiency, especially in trauma care and acute care. People are being saved whom only a short time ago would have expired. Western medicine uses a wide range of strategies to attack disease, while the eastern practitioner's strategy is to restore balance and harmony.

The issue of complementary medicine and brain injury is complex. The scientific literature clearly demonstrates that severe brain injury at the acute stage relies almost exclusively on traditional medicine with its emphasis on drugs, CT scans, intracranial pressure monitoring, respiratory therapy, and advanced technological monitoring following neurosurgery. The goal at this stage is to prevent death and to retain as many functions as possible with allopathic medicine. What happens next depends on where the person receives treatment, the prevailing philosophy of the post-acute care center, the resources available, the attitude of the doctor and the support received from the family. It is here that complementary medicine can play an important role.

Complementary/alternative medicine (CAM) has been described by Ernst et al.[2] as "diagnosis, treatment and/or prevention which complements mainstream medicine by contributing to a common whole, satisfying a demand not met by orthodoxy or diversifying the conceptual frameworks of medicine." Approximately 1500 articles on CAM are published annually in the literature covered by Medline.[3] To understand the growth of CAM is useful in determining the value of its use. For example, in the UK the market for herbal and homeopathic remedies and aromatherapy oils increased by 41% between 1992 and 1996.[4] In Germany, the herbal remedy St. John's Wort is now the most frequently prescribed drug for depression. In the USA the sales of St. John's Wort rose by 2800% between 1997 and 1998, and the total market for medicinal botanicals was worth US$3.7 billion in 1998.[4]

We will discuss each of the modalities identified by the Office for Alternative Medicine (OAM), National Institutes of Health as they pertain to brain injury. The US Congress established the OAM in 1992 to determine the effectiveness of alternative medicine treatment modalities and to integrate effective treatments into mainstream traditional medical practice.

OAM has identified seven categories of alternative practice that they will study:

- Diet/nutrition/lifestyle change.
- Mind/body intervention (dance therapy / guided imaging / yoga / meditation).
- Alternative systems (acupuncture, traditional Chinese medicine).
- Bioelectromagnetic applications in medicine.
- Manual healing methods (Feldenkrais methods, massage therapy, osteopathy, therapeutic touch).
- Pharmacological and biological treatments.
- Herbal medicine.

OAM has funded the following studies relevant to brain injury:

- Acupuncture for attention deficit hyperactivity disorder (ADHD) at the Medical College of Virginia with Neil Sonenclar, MD.
- Ayurvedic herbals for Parkinson's disease at Southern Illinois University School of Medicine in Springfield with Bala Manyam, MD.
- EEG normalization for mild head trauma at the Baylor College of Medicine in Houston Texas with Wayne Whitehouse, PhD.
- Homeopathy for mild traumatic brain injury at Spaulding Rehabilitation Hospital in Boston Massachusetts with Elaine Woo, MD.
- Music therapy for psychosocial adjustments after brain injury at Pennsylvania State University in Hershey Pennsylvania with Paul Eslinger, PhD.
- T'ai Chi for mild balance disorder at Northwestern University in Chicago Illinois with Timothy Hayes, MD.

According to Ullman,[5] homeopathic medicine is based on the principle of similars – that is, whatever symptoms and syndromes a substance causes in large or toxic doses, it can heal when given in specially prepared, exceedingly small doses. In fact, homeopathy derives its name from the Greek *homoios* meaning "similar" and *pathos* meaning "disease" or "suffering". Homeopathy was formally developed into a systemic method of applying the similars principle in the early 1800s. The use of this approach is an ancient pharmacological strategy that was used by the Egyptians, Chinese, Incas, Aztecs, and Native Americans. According to Ullman, persons sustaining severe to moderate head injuries should seek proper medical attention first. She suggests that in addition to such care, homeopathic medicines may be useful in decreasing the possibilities of complications from head injuries. Post-acute treatment of headache, fatigue, depression, sleeplessness, anxiety and other commonly described symptoms following a head injury may also be helped by the use of homeopathic remedies. It is suggested that prior to use of such practices the patient should consult with his or her physician and seek out a qualified practitioner of homeopathic medicine.

Methodology

Feldenkrais method

The Feldenkrais method was developed in the 1940s and 1950s by Moshe Feldenkrais, an Israeli physicist and electrical engineer. He began a study of human movement through his interest in judo and during his own recovery from an incapacitating injury.[6] Moshe Feldenkrais worked to enhance the function of athletes, musicians, actors and dancers, as well as students with orthopedic and neurological injuries. He began personally teaching the method to others and since his death the training and certification of Feldenkrais practitioners is administered by the Feldenkrais Guild.

The Feldenkrais method is a methodology of exploration and study of movement for the enhancement of human function. The method does not limit itself to cognitive learning but includes a vast array of sensory and psychological approaches to learning.[7-11] This is relevant to the neurologically injured person who has lost physical function and has an impaired ability to relearn movement due to CNS injury.

The normal neural pathways that allow a person to raise an arm may be lost and the ability to improve this movement may be dramatically impaired by damage to the central processing of information from the peripheral nervous system and from other areas of the CNS. The Feldenkrais method proposes new approaches to learning that stimulate new and existing parallel neural pathways and thus elicit return of physical function.[12] In the method, the neurologically impaired person becomes a student of the self in movement. The student is taught to understand and enjoy the process of exploring and learning about the use of himself. Rather than feeling himself as a collection of working and non-working parts, the student develops a sense of his whole self in function.[13] The focus shifts from an injured person trying to raise a hemiplegic arm to a student of movement who gains fascination and interest in the process of learning to use his arm, much like a violinist learning to make a particular sound.[14] Gaining the tools, interest and enjoyment in the process of learning will allow the student to continue to improve and refine his other functional movement outside the Feldenkrais lesson.

In the traditional mode of movement learning, a therapist/teacher shows and describes a movement and guides the learner to repeat and practice that movement using both verbal and tactile cues. Sometimes, muscles involved in the movement are stimulated by tapping, vibration, etc. For example, to learn to shift weight onto a hemiplegic leg, the therapist/teacher may inform the patient that the shifting of the hips over the leg is essential. The patient then practices this weight shift facilitated by the teacher/therapist using hands on the hips to cue the shift and through repeated demonstration. The patient must remember this movement to use in his life.

In the Feldenkrais method, the practitioner encourages and guides the student to enjoy exploration of movement choices so that the student becomes conscious of the wide range of choices that he then has access to use in his daily life.[8] To learn to shift weight over the injured leg, the practitioner/teacher first guides the student on a mat to become aware of the connections of the foot to the leg, to the hips, etc., and to become interested in these connections. As the student gains a clear kinesthetic understanding and image of these connections, the lesson shifts to actual weight bearing on the leg. In the upright position, the student is guided to become aware of the sensation of weight bearing through that leg at the feet, the knees, the hip, the trunk, the neck, the head and eyes and how he may subtly change these sensations through conscious movement. Even the emotional and psychological effect of weight bearing on that leg is explored and discussed. The method assumes that as the awareness of weight bearing over the hemiplegic leg produces clearer and more detailed peripheral feedback to the CNS, new pathways of control of weight bearing over the hemiplegic leg will develop.[12] The student is encouraged to explore and discover for himself the best way to weight shift during functional activities of dynamic standing and gait during his daily activities. The student does not need to remember a correct way to weight bear after a lesson. He only needs to remember to continue to expand his awareness of weight bearing through self-exploration.

The method makes use of numerous techniques of movement learning,[7,8,15] but the Feldenkrais practitioner is not limited to these techniques and is guided by the intention to enhance the ability of the student to continue the learning on his own. There are several accounts of how Feldenkrais movement learning techniques have been used with those with injury to the CNS. In "New Pathways in the Recovery from Brain Injury", Bach-y-Rita[12] describes the effects of the method used in a group setting with people with post-stroke hemiplegia. Rywerwant[16] describes the use of sensory substitution of auditory instead of kinesthetic feedback in order to train a flutist to regain fine motor control of his hand after a stroke. In *The Case of Nora*, Feldenkrais[7] relates a wide variety of approaches to improve the function of a woman who was disabled by a stroke.

Feldenkrais lessons are given in one-to-one sessions called Functional Integration (FI) lessons and group sessions called Awareness Through Movement (ATM) lessons. In an FI, the practitioner facilitates learning and exploration both verbally and through gentle tactile and movement cues. In an ATM, the practitioner verbally guides the group through gentle movement exploration.

The Alexander technique

The Alexander technique is an educational method of becoming aware of one's posture and movement during activities of daily living. It was founded in the late 1800s by F. M. Alexander, who was an actor in the British theatre. Alexander repeatedly lost his voice during performances, and the prescribed treatment was not helpful. He spent the next 9 years analyzing his posture, concentrating on the way his head moved on his spine in two different conditions: during everyday conversation, and while he intended to perform. Alexander discovered that when intending to perform, he pulled his head down and back, depressing his larynx. However, in everyday conversation he was able to maintain his head forward and up, enabling him to speak with a stronger voice.[17] In 1918 he published his self-study titled *The Use of Self*, with an introduction written by American philosopher and educator, John Dewey.

John Dewey began taking Alexander lessons in the 1920s. Dewey endorsed the technique in his books, and supported a fellow professor, Frank Pierce Jones, in pursuing scientific research of the technique. Jones had taken a 3 year leave of absence from his work to attend the Alexander training program given by F. M. Alexander's brother, A. R. Alexander. "My strongest impression when A. R. Alexander first demonstrated the Technique to me was that of a mechanism working against gravity . . . I was occupying more space; my movements were less jerky; and I had lost my customary feeling of heaviness."[18] Jones proceeded to conduct postural studies in the 1960s during sit-to-stand, using multiple-image photos in two conditions: guided and habitual.[19] In the guided condition, the experimenter guided the subject's head forward and up. He found that three indexes significantly improved in the guided condition: head thrust decreased, rise time from the chair decreased, and the head trajectory became closer to a straight line ($n = 36$, $p < 0.01$). Jones also studied the head–neck relationship using X-rays in three different postures: habitual relaxed, habitual erect, and experimental, or guided.[20] The results demonstrated that the distance between the first two vertebrae was greater in the experimental posture ($n = 20$, $p < 0.01$), thus improving skeletal alignment. The studies supported Alexander's theory of primary control.

Alexander studied the interaction of the head, neck, and torso, and believed that this relationship was primary in controlling movement. When the head is allowed to rotate forward, spinal lengthening occurs, which is necessary for movement to occur as efficiently as possible.[21] This balance of the head on the neck triggers a tractive force on the spine, guiding the torso upward. During a lesson, the Alexander teacher guides the student through simple movements, such as sitting, lying down, walking, and bending over. The teacher uses simple instructions, a gentle touch, and occasionally a mirror to guide the student. In the beginning, the teacher uses a gentle manual guidance during all of the activities, and eventually the student begins to monitor his or her own movement pattern. Alexander believed that this inhibition of habitual responses "opens the way for conscious direction and control".[18] The recommended course of the Alexander technique is 30 lessons, depending on the student's progress and goals.

The Alexander technique has been used for over 100 years by musicians, singers, and actors to enhance their performances. The technique is taught in several universities and conservatories, including the Yale School of Drama, the Julliard School, and the New England Conservatory of Music. Many of the artists that have used the technique say it has helped them with reducing tension, and improving concentration and vocalization. More recently, Austin and Ausubel's a study[22] has shown that the technique may enhance respiratory function by increasing the strength and endurance of the muscles of the abdominal wall, reducing the resting tensions of the chest wall muscles, and improving the coordination of the respiratory muscles in healthy subjects.[22] The technique seems to assist in maximizing the length–tension relationship of the respiratory muscles, to allow for optimal function.

The technique has also been studied in relation to stress, pain control, and balance. Nielsen's study[23] using the members of a symphony orchestra compared changes in heart rate and blood pressure (common measures of the stress response) in three groups: an exercise group, an Alexander technique group, and a beta-blocker group. Results indicated that the technique lowered systolic blood pressure a significant amount, similar to the effect of the beta-blockers. Pain is a more subjective variable, and therefore more difficult to study. A multidisciplinary pain management program conducted a study using patients with chronic pain, and concluded that the technique was a powerful component in improving disability ratings and activity levels in these patients.[24] Balance is another important factor that the technique may improve. Zuck's study[17] researched postural sway in the feet together and eyes closed position, and found that the Alexander-trained group had significantly less sway than the control group. Balance can also be measured using the functional reach test. Dennis[25] found that two groups instructed in the technique significantly improved their functional reach scores, as compared to the control group. More scientific studies need to be conducted in all of these areas; however, the preliminary research is promising.

Patients suffering from acquired brain injuries (ABI) often have difficulty maintaining good posture and balance, controlling pain, and managing stress following their injury. These patients tend to recruit improper neuromuscular movement patterns, which may lead to poor posture, muscular changes, pain, and balance deficits. The inappropriate movement may be related to the patients' changes in their muscular tone or strength, proprioception, sensation, and/or posture. The Alexander technique may assist physical, occupational, and speech therapists in the neuromuscular re-education process of the patients. The technique uses an educational process to help the patients relearn proper alignment, to reduce muscular tension, and improve kinesthetic awareness, similarly to the traditional therapies. The Alexander technique addresses the areas of dysfunction with repetitive, guided movements, allowing the patient to feel his or her movement in the proper alignment, followed by the patient attempting the movement on their own. The technique is a slow, individual, repetitive process, and the lessons incorporate verbal, manual, and visual feedback, which aid the patients in correcting their alignment during activities of daily living. This approach is useful with patients who may have difficulty following directions, maintaining attention, or understanding complex verbal commands. The Alexander technique can be a functional and effective approach for many people with posture, pain, and balance issues, and may be useful in addition to the traditional therapies for patients with acquired brain injuries.

Acupuncture

According to Duggan,[26] acupuncture is based on concepts of energy flowing through the body. Acupuncturists have developed a sophisticated and integrated healing system based on a longstanding tradition dating back to ancient China. In acupuncture therapy, the individual is treated as a unique and complex individual. The acupuncturist's goal is to restore "chi" (life force) of the individual that is blocked. In acupuncture, special needles are inserted into specific points/meridians of the body, thereby manipulating the flow of "chi" to restore the yin/yang balance of the individual. Yin/yang is an underlying philosophy of traditional Chinese medicine. The Chinese characters of yin and yang mean literally the sunny side of the hill and the shady side of the hill. Yin denotes the feminine qualities in the universe, yang the masculine. Yin relates to blood, yang to energy.

T'ai Chi

Robert Levine, director of the T'ai Chi Foundation, has used T'ai Chi to help persons with brain injury to improve balance, cognitive functioning and to reduce acting out behavior. T'ai Chi originated as a martial art embodying the Taoist principle of man being rooted in the earth. T'ai Chi is a fundamental component of traditional Chinese medicine for general health maintenance. It is seen as a means of cultivating harmony between the self and the external world by restoring the flow of "chi" or energy throughout the body by coordinating the human breadth with a series of defined specific body movements.

Hippotherapy

Hippotherapy is monitored horseback riding in which the movements of the horse simulate the walking movements on the pelvis of an able-bodied person. These movements improve balance and coordination in the rider. For many persons with brain injury, hippotherapy is used to foster self-confidence, concentration, attention, and a sense of well-being. Hippotherapy requires a trained team of specialists (monitors) as well as a trained horse.

Massage therapy

According to Martha Menard,[27] massage therapy is the oldest and largest system of natural therapy, dating back to the ancient Chinese as well as to the Greek physician Hippocrates. According to the practitioners of massage therapy, it has a major effect on muscle relaxation and may also improve blood circulation, remove accumulated toxins, stimulate nerve activity, increase lung activity, quiet and soothe the nervous system and stimulate lymphatic circulation. Massage therapy is being used in rehabilitation of persons with brain injury for relaxation, reduction of fatigue, and to assist in calming.

"Real world" therapy

Real world therapy is a neurorehabilitation intervention developed by Lynwood O. Gentry, OTR/L, Program Director of the John Jane Brain Injury Center at Martha Jefferson Hospital located in Charlottesville Virginia. Real world therapy as well as traditional medical rehabilitation is practiced at the John Jane Brain Injury Center. The center, which is located in a historic house in the the city, serves individuals with acquired brain injury. Real world therapy can be described as applying therapy in community-based settings, providing persons with brain injury the opportunity to relearn skills such as banking, shopping, using the post office, and other everyday tasks necessary to live and work independently in the community. Clients of the center practice dining out skills in local restaurants to assist them in socialization, conversation and listening skills. Beginning in the late 1960s, the community movement gained momentum. Creating community settings for persons with brain disability outside of large institutions began to take hold in places like New Haven, Connecticut.[28] Recreation is provided in local recreational centers along with exercise and fitness programs in community swimming pools and athletic clubs. In addition, clients enroll in T'ai Chi classes, yoga classes, music classes and participate in therapeutic riding (hippotherapy), massage and Feldenkrais classes. Clients also can enroll in the local community college for classes on computer training, French and Spanish language, and any other classes of interest to the individual. The center is staffed by physicians, occupational and physical therapists, neuropsychologists, family counselors and speech and language pathologists, all of whom provide traditional neurorehabilitation and medical intervention, as well as complementary medicine. Family members, along with the clients, participate in planning and developing their own rehabilitation plan. Family counseling and family support groups are provided to assist with family dynamics and to give families information and knowledge about brain injury. The goal of real world therapy is to improve outcomes in natural settings, and to maintain the individual in his/her family and community.

Biofeedback, visualization, imagery, stress reduction

These are techniques that have been used to treat those individuals with closed head injuries, attention deficit disorders, disorders marked by a relative surplus of slow wave activity and the relative absence of fast wave activity. Using a digitizing EEG can drive a feedback tone and help individuals alter theta/beta and delta/beta ratios and associated behaviors, thus supposedly improving attention span and impulse control.

These techniques, in addition to breathing techniques, can be useful in treating head injury associated with fatigue, pain and tinnitus. Stress management can help control anxiety and may help reduce symptomology.

Herbology

According to Henry C. Lee,[29] herbology has a long and ancient history in Chinese medicine. In clinical practice, herbs are used based upon the nature and capability of the herb, and the herbs used are based upon their energies, flavors, movements, and meridian routes.

The four energies of herbs are cold, hot, warm, and cool. For example, when a herb is effective in the treatment of a hot syndrome, that particular herb is considered to have cold energy, and vice versa. The five flavors refer to pungent, sweet, sour, bitter, and salty. Pungent herbs can disperse, sour herbs can restrict, sweet herbs can slow down, bitter herbs can harden, and salty herbs can soften up. Therefore, herbs were used to promote the flow of energy, tone up, harmonize, and dry up. The four movements of herbs are to push upward, to push downward, to float, and to sink. The meridian routes refer to the meridian a given herb is capable of traveling through. In clinical application, herbs are selected that travel through the meridian in the diseased region. Henry C. Lee, a noted practitioner of Chinese medicine, uses herbs to treat headache, fatigue, to calm a person, pain, insomnia, depression, behavioral disturbances and loss of memory of persons with head injuries. He uses a herbal formula to determine the proper formula for each individual.

Transcranial magnetic therapy

From a neurocognitive standpoint, mild to moderate head injury can be conceptualized as a sudden event that produces a pattern of initial generalized neurocognitive deficits, which have natural history of recovery in uncomplicated cases.[30–33] Recovery typically follows a negatively accelerating curve, with the majority of recovery occurring in the first year post-event, with meaningful recovery continuing to extend into the second year post-event. However, a significant number of individuals experiencing mild to moderate head injury exhibit persistent deficits in neurocognitive function, which do not improve.

The use of magnetism in the healing arts has been mentioned throughout the recorded history of medicine. Starting with the *Yellow Emperor's Book of Internal Medicine* (4000 BC), many early civilizations have considered magnetism as a significant aspect in the phenomenon of body health. Magnetism and electromagnetism are used in current medical practices. The prime example is magnetic resonance imaging (MRI) in diagnostic techniques. Other examples are in pain reduction, bone growth stimulation, Parkinson's disease, cancer, blood, cardiac studies and sleep.

The electromagnetic phenomena so prevalent in our culture today involves alternating current or pulsed direct current which produce frequencies not resonating at the natural rhythms or frequency of the human body (2–12 cycles/s). Interference with body resonance depends on the proximity to the field. The human body is electromagnetic by design, being composed largely of atoms, electrons, protons and ions, all vital to the function of life. It is understood that electron transfer is the basic action in all chemical reactions of the body. The induction (outward flow) of a magnetic field accelerates this natural process. This is validated by the quantum mechanical principle of precession. It has been theorized that the increase of magnetic fields on the human body would act as a catalyst to activate those chemical reactions already naturally occurring in the human body. This would infer the improvement of all body functions. Prime examples of these chemical reactions in which magnetic field induction may particularly affect their function are: oxygen-carrying capacity, assimilation of nutrients, manufacturing of enzymes, metabolic waste removal, reduction of free radicals, tissue regeneration and healing.

The hypothesis is that the natural healing process inherent in the human body can be accelerated by the induction of a high strength magnetic field based on the principle of precession. In an injured brain, Sandyk postulates, stimulation of neurotransmitter release may lead to a cascade of neuronal level activity, including improved hormone regulation, neuronal growth and vascular proliferation.[34] Sandyk suggests that these events might "energize" the spontaneous healing mechanism of the brain, leading to improved functional outcome following neurological insult. Bonlie (1995) developed the Magnetic Molecular Energizer (MME) to treat patients with neurological impairments related to stroke and brain injury, though never in a controlled study. The MME consists of two large electromagnets. In treatment, an individual lies on an open table between two magnets, and is subjected to steady direct current, negative magnetic field of 3000–5000 Gauss. This level of electromagnetic current is considered well within the safety limits established by the US Office of the Food and Drug Administration. It is hypothesized that this electromagnet treatment may have a facilitating effect on recovery and will limit the likelihood of persistent deficits.

Nutrition, wellness and lifestyle changes

Nutrition plays an important role in the recovery from a brain injury, from the acute stage, throughout life.[35] Nutrition is often overlooked in the rehabilitation process. Following the acute phase, persons with moderate to severe brain injury often lack the cognitive or physical skills to pay attention to nutrition, ranging from food shopping, food preparation and recognizing a nutritional diet. Home health aides, mentors or family members can play an important role here. Nutrition is more than eating the right food in the right amount and prepared in the proper way. Nutrition must be individualized to the person's health, activity level, lifestyle and special needs for those with headaches, fatigue, dysphasia, chewing problems or endocrine problems following their head injury. A nutritionist can be helpful in assessing the person with a brain injury for nutritional adequacy and plan corrective diets that are palatable and consistent with the person's capabilities. The nutritionist may also suggest ways to deal with the impact of disability on grocery shopping, cooking, etc. Adaptive programs are needed in many cases. Food shopping, preparation and serving are useful in rehabilitation programs to build self-confidence, assist with memory and for socialization skills.

There has been considerable interest in the use of antioxidants and vitamin supplements in the nutritional rehabilitation of persons with brain injury. Vitamin C, vitamin E, other vitamins, and foods that have well-known antioxidant characteristics, like beta-carotene, are being used as adjunct therapy.[36] As stated earlier in this chapter, the emphasis for physicians and other healthcare professionals has been expanded from the concentration on sickness and cure to the emphasis on the full continuum of wellness–illness. This is especially true where interdisciplinary teams make up the rehabilitation program.

Lifestyle is an often neglected area when accessing the needs of a person with brain injury. Is there a history of substance abuse, drugs or alcohol? Where and how does the person live? Who are the friends of the person with brain injury? Does the individual have an income? What were the premorbid factors that may influence lifestyle? These issues and the after effects of brain injury are pervasive, influencing not only the physical health, but also the emotional well-being of the individual. The Brain Injury Association conducted a survey that showed that a majority of brain injuries are caused by motor vehicle crashes related to alcohol. In addition, the survey showed that alcohol figures prominently in the high unemployment rate of people with mild traumatic brain injury. Substance abuse responds best to a combination of therapies, including 12-step programs such as Alcoholics Anonymous (AA) or Narcotics Anonymous (NA), and behavior modification therapy. Lifestyle change needs to be included in the individual's rehabilitation plan. This may mean moving to a new environment, preparing for a new job or career, and developing a new social network of support. Persons with brain injury are often lonely and report the loss of friends and the inability to make new friends. This may lead to unacceptable behaviors and association with individuals who use and abuse persons with brain injury. Developing social outlets and creating social opportunities is often needed.

Qui Gong

For centuries, Oriental medicine philosophy has believed that a mysterious and invisible energy exists throughout the universe. This vital energy drives and sustains life. In the view of the ancient philosophers, this energy permeates the human organism. There are certain vital activities that sustain life, such as breathing, eating, drinking, sleeping, thinking, choosing, exercising – any and all of which maintain all the vital structures and functions of the body. It is the vital force that nourishes the cells, tissues and interconnecting subsystems of the body. This life energy is what the ancient philosophers called Qui. Qui is the vital life force that sustains all living things. Qui is the energy of life: flowing throughout and over the whole body along minute and precise channels called meridians.[37] This basic concept of Qui flowing through a meridian system is closely related to the cosmic principle of "yin" and "yang". Yin and yang are inseparable tendencies of Qui. They coexist as opposite but complementary forces.

Gong refers to work or exercise that requires both study and practice. It also means a *method of training* designed to accomplish a certain skill or objective. Qui Gong is a general name for many different sets of exercise designed to strengthen and balance the life energy that connects body, mind and spirit. Common to all, Qui Gong exercise is the role of movement, proper breathing and concentration. Qui Gong may be practiced in either an active (yang dominant) or passive (yin dominant) form. Active Qui Gong is assertive and dynamic; it involves movement designed to get the Qui flowing freely through the body's energy pathways to promote vibrant health and longevity. Passive Qui Gong is more tranquil and static; it involves no movement (examples are different forms of meditation while sitting, standing or lying down).

Qui Gong is being used in neurorehabilitation for persons with acquired brain injury to promote balance, concentration, and to increase energy levels. Passive Qui Gong is used to help calm, to promote concentration and to improve memory.

Pal Don Gum, or Eight Silken Movements, is an active form of Qui Gong that consists of a sequence of eight gentle exercises. It is used as a method of training the body, breath and mind and the Qui to improve health and longevity. Because it is easy to learn, fun to do and takes only 6 minutes from start to finish, it is being successfully used in day programs for persons with brain injury.

Art, dance and music therapy

Art, dance and music therapy has been a standard adjunct therapy for persons with brain injury throughout recorded medical history. These therapies are in common use today in all major neurorehabilitation programs. They are used to assist in movement, balance, coordination and physical well-being and in neurorehabilitation and cognitive programs.

Pet therapy

The health benefits we get from helping others extend to caring for our pets. Several studies suggest that pet owners enjoy better health. One year after a heart attack, patients who have pets have one-fifth the death rate of the petless. Petting a dog has been shown to lower blood pressure, and bringing a pet into a nursing home or hospital can boost patients' moods and enhance their social interaction.[38] The relationship between pets and health can be explained in several ways. Pet owners often feel needed and responsible, which may stimulate the survival incentive. They feel that they need to survive to take care of their pets. Stroking a dog, watching a kitten play, observing the hypnotic exploration of fish can help elevate mood or make a stressful day less stressful.

Pets can also be a source of unconditional, non-judgmental love and affection. Pets can shift the narrow focus beyond self, helping us feel connected to a larger world. Persons with brain injury report a general improvement in mood and feeling needed and connected. In observation of interaction between the person with a brain injury and caring for a pet, it has been reported that self-esteem, concentration on task and memory have improved.

Aquatic therapy

With a large segment of the population having some degree of disability, it is important that all reasonable means be utilized to assist these individuals in their social, physical and mental functioning. Swimming offers some unique opportunities to persons with a disability and for persons with brain injury. The value of swimming falls into three categories: physiological, psychological and sociological. The physiological benefits of swimming are divided into two major areas: (1) organic development (physical fitness); (2) psychomotor performance (motor performance). Organic development consists of the following components:

- Cardiovascular endurance – the ability of the heart, lungs and circulatory system to sustain vigorous activity.
- Muscle endurance – the capacity for continued exertion; the ability of the muscles to sustain activity for increasing periods of time.
- Strength – the ability to exert force.
- Flexibility – the ability to bend, stretch and move through a normal range of motion.

The factors that contribute to psychomotor performance are:

- Speed – the ability to act or move quickly.
- Agility – the ability to change direction with concentrated body movements.

The factors that contribute to perceptual motor performance are:

- Balance.
- Kinesthetic sense.
- Laterality.
- Dominance.
- Spatial relationships.
- Directionality.
- Visual discrimination.
- Auditory discrimination.
- Eye–hand coordination.
- Eye–hand–foot coordination.

Research studies published by the American Red Cross[39] have indicated that a well-planned physical activity program contributes to organic and motor development. For the person with a disability, participation in swimming activities where the water supports much of the body weight may be the only opportunity for development of these areas. Because of the lessened effects of gravity, there is less weight on the joints, less strength is required for movement, and an independent upright position may be more easily attainable. This is helpful when working with a person with a brain injury that has affected the motor cortex. As a consequence, the overall activity level can be raised. It is often true that in warm water individuals can achieve greater relaxation and increase their range of motion and flexibility. Although there are many psychological benefits in swimming activity for persons with brain injury, it is important to realize that these benefits are of the same type experienced by all persons. Some of the psychological benefits of swimming activities are as follows:

- Experiencing success – the opportunity to do something well and to enjoy the feeling of success is important and can be experienced by well-planned aquatic activity.

- Enhancing the individual's self-image – being successful in any endeavor enhances the individual's self-image and persons with brain injury often have poor self-image. Success in the eyes of other people, especially peers, is possible with a structured aquatic activity.
- Providing positive emotional outlets – swimming is fun and for some people with brain injury one of the few activities in which they can engage with ease. Aquatic activities provide an environment in which anyone can release frustration safely.
- Lessening the evidence of disability – many impairments are far less evident when the individual is in the water. Wheelchair users often report improved sense of well-being when in the water and freedom of movement.

The effects of an impairment can be either increased or diminished by the environment. The Red Cross[39] current emphasis on normalization and full participation in all of society's activities by persons with disability is an attempt to aid the individual in entering the mainstream of society. Swimming is an activity that may contribute to this process.

When beginning an aquatic therapy program for persons with brain injury, it is important that the instructors are trained and certified adaptive aquatic instructors. In addition, the trained instructor should understand the general characteristics of persons with neurological dysfunction. It is important to understand that some individuals with brain injury may experience neurobehavioral problems, perceptual deficits, distractibility, perseveration, and emotional instability/behavior disorientation. When beginning a swimming program for persons with brain injury, the instructor needs to account for these factors since they will influence the outcome.

Supervision and safety are prime considerations in an aquatic therapy program, especially where the disability may interfere with understanding instructions, or in participating without one-to-one supervision.

Summary and conclusion

The more we learn about the brain, the clearer it becomes that the structure of an individual's brain is the result of a complex interplay between nature and nurture, with the two forces working together and modifying each other's messages to an extent that it becomes meaningless to talk about the individual contribution of one or the other. To the same end scientists have now begun to look at stem cell repair of the damaged brain but realize that without the contribution of relearning and rehabilitation the individual will not become whole. As discussed throughout this chapter, traditional medicine and complementary medicine are both needed if a person with a brain injury is going to be able to cope with life demands. One without the other is meaningless. In the world today, medical rehabilitation of a person with a brain injury depends on having available a full range of services: at the acute stage, surgery, drugs, diagnostic imaging, various machines to monitor intra-cranial pressure, to regulate breathing, etc.; at the community re-entry stage, physical therapy, speech/language therapy, occupational therapy, neuro-psychological therapy, and social/recreational services. Upon closer examin-ation at the acute stages you find, for example, therapists using aromatherapy, massage therapy and other complementary therapy, while at the community re-entry stage you find therapists, for example, performing therapy in a natural setting, employing Tai'Chi for balance, aquatic therapy and hippotherapy for balance, coordination, etc. In other words, there is recognition that traditional medicine and complementary medicine support one another and are needed to help the patient regain cognitive, emotional and physical functioning.

In conclusion, it is important to embrace medicine and complementary medicine when treating people with brain injury.

References

1. Landis, S. (1991). *Maximizing human potential: Decade of the brain report.* Washington, DC: Office of Science and Technology Policy, US Department of Health and Human Services.
2. Ernst, E., et al. (1995). Complementary medicine – a definition. *Br. J. Gen. Pract., 1*, 10–15.
3. Barnes, J. (1999). Article on complementary medicine in the mainstream medical literature. *Arch. Int. Med., 1*, 122–133.
4. Brevoort, P. (1980). The booming US botanical market: a new overview. *Herbal Gram.*, 79–81.
5. Ullman, D. (1995). *The consumer guide to homeopathy.* New York: Tarcher and Putnam.
6. Alon, T. (1980). First encounter with Feldenkrais: a reminiscence. *Somatics, 3*, 1.
7. Feldenkrais, M. (1977). *The case of Nora.* New York: Harper and Row.
8. Goldfarb, L. (1990). *Articulating changes.* Berkeley, CA: Feldenkrais Resources.
9. Feldenkrais, M. (1949). *Body and mature behavior.* New York: International Uni-versities Press.
10. Feldenkrais, M. (1985). *The elusive obvious.* Cupertino: Meta Publications.
11. Feldenkrais, M. (1985). *The potent self.* New York: Harper and Row.
12. Bach-y-Rita, E. (1981). New pathways in the recovery from brain injury, Part 1 and Part 2. *Somatics.*
13. Feldenkrais, M. (1966). Image, movement and actor: restoration of potentiality. *Tulane Drama Rev., 10*, 3..
14. Taylor, P. (1981). The magic of Moshe. *New Age*, December.
15. Zermach-Bersin, D. (1999). resources for awareness through movement. *In Touch*, November.
16. Rywerwant, Y. (1979). *Somatics*, Autumn.
17. Zuck, D. (1997). The Alexander technique. In C. M. Davis (Ed.), *Complementary therapies in rehabilitation.* New Jersey: Slack.
18. Jones, F. P. (1997). *Freedom to change* (3rd ed., pp. 2, 139). London: Mouritz.
19. Jones, F. P. (1965). Method for changing stereotyped response patterns by the inhibition of certain postural sets. *Psychol. Rev., 72*, 196–214.

20. Jones, F. P., & Gilley, P. F. M. (1960). Head balance and sitting posture: an X-ray analysis. *J. Psychol., 49*, 289–293.
21. Caplan, D. (1984). Skeletal appreciations inspired by Alexander. *The Alexandrian, 3*, 3.
22. Austin, J., & Ausubel, P. (1992). Enhanced respiratory muscular function in normal adults after lessons in proprioceptive musculoskeletal education without exercises. *Chest, 102*, 486–490.
23. Nielsen, M. (1994). A study of stress amongst professional musicians. In C. Stevens (Ed.), *The Alexander technique: Medical and physiological aspects.* London: STAT Books.
24. Fisher, K. (1988). Early experiences of a multidisciplinary pain management programme. *Holistic Medicine, 3*, 47–56.
25. Dennis, R. J. (1999). Functional reach improvement in normal older women after Alexander technique instruction. *J. Gerontol. Series A, Biol Sci Med Sci, 54*, M8–11.
26. Duggan, R. (1996). Traditional Acupuncture Institute, Maryland. Paper presented at a seminar on Complementary Medicine and Neurotrauma: A Discussion on Health Care in America, Charlottesville, VA.
27. Menard, M. (1996). Use of auditory feedback after stroke. Paper presented at a seminar on Complementary Medicine and Neurotrauma: A Discussion on Health Care in America, Charlottesville, VA.
28. Sarason, G., & Zitnay, G. (1970). *Creation of a community setting.* New York: Syracuse University Press.
29. Lee, H. C. (1999). *Chinese natural cures.* New York: Black Dog and Leventhal Publishers.
30. Barth, J. T., Diamond, R., & Errico, A. (1996). Massage therapy with TBI patients. *Clin. Encephal., 27*, 183–186.
31. Broshek, D. K, Seemiller, R. A., Diamond, R., & Barth, J. T. (1999) *Disability analysis in practice.* Iowa: Kendall-Hunt.
32. Filley, C. M. (1995). *Neurobehavioral anatomy.* Colorado: University of Colorado Press.
33. Sohlberg, M., & Mateen, C. A. (1989). *Introduction to cognitive rehabilitation: Theory and practice.* New York: Guilford Press.
34. Sandyk, R. (1994). Improvement in word fluency performance in patients with multiple sclerosis by electromagnetic fields. *Int. J. Neurosci., 79*, 75–90.
35. Ramsdell, J. W. (1990). *A rehabilitation orientation on the workup of general medical problems.* Texas: ProEd.
36. Weinreb, R., Freeman, R., & Selezinka, W. (1990). *Geriatric rehabilitation.* Texas: ProEd.
37. Wilson, S. D. (1997). *Qui Gong: Eight easy movements for vibrant health.* Portland, OR: Rudra Press.
38. Sobel, D., & Ornstein, R. (1996). *The healthy mind, healthy body handbook.* New York: Time Life Medical.
39. American Red Cross. (1977). *Adaptive aquatics.* New York: Doubleday.

23 The role of family in the rehabilitation of traumatic brain injury patients

Advocate or co-therapist

José León-Carrión, Claudio Perino, and George A. Zitnay

Introduction

This chapter explains the role that the family should play in the rehabilitation process of a person with brain injury. Authors and family groups propose different roles for families in the process of brain injury recovery.[1-5] Frank[6] suggests that effective rehabilitation may depend on the ability of professionals to understand the dynamics of the family system. Different approaches range from affirming that the family should participate in the rehabilitation process, even being physically present during therapy sessions, to thinking that the family should have a limited role in the process. Not all families are the same, nor are all the environments and contexts in which the different types of families move. In countries with limited resources, families sometimes play an important role in rehabilitation because they are the ones who assist the patient due to the lack of caretakers and specialized personnel in hospitals or because of a lack of finances. Thus, what appears to function in one place may not function in another since the demands of the families depend very much on the socio-economic and cultural status and the level of progress in the country where they live. Furthermore, it is not the family but rather the rehabilitation center where the patient receives treatment that usually has the legal responsibility for the rehabilitation treatment. Therefore, this chapter analyses the role that a given family should play in its environment, rather than the type of family intervention in a highly specialized and complex treatment center, where multidisciplinary methods are used. The question that we are asking is whether the family should be the therapist or the advocate, or somewhere in-between.

The family and brain injury

A person with a traumatic brain injury (TBI) normally lives in a family setting, but many people live alone, by choice or circumstance. In most cultures, family plays a central role in personal development and individual-ization. Family is the support and base where affection leads to progress, where one learns to love, be loved and express feelings. Family is stable, always there, through good or bad. Within the family one learns to under-stand and to tolerate difference. Family is a bond that ties each of its mem-bers together. What happens to one of its components happens to the whole family. A knot is made tying all the ends together. If one of the ends is broken the knot can come undone. The same occurs in a family when one of its members is affected by traumatic brain injury.

However, when a family member has sustained a traumatic brain injury, life continues. Perhaps we should say "fortunately" life goes on and requires participation by all family members. The fact that life goes on is therapeutic, it demands that people go on living. But this does not avoid the sensation that a bomb has exploded in the family during the first moments, days or even months after one of its members sustains a brain injury.

One must keep in mind that TBI occurs as a consequence of an unintentional injury, it is something that cannot be predicted. Therefore it catches the family completely off guard, without any preparation at all. A study by Kreutzer and colleagues[7] investigated the prevalence of psycho-logical distress and unhealthy family functioning among primary caregivers of adult persons with TBI. Approximately half of the caregivers reported elevated distress. High anxiety was found among one-third of the sample, and depression in one-fourth. Some of the caregivers reported paranoid ideation and psychotic answers. Spouses were significantly more likely to report depression and unhealthy family functioning compared to parents. Tranquil-izers or sleeping pills were used by 61% of relatives.[8] But, as Camplair et al.[9] suggested, family members of persons with severe injuries are not universally distressed. Positive influences, including familial, community and profes-sional resources, can help preserve and maintain adaptive family functioning.

Family life is completely disrupted during and after TBI. All normal behavioral patterns change. A lot of time is spent in the hospital with the patient or in the waiting room expecting to hear about the evolution of the injury. Fear of the unknown, of what can occur, is an inevitable outcome. It is hard to accept that what is happening is real and that it is happening in my family; it is something no one wants to believe or accept. No one wants to know anything about what is happening in the outside world or in the home. Families pay all of their attention to this new situation: a loved one whom they feel is a part of them has sustained an injury that has affected his or her brain. For all these reasons, 1 month after injury 39% of relatives suffer clinical depression,[1] and 25% of relatives are clinically anxious and depressed.[10] Standardized measures of psychological distress seem to con-firm the clinical impression that family caregivers of people with TBI feel alienated, isolated, overwhelmed, and mentally preoccupied, according to a study done by Gervasio and Kreutzer.[11] Spouses experience more distress, suggesting that earlier marital intervention may be needed and helpful.

Perino[12] shows that spouses seem to need more "personal time" to cope better, and that parents consider physical problems more than spouses do. But at the same time there is a tendency for families to deny disability, fantasize about noticeable improvements even though none have actually occurred, and express unrealistic optimism for patient recovery.[5,13,14] Many family members, especially spouses and/or parents, experience chronic sorrow,[15] in which the family member goes through grieving of the loss of the person that was, while trying to understand the new person. Chronic sorrow is often expressed over a lifetime, especially at important milestones, such as birthdays, wedding anniversaries, etc.

Family systems

All families are not the same

Not all families are the same in their internal organization or in socio-economic and cultural levels. Sociologists, social psychologists, and family therapists have demonstrated that the history of the family is a story of diversity and complexity.[16-19] Even so, in general, facing the impact of brain injury in a family depends on the type of family to which the person with TBI belongs. A study by Perino[12] found that socio-cultural bias must be considered when coping with TBI. There exist, in a simplified manner, at least two forms of family organization, nuclear and extended, and within these are structured and unstructured, and other types of non-conventional and at-risk families, as illustrated in Figure 23.1.

Both nuclear and extended families have their own resources for confronting the sudden crisis when one of their members sustains a traumatic brain injury. The greater or lesser impact will depend on the family organization. In structured families, the affective and organizational shock will be greater than in unstructured families, at least in the first phase. In non-structured families, the problems of one of its members have never had as strong an impact on the rest of the family, for which TBI will alter the situation somewhat, but not as substantially. The functioning of a structured family depends on where each of its members fits in. However, in a short time the structured family will be more capable of confronting the new situation positively for the patient and, in a short time, being in a position to use their own resources and those offered by the community to move forward into the post-acute phase.

In non-conventional family contexts (NCF) the appearance of brain injury in one of its members is an event that complicates the difficult situation in which, in many cases, NCF are living. In *at-risk families*, the situation is often worse given the relationships between the members and lifestyles (drugs, alcohol, prison, delinquency, etc.). Their own current individual survival is already difficult, and the fact that one of them sustains a TBI is a factor that may lead to further disintegration. At-risk families do not have the resources to properly face the complexity of a TBI. On the other hand, many of its

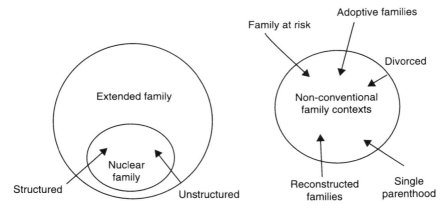

Figure 23.1 TBI can appear in any kind of family. Coping mechanisms are not the same for every family context. Family cohesion, traditions of coping and caring all play a role in how the family will handle the advent of the sudden onset of a TBI. Family financial conditions play a significant role in recovery and coping.

members support each other physically and psychologically in their own ways, being the only thing they have and each other's only resource. The biggest factor influencing how these families cope with a TBI is financial. Without financial means stress, guilt, anger, fear and a sense of hopelessness often lead to further family breakdown. Family support is needed to help these families through the rehabilitation process.

In *adoptive families*, the impact of TBI within tends to be very similar to nuclear families, if they follow that type of organization. In general, in our experience, coping mechanisms may be better depending on two factors: the child's age when adopted (better coping when adopted at a younger age), and the mechanism of injury. The family copes better when the TBI patient is not responsible for his or her TBI. That is, when TBI is the result of an unintentional injury rather than the lifestyle of the adopted person.

Divorce is devastating for the recovery of a married person with TBI. Some couples whose relationship was not very strong before the accident are not able to handle the different evolving phases of TBI, and the non-injured partner tends to be unable to deal with an additional difficult situation and ends up asking for a divorce. Within 7 years of a severe head injury to one partner, 30% of marriages end in divorce (14–18% in normal population).[20] Other authors have found an incidence of separation and divorce in nearly half of the couples when one of the partners sustains a brain injury, regardless of whether they have children or not. The longer they have been married, the less the possibility of separation or divorce. According to Webster et al.,[21] the difficulty of coping with a spouse's head injury is reported to differ from that of adjusting to other injuries (e.g., spinal cord injury) because of the added neurobehavioral sequelae. These are reported by spouses as harder to live with than physical disability and can adversely affect most aspects of the relationship. Often the non-injured spouse must assume roles within the family that he/she is unprepared for, such as managing finances.

For children, researchers tend to show mainly the negative aspects of parent–child relationships during and after divorce: eroding discipline, parenting stress, or problems in children's adjustment.[22,23] However, people seem to agree that divorce does not greatly impair or damage the children's relationship with the custodial parent.[24,25] Other research indicates that parental support is multifaceted in nature and contributes to life satisfaction and well-being for children and young adults. After divorce, more positive feelings towards parents, especially mothers, were associated with better psychological functioning for adolescents. In the cases of children with TBI involved in the process of their parents' divorce, it is very necessary to take care of the divorced parent–child relationship. First, emphasize closeness, appreciation, tenderness, support, and making the child feel both parents are available when needed. All of this has a positive effect on the recovery of the child, especially in the emotional aspect of recovery. Children with TBI need to learn that they are not the cause of the divorce. This is important, since children often blame themselves.

Single parenting is an ever more common situation in many developed countries. According to the 1996 US Bureau of Census report,[26] by 1994 in the US family profile 37.8% of all births were to unmarried women. Of these, 20.6% were births to unmarried women aged 30–44 years. Some authors express concern about the family decline,[27] while others write that it is only a change in the family configuration emerging from new social patterns and economic factors.[28] For others, single motherhood's choices are influenced by economic aspects and by men's new attitudes and commitment to family.[18,29]

The family structure in single-parent families is very different from families with a father and a mother. In the first case, all of the educational responsibilities, including emotional and social aspects, fall on only one adult. When single parenting is voluntary or is accepted, the care of children with TBI is not compromised, and the parent copes well enough with his/her resources to support the recovery of the child with TBI. But this is not true for teenage mothers or mothers dealing with poverty. One of the biggest problems appears when a single parent has to work every day in order to survive, and if he/she does not work they have no income. In 1994, according to the US Labor Department, there is an increasing number of women in the formal labor market resulting from a variety of social and demographic factors. At the same time there is a growing number of adult persons in need of long-term care assistance, and more people than ever before are combining family care and employment responsibilities. Today, nearly 60% of mothers and 80% of fathers with children under the age of 6 are employed in the USA. In addition, more than 80% of the long-term care assistance needed by older adults is provided by family members, of whom approximately one-half are employed full time,[30] and there is an increasing number of people working who have multigenerational (children and disabled old parents) caregiving responsibilities.

The need of single parents to work not only has repercussions on the child's care, but also on the single parent's emotional life. Single parenthood and TBI are very difficult to combine, and economical and emotional problems for the mother or father will arise. A single mother or father is going to need social as well as professional support. Many of these families have no social network, so it will be more difficult, but if the child with TBI is going to recover, a social network will need to be created.

Reconstructed families

Present divorce rates mean that a significant number of children are being co-parented in reconstructed families. Many studies show that, in spite of legal reforms in past years (joint legal custody, mediation, and so forth), many parents find the co-parenting role very difficult.[31,32] Coping with TBI in a reconstructed family depends on the quality of co-parenting relationships. The more inherent aspects on how reconstructed families cope with this situation are related to the conflict with the other spouse, how responsibilities are shared, the frequency of contact with the former spouse, the child's satisfaction with his or her mother/father's new partner, and the new couple's satisfaction and acceptance of the child who may, as a result of the TBI, be a different child.

Socio-economic and cultural status related to TBI outcome

In our experience, a family's socio-economic and cultural status has a definitive impact on the prognosis and course of rehabilitation of persons with TBI. Even when the prognosis is worse for a patient with a high socio-economic and cultural (SECS) level than a patient from a low SECS, recovery may be better in the first case. That is, patients that come from a high economic and cultural status will often recover better than patients belonging to a low level, even when the prognosis was worse for the high SECS.

This is true mainly because families with high SECS know how and are accustomed to better using their resources and those of the community in their own interest, and in this case, in the interests of the person with a brain injury. Also, these families are used to making decisions and not conforming to and accepting reports, advice or points of view given to them by others. High SECS families are accustomed to making their own decisions after collecting information and their decisions are directed toward resolving the problem in the best possible way quickly and using the most possibilities. They do not give up easily, and try to use all of the keys of the system to obtain the searched for results.

On the other hand, families with low SECS are more accustomed to letting others decide for them in different aspects of their lives, since the medical model supports this kind of compliance, especially when a professional gives them a report on a situation or a health treatment plan to follow. They are highly unlikely to do the contrary and simply do what they have been told. Often information that is understandable and useful is not available to help them with decision making. They accept the facts as they are presented. Also, many of them do not know how to use resources available in the community to help them solve social and health problems, and they may not even be familiar with the laws in their favor.

All of this is very important when a patient arrives at a rehabilitation center for the first time seeking treatment. When giving information to the family members about treatment possibilities, the socio-economic and cultural level to which the family belongs should be considered. The quality and quantity of information given to the families and how they treat this information will influence the resources they use in the patient's recovery process, and even the possibility of the patient's being treated. In the USA, the Brain Injury Association has developed multimedia venues for families to assist them with answering questions about TBI. Headway in the UK offers families a support network as do other family associations.

Influence of legal issues in the recovery of TBI patients

The role of the family

The role of the family when taking on the legal aspects of TBI is very important for getting economic and healthcare resources for correct and proper treatment of the patient. As Voogt reports,[33] TBI has created a multitude of legal issues. After an accident, blame is often sought so that a party can be found responsible for the cost of care for the injured party. In the USA, and increasingly in many European countries, this contributes to the rise of third-party lawsuits. For people sustaining TBI there is a direct relationship between quality of life and financial resources. As such, healthcare issues become part of legal complications and the individual's quality of life is compromised. One problem is the lack of lawyers who are trained in the complex nature of representing individuals with TBI. Often, lawyers do not have expertise in TBI and lack the resources to obtain the services of those who do.

In this aspect, the family's role is primary. They must try to obtain all the economic and social resources available in order to make the patient's recovery possible, with the final objective of trying to obtain maximum physical and psychological independence for the patient, and the best possible quality of life. At the same time, as León-Jiménez reports,[34] it is crucial to confront the ethical and legal aspects of this matter in order to ensure that the results of the recovery process are as satisfactory as can be deemed possible. Along these same lines, it would be especially useful to establish a series of general ethical principles to be adopted by those professionals, who, for different reasons, might have influence over the patient's life during this process.

In a study by León-Jimenez, León-Carrión and colleagues,[35] they conclude with the following proposals:

1   The European legal system of compensation for personal damage is reasonable and acceptable in very general terms, although it could be improved, especially when referring to compensatory amounts. However, there are many defects and malfunctions in the legal treatment of traumatic brain injury caused by culpable actions resulting from motor vehicles.
2   Neuropsychological and physical rehabilitation of patients should be the main objective to satisfy. Public powers have an obligation; the objective of the judicial process should focus on recovery more than on economic compensation, trying to avoid serious injustices.
3   It is necessary for judges and prosecutors to be aware of the special incapacitation of this type of injured person. These professionals should promote directing the compensation towards rehabilitation, and not only granting economic compensation to family members. In this way it is necessary to articulate formulas to follow and to direct rehabilitation, both during the process and after settlement.
4   A mindset of agreement should be promoted in judicial processes involving TBI. The agreements should be centered on favoring the expectations of the patient's recovery. This attitude will not only benefit the patient's rehabilitation, but also the economic interests of payors.

The role of the family should be centered on helping find the legal means to achieve maximum recovery of the patient. Compensation must be directed to helping with the rehabilitation and quality of life for the person with the TBI as well as for the family. Family associations play an important role in helping families find proper legal support, and later proper rehabilitation in community-based, post-acute rehabilitation programs.

Desired and undesired conditions for family intervention

Everything written to this point suggests that the family's intervention in the rehabilitation process of persons with brain injury is desirable under most conditions but not under others. In a survey conducted in Italy on family presence in an acute rehabilitation ward asking if family presence is helpful for the patient, results showed disagreement between families and staff. While 95% of the families consider their presence helpful during rehabilitation, this is only considered helpful by 75% of the staff. In addition, 85% of the staff recommended regulation of the possible presence of the family. Also 15% of the staff said that the presence of family members should be avoided (see Table 23.1). These figures suggest that there are favorable and non-favorable conditions for family participation according to this study (see Table 23.2). Table 23.3 sums up the advantages, disadvantages and conflicts of desirable family participation. Table 23.4 displays practice guidelines for family participation adapted from the Italian Rehabilitation Medicine Society TBI Section Group Seminars 1997–1998.

Intervention with the families

In general, family participation is desirable in the patient's rehabilitation process, and families should be an integral part of the rehabilitation team.[36] Centers should include family members in their programs, training opportunities and educational programs. Family support groups play an important role in the rehabilitation process. Many centers offer family members the opportunity to meet with the patient in group sessions with other families to provide emotional support and help in working through family issues. It is important for centers to have established procedures for the family during the whole rehabilitation process. The family should be included in the

Table 23.1 Consideration of family presence during acute rehabilitation

	Families (%)	Staff (%)
Helpful	95	75
Difficult to sustain	22	28
Need to be regulated	34	85
Should be avoided	0	15

Table 23.2 Favorable and non-favorable conditions for family participation in the rehabilitation process of a TBI patient

Desirable	Non-desirable
When it is included in the rehabilitation center's program	When it is not included in the rehabilitation center's program
In the process of emotional recovery as presented by the team	during the cognitive rehabilitation program in the center
In returning to the community	during physical rehabilitation
In the legal process	during medication
	When the family is very sensitive to the new situation
	When the family is seeking mainly economical compensation
	When the patient had a bad prior relationship with the family or previous legal conflict with them
	In families at-risk

Table 23.3 Advantages and conflicts of family participation in the TBI rehabilitation process

Advantages	Family education and adaptation
	Patient monitoring
	Positive/loving environment for the patient
	Patient reassurance and care continuity
	Family orientation to reality
	Evaluation of family roles and dynamics
Disadvantages	Additional staff work
	Staff/family conflicts
Conflicts	Different cultural and educational backgrounds
	Different institutional roles
	Healthcare providers unable to tolerate projection of family crisis onto staff member

Table 23.4 Family participation practice guidelines of the Italian Rehabilitation Medicine Society TBI Section Group Seminars, 1997–1998

Intervention with the family in the acute rehabilitation period	Assess level of information and misunderstanding
	Evaluate attitude and expectations
	Inquire about premorbid situation and accident circumstances
	Find a primary referent in the family
	Illustrate facility organization and therapies
	Communicate about ongoing clinical changes
	Inform on behavior with patient and staff
	Find out about socio-cultural and religious background
Family participation in the rehabilitation process	Discuss presence in the unit
	Possibly identify and educate a primary caregiver
	Regulate all visits of family and friends
	Involve in therapy observation (not direct participation at this time)
	Educate on specific tasks with the patient during meals, rest, night, weekends
Family education before discharge	Find out about logistics at home
	Solve practical problems and prescribe disability equipment if needed
	Organize family psychological support if necessary
	Organize patient home visits before discharge
	Find social support in the community

development of the rehabilitation plan and involved in setting goals for the patient as well as for the family. Persons with TBI can, in most instances, set their own goals with support from the team. The most traditional methods for family intervention have been: counseling, education and support,[5,37,38] and recently telerehabilitation has been included to support families caring for individuals with prolonged states of reduced consciousness at home.[39]

The family plays an especially relevant role in the person with TBI's reintegration in society. This intervention is fundamental because the person with TBI must return to his or her own family and community, and it is predictable that the family members know the patient better than anyone else. The family should be involved in the established plan of social integration to make it possible for the person with TBI again to lead a normalized social life and adapt to their new situation.

When a family cannot cope with or does not want to accept the new person who has emerged from a TBI, it is necessary to establish a surrogate support system or family.[40] This can be through a friend, a student or family association. Not all families can, or want to, participate in the rehabilitation process. This is important to ascertain when developing the rehabilitation treatment plan. Regular family conferences need to be scheduled to make sure that the families are following the rehabilitation treatment plan. Case managers need to be aware of problems with compliance or denial of problems. Family issues should be included in staff conferences and where possible family members should be included so that they understand, accept and support the plan.

The rehabilitation team must pay special attention when they detect that the family is more interested in monetary compensation than the patient's cure or rehabilitation. These cases are especially disruptive for the rehabilitation process because in many cases both the family and the legal team do not want the patient to obtain significant and noticeable improvements, since these improvements can substantially diminish the compensation being pursued. In these rare cases the rehabilitation team must be aware that therapeutic achievements obtained by the patient observed by the family can be cause for discussion and problems in their relationship with the patient's family. We have seen how families have asked the patient to be discharged from the rehabilitation center to avoid forensic examiners noticing any type of recovery in the patient. This type of family seeks medical and neuro-psychological reports informing about the most severe damages and sequelae to present in court to guarantee maximum economical compensation. While this type of family is rare, it does exist.

The other condition when it is better for the family not to participate is knowledge that the prior family–patient relationship was disruptive and even damaging, and dangerous for the person with TBI. In these cases, the team of specialists must be very cautious. It may be important for a case manager to pay special attention to this kind of situation and to find other surrogate family supports.

Concluding remarks

One of the great controversies in the rehabilitation of brain injury patients is the role of the family in the rehabilitation process. Some authors say that the family should actively participate in this process, but others believe the role should only be to find resources so the patient can be treated in the best conditions. In the first case the family acts voluntarily as non-specialized co-therapists, while the role of the second group is to advocate in order to cope with this new situation after TBI.

However, both the role of the co-therapist and that of the advocate depend on the type of family of the person with TBI, the socio-economic and cultural level, and the legal issues. Therefore not all families can be prepared to act as co-therapists or to actively participate in the patient's recovery process. In a few cases family participation may even be undesired. It is also true that not all families have appropriate mechanisms to cope with or, in other cases, to act as advocates for the patient in the new situation created by brain injury.

Each family has its own role depending on how it functioned before the injury. Under no circumstance should members of the family unit substitute the role of professionals specialized in the rehabilitation of person with TBI. This only impedes the cognitive and emotional progress of the patient. It can be good, at times, to give the family a break and put all the responsibility for rehabilitation in the hands of the professionals. Breathing space and rest intervals should be available to family members.

In all cases, unless contraindicated, in the design of the patient's rehabilitation program, family members should be included as part of the rehabilitation. Their role must be specifically and precisely defined. The design for the rehabilitation plan should include therapeutic techniques for managing the feelings and emotional reactions of the family during the rehabilitation program.

The role of the family after discharge from the specialized rehabilitation center is critical since successful re-entry into the family and community is a large part dependent on family support. Therefore this needs to be planned for from day one of the rehabilitation process. TBI not only affects the person with the injury but the whole family. Families are an important resource that can be mobilized through education and support.

References

1. Oddy, M., Humphrey, M., & Uttley, D. (1978). Stresses upon the relatives of head-injured patients. *Br. J. Psychiatry, 133*, 507–513.
2. Livingston, M. G., Brooks, D. N., & Bond, M. R. (1985). Three months after severe head injury: psychiatric and social impact on relatives. *J. Neurol. Neurosurg. Psychiatry, 48*, 870–875.
3. Frank, R. G., Haut, A. C., Smick, M., Haut, M. W., & Chaney, J. M. (1990). Coping and family function after closed head injury. *Brain Inj., 4*, 289–295.
4. Moore, A., Stambrook, M., & Peters, L. (1993). Centripetal and centrifugal

family life cycle factors in longterm outcome following traumatic brain injury. *Brain Inj., 7,* 247–255.

5. León-Carrión, J. (1994). *Brain injury: Guide for families and caregivers.* Madrid: Siglo XXI.
6. Frank, R. G. (1994). Families and rehabilitation. *Brain Inj., 8,* 193.
7. Kreutzer, J. S., Sander, A. M., & Fernandez, C. (1997). Misperceptions, mishaps, and pitfalls in working with families after traumatic brain injury. *J. Head Trauma Rehabil., 12,* 63.
8. Panting, A., & Merry, A. (1972). The long-term rehabilitation of severe head injuries with particular reference to the need for social and medical support for the patient's family. *Rehabilitation, 38,* 33.
9. Camplair, P., Kreutzer, J. S., & Doherty, K. (1990). Family outcome following adult traumatic brain injury: a critical review of the literature. In J. S. Kreutzer and P. Wehman P. (Eds.), *Community integration following traumatic brain injury.* Baltimore, MD: Paul H. Brookes.
10. Brooks, N. D. (1991). The head-injured family. *J. Clin. Exp. Neuropsychol., 13,* 155.
11. Gervasio, A. H., & Kreutzer, J. S. (1997). Kinship and family members' psychological distress after traumatic brain injury: a large sample study. *J. Head Trauma Rehabil., 12,* 14.
12. Perino, C., et al. (1999). La riabilitazione del traumatizzato cranioencefalico. In G. N. Valobra (Ed.), *Trattato di Medicina Fisica e Riabilitazione,* 1515–1544. Ed. UTET, Turino, Italy, 2000.
13. Romano, J. L. (1974). Family response to traumatic head injury. *Scand. J. Rehabil. Med., 6,* 1.
14. Springer, J. A., Farmer, J. E., & Bouman, D. E. (1997). Common misconceptions about traumatic brain injury among family members of rehabilitation patients. *J. Head Trauma Rehabil., 12,* 4.
15. Sarason, S., Zitnay, G., & Kaplan Grossman, F. (1972). *Creation of a community setting.* New York: Syracuse University Press.
16. Hareven, T. K. (1994). Historical perspectives on the family and aging. In R. Blieszner and V. H. Bedford (Eds.), *Handbook of aging and the family* (pp. 13–31). Westport, CT: Greenwood Press.
17. Glenn, N. D. (1997). A critique of twenty families and marriage. *Family Relations, 46,* 197.
18. Stacey, J. (1990). *Brave new families.* New York: Basic Books.
19. Coontz, S. (1997). *The way we really are.* New York: Basic Books.
20. Stilwell, P., Stilwell, J., Hawley, C., & Davies, C. (1997). *The national traumatic brain injury study* (p. 80). Coventry: Centre for Health Services Studies, University of Warwick.
21. Webster, G., Daisley, A., & King, N. (1999). Relationship and family breakdown following acquired brain injury: the role of the rehabilitation team,. *Brain Inj., 13,* 593–603.
22. Capaldi, D. M., & Patterson, G. R. (1991). Relation of parental transitions to boys' adjustment problems: I. A linear hypothesis. II. Mothers at risk for transitions and unskilled parenting. *Dev. Psychol., 3,* 489.
23. Hetherington, E. M. (1989). Coping with family transitions: winners, losers and survivors, *Child Dev., 60,* 1.
24. Acock, A., & Demo, D. (1994). *Family diversity and well being.* Thousand Oaks, CA: Sage.

25. Aquilino, W. S. (1994). Impact of childhood family disruption on young adults' relationships with parents. *J. Marriage and the Family, 56*, 295.
26. US Bureau of Census (1996). *Statistical abstracts of the US: 1996* (116th ed.). Washington, DC: US Government Printing Office.
27. Blankenthorn, D. (1995). *Fatherless America: Confronting our most urgent social problem.* New York: Basic Books.
28. Stacey, J. (1996). *In the name of the family.* Boston, MA: Beacon.
29. Gerson, K. (1997). The social construction of fatherhood. In T. Arendell (Ed.), *Contemporary parenting: Challenges and issues.* Thousand Oaks, CA: Sage.
30. Fredriksen, K., & Scharlach, A. (1999). Employee family care responsibilities. *Family Relations, 48*, 189.
31. Maccoby, E. E., Depner, C. E., & Mnookin, R. H. (1990). Coparenting in the second year after divorce. *J. Marriage and the Family, 52*, 141.
32. Ahrons, C. R., & Rodgers, R. H. (1987). *Divorced families: An interdisciplinary developmental view.* New York: Norton.
33. Voogt, R. (1997). Economic and legal aspects of neuropsychological rehabilitation. In J. León-Carrión (Ed.), *Neuropsychological rehabilitation: Fundamentals, innovations and directions.* DelRay Beach, FL: St. Lucie Press.
34. León-Jiménez, F. (1998). Ethical and legal issues in brain injury rehabilitation. *NeuroRehabilitation: An Interdisciplinary Journal, 11*, 107.
35. León-Jiménez, F., León-Carrión, J., Murga, M., Domínguez-Morales, M., Lucena, R., & Vela-Bueno, J. Y. (1999). Economic impact of intensive treatment of brain injury derived from traffic accidents: an economic–legal perspective. *Revista Española de Neuropsicología, 1*, 99–118.
36. León-Carrión, J. (1998). Rehabilitation models for neurobehavioral disorders after brain injury. *Brain Inj. Source, 2*, 16.
37. Sachs, P. R. (1991). *Treating families of brain injury survivors.* New York: Springer.
38. Dell Orto, A. E., & Power, P. W. (1994). *Head injury and the family: A life and living perspectives.* Winter Park, FL: PMD.
39. Hauber, R. P., & Jones, M. L. (2002). Telerehabilitation support for families at home caring for individuals in prolonged states of reduced consciousness. *J. Head Trauma Rehabil., 17*, 489–496.
40. Frank, R. G., Leach, L. R., Bouman, D. E., & Farmer, J. (1994). Family functioning, social support and depression after traumatic brain injury. *Brain Inj., 8*, 599–606.

24 Return to work after brain injury

Davide Vernè, Tiziana Mezzanato, and Elina Caminiti

Introduction

Return to work is considered one of the most important variables of patients' psychosocial outcome after brain injury.[1–3] Studies investigating employment outcome generally revealed a high unemployment rate, ranging between 50 and 78%, that can persist a long time post-injury.[4–8] The majority of TBI survivors are young adults, hence brain injury results in economic hardship on them and on society. Wehman et al.[9] report a social cost of $71,000/year per person for those who survived after head injury in the USA in 1985, including lost productivity and wages, health maintenance and long-term care.

The reasons for failure in work reintegration frequently reported by co-workers and employers are difficulty in social contacts with colleagues, low productivity and irregular presence at work. Subjects often report lack of motivation, fatigue, fears of failure, and difficulty in interaction with co-workers.[10]

Generally TBI patients exhibit physical, cognitive and/or psychosocial impairments that limit employment and other activities of daily living, and people who return to work often do so in sheltered employment or voluntary work.[11] Many other "external" variables affect the employment rates of these people, like community labor market or eventual welfare facilities. Furthermore, traditional placement agencies are in trouble with TBI survivors because their goal is to have clients maintaining their workplace as long as possible, regardless of the individuals' level of satisfaction and motivation. So individuals with severe TBI often receive little or no help with their return to work in a productive position.

Many different training methods can be developed to help TBI survivors return to work, but all efforts must be integrated in a rehabilitation model that copes with the complexity of the individual situation of any particular subject.

This chapter tries to analyze the most important factors involved in designing such a model, discussing data from literature and presenting some interventions already realized. First, we present in a systematic way results of outcome studies looking for those predictive factors that can explain the high number of failures suffered by TBI subjects returning to work. Then, we suggest a three-step framework to achieve the goal of work reintegration in the best way:

1   A functionally oriented assessment of subjects' abilities, directed towards entering a work environment.
2   The job-finding process, which must contemplate participants' interests and abilities as well as employers' requirements.
3   The step of work adaptation, using assistive technology and compensatory strategies taking into account the needs of each single subject.

Inside this general framework, we discuss two types of vocational training, the first defined as *client-centered*, the other one as *job-centered*. A job-centered program puts the emphasis on preparing people for a specific job, and it is appropriate for clients with high performance and limited neurobehavioral or cognitive problems. A client-centered program is characterized by a holistic assessment of the subject, looking for a job that meets his or her characteristics, abilities and residual deficits. Examples of specific programs are provided.

Finally, we present a case study of L, a 40-year-old married man working as a business executive in a multinational corporation, who returned to work after a global outpatient rehabilitation program, the Kite project at the Presidio Ausiliatrice of Turin.

Predictive factors

Outcome studies centered on TBI patients' return to work pointed out a high number of variables involved in this topic.[7,12–18] First, we have to consider some demographic factors. Age is considered important for general outcome: the younger the patient, the better the prognosis. This correlation is not so clear when we specifically consider return to work. It seems that sometimes older people can benefit from their premorbid experience and skills. Furthermore, we have to take into account other concomitant factors; for example, Greenspan et al.[17] reported a lower employment rate for unmarried people, who are expected to be younger than married ones. Other studies[19,20] could not find a significant age difference between employed and unemployed subjects. Crepeau and Scherzer,[13] in a meta-analysis of previous outcome studies, found that the age factor gains a significant role when subjects older than 60 are included.

Also, gender is considered a variable involved in return to work. Mazaux et al.[21,22] found a lower employment rate in a group of women who suffered TBI. Brooks et al.[5] and Schmidt et al.[23] included gender among significant independent variables, but this result is not shared in other studies.[19]

The majority of outcome studies investigated the education level, which is generally considered a predictive factor for global outcome. Greenspan et al.[17] reported an unemployment rate of 27% among patients who have completed high school. The rate is significantly higher in a low education group (56%). The level of education in the healthy population is associated with different status of occupation, but TBI subjects who return to work frequently find a less demanding position despite their education. Success in high status occupations is more difficult because of lower error tolerances, and people who suffer severe brain injury often cannot cope with high production standards. Rappaport et al.,[6] in a 10-year post-injury follow-up, found an overall unemployment rate of 61% (in a fully employed pre-injury group); 11% of the sample was constituted by professionals, and no one returned to his or her previous job. It is probably easier to re-enter competitive work for higher educated TBI subjects, but the loss of vocational status can cause frustration and a low level of motivation.

Alcohol and illicit drug use is another variable normally considered in evaluating outcome in a TBI population, (Witol, Sander, Seel, Kreutzer[24], Wehman et al.[25]) This factor negatively affects the overall cognitive performance and social behavior, and can also be considered an index of the presence of psychiatric symptoms or of an unfavorable social condition.

Level of trauma severity is considered a powerful predictor of return to work and of global outcome in general.[26] When searching for clear and valid criteria to quantify this factor, investigators used many variables as a severity index in their studies, such as length of coma, length of acute hospital stay, length of stay in a rehabilitation unit, Post-Traumatic Amnesia (PTA), Glasgow Coma Score (GCS), TC or MR scan results. The etherogeneity of these measures causes difficulties when comparing different studies. Nevertheless, there is an obvious relationship between clinical status after trauma and general outcome, (Rao et al.[7], Cattelani et al.[27]).

Many authors studied cognitive impairments and behavioral problems after TBI, and their consequences in regard to return to work. Brooks et al.[5] observed lower scores in attentional, verbal, memory and visuo-spatial tests among unemployed TBI subjects. Similarly, Ip et al.[28] studied a group of TBI patients 3 years after trauma and correlated unemployment status with deficits of attention, spatial memory and perceptual/motor skills. Zoccolotti,[29] in a multicentric investigation of 98 Italian TBI patients, pointed out the high significance of attentional disorders as an obstacle to returning to work. The two groups (employed/unemployed subjects) were not different in intelligence test scores, and the author emphasized the specific characteristics of neuropsychological impairments of unemployed subjects.

European researchers documented family members' complaints of cognitive, emotional and behavioral problems in TBI patients. Brooks et al.[30] reported emotional and behavioral problems as well as memory impairment and slowness at 5 years post-injury: personality changes, irritability and bad temper. Thomsen,[8] at 10–15 years post-injury, found that a majority of symptoms reported in the initial evaluation continued to be problematic, such as slowness, poor memory, lack of social contact and irritability. Furthermore, significant worsening was reported in tiredness, lack of interest and sensitivity to distress. One of the most important consequences of behavioral problems is a progressively decreasing size of the patients' social network, with a concomitant increasing reliance on family for emotional support and recreation.[31] People with severe injuries engage in fewer leisure activities and have fewer friends than before trauma.

Brooks et al.[5] tried to identify patients' personality characteristics that could differentiate between employed and unemployed groups at 2–7 years post-injury, and they found that many behavioral factors were significant, such as temper, immaturity, insensitivity, reasonableness, and self-reliance. Serio and Devens[32] identified motivation and temper difficulties as employment obstacles in more than 10% of a sample of relatives' reports.

The description of brain injury sequelae in an unemployed TBI population in the USA depicted by Witol et al.[24] is consistent with that reported by European researchers. Slowness was a pervasive problem affecting reading, writing, thinking and motor skills. Authors reported cognitive problems related to decision making, learning and memory, attention/concentration and lack of coordination. Regarding neurobehavioral impairments, relatives reported impatience, feeling misunderstood by others, boredom and frustration. Substance abuse, arrest and criminal records indicated a high level of psychosocial adjustment difficulties: 25% of the sample was described as moderate or heavy drinkers, and in the subgroup studied more than 10 years post-injury, 22% reported an arrest history and 19% were convicted. In addiction, a history of post-injury psychiatric treatment was reported by approximately two-thirds of the subjects in the same group.

Limited self-awareness is another common impairment in TBI patients which can cause subjects to fail to gain or maintain employment. In fact, they can have overly optimistic expectations or overestimate their skills and suitability for jobs. The problem of self-awareness was already described by Schilder[33] in the acute post-traumatic stage, and it is well known by all rehabilitation staff members, who often experience failure because of low compliance of their TBI patients. Prigatano and Fordyce,[34] and Fordyce and Roueche[35] used their Patient Competency Rating Scale (PCRS) submitted to TBI subjects and their relatives to assess and quantify this symptom, and proposed specific training to cope successfully with the problem. Zettin et al.[36] found that not only patients, but also family members tend to underestimate subjects' deficits. This observation leads to the necessity of involving both patients and their relatives in a rehabilitation program centered on reduction of anosognosia. This training includes strategies such as educating patients about the consequences of brain injury, asking them to discuss their difficulties in groups, and reinforcing all behavior related to an increasing acceptance of their deficits. Family members are involved in some group sessions which discuss correct behavioral strategies to limit patients' denial of deficits.

Recent research is oriented towards investigating the overall functional outcome after brain injury, i.e., Wagner and colleagues.[37] This trend can be very helpful in trying to understand the real impact of residual disabilities on everyday lives of patients. The ultimate goal of rehabilitation is to optimize patients' functioning in their own environments. From this statement it follows that all rehabilitative efforts and programs have to be highly individualized and they must also take into account social, economic, and other environmental factors. The Community Integration Questionnaire (CIQ),[38-40] is a useful quantitative measure of community reintegration after TBI, composed of 15 items related to three independent factors: Home Integration, Social Integration and Productive Activity. Corrigan and Deming[40] found an overall lower level of community integration in a group of brain injured people 3 months after rehabilitation discharge, comparing these scores to retrospective ones for pre-injury functioning. The worsening was due to lower Social Integration and Productive Activity scores, while no significant difference was found for the Home Integration factor.

Sander et al.[19] studied a sample of TBI subjects previously admitted to rehabilitation via a longitudinal research design. Data were available about pre-injury productivity status, and 1, 2, 3 or 4 years post-injury follow-up. CIQ was submitted directly to patients or to close relatives. Results showed scores on the Home Integration and Social Integration scales similar to those for Willer's[38] sample without disabilities, but lower Productive Activity scores. Evidence is not provided for changes over time. The employment rates of this sample were dynamic. 25% of subjects employed at first follow-up had lost their work by the final follow-up, and 50% of unemployed people at the first follow-up did not change their status at the end. Only three of these subjects obtained competitive work; the others were engaged in other productive activities, like academic activity, voluntary work and homemaking. Authors pointed out the necessity of collecting information regarding wages, numbers of hours worked, level of employment, supervisor's ratings and level of satisfaction in order to clearly understand employment patterns. In summarizing conclusions about studies of predictive variables of return to work, we can outline some points:

1   One of the most powerful predictors of general outcome and post-traumatic employment seems to be the severity of injury. This factor can be measured by many parameters, such as length of hospital stay, length of rehabilitation and length of coma. GCS at admission, PTA length, MR or TC scan results are other clinical tools that can also be used. Researchers should try to reduce the etherogeneity of these indexes.

2   Demographic variables like age, gender or level of education can be useful in understanding global outcome, but they should be considered in a wider context to evaluate their real impact and mutual relationships.

3   Neuropsychological and neurobehavioral problems are strictly related to social and vocational outcome; the evaluation of these variables increases its usefulness when their functional consequences are measured.
4   Pre-injury activity and family and social environment of the sample group must be carefully considered in order to fully understand employment patterns in outcome studies.
5   The CIQ or other similar instruments may be helpful when trying to evaluate functional outcome of a given TBI population. Any rehabilitation framework in which social and vocational reinsertion is promoted should be based on real functioning in everyday life.

First step: patient assessment

The necessity of adequate vocational assistance to return to work is widely recognized by all authors involved in rehabilitation of TBI patients. The purpose of any vocational training is to match a specific subject to a specific job, and the key elements for obtaining this result are the trainee (or client) and the available job. Trainees' skills must be determined through vocational profiling, and job characteristics have to be determined through job analysis. Different models of vocational rehabilitation are available but, in any case, the first step is to assess residual skills and abilities of TBI subjects and their mutual interaction with "external" variables such as social condition, disability income and family relationships. The goal is to determine if the subject is able to return to work and then to decide what kind of job this particular individual can do. Three different choices are available regarding return to work after brain injury:

1   The possibility of not returning to work.
2   Non-competitive participation in a sheltered workshop.
3   Return to competitive work, in the previous position or in a new one.

The second or third choices imply the implementation of a vocational training program based on specific residual abilities of the patient.

A global assessment must take into account different elements that can be collected when interviewing patient and family members, observing the subject in different environments and reviewing records and evaluations about previous work experience. Clinical data about injury and ratings of the neuropsychological, neurobehavioral situation and motor skills must be available.

If the patient is currently involved in a rehabilitation program, this data can easily be obtained by rehabilitators, but if the patient has been previously discharged from a rehabilitation service or no rehabilitation was available before, collecting all information could be difficult and the intervention of different professionals (such as neuropsychologist, occupational therapist, physician, and so on) should be taken into account.

At any rate, the goal of assessment is to determine how subjects function in their environment, and available data must be considered accordingly. We will now analyze a possible framework for global evaluation of TBI survivors.

Motor skills

It is difficult to define one or more "typical" frameworks of motor disability due to traumatic brain injury. Roberts[41] reported that 40% of his TBI population was hemiplegic and 20% suffered a "mixed" syndrome with hemiparesis and cerebellar symptoms. Also, the level of severity of motor disability can vary widely, with different impact on ADLs. In any case, a large number of severe TBI patients show motor slowness, low levels of coordination and difficulty in fine movements, especially of hands.

The impact of damaged motor skills on return to work differs widely according to the type of job and, for this reason, it is very useful to express residual motor abilities in terms of global autonomy in daily life activities.

Cognitive abilities

A complete neuropsychological assessment can give essential information about residual cognitive abilities not only for severe injuries, but also for mild and moderate ones. Brain damage in TBI is often global and diffuse and, consequently, cognitive functions can be impaired at any level. In a TBI population we can very often find attentional disorders and memory and executive function impairments, plus loss of verbal skills or poor vision. Cognitive abilities have to be measured in a quantitative way by neuropsychological tests, and also by "ecological" trials that are frequently sensitive to complex functions such as planning or problem solving. Family members can often give important feedback about real cognitive potentialities of patients in everyday life, and these observations can be useful in completing the picture designed by neuropsychological testing. Finally, we should remember that neuropsychological evaluation must provide information about global functional outcome of the patient, and must be oriented towards answering rehabilitation questions and goals.

Neurobehavioral deficits

Behavioral and emotional consequences of TBI are very often reported by relatives, even years post-injury. These symptoms are the result of neurological lesions and of emotional distress caused by consequences of the traumatic event on everyday life. It is often very difficult to distinguish between the direct effects of the injury and the psychodynamic response of the subject to his or her trauma. Thomsen[8] reported a significant worsening of some symptoms like tiredness and sensitivity to distress 10–15 years post-injury.

Residual neurobehavioral problems and social skills can be assessed only by directly observing the behavior of the patient, for example in a rehabilitation group setting, and by collecting information from interviews with relatives and friends. To do that in a systematic way, it is very helpful to use a quantitative instrument like the Neurobehavioral Rating Scale (NRS) or the Neurologically-related Changes in Personality Inventory (NECHAPI).[42,43] These are checklists of the most common behavioral problems of TBI subjects expressed by simple sentences that can be easily understood by non-specialists. These questionnaires can be submitted directly to patients and their relatives, but the ratings have to be matched with operators' observations, because of the patients' tendencies to underestimate their own behavioral problems. We should not forget that the same bias can sometimes be revealed by relatives' ratings.[36,44] Differences in evaluation between professionals, family members and patients can be used as a measure of the level of deficit awareness.

Pre-injury and post-injury alcohol and illicit drug use has to be recorded, because this factor heavily affects social behavior, and can also be considered an index of the presence of psychiatric symptoms. A history of drug abuse is sometimes associated with arrest or conviction, and these data often prevent return to work in a competitive environment.

Demographic and social variables

Demographic variables, as presented in the previous paragraph, and premorbid work activity are involved in return to work and mutually interact. For example, let us analyze the importance of age. The majority of the TBI population is composed of young people who did not work consistently before trauma. This situation can also be favorable because it allows more flexibility in planning specific training before employment. On the other hand, young people are not very frequently able to express vocational aspirations because they had not experienced them before in any work situation. In the case of adults with TBI, work performed pre-injury is often not feasible post-injury, and patients cannot give consistent feedback about their preferences. People who pre-injury had higher status occupations frequently have to change their employment and find a less demanding job. This experience can lead to failure because of a low satisfaction rate.

A high educational status is normally considered to be a good predictor of global social and occupational outcome, because of better pre-injury cognitive instruments: at the same time, people with higher education have high work aspirations that are often frustrated by current post-injury limitations in working skills. These individuals are expected to experience frustration when a lower occupational status is proposed post-injury, and this situation can lead to poor acceptance of the new condition.

Finally, TBI survivors returning to work can be afraid of losing disability income or medical insurance, especially when these constitute a significant part of the total amount of family income.

Family situation

It is essential to evaluate the role of the subject in his or her family and the change that return to work of the subject can produce. Recovery of a productive status can modify the position of the subject in a radical way, and the evaluation of a patient's expectation and that of his or her relatives is important in trying to understand what kind of feedback family can give.

When the subject lives with his or her parents, the family sometimes accepts loss of autonomy due to injury. They may respond with an overprotective attitude to the new condition, unconsciously reinforcing childish behavior of the subject. In this case, return to work can be associated with an increasing autonomy and, consequently, with the partial loss of parental role. This situation can cause a low collaboration rate of the family with the rehabilitation staff, and possibly a failure of the rehabilitators' goals.

The attitude of spouses is normally different, and rarely they are inclined to overprotect the injured individual assuming a parental role. The rate of divorce or separation after TBI is high because of the difficulty of spouses to accept autonomy loss and modifications of the role of the subject in the family. In these cases, return to work is normally considered a good opportunity to partially recover the pre-injury productive position and to increase level of responsibility.

At the end of this assessment, which could engage professionals for a long time, the staff should be able to give adequate suggestions about further steps in educational/vocational training of the patient according to his or her global level of autonomy. Decisions about returning to work must be reached by rehabilitators, the subject and his or her relatives together, with a high level of agreement if possible, taking into account all elements of the assessment. To do that, a good level of cooperation and adequate feedback on residual abilities are very important to the individual and the family, with the aim of obtaining a high level of acceptance. It is quite difficult for the subject and family members to understand the connections between specific cognitive and neurobehavioral impairments and consequent functional problems. The rehabilitation staff has to clarify this connection throughout the whole rehabilitation program.

If assessment results are compatible with return to work, the following step is to check existing resources that are able to meet patients' needs.

Second step: finding a job

Job finding is the identification of suitable organizations and types of work for individuals. The job finding process can be conducted in two different ways: first, we can look for a particular type of placement that meets the needs of a subject; second, we can look for subjects who can successfully meet placement opportunities held on file. In any event, identified jobs must reflect interests and abilities of participants as well as employers' needs.

In previous paragraphs we emphasized the necessity of global assessment for return-to-work candidates; in the same way, a careful analysis of suitable resources is needed. There are thousands of different types of jobs that people with disabilities can perform well. Wehman et al.[9] identified six main categories:

1   Cleaning and laundry services.
2   Clerical services.
3   Grounds and greenhouse work.
4   Food service.
5   Warehouse, distribution and factory work.
6   Retail work.

An exact identification of job components, such as position title, work site description, specific tasks needed, equipment and supplies is important to have. Another variable to control is the level of communication and interpersonal skills necessary to perform a specific job. It depends in part on particular tasks that are required, and also on specific work sites. All this information can help professionals to check a list of available opportunities for any specific subject, and it can also encourage the individual to choose one or more possible jobs.

Sheltered workshops or pre-vocational training services can be proposed when professionals believe that an individual cannot successfully face a competitive job, or that further specific training is necessary. Nevertheless, these solutions have to be considered at the same time; the subject must meet inclusion criteria and he or she must actively choose a specific proposal. Sheltered workshops are not necessarily a definitive choice, but they can be an intermediate step to competitive employment and an opportunity to observe subjects' work skills.

Pre-vocational training programs have been developed to answer patients' rehabilitative needs and are not necessarily restricted simply to vocational assistance. These programs can be considered part of a global rehabilitation project. An example is TORNEO, a program developed by the Don Calabria Foundation in Ferrara, Italy.[45] TORNEO focuses on four curricular areas: (a) personal profiling and assessment of training needs (global assessment, see previous paragraph); (b) cognitive skills; (c) social skills, such as communication and interpersonal skills; (d) educational/vocational skills. Pre-vocational provision also offers a wide range of supported training options such as decision-making skills, stress management, time management, assertiveness, basic adult education, life skills and work essays.

In the same way, the Kite project of the Presidio Ausiliatrice of Turin, Italy,[46] is a global outpatient rehabilitation program, based mainly on the therapeutic milieu approach,[47] and utilizing mainly group treatment sessions. This project cannot be considered only a pre-vocational training experience, but also a rehabilitative instrument created to link traditional inpatient treatments with patients' social environments.[46,48] The basic assumption of this kind of program is to point out and reinforce patients' residual skills, giving continuous feedback to subjects about their own abilities. It allows the participants to reach a higher level of self-awareness and to reconsider themselves in a more realistic way after trauma. Better self-awareness leads subjects to actively research their own compensatory strategies for coping with everyday life problems and challenges. In a therapeutic milieu approach, return to work can be considered one of the goals to reach in the direction of the best global outcome, and job finding is a step in that process conducted by the rehabilitation staff working with the individual in the context of social reintegration into a natural environment. In another part of this same chapter we will describe a case study relative to the results of this program.

In the USA a number of global rehabilitation programs are available. Independent Living Centers (ILCs) are an interesting example of this kind of framework. ILCs are funded under Title VII of the Rehabilitation Act, and they include counseling, housing, transportation, work placement, attendant and healthcare and recreation. Johnston and Lewis[49] found that 1 year after discharge the percentage of people requiring constant supervision lowered from 72.8% to 13%. In addition, a large number of ILCs have started specific brain injury support groups to expand the social network of TBI patients.[50] Furthermore, ILCs provide information to patients and relatives about the available services in the community.

Third step: work adaptation

Re-entering a productive environment is a challenge that people who suffer from TBI can only face by highly individualized adaptation. The subject's assessment should provide data about global functioning of the individual in a social context. Moreover, a careful analysis of residual motor, cognitive and behavioral disorders that can affect return to work should be carried out. Professionals and individuals together can find helpful tools for adaptation in three different areas: assistive technology, compensatory strategies, and natural supports.

Assistive technology can supply individuals who suffered severe head injuries with a large number of devices that help people in many everyday activities, such as touch talkers, environmental control units, cars with adaptive driving controls, electric wheelchairs, etc.[51] Furthermore, in the last 15 years the rapid improvement of computer technology has given new tools characterized by high flexibility to disabled people. The need for an assistive technology device must be determined by the functional assessment of the individual's environment, and it is important that the user participates in selecting and evaluating different available resources. Furthermore, the subject should learn the practical use of any device and test its effectiveness in daily life. Long-term follow-up should be provided to test new improved devices and determine the possible need for changes over the years.

Compensatory strategies are the adjustments that an individual makes to solve a problem and succeed in a specific task using unconventional procedures. People with TBI need compensatory strategies not only at the workplace, but also in everyday life at home, to cope with their physical, cognitive and behavioral problems. Any strategy is highly individualized because effectiveness has to be evaluated directly by the user, who is directly involved in the development of needed instruments. Professionals help the subject's search for right strategies, taking into account information that comes from family members and co-workers. We have to remember that compensatory strategies, in order to be effective, must be self-initiated and, consequently, comfortable and well-accepted by the user. Modifications of work environment, reorganization of necessary equipment, use of checklists or written cues can compensate well for limitations when performing problematic tasks.

To enhance functional performance in community and workplace, disabled people often develop an informal support network formed by family members, friends and co-workers. This network is called *natural support*, and can be successfully used in return to work programs: West and Parent[52] investigated the effect of the presence of natural support in a group of people involved in a supported employment program. Physical proximity to co-workers, the presence of common areas for meals and opportunities for social interaction inside and outside the work environment were significant factors in successful placement, and the authors concluded that social aspects can be important in promoting return to work for disabled people. Curl et al.[53] described a program in which co-workers, trained and monitored by rehabilitation professionals, were used as trainers of TBI individuals. The program proved effective for one-third of an experimental group.

Looking for an effective model

Which are the characteristics of a truly effective vocational rehabilitation program? Can we design a general framework to cope with all the variables involved in a patient's outcome? First, we have to distinguish between two types of vocational training. We can define the first as *job-centered* and the second as *client-centered.*

A job-centered program puts the emphasis on preparing clients for a specific job and most effort is spent before placement in helping the client to develop abilities in an extensive manner under close supervision. This kind of intervention normally offers sheltered workshops before placement and limited intervention of follow-up after placement. Candidates for these programs are normally selected by excluding people who encountered problems like substance abuse, depression, apathy, disinhibition and aggressiveness. For this reason, this kind of program is appropriate for people with high performance and limited neurobehavioral or cognitive problems.

A client-centered program is characterized by a holistic assessment of the client involved in the choice of a job that meets his or her characteristics, abilities and residual deficits. This kind of program provides for long-term intervention after placement and long-term follow-up. Clients are rarely excluded on the basis of behavioral or medical problems. This second option does not exclude the possibility of intensive training, adaptation and accommodation provided *before* the placement. The Supported Employment model is an example of implementation of this second framework

The Supported Employment model

Supported Employment was first developed in the USA in the late 1970s, with federally funded research, particularly in Virginia, Oregon and Illinois.[9] The initial focus of the research was on people with learning disabilities, but subsequently the project was opened up to the full spectrum of disabilities. The idea of these first programs was that people with severe physical, cognitive or behavioral impairments, normally addressed to sheltered workshops or considered unable to work, could be employed in a competitive environment if given adequate support.[54]

Only in recent years this model has been applied to the brain-injured population, traditionally considered a group with very low rates of return to work, especially after severe injury. Data collected in the USA show good results for this model over a long-term period, with employment ratio increased from 13% to 67%.[15] The Supported Employment model is a service option included in the US vocational rehabilitation service system via the Rehabilitation Acts Amendments of 1986 (Federal Register, 1987). Now, Supported Employment has spread across Europe, and a European Union Supported Employment program has been constituted with individuals working in each member state.

First, it is important to distinguish between *supported employment* and *job support*, two terms that are often confused and used in alternative ways. Supported Employment refers to subjects who are supported in a paid job in a competitive situation. Job support is when somebody, usually voluntary, is supported to train at the workplace. Nevertheless, these two models both share the same principles and also the same key practices.

As any other vocational rehabilitation training, Supported Employment needs vocational profiling of the trainee, and then a subsequent job analysis. Wehman et al.[9] emphasized the necessity of the subject actively choosing the desired employment. In fact, motivational elements are very important in preventing subsequent failure in placement of trainees.

This model suggests that training should be conducted in a competitive position and in a real work environment. The basic idea is that placement should occur *before* training, and then the professional follows the trainee on a long-term basis, supporting him or her in learning and performing the job. According to the principles of this kind of program, job analysis has to be conducted *after* placement, developing a task analysis for each job task that the individual is not able to perform independently. Task analysis is conducted by studying each partial step necessary to achieve the goals. Then systematic instruction is given to the trainee on the job site, using prompts, reinforcing and other training techniques. The operator chooses the necessary tools suitable for the patient's existing cognitive strengths and abilities, in order to maximize the effect of the training.

The Supported Employment model has been developed to promote returning to work in a competitive environment. Therefore people involved in such a project have to maintain a certain production standard. Professionals should find out if a company standard exists, or if they have to determine it by collecting information on how long a worker takes to perform a specific job. The trainer can also do it by observing co-workers and taking an average of production rates based on several samples on different days. The same observations must be made on the trainee, to determine the individual's current production rate and to establish possible differences between company standards and the trainee's performance. A careful analysis of the individual's performance can lead to identifying weaknesses and problems to cope with and therefore, try to implement adequate adaptations.

Another basic characteristic of the model is *follow-along*, defined as ongoing assessment and monitoring of an individual's work performance. It can also be considered a helpful instrument to cope with severe TBI patients' problems with job retention. The aim of follow-along is collecting data, making observations, providing advocacy, and maintaining the availability of additional intervention and support services as needed. Wehman et al.[9] identified some areas in which providing ongoing assessment is needed: (a) level of dependability; (b) current job performance; (c) adherence to company policies; (d) appropriateness of compensatory strategies; (e) dynamics of interpersonal job site relations; (f) changes in work routine or work environment; (g) level of job satisfaction; and (h) "external" factors affecting job performance. The outcome of this data collection allows defining the level of follow-along to be provided and the number of professional contacts, which can fluctuate over time, based on overall job performance of the individual. Follow-along can be implemented using formal and informal methods. Formal methods include the trainee's assessment in task performance, production and quality areas. Informal methods include conversations with the subject, his or her relatives, supervisors and co-workers.

Finally, the Supported Employment model takes into account typical patterns of severely disabled people: frequent job changes due to their deficits, the need to relearn work skills, and the difficulty of successfully identifying job preferences. This model provides long-term support during unemployment periods as well, and the success of the project is determined by the overall participation of the workforce, not by the retention of a single job. In fact, Wehman et al.[16] reported that, on the average, one-third of the entire time of the program is spent between jobs, in an unemployed position. For many people, job keeping tends to improve only with their second or third placement.

The multi-regional project for TBI patients' return to work

An interesting experience of vocational training specifically designed for TBI survivors was carried out in 1997 in three regions in Northern Italy (Piedmont, Veneto and the Autonomous Province of Bolzano) involving 44 persons. The project was funded by the EEC Social Fund and Italian Ministry of Labor and Social Security.[55] The program was reserved for young people who had suffered TBI and were unemployed for over a year. It lasted 700 training hours and the goal was to provide effective training in office automation; 320 h were dedicated to learning the software used in clerical work. Additional specific software was previously developed to provide an instrument for training attention, memory and problem-solving; 240 h were dedicated to these rehabilitative issues. Finally, trainees experienced 140 h of training in private companies and public corporations involved in the project. Cognitive rehabilitation sessions and specific office automation training were carried out side by side, and trainees were engaged in course activity for 6 h every day for the first 3 months, and 8 h subsequently.

Educational enterprises involved in the project supplied office automation teachers, and cognitive training was supervised by rehabilitation professionals, such as occupational therapists, speech therapists and neuropsychologists. There were four different course centers, and a tutor was responsible for the general coordination of each course. All teachers and professionals had attended some preliminary meetings to ensure a common background of knowledge about TBI subjects and their problems, and to define guidelines about teaching and rehabilitation issues. Possible behavioral problems of TBI subjects were discussed with special emphasis, so that teachers could successfully deal with management of group interaction in classrooms and collect data about the social skills of each trainee. Possible candidates were selected on the basis of the following requirements:

- Age 17–35 years.
- Time post-injury, 6 months–10 years.
- Documented unemployed status of more than 1 year.
- Stabilized health conditions, compatible with class attendance.
- Absence of severe motor impairments, with sufficient autonomy in ADLs.
- Absence of severe cognitive and speech impairments.
- Absence of severe behavioral problems in social situations.
- Documented previous attendance at a rehabilitation program.
- Adequate level of individual's motivation.
- Adequate collaboration of family members.

All post-traumatic sequelae were carefully considered: every candidate was submitted to an examination by a physical medicine and rehabilitation specialist; an interview took place with each candidate and his or her family members together, to assess level of autonomy in ADLs, possible behavioral problems, level of motivation and level of family involvement in the project.

Before the beginning of the course, all 44 selected subjects (38 males, 6 females) were submitted to a brief neuropsychological examination by the same psychologist (not otherwise involved in the program), supported by a specialized physician who carried out a behavioral observation. Mean age of our population was 23.9 years (SD 4.9), with a mean education of 10.1 years (SD 2.4). All subjects had suffered a TBI that could be classified as "severe". The neuropsychological battery consisted of six tests:

- Raven colored matrices.
- Digit span forward and backward.
- Corsi's visuo-spatial span, forward and backward.
- Rey's complex figure, copy and memory recall trials.
- Stroop test.
- California Verbal Learning Test (CVLT).

The results of this first baseline cognitive assessment were subsequently compared to the same test battery submitted at the end of the course, to evaluate the effect of the cognitive training included in the project.[56]

At the end of the first part of the course, the tutor and professionals completed a qualitative assessment of each individual, taking into account not only the competence level in the use of the software, but also the overall cognitive performance and social skills. These data allowed an individualized choice of placement for the last 140 hours of real workplace training.

There was a wide range of companies and public corporations involved in this project. Tutors had previously analyzed the kind of specific tasks requested of trainees and other workplace variables "external" to the job, such as proximity with co-workers, necessity of coordination with them in task completion, physical environment, required level of productivity and natural support availability. Tutors met with trainees' supervisors before placement to explain the specific characteristics of the trainee and to plan an individualized training program that could cope with each subject's weaknesses and strengths. For example, one individual showed a high level of anxiety in social contacts in the classroom, and a low rate of endurance to frustration. For this reason, he was placed in a company where he could complete most of the tasks alone, even if under the strict and direct supervision of a co-worker who had previously worked with disabled people having similar behavioral problems.

Tutors visited the subjects regularly at the workplace during the 140 h period, collecting qualitative data about the performance and quality of social skills of the trainees, and eventually providing compensatory strategies to cope with specific difficulties encountered by the subjects. Constant feedback was asked to supervisors, who provided a final evaluation of the training period.

Of the 44 subjects, 39 completed the course successfully, got through an examination and obtained a certificate of vocational qualification. Six months after the end of the program, the level of employed people was verified. The overall employment rate was 46% (18 subjects), and varied from 42% in Piedmont, 46% in Veneto, and 50% in the Autonomous Province of Bolzano. These differences can be due to various social and economic factors. Piedmont is a region with a higher general unemployment rate because of an economic recession. On the other hand, the Province of Bolzano has a special welfare system (22% of employed people in this area work in public companies).

As we explained before, 39 subjects who completed the program were submitted to a final neuropsychological assessment again, with the aim of evaluating the effectiveness of cognitive training implemented during the course. Comparing the results of the first evaluation (pre-training) and the second one (post-training), some differences were found to be statistically significant.[56] The overall performance of subjects in Rey's complex figure memory recall was better in post-training evaluation, both for short-term memory trial ($p = 0.006$) and long-term memory trial ($p = 0.006$). The stimulation of visuo-spatial abilities by cognitive training tools and by working with a specific software application can explain this result. Another interesting result is improvement in the clustering ability of our population in CVLT. These differences reached statistical significance only in the first and last of five recall trials ($p = 0.03$ and $p = 0.01$). Nevertheless, the overall performance of this sample of TBI survivors after intensive rehabilitative training remained under the normal scores both in verbal memory and clustering abilities.

This multi-regional project can be considered a *job-centered* program, due to some of its characteristics. In fact, the participants are selected by inclusion criteria, the emphasis being on training for a specific job, and a workshop was offered before placement. At the same time, we can recognize some peculiarities of a *client-centered* program; first, the role of the tutor in the last part of the training was centered on highly individualized placement. Furthermore, the implementation of cognitive training and the particular care to recognize behavioral problems offered opportunities for a global assessment and adjustment of individuals involved in the project.

From rehabilitation to return to work: a case study

In a previous paragraph we wrote about the Kite project at the Presidio Ausiliatrice of Turin, a global outpatient rehabilitation program aimed at linking traditional inpatient treatment to return to subjects' social environments. We explained that, using a therapeutic milieu approach, return to work can be considered one of the goals to optimize global outcome. In this paragraph we shall describe the story of L, a 40 year-old married man working as a business executive in a multinational corporation. In December 1997, L had an accident driving his car and suffered a severe brain injury. The length of coma was 5 days and the GCS score at hospital admission was 7. TC scans revealed bilateral fronto-basal and left temporal cerebral contusions and a diffuse subarachnoidal hemorrhage. At the beginning of February 1998, L was admitted to Ausiliatrice's inpatient rehabilitation ward, where he rapidly improved his motor and cognitive skills. In March, when L achieved a good level of independence in ADLs measured by the FIM/FAM scale, the rehabilitation team decided to start him in the outpatient program. At that time, neuropsychological assessment revealed slow reaction times, a deficit in working memory, poor verbal learning abilities and problems in planning complex activities. Speech abilities, reading and writing were mostly preserved, but a formal examination detected anomia and poor verbal fluency. L exhibited some behavioral problems, such as unawareness of deficits, logorrhea, verbal perseveration, irritability, depression and anxiety. The psychologist interviewed L's wife, who confirmed data observed by rehabilitation professionals and stressed a poor level of tolerance towards his two sons.

The rehabilitation program included physical therapy (to cope with residual motor coordination deficits), speech therapy and neuropsychological treatment 3 days per week. Individual cognitive training took place with the use of a computer to enhance attentional capacities and to improve memory and problem-solving abilities. At the same time, L met every week with a psychologist to discuss behavioral problems and to reinforce self-awareness and motivation, while looking for adaptive behavioral strategies. L was also included in group sessions with other patients, to discuss difficulties and obstacles in reintegrating into family and social context. The goal of group treatment is to enhance relational and emotional abilities by increasing the control of impulsivity, tolerance and respect for individual differences. This group was subsequently involved in the production of a "magazine" about interests and hobbies of the patients. This work also included some tales and autobiographical short stories in which authors' memories, feelings and fantasies emerged, permitting a higher awareness of patients' own emotions and, as a consequence, a better re-elaboration of emotions. Furthermore, this kind of task stimulated memory, attention, problem-solving and planning abilities in a unconventional way.

Ten months after the beginning of rehabilitation, L and the staff both decided that he was able to return to his previous job. The psychologist interviewed L's co-workers and managers to plan a gradual re-entry in the work environment, while natural supports were identified. L started working part-time (5 h, 5 days/week) and support sessions with the neuropsychologist were established weekly for 3 months, looking for further compensatory strategies for specific cognitive and relational problems. At present, L is successfully employed full-time in the same pre-traumatic position, and a follow-up session is provided twice a year.

This highly individualized project can be considered a *client-centered* program. Intensive training was carried out *before* placement, treating behavioral and cognitive deficits, but a follow-along intervention was planned *after* return to work to give adequate answers to specific adaptation problems in an ecological perspective.

Conclusions

The high unemployment rate of TBI survivors due to the complexity of their physical, cognitive and psychosocial impairments shows that return to work for these subjects is a demanding challenge for rehabilitators. Outcome studies pointed out a high number of variables involved, such as demographic factors, alcohol and illicit drug use, severity of trauma, cognitive impairments, behavioral problems, and limited self-awareness.

The rehabilitation goal is to optimize patients' functioning in their own environments, and it is necessary that all rehabilitation programs be highly individualized. To do that, any vocational training must match a specific subject to a specific job in three steps:

1 *Patient assessment*, which must take into account the clinical data, motor skills, cognitive and neurobehavioral impairments and family and social situation. The ultimate goal is to determine the real global functioning of the subjects in their environment.
2 *Finding a job*, which implies a careful analysis of suitable resources with the exact identification of job components, such as position title, work site, specific tasks needed and equipment. At the same time, jobs identified must reflect candidates' interests and abilities as well as employers' needs.
3 *Work adaptation*, using assistive technological devices and compensatory strategies that have to be well accepted by the user. An informal support network formed by friends, co-workers and family members can be very helpful.

Authors proposed many different models of vocational training, and we can distinguish between *job-centered* and *client-centered* programs. In a job-centered model, most efforts are expended *before* placement offering sheltered workshops and limited follow-up after placement is provided. On the other hand, the client-centered model provides a holistic assessment of the patient and long-term intervention *after* placement. The Supported Employment model is a good example of this second kind of vocational rehabilitation.

Our experience teaches us that both of these models give interesting suggestions for the implementation of different effective vocational training. Rehabilitation professionals can choose among a wide variety of interventions on the basis of their ultimate goals, the types of subjects involved and suitable environmental resources. We hope that the increasing knowledge about functional outcome of TBI survivors and the efforts of many rehabilitators all over the world can raise the number of successfully re-employed individuals in productive positions.

References

1. Kreutzer, J. S., Wehman, P., Morton, M. V., & Stonnington, H. H. (1988). Supported employment and compensatory strategies for enhancing vocational outcome following TBI. *Brain Inj., 2,* 205–223.
2. Buffington, A., & Malec, J. (1997). The vocational rehabilitation continuum: maximizing outcomes through bridging the gap from hospital to community based services. *J. Head Trauma Rehabil., 12,* 1–13.
3. Klonoff, P. S., Lamb, D. G., Henderson, S. W., & Shepherd, J. (1998). Outcome assessment after milieu-oriented rehabilitation: new considerations. *Arch. Phys. Med. Rehabil., 79,* 684–690.
4. Weddell, R., Oddy, M., & Jenkins, D. (1980). Social adjustment after rehabilitation: a two-year follow-up of patients with severe head injury. *Psychol. Med., 10,* 257–263.
5. Brooks, N., McKinlay, W., Symington, C., Beattie, A., & Campsie, L. (1987). Return to work within the first seven years of severe head injury. *Brain Inj., 1,* 5–19.
6. Rappaport, M., Herrero-Backe, C., Rappaport, M. L., & Winterfield, K. M. (1989). Head injury outcome up to ten years later. *Arch. Phys. Med. Rehabil., 70,* 885–892.
7. Rao, N., Rosenthal, M., Cronin-Stubbs, D., Lambert, R., Barnes, B., & Swanson, B. (1990). Return to work after rehabilitation following traumatic brain injury. *Brain Inj., 4,* 49–56.
8. Thomsen, I. V. (1984). Late outcome of very severe blunt head trauma: a 10–15 year second follow-up. *J. Neurol. Neurosurg. Psychiatry, 47,* 260–268.
9. Wehman, P., West, M., Johnson, A., & Cifu, D. X. (1999). Vocational rehabilitation for individuals with traumatic brain injury. In M. Rosenthal, E. R. Griffith, J. S. Kreutzer, and B. Pentland (Eds.), *Rehabilitation of the adult and child with traumatic brain injury.* Philadelphia: F. A. Davis.
10. Cook, J. (1990). Return to work after TBI. In M. Rosenthal, E. R. Griffith, J. S. Kreutzer, and B. Pentland (Eds.), *Rehabilitation of the adult and child with traumatic brain injury.* Philadelphia: F. A. Davis.
11. McMordie, W. R., Barker, S. L., & Paolo, T. M. (1990). Return to work (RTW) after head injury. *Brain Inj., 4,* 57–69.
12. Melamed, S., Groswasser, Z., & Stern, M. J. (1992). Acceptance of disability, work involvement and subjective rehabilitation status of traumatic brain injury patients. *Brain Inj., 6,* 233–243.
13. Crepeau, F., & Scherzer, P. (1993). Predictors and indicators of work status after traumatic brain injury. A meta-analysis. *Neuropsych. Rehabil., 3,* 5–35.
14. Wehman, P. (1981). *Competitive employment: New horizons for severely disabled persons.* Baltimore, MD: Brookes.
15. Wehman, P., Kregel, J., Sherron, P., et al. (1993). Critical factors associated with the successful supported employment placement of patients with severe traumatic brain injury. *Brain Inj., 7,* 31–44.
16. Wehman, P., Sherron, P., Kregel, J., Kreutzer, J. S., Tran, S., & Cifu, D. X. (1993). Return to work for persons following traumatic brain injury. *Am. J. Phys. Med. Rehabil., 72,* 355–363.
17. Greenspan, A. I., Wrigley, J. M., Kresnow, M., Branche-Dorsey, C. M., & Fine, P. R. (1996). Factors influencing failure to return to work due to traumatic brain injury. *Brain Inj., 10,* 207–218.

18. Keyser-Marcus, L. A., Bricout, J. C., Wehman, P., et al. (2002). Acute predictors of return to employment after traumatic brain injury: a longitudinal follow-up. *Arch. Phys. Med. Rehabil., 83*, 635–641.
19. Sander, A., Kreutzer, J. S., Rosenthal, M., Delmonico, R., & Young, M. (1996). A multicenter, longitudinal investigation of return to work and community integration following traumatic brain injury. *J. Head Trauma Rehabil., 11*, 70–84.
20. Perini, P., & Cantagallo, A. (1998). Trauma cranico e ritorno al lavoro: uno studio sui predittori socio-demografici [Traumatic brain injury and return to work: A study on social and demographic predictors]. Paper presented at the symposium Reinserimento lavorativo e sociale di soggetti con esito di trauma cranio-encefalico, Ferrara, Italy.
21. Mazaux, J. M., Dartigues, J. F., Daverat, P., et al. (1989). La réinsertion professionelle des traumatises craniens légers et modérés en Gironde [Vocational reintegration of mild and moderate TBI in Gironde]. *Annales de Réadaptation et de Médecine Physique, 32*, 699.
22. Mazaux, J. M., Levin, H. S., & Vanier, M. (1990). Évaluation des troubles neuropsychologiques et comportamentaux des traumatises craniens par le clinicien: Proposition d'une echelle neurocomportamentale et premiers résultats de sa version française. [Assessment of TBI neuropsychological and behavioral disorders by the clinician. The proposal of a neurobehavioral scale and first results of French edition]. *Annales de Réadaptation et de Médecine Physique, 33*, 35.
23. Schmidt, M. F., Garvin, L. J., Heinemann, A. W., & Kelly, J. P. (1995). Gender and age-related role changes following brain injury. *J. Head Trauma Rehabil., 10*, 14–27.
24. Witol, A. D., Sander, A. M., Seel, R. T., & Kreutzer, J. S. (1996). Long term neurobehavioral characteristics after brain injury: implications for vocational rehabilitation. *J. Vocational Rehabil., 7*, 159–167.
25. Wehman, P., Targett, P., Yasuda, S., & Brown, T. (2000). Return to work for individuals with TBI and a history of substance abuse. *NeuroRehabilitation, 15*, 71–77.
26. Dikmen, S. S., Temkin, N. R., Machamer, J. E., Holubkov, A. L., Fraser, R. T., & Winn, H. R. (1994). Employment following traumatic head injuries. *Arch. Neurol., 51*, 177–186.
27. Cattelani, R., Tanzi, F., Lombardi, F., & Mazzucchi, A. (2002). Competitive re-employment after severe traumatic brain injury: clinical, cognitive and behavioural predictive variables. *Brain Inj., 16*, 51–64.
28. Ip, R. Y., Dornan, J., & Schentag, C. (1995). Traumatic brain injury: factors predicting return to work or school. *Brain Inj., 9*, 517–532.
29. Zoccolotti, P. (1998). Fattori prognostici per il ritorno al lavoro dei pazienti traumatizzati cranici [Prognostic factors in return to work of TBI patients]. Paper presented at the symposium Reinserimento lavorativo e sociale di soggetti con esito di trauma cranio-encefalico, Ferrara, Italy.
30. Brooks, N., Campsie, L., Symington, C., Beattie, A., & McKinlay, W. (1986). The five year outcome of severe blunt head injury: a relative's view. *J. Neurol. Neurosurg. Psychiatry, 49*, 764–770.
31. Kozloff, R. (1987). Networks of social support and the outcome from severe head injury. *J. Head Trauma Rehabil., 2*, 14–23.
32. Serio, C. D., & Devens, M. (1994). Employment problems following traumatic brain injury: families assess the causes. *NeuroRehabilitation, 4*, 53–57.

33. Schilder, P. (1934). Psychiatric disturbances after head injuries. *Am. J. Psychiatry,* *91*, 155–158.
34. Prigatano, G. P., & Fordyce, D. J. (1986). The neuropsychological rehabilitation program at Presbyterian Hospital. In G. P. Prigatano, et al. (Eds.), *Neuropsychological rehabilitation after brain injury.* Baltimore, MD: Johns Hopkins University Press.
35. Fordyce, D. J., & Roueche, J. R. (1986). Changes in perspectives of disability among patients, staff and relatives during rehabilitation of brain injury. *Rehabil. Psychiatry, 31,* 217–229.
36. Zettin, M., Vernè, D., Perino, C., & Rago, R. (1993). Il traumatizzato cranio-encefalico e la negazione della disabilità [TBI patients and unawareness of disability] (abstract in English). *Eur. Med. Phys., 29,* 177–185.
37. Wagner, A. K., Hammond, F. M., Sasser, H. C., & Wiercisiewski, D. (2002). Return to productive activity after traumatic brain injury relationship with measures of disability, handicap and community integration. *Arch. Phys. Med. Rehabil., 83,* 107–114.
38. Willer, B., Rosenthal, M., Kreutzer, J. S., Gordon, W. A., & Rempel, R. (1993). Assessment of community integration following rehabilitation for traumatic brain injury. *J. Head Trauma Rehabil., 8,* 75–87.
39. Willer, B., Ottenbacher, K. J., & Coad, M. L. (1994). The Community Integration Questionnaire: a comparative examination. *Am. J. Physical Med. Rehabil., 73,* 103–111.
40. Corrigan, J. D., & Deming, R. (1995). Psychometric characteristics of the Community Integration Questionnaire: replication and extension. *J. Head Trauma Rehabil., 10,* 41–53.
41. Roberts, A. H. (1979). *Severe accidental head injury: An assessment of long term prognosis.* Basingstoke: Macmillan.
42. Levin, H. S., Goethe, K. E., Sisson, R. A., et al. (1987). The Neurobehavioral Rating Scale: assessment of the behavioral sequelae of head injury by the clinician. *J. Neurol. Neurosurg. Psychiatry, 50,* 183–193.
43. León-Carrión, J. (1998). Neurologically-related Changes in Personality Inventory (NECHAPI): a clinical tool addressed to neurorehabilitation planning and monitoring effects of personality treatment. *NeuroRehabilitation, 11,* 129–139.
44. Romano, M. D. (1974). Family response to traumatic brain injury. *Scand. J. Rehabil. Med., 6,* 1–4.
45. Binder, C., & Perini, P. (1998). Reinserimento lavorativo e sociale di soggetti con esito di trauma cranio-encefalico. Paper presented at symposium, Ferrara, Italy.
46. Perino, C., & Rago, R. (1995). *Riabilitazione e reinserimento sociale negli esiti di trauma encefalico [Rehabilitation and social reintegration of TBI survivors].* Rome: Marrapese.
47. Ben-Yishay, Y., & Gold, J. (1990). Therapeutic milieu approach to neuropsychological rehabilitation. In R. L. Wood (Ed.), *Neurobehavioral sequelae of traumatic brain injury.* London: Taylor & Francis.
48. Zettin, M., Vernè, D., Perino, C., & Rago, R. (1995). Il reinserimento sociale: Follow-up a lungo termine [Social reintegration: long term follow-up]. In M. Zettin and R. Rago (Eds.) *Trauma cranico: Conseguenze neuropsicologiche e comportamentali.* Turin: Bollati Boringhieri.
49. Johnston, M., & Lewis, F. (1991). Outcomes of community re-entry programmes

for brain injury survivors. Part 1: Independent living and productive activities. *Brain Inj., 5*, 141–154.

50. Matthews, R. (1990). Independent living as a lifelong community service, *J. Head Trauma Rehabil., 5*, 23.
51. Inge, K., Flippo, K., & Barcus, M. (1995). *Assistive technology*, Baltimore, MD: Paul Brookes.
52. West, M. D., & Parent, W. S. (1995). Community and workplace supports for individuals with severe mental illness in supported employment. *Psychosocial Rehab., 18*, 13–24.
53. Curl, R. M., Fraser, R. T., Cook, R. G., & Clemmons, D. (1996). Traumatic brain injury vocational rehabilitation: preliminary findings for the co-worker as trainer project. *J. Head Trauma Rehabil., 11*, 75–85.
54. Wehman, P., West, M. D., Kregel, J., Sherron, P., Kreutzer, J. S. (1995). Return to work for person with severe traumatic brain injury: a data-base approach to program development. *J Head Trauma Rehabil., 10*, 27–39.
55. Zappalà, G. (1998). Reinserimento sociale e lavorativo negli esiti di trauma cranio-encefalico [Social and work reintegration of TBI survivors]. Paper presented at a symposium, Vicenza, Italy.
56. Zappalà G. (1998). Valutazione dei risultati [Results discussion]. Paper presented at a symposium, Vicenza, Italy.

Index

Note: Page numbers in *Italics* refer to figures and tables.

Millon Clinical Multiaxial Inventory-III, 302
Milner, B., 292
Minderhound, J.M., 129
Mini Mental Status Examination, 290
minimally conscious states (MCS), 134, 137–8, *138, 416*
  pediatric, 415–20
  therapy during, *480*
minimally responsive state *see* minimally conscious states (MCS)
Ministry of Labor and Social Security, Italy, 541
Minnesota Multiphasic Personality Inventory–2 (MMPI–2), 151, 301
  correction factor for CHI, 301
Mintz, M.C., 429
miopathy, 45
miotonometer, 477
Mirsky, A.F., 281–2
Mitchell, S., 125
mnesia, 297
mnesic contamination, 322
mnesic gain, 322
mobility, after stroke, 41
mobilization, in hydrotherapy, 267–70, *269*
modafinil, 176, 210
Modified Ashworth Scale (MAS), 232–3
monitoring techniques
  for CBF and metabolic activity, 52–5
  cerebral, 48–55
monoamine, 206–8
  oxidase inhibitors (MAOs), 153–4
mood disorders, 147–50, 177, 474
mood stabilizers, 154
moodiness, 152
Moran, S.G., 20, 22
Moria syndrome, 480
Moriya, T., 92–3
morphine sedation, 97–8
Mortimer, J., 81
Motion Analysis, 232
motivation assessment profile (MAP), 373
  neuropsychological assessment (MAP-NA), *368–73*
motor control
  classic theory of, 189
  cognitive involvement in, *193*
  components of, 188
  hierarchical theory of, 189–90
  programming theories of, 190
  and stability, 188–90, *189*

system theories of, 190
  task-oriented theories of, 190
motor impairments, pharmacologic treatment of, 216–17
motor skills, 533
movement, 208
  disorders, pharmacologic treatment of, 217–18
  stereotypic, 130
Muller, R.A., 432
Mullie, A., 122
Multi-Society Task Force on Persistent Vegetative State, 415, 417–20
Multimodal-Early-Onset-Stimulation (MEOS), 126
multiple sclerosis, 217, 241
Multiple Sleep Latency Test (MSLT), 171
Murray, G.D., 66
Murshid, W.R., 22
muscarinic receptors, 206–7
muscles
  activation of, 196–8
  hydrotherapeutic strengthening excercises for, 260–5
  involved in spasticity, 233–8
  measurement of tone, 477
  paralyzed, 81
  relaxants for, 49
music therapy, 493, 497, 508
mutism, 221
  akinetic, 134–5, 138
myasthenia gravis, 45
myocardial infarction, 29
myoclonus, 217–18

Nagib, M.G., *122*
Najeson, T., 130
naloxone, 213
naltrexone, 213–14
narcolepsy, 170, 175–7, 220
  post-traumatic, 176–7
narcoleptic tetrad, 175
Narcotics Anonymous (NA), 507
nasal-CPAP, 173
nasogastric tube, 254
National Brain Injury Research, Treatment and Training Foundation (NBIRTT), 75
National Institute of Health (NIH), USA, 43
  Stroke Scale (NIHSS), 44
National Institute for Neurological Disorders and Stroke (NINDS), 42–3, 98